Fundamentals of
Critical Care

Fundamentals of
Critical Care
A Textbook for Nursing and Healthcare Students

EDITED BY

IAN PEATE

Senior Lecturer, Roehampton University; Visiting Professor of Nursing, St George's University of London and Kingston University London; Visiting Professor, Northumbria University; Visiting Senior Clinical Fellow, University of Hertfordshire, and Editor-in-Chief of the British Journal of Nursing

AND

BARRY HILL

Director of Education (Employability) and Assistant Professor, Northumbria University; Clinical Series and Commisoning Editor of the British Journal of Nursing

WILEY Blackwell

This edition first published 2023
© 2023 John Wiley & Sons Ltd

Registered Offices
John Wiley & Sons, Inc., 111 River Street, Hoboken, NJ 07030, USA
John Wiley & Sons Ltd, The Atrium, Southern Gate, Chichester, West Sussex, PO19 8SQ, UK

Editorial Office
9600 Garsington Road, Oxford, OX4 2DQ, UK

For details of our global editorial offices, customer services, and more information about Wiley products visit us at www.wiley.com.

Wiley also publishes its books in a variety of electronic formats and by print-on-demand. Some content that appears in standard print versions of this book may not be available in other formats.

Library of Congress Cataloging-in-Publication Data applied for

Paperback ISBN: 9781119783251, LCCN 2022035756 (print)

Cover Design: Wiley
Cover Image: © Grafton Marshall Smith/Getty Images

Set in 10/12pt MyriadPro by Straive, Pondicherry, India

Contents

Contributors   xix
Preface   xxv
Acknowledgements   xxvii
How to use your textbook   xxix
About the companion website   xxxi

Chapter 1   The critical care unit   1
Vikki Park

Introduction   2
Levels of care   2
The critical care environment   2
Critical care patients   3
Level 1 care   4
Level 2 care   4
Level 3 care   4
Critical care competence   5
The interprofessional team   6
Communication   7
Ways of working   7
Understanding philosophies of care   8
Humanising critical care   8
Surviving critical care   9
Death in critical care   9
Resilience   9
Nursing considerations and recommendations for practice   11
Future challenges   11
Conclusion   11
References   12

Chapter 2   Organisational influences   14
Vikki Park

Introduction   15
The four UK nations   15
Legislation   15
Professional Statutory Regulatory Bodies (PSRBs)   15
Shared decision making   16
Capacity for shared decision making   16
Confidentiality   17
Decisions relating to end-of-life care   17
Risk management   18
International influences   18
National influences   18
UK government organisations   18
Networks   19
National guidelines   20

Quality assurance   20
Local policies   21
Nursing considerations and recommendations for practice   21
Conclusion   21
References   22

Chapter 3   Legal and ethical issues   **24**
Leonie Armstrong, Tracey Carrott, and Jacqueline Newby

Introduction   25
Confidentiality   25
End-of-life care and best interest decisions   26
Ethical themes   27
Mental Capacity Act   27
Organ donation   29
Consent (authorisation in Scotland) for organ donation   30
First person consent   31
First person opt-in   31
First person opt-out   31
Appointed/nominated representative (not Scotland)   31
Deemed consent   31
The ethics of deemed consent   32
Consent from a person in the highest-ranking relationship   32
Cadaveric organ donation   33
The organ donation process   33
Post organ retrieval   34
Organ allocation   34
Conclusion   35
References   35

Chapter 4   Professional issues in critical care   **37**
Aurora Medonica

Introduction   38
Opportunities for learning   38
NMC Code in critical care units: journey to independent,
safe practice   38
The core principles   39
UK National Competency Framework: critical care   41
Development of critical thinking in healthcare   42
The prioritising process   42
Support systems: the student   44
Conclusion   44
References   45

Chapter 5   Using an evidence-based approach   **46**
Sadie Diamond-Fox and Alexandra Gatehouse

Introduction   47
What is evidence-based practice (EBP)?   47
Step 1: formulating a clinical question – the PICO method   48
Step 2: locating the evidence/research: performing a systematic literature review 48
Step 3: critical appraisal and the hierarchy of evidence   49
Step 4: extracting the most relevant and useful results   51

Step 5: implementing research into practice   52
Quality healthcare in critical care   53
Clinical audit and quality improvement   53
Research and development in critical care   55
Conclusion   56
References   56

Chapter 6   Nursing care   **58**
Sarah Crowe and Fiona McLeod

Introduction   59
Standards of care   59
Physical care   63
Mobility   66
Critical care bundles   67
Conclusion   67
References   68

Chapter 7   Skin integrity   **70**
Victoria Clemett

Introduction   71
Anatomy and physiology of the skin   71
Impact of ageing on skin and tissue integrity   71
Pressure ulcers   71
Nursing assessment   75
Prevention of pressure ulcers   76
Management of pressure ulcers   79
Wound healing   79
Patient factors that affect wound healing   79
Nursing assessment   79
Recognising wound infection   81
Management of non-healing wounds   83
Conclusion   83
References   84

Chapter 8   Shock   **86**
Barry Hill

Introduction   87
Shock   87
Hypovolaemic shock   87
Blood analysis   88
Multiple organ dysfunction syndrome   89
Staging of hypovolaemic shock   89
Principles of managing hypovolaemic shock   90
Fluid resuscitation   91
Training and education for Registered Nurses   91
Cardiogenic shock   91
Obstructive shock   93
Altered pathophysiology   93
Tension pneumothorax   94
Cardiac tamponade   94
Pulmonary embolism (PE)   94

Distributive shock   95
Conclusion   96
References   97

Chapter 9   Communication   **98**
               Paul Jebb

               Introduction   99
               Communicating effectively with patients   100
               Communicating during a pandemic   100
               Communication with families   102
               Conclusion   103
               References   103

Chapter 10   Electronic health records   105
               Timothy Kuhn

               Introduction   106
               Digitisation within healthcare   106
               Understand your responsibilities and the law in relation to record keeping   107
               Intensive Care Society Guidelines   107
               Understanding the different types of EHRs in critical care and how they are used   108
               Understanding what patient data is available within the critical care unit and how this is
               recorded in an electronic health record   109
               Understanding how EHRs are used in critical care audit and research   110
               Understanding the benefits and barriers to EHRs   112
               Conclusion   113
               References   113

Chapter 11   Pharmacology   115
               Sadie Diamond-Fox and Alexandra Gatehouse

               Introduction   116
               Principles of pharmacology and pharmacotherapy   116
               The processes of drug therapy   116
               Medication safety in critical care   119
               Drugs and dialysis   120
               Core drugs utilised within critical care   120
               Respiratory drugs   120
               Cardiovascular drugs   122
               Haematological drugs   126
               Renal drugs   126
               Fluids and electrolytes   127
               Gastrointestinal drugs   128
               Insulin   129
               H_2-histamine antagonists and proton pump inhibitors (PPIs)   129
               Anti-emetics   129
               Laxatives and anti-diarrhoeal drugs   130
               Neurological drugs   130
               Analgesics   130
               Opioids   130
               Non-opioid analgesics   130
               Epidural and regional anaesthesia   130
               Sedatives and anxiolytics   131
               Muscle relaxants   131

Anticonvulsants   132
Antideliriogenics   132
Immunomodulatory drugs   132
Antibacterial agents   132
Antifungals   133
Antiviral drugs   134
Corticosteroids   134
Immunoglobulins   134
Toxicology   134
Conclusion   135
References   135

Chapter 12   Anaesthesia and sedation   138
Lorraine Mutrie and Iain Carstairs

Introduction   139
Indications for sedation and anaesthesia   139
Anaesthetic and sedative medications   142
Sedative drugs   142
Neuromuscular blocking agents and reversal agents   143
Sedation management   145
Conclusion   147
References   148

Chapter 13   Medicines management and drug calculations   150
Jan Guerin

Introduction   151
Purpose of pharmacological interventions in the critically ill adult patient   152
Legal and professional issues   152
Collaborative multidisciplinary team working   154
Medication errors   154
Overview of routes and methods of administering medications in CCU   155
Rights of medication administration   158
Managing and reporting a medication error   159
Anaphylaxis   160
Pathophysiology and clinical manifestations of DIA   160
Management for DIA   160
Medication calculation formulae   160
Displacement   165
Conclusion   165
References   166

Chapter 14   Neurological critical care   167
Samantha O'Driscoll

Introduction   168
Neurological anatomy and physiology   168
Central nervous system   169
Neurological assessment   174
Signs and symptoms of increasing ICP   179
Primary and secondary brain injury   180
Management of raised ICP   180
Nursing care   181

Transfer   182
Conclusion   184
References   184

Chapter 15   Cognition   186
Barry Hill and Sadie Diamond-Fox

Introduction   187
Cognitive impairment   187
Causes of cognitive impairment   187
Signs of cognitive impairment   188
Delirium   188
Risk factors   190
Management of delirium   191
Sleep   193
Assessment of sleep in ICU   193
Conclusion   195
References   195

Chapter 16   Respiratory care: intubation and mechanical ventilation   197
Barry Hill and Lorraine Mutrie

Introduction   198
Respiratory failure   198
Hypoventilation   198
Ventilation/perfusion (V/Q) mismatch   199
Work of breathing   199
Arterial blood gases (ABGs)   200
Non-invasive ventilation (NIV)   201
Continuous positive airway pressure (CPAP)   204
High flow nasal oxygen   204
Intubation   204
Mechanical ventilation   206
Artificial ventilation   207
Minute ventilation (Vm)   207
Fraction of inspired oxygen   207
Positive end-expiratory pressure (PEEP)   207
Volume control   207
Pressure control   207
Inspiratory:Expiratory (I:E) ratio   208
Inverse ratio   208
Synchronisation   208
Humidification   208
Benefits of mechanical ventilation   208
Risks of mechanical ventilation   208
Ventilator care bundles   209
Prone positioning   209
Prone positioning in COVID-19   209
Weaning from mechanical ventilation   210
Conclusion   210
References   211

Chapter 17 Lung function in critical care   **213**
Rana Din and Joyce Smith

Introduction   214
Anatomy and physiology   214
Composition of air   215
Alveolar gas   215
Expired air   216
Lung volumes   216
Pulmonary ventilation   216
External respiration   217
Ventilation/Perfusion   217
Transport of gases   217
Internal respiration   218
Assessment of lung function   220
Normal breath sounds (vesicular)   221
Absent Sounds   221
Wheeze   222
Crackles   222
The work of breathing   222
Compliance   222
Resistance   222
Emphysema   222
Asthma   223
Obstructive sleep apnoea   224
Prone positioning   224
Conclusion   225
References   226

Chapter 18 Cardiac physiology   **227**
Paul Sinnott

Introduction   228
Functions of the cardiovascular system   228
Anatomy of the heart and great vessels   228
Pericardium   229
Layers of the heart   229
Chambers of the heart   230
Valves of the heart   230
Coronary circulation   232
Cardiac conduction system   235
The cardiac cycle   236
Cardiac output and blood pressure   237
Regulation of heart rate   238
Stroke volume   239
The regulation of blood pressure   240
The microcirculation   242
Capillary exchange   243
Effects of ventilation on the cardiovascular system   245
Conclusion   245
References   246

Chapter 19   Cardiovascular critical care   247
             Alice Shaw and Paul Sinnott

             Introduction   248
             Cardiovascular assessment   248
             Heart rate and rhythm   248
             Atrial ectopic beats   249
             Ventricular ectopic beats   253
             Blood pressure   254
             Invasive blood pressure monitoring   255
             Central venous catheters (CVCs) and central venous pressure (CVP)   256
             Markers of organ and tissue perfusion   258
             Neurological status   258
             Urine output   258
             Blood results   259
             Advanced haemodynamic monitoring   260
             Cardiac pacing   262
             Nursing considerations and recommendations for practice   263
             Conclusion   263
             References   263

Chapter 20   Fluids and electrolytes in critically ill patients   265
             Barry Hill

             Introduction   266
             The role of the critical care nurse   266
             Intravenous fluids   266
             Crystalloids versus colloids critical care   267
             Fluid management   268
             Third spacing   269
             Assessment and monitoring   269
             Training and education   271
             Electrolyte replacement therapy   271
             Management of hyperkalaemia   272
             Oral sodium and water   272
             Oral rehydration therapy (ORT)   272
             Oral bicarbonate   273
             Parenteral preparations for fluid and electrolyte imbalance   273
             Plasma and plasma substitutes   276
             Plasma substitutes   276
             Fluid overload   276
             The four Ds of fluid management   276
             Hyponatraemia   277
             Hypernatraemia   277
             Hypokalaemia   277
             Hyperkalaemia   277
             Hypophosphataemia   278
             Hypocalcaemia   278
             Hypomagnesaemia   278
             Conclusion   279
             References   279

Chapter 21 Critical care emergencies 280
Alexandra Gatehouse and Sadie Diamond-Fox

Introduction 281
A – Airway 282
B – Breathing 290
C – Circulation/Cardiovascular 291
D – Disability 298
E – Everything else (exposure, endocrine, electrolytes and environmental) 301
Care of the patient post return of spontaneous circulation (ROSC) 307
Critical care emergencies and human factors 307
Debriefing 309
Do-not-attempt-cardiopulmonary-resuscitation (DNACPR) and Recommended Summary
Plan for Emergency Care and Treatment (ReSPECT) 309
Conclusion 310
References 310

Chapter 22 **Gastrointestinal critical care** 313
Anna Riley, Joe Box, and Aileen Aherne

Introduction 314
Anatomy and physiology 314
GI monitoring and investigation in the critically ill 317
Imaging and endoscopy 318
Bowel charts and abnormal GI motility 320
The acute abdomen in critical care 322
Common surgical procedures cared for in critical care 325
Post-operative monitoring 325
Abdominal surgical drains 326
Anaesthetics 326
Post-operative complications 326
Wound dehiscence 327
GI pharmacology 327
Conclusion 328
References 328

Chapter 23 **Nutrition in critical care** 330
Barry Hill and Lorraine Mutrie

Introduction 331
Pathophysiology 331
Fight or flight 332
Resistance 332
Exhaustion 332
Nutritional screening and assessment 333
Indirect calorimetry (IC) 333
Routes of administration 334
Nursing considerations and recommendations for practice 336
Care of people with feeding tubes 336
Glycaemic control 337
Refeeding syndrome 338
Discontinuing feed 339

Nutritional guidance   339
Conclusion   340
References   341

Chapter 24   Renal critical care   343
                Alexandra Gatehouse and Sadie Diamond-Fox

Introduction   344
Anatomy and physiology of the renal tract   344
Vascular supply   344
Renin-angiotensin-aldosterone system (RASS)   344
The nephrons   345
Control of plasma osmolality   346
Electrolyte balance   346
Acid-base balance   352
Renal failure   352
Acute kidney injury   353
Classification of AKI   353
Pathophysiology   353
Organ cross-talk   354
Risk factors for AKI   355
Clinical features and examination   355
Investigations   355
Specific disorders associated with AKI   357
Drug-induced renal damage   357
Management of AKI   359
Clinical features and examination   361
Management   361
Chronic kidney disease   362
Management   362
Diabetic nephropathy   362
Continuous renal replacement therapy (CRRT)   364
Dosing of CRRT   364
Anticoagulation   364
Drug dosing and RRT   367
Kidney transplantation – critical care considerations   367
Conclusion   368
References   368

Chapter 25   Endocrine critical care   370
                Geraldine Fitzgerald O'Connor and Emma Long

Introduction   371
Thyroid and parathyroid glands   371
Disorders of the thyroid gland   371
Thyroid crisis   372
Parathyroid glands   372
Disorders of the parathyroid glands   372
Hypocalcaemia   373
Pituitary gland   373
Disorders of the pituitary gland   373
Diabetes insipidus   374
Pathophysiology   375

Hyperglycaemia in the critically ill   376
Diabetic emergencies   376
Pathophysiology   380
Conclusion   383
References   384

Chapter 26   Haematological and immunological critical care   385
              Barry Hill, Gerri Mortimore, and Pamela Arasen

Introduction   386
Normal physiology   386
Blood components   386
Haematopoiesis   387
Disorders of erythrocytes   387
B12 vitamin deficiency   387
Sickle cell anaemia   388
Genetic haemochromatosis   389
Haemostasis   390
Lymphoma   390
Disseminated intravascular coagulation   393
Thrombocytopenia   394
Neutropenia and sepsis   394
Vasculitis   396
Blood transfusions in adults   397
Blood sample collections   398
Blood groups   398
Compatibility   399
Indications for blood transfusions   399
Platelets   400
Fresh frozen plasma (FFP)   400
Cryoprecipitate   400
Granulocytes   400
Procedural safety   400
Pre-procedure and sampling   400
Administration of the blood product   400
Post-procedural care   401
Traceability   401
Patient information   402
Alternatives to blood transfusions   403
Summary of SaBTO recommendations on consent   403
Conclusion   408
References   408

Chapter 27   Musculoskeletal considerations in critical care   411
              Clare L. Wade and Helen Sanger

Introduction   412
Trauma   412
Management of traumatic injury   413
Intensive care unit-acquired weakness   415
Assessment of musculoskeletal impairment or injury   418
Management of musculoskeletal injury and impairment   419
Conclusion   424
References   424

Chapter 28 Burn care within a critical care setting 426
Nicole Lee

Introduction 427
Classification of burn wound depths 427
Pathological considerations 429
Burn size estimation 430
An ABCDE approach to burn care 432
Breathing 433
Cardiovascular 433
Disability (neurological assessment) 434
Exposure (and everything else) 434
Psychological support 434
Acknowledgement 436
References 436

Chapter 29 Maternal critical care 438
Wendy Pollock

Introduction 439
Epidemiology 439
Adapted physiology 439
Recognising clinical deterioration 441
Nursing considerations and recommendations for practice 442
Conclusion 448
References 449

Chapter 30 **Critical care transfers** 451
Kirstin Geer, Mark Cannan, and Stuart Cox

Inter-hospital and intra-hospital patient transfers 452
Transfer of the critically ill adult 452
Critical care bed and repatriation 456
The risks of critical care transfer 457
Preparation for transfer 458
ABCDE process during critical care transfer 458
Conclusion 469
References 469

Chapter 31 **Rehabilitation after critical illness** 470
Helen Sanger and Clare L. Wade

Introduction 471
The impact of critical illness – what do we mean by morbidity? 471
Describing physical functioning and morbidity 472
Models of post-critical care morbidity 473
Assessment 473
Goals 475
Key timepoints in RaCI 477
Treatment 478
National guidelines and standards 480
Conclusion 481
References 481

Chapter 32 **Dying and death**   **484**
Helen Merlane and Leonie Armstrong

Introduction   485
End-of-life care   485
Palliative care   486
Dying   486
Recognising Dying   486
Advance care planning   488
Involve and support   489
Nursing the dying patient   489
The critical care environment   489
Symptom management   490
End-of-life care discharges from a critical care setting   491
Care after death   494
Conclusion   495
References   495

Index   *497*

Contributors

Aileen Aherne, RN, Dip HE (Nursing), BHSc Nursing, MSc Nursing Studies, MSc Advanced Clinical Practice, V300
Central Manchester University Hospitals NHS Foundation Trust

Aileen's interests lie in hepatology, nursing Science and Oncology Aileen has skills and expertise in nursing, palliative medicine, and clinical nursing. She works in the Department of General Surgery at Manchester Royal Infirmary.

Pamela Arasen, RN, FHEA, BScN in Cardiorespiratory Care, MSc in Advanced Practice in Critical care, PGCE
Senior Lecturer in Critical Care Nursing, University of West London (UWL).

Pamela started her career as a registered nurse after completing a Diploma in Nursing at St Bartholomew School of Nursing, City University in 2005. She spent a few years working in Acute Medical/Surgical wards and A&E, continued her education pathway in a BSc in Cardiorespiratory Care, before moving to Critical Care at West Middlesex University Hospital. She specialised in the Critical Care Outreach Team at King's College Hospital, after completing her MSc in Advanced Practice in Critical Care in 2015. In 2018, she was appointed as a Lecturer Practitioner in Intensive Care at UWL teaching on the ITU course. She had a joint appointment at the London Northwest Healthcare Trust as the Lead in Education in Intensive Care Nursing, where she introduced the inhouse Intensive Care Adult course with UWL partnership during the COVID 19 pandemic. After the completion of the Academic Professional Apprenticeship, she works as a Senior Lecturer in Critical Care at the UWL, teaching in the Continuous Professional Development modules. Pamela's special interests are Critical Care, Education and Career Development in Nursing.

Leonie Armstrong, RGN, NMP, Ma Ethics in Cancer and Palliative Care

Leonie qualified as a registered general nurse in 1994. She has worked in the speciality of palliative care for over 25 years in hospices and hospital palliative care services in the North East. Her current role is clinical lead nurse for hospital palliative care at Northumbria specialised emergency care hospital.

Joe Box, RN, BSc, MSc (Advanced Clinical Practice), V300

Joe has worked in emergency surgical admissions for 15 years, initially in Liverpool and Melbourne, before settling in Manchester. Whilst a ward-based nurse, he facilitated the student nurse programme and received multiple award nominations for mentor of the year and then placement provider of the year. Going back to university to complete a MSc in Advanced Clinical Practice after 10 years of experience, he now works in a Nursing Times award winning team of emergency general surgical Advanced Nurse Practitioners and retains his passion for educating existing staff and the next generation of nurses.

Mark Cannan, MSc, BSc (Hons), Dip HE
Advanced Critical Care Practitioner, Intensive Care, North Cumbria University Hospitals Foundation Trust, UK

Mark entered the health care profession as an Operating Department Practitioner (ODP) in 2013 with the University of Central Lancashire (UCLan), having witnessed the work of an ODP first hand in the theatres of Camp Bastion, Afghanistan. On qualification, he rotated through anaesthetic and scrub practice, in both elective and emergency surgical procedures in two busy district general hospitals. Whilst qualifying with a diploma, he continued in education by completing an Honours Degree in Acute and Critical Care at the University of Cumbria, which is where he discovered the Advanced Critical Care Practitioner (ACCP) role. Having excluded career progression in managerial or educational roles, the ACCP role seemed to best fit his aspirations by being retained at the bedside, performing clinical duties. Mark started his ACCP training with Northumbria University in 2017 and qualified in 2019 with a Post Graduate Diploma and works across two general intensive care units, which increased to four during the COVID-19 pandemic. Mark has since completed his Master's Degree and has specialist interests in advanced airway management, regional anaesthesia and transfer of the critically ill patient. He is also on the national working group for legislation change in allowing ODPs who have progressed into advanced practice the ability to undertake non-medical prescribing.

Tracey Carrott, MA, RGN

Tracey qualified as a Registered General Nurse some 40 years ago (1982) and she has worked in the Northeast of England the entire time. Tracey have witnessed many changes to the provision of health care during this time, however, she is still as passionate about the role as a nurse as she was and when she began nurse training. Tracey's nursing background and clinical expertise is that of scientific paradigm having predominantly worked within the biomedical domain of critical care. Her current role is that of a Specialist Nurse in Organ Donation (SNOD). This niche role involves promoting and raising awareness about the value of organ and tissue donation. Fundamentally, she has the opportunity to be able to empower a family and to support them should their loved one become an organ and tissue donor. She has been in this role for 12 years although now work part-time. Prior to becoming a SNOD she worked as a nurse in Cardio-thoracic critical care and as a nurse practitioner in an accident and emergency department. She also managed a Coronary Care Unit for several years. Tracy has always had an avid interest in education and posess an MA in Advanced Practice. She is also a Registered NMC Lecturer Practitioner, having achieved a Post Graduate Diploma with Commendation in Health and Social Care Practice, Education and Development.

Iain Carstairs, MBBS, BSc (Hons) Pharmacology and Neuroscience

Specialist Grade Doctor in Anaesthetics.

Iain studied medicine at Newcastle University and practiced his early career in the speciality of Emergency Medicine at Edinburgh Royal Infirmary. In 2009 he transferred to the speciality of anaesthesia within the Northern Deanery and currently works as a Specialty Grade Anaesthetist at Northumbria Healthcare NHS Foundation Trust. In his current role Iain provides planned and emergency care across a range of clinical settings that includes theatres, obstetrics, pre-assessment and CPEX, and critical care to patients of all age ranges. He supports the clinical education and development of many members of the multidisciplinary team including trainee doctors, ODPs and Physician Associates. Iain is a member of the Association of Anaesthetists of Great Britain and Ireland and an SAS member of the Royal College of Anaesthetists.

Victoria Clemett, PhD, RN (adult), BNurs, FHEA

Victoria began her nursing a career as a healthcare assistant before completed her registered nurse (RN) training at The University of Birmingham, UK in 2005. Following her junior staff nurse rotations at The University Hospital Birmingham, she specialised in burns and reconstructive practice surgery. Victoria relocated to the southeast and moved into research and education. Victoria is an NMC registered teacher and has several years' experience in nurse education. Special interests include wound care, clinical decision making, translational research and simulated learning.

Sarah Crowe, MN, PMD-NP(F), CNCC(C), NP

Critical Care Nurse Practitioner, Surrey Memorial Hospital, Fraser Health
Adjunct Professor, School of Nursing, University of British Columbia
Instructor, Critical Care Speciality Nursing Program, British Columbia Institute of Technology
President, Canadian Association of Critical Care Nurses
Adjunct Professor, UBC School of Nursing

Sarah began her nursing career at Surrey Memorial Hospital in 2000 in the Emergency department before transitioning to critical care in 2004. She completed dual specialty certification in both Emergency and Critical Care Nursing. She went on to complete a Master's of Nursing in 2010, and a post-Master's graduate diploma in Nurse Practitioner in 2018. Her key areas of research and interest are in ICU survivorship, chronically critically ill patients, and supporting the mental health and practice of critical care nurses. She has received several research grants for her work. Sarah is currently the Vice President of the Canadian Association of Critical Care Nurses.

Stuart Cox, BSc (Hons), MSc (ACCP), mFICM

Advanced Critical Care Practitioner, University Hospitals Southampton NHS & Dorset and Somerset Air Ambulance.

Stuart works as an Advanced Critical Care Practitioner (ACCP) at University Hospitals Southampton NHS & Dorset and Somerset Air Ambulance. Prior to this he was employed as a Senior Charge Nurse ICU at Southampton and Senior Nurse CEGA Air Ambulance. He graduated with a BSc (Hons) in Nursing Science and completed his MSc in ACCP in 2018. Stuart is a Registered Nurse with the Nursing and Midwifery Council (NMC), and an ACCP with membership with the faculty of intensive care medicine (FICM).

Sadie Diamond-Fox, MCP ACCP (mFICM), BSc (Hons) RN, PGCAHP, NMP (V300), FHEA

Sadie Diamond-Fox graduated from Northampton University in 2008 with a BSc (Hons) Adult Nursing and immediately began her critical care career, initially working at Papworth and Cambridge Hospitals. In 2012 she moved to Newcastle upon Tyne Hospitals to commence training as an Advanced Critical Care Practitioner, completing a Masters of Clinical Practice in Advanced Critical Care Practice (ACCP) in 2015 and was awarded ACCP membership to the Faculty of Intensive Care Medicine in 2016. Sadie has since continued to work clinically as an ACCP alongside developing an extensive teaching portfolio with Northumbria University, and is currently studying a PhD (The 'ImpACCPt' study). Sadie has several national roles in the fields of advanced practice and critical care, including her more recent appointments with Health Education England (HEE) as Regional Advancing Practice Supervision and Assessment Lead for North East & Yorkshire, the Intensive Care Society as Council Member, Education Committee Member and Chair of the Professional Advisory Group for Advanced Practitioners in Critical Care (APCC PAG). Sadie also co-chairs the Advanced Clinical Practitioners Academic Network (ACPAN).

Rana Din, RGN BSc (Hons) Nursing (Manchester Metropolitan University), MSc Advance Clinical Nursing Skills (University of Huddersfield), PGCE

Lecturer, University of Salford

Rana began his nursing career at Birch Hill Hospital in Rochdale working within Medicine/Surgery and ICU. The majority of his career has been based in Critical Care in the

North West of England in various roles as Practice Educator, Charge Nurse and Matron. Also he has had extensive experience of working in nurse education at the University of Chester, University of Bolton and currently at the University of Salford.

Alexandra Gatehouse

Alexandra Gatehouse graduated from Nottingham University in 2000 with a BSc (Hons) Physiotherapy. Following Junior Rotations in the Newcastle Trust she specialised in Respiratory Physiotherapy in Adult Critical Care, also working within New Zealand. In 2012 she trained as an Advanced Critical Care Practitioner, completing a Masters in Clinical Practice in Critical Care and qualifying in 2014. Alex subsequently completed her non-medical prescribing qualification and continues to rotate within all of the Critical Care Units in Newcastle Upon Tyne, also enjoying teaching on the regional transfer course. She is a co-founder of the Advanced Critical Care Practitioner Northern Region Group and is a committee member of the North East Intensive Care Society. Alex has presented abstracts at the European Society of Intensive Care Medicine and the North East Intensive Care Society conferences.

Kirstin Geer, BSc (Hons) MSc (Advanced Clinical Practice) PGDip (Advanced Critical Care Practice) mFICM. Advanced Critical Care Practitioner, North Cumbria Integrated Care, UK

Kirstin qualified as a nurse in 2005 and has worked in Emergency Admissions, Critical Care Outreach and qualified as an Advanced Critical Care Practitioner in 2016.

Special interests include Critical Care Transfer and Simulation.

Jan Guerin, Dip General Nursing (RSA), BSc Nursing Education (RSA), PGD ANP(UK), Diploma General Adult Critical Care (RSA), Diploma Trauma and Emergency Nursing Science (RSA). Certified Lifestyle Medicine Practitioner (UK)

Jan is currently in a role as a General Manager of a residential adult care home, working for Signature Senior Lifestyle in the UK. Jan qualified as a General Registered Nurse in South Africa in 1992. She gained 12 years of accumulative experience working in acute care settings within the field of adult emergency and critical care including 4 years as a lead lecturer for Trauma and Emergency Nursing. Jan moved to the UK in 2006 and joined Hammersmith Hospitals NHS Trust as a Senior Staff Nurse in adult General ITU which included a year of secondment experience in Critical Care Outreach at Charing Cross Hospital. In 2017, Jan worked for the Hillingdon Hospitals NHS Trust and in the roles as an ITU Nurse Educator and Practice Nurse Educator as lead for Clinical skills. Jan moved to adult social care nursing in 2020, and is in a role as a Quality Business Partner with Sunrise-Gracewell Senior Living. Jan has a special interest in health promotion and prevention of chronic disease and is a certified Lifestyle Medicine Practitioner.

Barry Hill, MSc, ANP, PGCAP, PGCE, BSc (Hons), DipHE, O.A. Dip, Fellow (FHEA), NMC RN & TCH & V300

Barry completed his Registered Nurse (RN) training at Northumbria University and Buckinghamshire Chilterns University College (BCUC). Barry's clinical experience is within critical care nursing which has been gained at Imperial College NHS Trust, London, UK. Barry is critical care certified, has a clinical master's in advanced practice (clinical), and has a PGC in Academic Practice. Barry is registered with the NMC as a Registered Nurse, independent and supplementary prescriber (V300), and Registered Teacher (TCH). Barry is currently the Director of Education (Employability) and Assistant Professor at Northumbria University. He teaches undergraduate and postgraduate students from all clinical healthcare disciplines. His key areas of interest are clinical education, acute and critical care, clinical skills, prescribing and pharmacology, and advanced-level practice. Barry has published books, book chapters, and peer-reviewed journal articles. He is a Senior Fellow with the Higher Education Academy (SFHEA) and Clinical Series and Commissioning Editor of the British Journal of Nursing.

Paul Jebb, OStJ MA, BSc(Hons), DipHE RN

Paul qualified as a nurse in 1996 and worked in numerous posts within nursing, operational management and a national role within NHS England.

In December 2016 Paul returned to an NHS Trust and is now Associate Chief Nurse Experience, Engagement & Safeguarding at Lancashire & South Cumbria NHS FT.

Paul has been involved and led on numerous quality improvement initiatives throughout his career, and has gained several awards and accolades.

Paul is also a member of an NMC Professional Standards advisory panel, and has represented the Royal College of Nursing at local, regional, national and international levels, and is currently a member of the RCN Nurses in Leadership & Management Forum steering group as well as a member of RCNi Editorial Advisory Board.

Paul also holds an Honorary Senior Lecturer post at the University of Central Lancashire.

Paul is also chair of the board of Trustees at Blackpool Carers Centre, and a passionate supporter of Cavell Nurses Trust.

Timothy Kuhn, RN, MSc, PgDip, BSc (Hons), Senior Lead Nurse Critical Care and Critical Care Outreach, Advanced Critical Care Practitioner

Timothy is a Registered Nurse educated to Master's level. He has extensive experience in critical care nursing with both senior clinical and senior management skills and experience. Timothy is also a Faculty of Intensive Care Medicine (FICM) accredited Advanced Critical Care Practitioner. In addition to his professional experience, he has a wealth of experience in the voluntary sector. Some of his interests include - nurse development and education, management, team development, clinical governance, vascular access, extracorporeal organ support, first aid teaching/training and voluntary sector work.

Nicole Lee, RN, BSc, PGCE

Nicole Lee, Burns Matron Chelsea and Westminster hospital, Lead Nurse London and South East Burns Network and Co course Lead Advanced Burns Module, University East Anglia. My Burns History takes me back to starting within the burns speciality in 2008 in St Andrews (Chelmsford) Burns ITU, where I worked for 15 Years from band 5 up to band 7 clinical facilitator looking after the large burns that required burns ITU multi organ support. I took on the burns lead nurse role for the network in 2019 where I am able to support regional and national change to our specialist burns services. In 2020 I took on the Burns Matron role at Queen Victoria Hospital for one year and moved on to Burns Matron at Chelsea and Westminster in 2021. Additional Specialist interests are Simulation training, Burns education, Burns prevention and supporting burns and critical care charities.

Emma Long, BSc (Hons) Nursing, Msc Advanced Nursing.
Practice Development Sister, Intensive Care, Chelsea & Westminster Hospital, London

Emma qualified in 1997. She started her Critical Care Nursing Career in 1998. She has worked not only in the UK (in London and Belfast) but also within the field in Australia. Emma has an interest in nursing education and is currently studying to become one the first Professional Nurse Advocates.

Fiona McLeod, RN, BScN, BSc, CNCC (C)
Manager of Clinical Operations, Critical Care and Biocontainment, Surrey Memorial Hospital.

Fiona began her nursing career at Surrey Memorial Hospital in 2007 in the ICU after graduating with a BScN from British Columbia Institute of Technology with Honours and winning the Associate Dean's Prize for Excellence in Clinical Nursing. Shortly after graduation she went on to complete her specialty certification in Critical Care. Fiona has spend her entire career in Critical Care starting as a bedside nurse and transitioning into many leadership roles throughout her time at Surrey Memorial Hospital. Fiona is also a member of the Canadian Association of Critical Care Nurses.

Aurora Medonica, PG Cert, BSc (Hons), MSc, NMC V300, mFICM
Advanced Critical Care Practitioner, Oxford University Hospitals Foundation Trust

Aurora began her nursing career in Italy with a BSc in Adult Nursing. She then moved to Oxford (UK), where she worked as registered intensive care nurse, deputy sister and advanced critical care practitioner in the cardiac and thoracic intensive care unit.

She also collaborated with Oxford Brookes University as a Specialist Lecturer and with the British Association of Critical Care Nurses, where she presented her MSc dissertation findings at the latest conference.

Her key areas of interest are intensive care and advanced practice.

Helen Merlane, MSC, BA (Hons), PGCE, PGDip HE, FHEA

Helen began her nursing a career at St James University Hospital, Leeds working on a medical and surgical ward, before becoming a Macmillan Clinical Nurse Specialist in Palliative Care in 1994. She worked as a Macmillan Nurse for 21 years at St James's University Hospital Leeds & the Freeman Hospital, Newcastle upon Tyne. Helen took up the role of a senior lecturer at Northumbria University in 2015, and teaches on the preregistration, apprenticeship and master's adult nursing programmes. She is currently undertaking a PhD, looking at what factors prepare student nurses to care for dying patients. Her key interests are palliative and end of life care.

Gerri Mortimore, PhD, MSc Advanced Practice; PgCert (IPPE); Ba(Hons) Health Studies; iLM, RGN, NMP, FHEA

Gerri is a RGN, with over 40 years' experience, spanning both acute medical and surgical nursing, within the UK and abroad. This nursing expertise, especially within the field of liver disease has enabled her to be selected as an expert advisor on three National Institute of Health and Care Excellence (NICE) Clinical Guidelines and two Quality Standards and be a specialist member of an Advisory Committee in patients with suspected alcohol related liver disease. In 2015, in recognition of her contribution to NICE, Gerri was awarded the title, Nurse Expert Advisor.

In 2020, along with her co-authors Gerri successfully authored the Venesection Best Practice Guidelines, endorsed by the Royal College of Nursing. This publication has assisted in standardising the care of thousands of UK patients undergoing venesection every year and culminated in Gerri winning the prestigious British Journal of Nursing, Nurse of the Year Award in 2021, nominated by the NMC.

Currently, Gerri is employed as an Associate Professor in Advanced Clinical Practice at the University of Derby and is also a Government Commissioner for the Commission of Human Medicines.

Lorraine Mutrie, Ma, PGC, BSc (Hons), DipHE, RN, FHEA
Assistant Professor and Programme Leader for Adult Critical Care Nursing and Advanced Practice.

Lorraine completed her registered nurse training at Leeds University and her early career was in surgical nursing. In 2005 she returned to the Northeast and continued her nursing career in critical care roles.

Since 2015 Lorraine has worked at Northumbria University leading on post registration programmes and modules in acute and critical illness and advanced practice. She also contributes to teaching on pre-registration healthcare programmes. Lorraine has published on topics related to critical care in textbooks and peer reviewed journal articles. Her research interests include the critical care workforce, and she is currently undertaking a PhD on this topic.

Lorraine was former chair of the Northern Region BACCN committee, is a current member of the NoECCN Education Group, and contributed to the development of the NoRF Level 1 Competence Framework.

Jacqueline Newby, BA

Jacqueline Newby is a specialist nurse in organ donation for NHS Blood and Transplant. She has been a nurse for 32 years working in intensive care or organ donation where she has been involved in developing and managing change in the dynamic field of donation and transplant.

Geraldine Fitzgerald O'Connor, BA (Hons)

Practice Development Sister, Intensive Care, Chelsea & Westminster Hospital, London

Geraldine began her nursing career studying at both Oxford Brookes University and at the University of Pennsylvania, Philadelphia. She followed a Specialist Nursing rotation following graduation and has continued working within Intensive Care since.

Geraldine has an interest in nursing education and is one of the first Professional Nurse Advocates.

Samantha O'Driscoll, RN (Adult), PGDip, BSc (Hons)
Senior Clinical Educator, Critical Care, Imperial College NHS Trust

Samantha studied Physiological Sciences at Bristol University. Whilst undertaking this degree she worked as an HCA at the Bristol Royal Infirmary, sparking a desire to pursue a career in nursing. She achieved a Post Graduate Diploma in Nursing from King's College, London. During her nursing training she developed a love for critical care nursing, blending her human sciences background with compassionate care. She worked as a Staff Nurse in Adult Intensive Care at St Mary's Hospital, Paddington, before moving into Emergency Department nursing and working as an Outreach Practitioner. She holds a postgraduate certificate in critical care and is an ALS instructor. Throughout her career she developed her skills in practice-based coaching and teaching. She now works in clinical education, with an interest in clinical development and the use of simulated practice to support learning.

Dr Vikki Park, PhD, PG Dip., PG Cert., BSc (Hons), FHEA, HEA Mentor, RN, RNT

Assistant Professor in Nursing & IPECP (Interprofessional Education & Collaborative Practice), Northumbria University, UK

Vikki has worked in healthcare since 1999 in nursing homes, acute medical admissions, and adult critical care. Vikki has been awarded a Doctor of Philosophy, Post Graduate Diploma in Academic and Professional Learning, Post Graduate Certificate in Practice Development, and BSc (Hons) in Nursing Studies. She is a Fellow and Mentor of the Higher Education Academy and an NMC Registered Nurse Teacher. Vikki has worked within education since 2010 with experience in Further Education and Higher Education. Principal areas of scholarly interest include interprofessionalism, critical care, simulation-based education, patient safety and clinical skills development. Vikki is an Adult Intensive Care Reviewer for the Nursing in Critical Care Journal, Treasurer & Trustee of the Northern Regional BACCN Committee (British Association of Critical Care Nurses), and elected National Board member of CAIPE (Centre for the Advancement of Interprofessional Education). Vikki is also an active member of several international working groups, including IP.Global and IPR.Global.

Wendy Pollock, RN(Aust), RM(Aust), GCALL (Melb), GD Crit Care Nsg (RMIT), GD Ed (Hawthorn-Melb), PhD (Melb)

Associate Professor, School of Nursing and Midwifery, Monash University, Australia; Visiting Scholar, Department of Nursing, Midwifery and Health, Northumbria University, UK.

Wendy began her nursing career at The Royal Melbourne Hospital (Australia), where she completed a general nursing certificate to become a Registered Nurse, followed by a critical care nursing certificate. After some time working in an intensive care unit, she completed a midwifery certificate at Mercy Hospital for Women to become a Registered Midwife. A number of university studies followed, culminating in a PhD on 'Critically ill pregnant and postpartum women in Victoria', conferred in 2008. Wendy has extensive clinical, education and research experience, primarily in the critical care context, with a focus on severe maternal morbidity, and she is widely published in this area. She has made long-standing active contributions to the Australian College of Critical Care Nurses and the Australian College of Midwives, and sat on the Consultative Council of Obstetric and Paediatric Mortality and Morbidity sub-committee reviewing all maternal deaths in Victoria, Australia for nearly 20 years.

Anna Riley, RGN, BNurs (Hons), PGCert, MSc, INP V300

Lead Advanced Clinical Practitioner, General and Emergency Surgery, Manchester Royal Infirmary, UK
Royal College of Nursing Strategic Alliance PhD student, University of Sheffield, UK

Anna began her career in central Manchester and after working immediately post qualification in urology surgery, moved on to work in the Critical Care Unit at Manchester Royal Infirmary as a staff nurse. After working here for four years and completing a PG Cert in Health Ethics in Law in her spare time, she left to pursue a career in advanced clinical practice within general surgery, completing her Master's degree at the University of Chester and qualifying in 2014.

Anna has worked across Wirral University Hospitals Foundation Trust before returning to Manchester Royal Infirmary in 2016 and has since been appointed as Service Lead. In 2019, Anna was awarded funding for PhD research study at the

University of Sheffield, as part of their five-year strategic alliance with the Royal College of Nursing. She continues to present at local, national and international congress, contribute to local and national research and policy and has strong links with local higher education institutes, with a true passion for her profession, education and development.

Helen Sanger, BSc (hons), PgCert MSc, MCSP

Helen Sanger is a clinical specialist physiotherapist in critical care at Newcastle Upon Tyne Hospitals NHS Foundation Trust. She qualified as a physiotherapist in 2010 and has worked in critical care since 2013. Her particular area of interest is rehabilitation during and after critical care. In addition to her NHS role, Helen has held numerous national posts, including newsletter editor for the association of chartered physiotherapists in respiratory care, and elected member of the physiotherapy professional advisory group for the Intensive Care Society. She completed a postgraduate certificate in advanced clinical practice (critical care) in 2020.

Alice Shaw, BN (Hons), PG Cert, FHEA

After completing her nursing degree at The University of Birmingham, Alice began her Critical Care career at Good Hope Hospital, Sutton Coldfield. She later moved to London where she spent nine years as a Staff Nurse, Team Leader, Practice Development Nurse and later Senior Practice Development Nurse on the Critical Care Units belonging to Kings College Hospital NHS Foundation Trust. Alice has been in clinical nurse education since 2013 and completed a PG Certificate in Clinical Education at Kings College London in 2019. She has a strong passion for critical care and clinical nurse education and currently works as an Education Development Practitioner, on the Cardiac Intensive Care Unit at Manchester Royal Infirmary, Manchester University NHS Foundation Trust. Alice is also a Practice Based Educator at the Greater Manchester Critical Care Skills Institute.

Paul Sinnott, RGN, BSc (Hons), M.Ed., MSc, ACCPFICM

Paul started his nursing career as a staff nurse working in the field of gastroenterology in 1996. Moving to the intensive care unit at Manchester Royal Infirmary in 1998 kindled a lifelong passion for critical care nursing. Over the last 23 years Paul has worked in a number of roles in both general and cardiac critical care. In 2016 Paul completed a masters in advanced clinical practice and took up post as an Advanced Critical Care Practitioner on the Cardiac Intensive Care Unit within the Manchester University NHS Foundation Trust. He subsequently achieved ACCP membership of the Faculty of Intensive Care Medicine in 2017. In addition to his clinical role, Paul holds an associate lecturer post at the University of Salford and supports the development of advanced clinical practitioners/advance critical care practitioners across Greater Manchester.

Joyce Smith, RN, EN(G), BSc (Hons), MSc, PGCE, ENB 100
Lecturer in Adult Nursing, School of Health and Society, University of Salford.

Joyce began her nursing career at Bury School of Nursing becoming an Enrolled nurse working in Intensive Care and later completing the conversion course and continuing to work in Intensive Care as a Sister and Practice Educator. In 2006 became a lecturer in nurse education at the University of Salford. Joyce's key areas of interest are in critical care nursing and recognising and responding to signs of deterioration. Joyce has published a book and also published in several peer-reviewed nursing journals. Joyce is on the Greater Manchester Critical Care Advisory Board and implemented the Acute Illness Management Course for student nurses in 2008.

Clare L. Wade, BSc (Hons), PGCAP, FHEA, MCSP
Lecturer in Physiotherapy, Northumbria University; Advanced Physiotherapist, The Newcastle upon Tyne Hospitals NHS Foundation Trust

Clare is an Advanced Physiotherapist at The Newcastle upon Tyne Hospitals NHS Foundation Trust and PhD candidate and Lecturer at Northumbria University. Qualifying as a physiotherapist in 2010, Clare went on to specialise in respiratory physiotherapy before becoming an advanced critical care physiotherapist in 2015. She has keen interests in intensive care unit-acquired weakness and rehabilitation after critical illness, with a particular research interest in culture of physical activity and rehabilitation in the critical care environment. Clare also has a keen interest in pre-registration and post-graduate cardiorespiratory physiotherapy education and has worked in higher education since 2018. She sits on the editorial board for the Association of Chartered Physiotherapists in Respiratory Care and is an elected member of the Physiotherapists Professional Advisory Group for the Intensive Care Society.

Preface

The emergence of the SARS-CoV-2 (severe acute respiratory syndrome coronavirus 2) virus and the disease COVID-19 (coronavirus disease) along with the World Health Organization's declaration of a pandemic in March 2020 has changed how we live. The health and wellbeing of all nations have been upended.

Nurses and other health and social care professionals have been in the headlines day in and day out. Those providing high-quality, safe and effective care in critical care settings have felt the brunt of the challenges that COVID-19 has brought. Critical care units continue to take every precaution available to ensure that patients and staff are safe from COVID-19. Critical care nurses have not let the fear of one disease keep them from doing what they need to do to keep people alive and stay healthy. Nor have they lost sight of the care required for people with other diseases and conditions that needed skilled, compassionate critical care nursing.

Fundamentals of Critical Care: A Textbook for Nursing and Healthcare Students has been written for a wide-ranging audience, for those who care for acutely ill adults. This comprehensive text contains information that a student may require in order to successfully complete their clinical placement in this dynamic, fast-changing and often highly charged care environment.

The book draws on the latest available evidence reflecting contemporary best practice and is compliant with Nursing and Midwifery Council (NMC) proficiencies (NMC, 2018a; NMC, 2018b). The standards enshrined in the NMC's Code (2018c) are evident throughout as the nurse provides care that:

- prioritises people
- is effective
- is safe
- promotes professionalism and trust.

The student nurse allocated to a critical care placement is the key focus. We aim to provide you with insight into the critical care environment. Healthcare students, for example those studying paramedicine, physiotherapy, operating department practice, midwifery and medicine, will also find the content of this text of value should they find themselves in a clinical placement in the critical care arena. This comprehensive resource can also meet the needs of the novice registered nurse who is commencing their professional career in this complex and dynamic area of care provision.

It is not possible, in any one text, to cover all conditions that may present in the critical care arena, but this text considers the more common disorders that you may come across. The further reading/resource sections at the end of chapters and the provision of a glossary may be useful as you delve deeper in order to expand your knowledge and develop your understanding further.

For most people (and remember, this includes patients and their families) the critical care environment can seem intimidating and complex, with a language that is highly sophisticated with the use of high-level and advanced technology. The overarching aim is to support your learning and ease your journey. The text provides you with access to an amazing care setting that requires a cutting-edge and knowledgeable response to the changing needs of patients and their families, all underpinned by a sound evidence base.

The text offers 32 chapters written by a range of clinical experts and academics with a strong clinical background in critical care nursing and experience of teaching nursing and health care subject matter. There is a wealth of content that will guide you as you develop and hone your critical care nursing skills and knowledge, so as to meet the many exciting challenges that this speciality brings. A holistic and caring approach has been adopted throughout. The patient, not the technology, is at the heart of all we do. This text emphasises that the critical care nurse offers care to the patient and not the technology. The technology is used to assist in this key role of caring and it should never be used the other way around.

Fundamentals of Critical Care: A Textbook for Nursing and Healthcare Students has been organised in user-friendly sections. Each chapter outlines the essential knowledge that is needed to understand key concepts, and high-quality, full-colour artwork is used to enhance learning and to encourage recall. Implications for practice boxes, further reading and resources and learning events are features that have been used to encourage revision and recall. Clinical scenarios are included, along with red and orange flags (physiological and psychological alerts respectively), with the aim of linking theory to practice.

The text considers patient-focused issues, ensuring that the patient is at the centre of all that is done. The technical knowledge necessary to care safely for people being nursed in a critical care setting is discussed. A range of common and specialised disease processes and treatments that require critical care have been described. The contribution that nurses and other health care practitioners make to care as they use their knowledge and skills when developing their own and others' practice is evident.

Generally, a systems approach has been adopted. It is likely that readers will dip in and dip out of the chapters depending on their needs. We have used the term Critical Care/Critical Care Units (CCU) throughout; this is an often-used term (the abbreviation should not be confused with Cardiac Care Units).

We have very much enjoyed the challenge of writing this book for you. We sincerely hope that it will help you deliver high-quality safe and effective care not only in the critical care unit but further afield.

References

Nursing and Midwifery Council (2018a). *Future Nurse: Standards of Proficiency for Registered Nurses*. https://www.nmc.org.uk/globalassets/sitedocuments/education-standards/future-nurse-proficiencies.pdf (accessed July 2022).

Nursing and Midwifery Council (2018b). *Standards of Proficiency for Nursing Associates*. https://www.nmc.org.uk/standards/standards-for-nursing-associates/standards-of-proficiency-for-nursing-associates/ (accessed July 2022).

Nursing and Midwifery Council (2018c). *The Code. Professional Standards of Practice and Behaviour for Nurses, Midwives and Nursing Associates*. https://www.nmc.org.uk/standards/code/ (accessed July 2022).

Acknowledgements

Ian would like to thank his partner Jussi Lahtinen for his continuous encouragement and enthusiasm and to his friend Mrs Frances Cohen for her time and generous support. Barry would like to thank his family and friends for their continued love and support. A special thanks goes to Imperial College NHS Trust and critical care academics Helen Dutton and Jaqueline Finch for his development as an ICU nurse in practice and in teaching and learning. He would like to dedicate this book to his dad Ray Hill who died December 2021, this is for you dad. Barry would also like to acknowledge his dear friends who were both nurses, Jackie Mullady and Helen Jackson, who both lost their young lives' to cancer.

We are grateful to the contributors, many of whom were providing critical care to patients during the COVID-19 pandemic while contributing to this text. Your dedication and commitment deserves much more than an acknowledgement. Our thanks also go to the team at Wiley headed up by Magenta Styles, who supported us throughout and helped us bring the concept to fruition.

How to use your textbook

Features contained within your textbook

Every chapter begins with **test your prior knowledge** questions.

Test your prior knowledge

- Describe critical care considering the environment, patient care, and underlying care philosophies.
- In hospital, how many levels of care can patients be categorised into and of these, at which level(s) would patients receive critical care provision?
- Name different members of the interprofessional critical care team and describe their professional roles.
- Based upon current evidence, critically discuss the holistic care needs of critically ill patients.
- Differentiate between the following terms: personal resilience, team resilience and organisational resilience.

Learning outcome boxes give a summary of the topics covered in a chapter.

Learning outcomes

After reading this chapter the reader will be able to:

- Describe the critical care environment.
- Appreciate the complexities and ways of working within critical care.
- Understand the holistic care needs of critically ill patients.
- Consider the theory of humanisation in care for critically ill patients.
- Discuss the emotional influence of critical care experiences on the workforce.

Red and Orange flag boxes:

- Red flags identify or draw the reader's attention to issues of importance that need to be dealt with. flags may highlight indicators of possible serious pathology.
- Orange flags are used to encourage the reader to give further thought to the wider scenario, drawing attention to any psychological impact on a person's health and wellbeing.

Red Flag

New-onset confusion is an indicator of acute illness and requires urgent clinical assessment. Acutely altered consciousness and cognition can be caused by sepsis, hypoxia, hypotension, or metabolic disturbances.

RCP (2020)

Orange Flag

Patients admitted to critical care can experience sensory overload, sleep deprivation and can develop delirium and PTSD during their recovery. Rehabilitation support for critical care survivors is advocated, including the utilisation of outside spaces to promote critical care patient recovery. Increased evidence is needed to support critical care patient recovery, such as consideration of the role of psychologists in critical care.

6Cs boxes focus on the delivering of high quality of care as well as treatment. They emphasise a set of common values that help to ensure that all patients receive care that is compassionate and respectful.

6Cs: Competence

To provide high-quality, safe and effective care, healthcare professionals must recognise and work within the limits of their competence for their professional field.

Take home points bring together succinctly the main points of the chapter.

Take home points

1. The critical care unit tends to be large, fast-paced and highly technological.
2. Critically ill patients have complex needs.
3. It takes many different professions to provide holistic critical care.
4. It is important to understand professional roles in critical care.
5. Clear effective communication is needed.
6. Care must be humanised and holistic in approach.
7. The critical care unit can be an emotionally demanding environment.
8. The critical care team must find ways to develop resilience.
9. Critical care patients may require rehabilitation after critical illness.
10. Families require information and support.

About the companion website

Don't forget to visit the companion website for this book:

www.wiley.com/go/peate/criticalcare

There you will find valuable material designed to enhance your learning, including:

- Interactive multiple choice questions
- Interactive true or false questions
- Self test and case studies
- Glossary
- Further reading/Web links

Scan this QR code to visit the companion website:

Chapter 1

The critical care unit

Vikki Park

Aim

This chapter introduces the critical care unit, giving insight into the complex nature of providing holistic patient-centred care to critically ill patients and their families. By reading this chapter, the complexity of care given to critically ill patients will be highlighted and the extensive roles and experiences of nurses and interprofessional team members will be considered.

Learning outcomes

After reading this chapter the reader will be able to:

- Describe the critical care environment.
- Appreciate the complexities and ways of working within critical care.
- Understand the holistic care needs of critically ill patients.
- Consider the theory of humanisation in care for critically ill patients.
- Discuss the emotional influence of critical care experiences on the workforce.

Test your prior knowledge

- Describe critical care considering the environment, patient care, and underlying care philosophies.
- In hospital, how many levels of care can patients be categorised into and of these, at which level(s) would patients receive critical care provision?
- Name different members of the interprofessional critical care team and describe their professional roles.
- Based upon current evidence, critically discuss the holistic care needs of critically ill patients.
- Differentiate between the following terms: personal resilience, team resilience and organisational resilience.

Fundamentals of Critical Care: A Textbook for Nursing and Healthcare Students, First Edition. Edited by Ian Peate and Barry Hill.
© 2023 John Wiley & Sons Ltd. Published 2023 by John Wiley & Sons Ltd.
Companion website: www.wiley.com/go/peate/criticalcare

2

Introduction

Chapter 1 explores the critical care unit, where the interprofessional team work together caring for critically ill patients and their families. The critical care unit is recognised as a complex demanding clinical environment (Rothschild et al., 2005), which aims to provide safe and effective care (Paradis et al., 2013) to the most severely ill patients in hospital making it one of the most expensive, resource demanding and stressful areas (Ervin et al., 2018), with staffing the greatest cost (Leon-Villapalos et al., 2020).

In the adult critical care unit, Park (2019, p. 24) defines critical care as:

> the complex and acute care provided to adults, with single or multiple organ failure, . . .and there should be the prospect of recovery or improvement in the patients' condition at the time of their admission.

This definition outlines intentions to improve patients' situations, and the Faculty of Intensive Care Medicine (FICM) and Intensive Care Society (ICS) (2019, p. 11) view critical care admissions from the focus of achieving patient-centred outcomes, based on the balance of 'burdens and benefits'. The FICM & ICS (2019) advocate flexible use of resources, including organ donation and end-of-life care for patients outside the critical care unit. This is a perceptible shift away from historical treatment of reversible patient illnesses previously identified by the Department of Health (DH, 1996, p. 6), which indicated that critical care was for patients with 'potentially recoverable conditions'. Definitions influence patient admissions and these decisions are complex and multifaceted, based upon patient need, patient wishes, philosophies of care, critical care resources such as bed capacity, specialist equipment, staff expertise, staffing levels, policies, and guidelines.

6Cs: Care

Critical care provision needs to be safe, effective, and evidence-based, and must be underpinned by ethical, person-centred, holistic, and humanistic principles.

'Critical care' as an umbrella term includes High Dependency, Intensive Care and the Post-Anaesthetic Care Unit (Albarran and Richardson, 2013). However, critically ill patients outside of these units can require critical care provision, and this was recognised within the DH (2000) modernisation policy entitled 'Comprehensive Critical Care' which re-envisaged the delivery of critical care services. The concept of 'critical care without walls' was created and patients were categorised by the level of care they required regardless of their location within hospital.

Levels of care

The four levels of care shown in Box 1.1 categorised by the DH (2000) are based upon the extent of patient illness and the intensity of care interventions required. The classification of levels of care provides a 'blueprint' for critical care provision along a continuum of care (Albarran and Richardson, 2013). The FICM & ICS (2019) integrated the care levels within their United Kingdom (UK) guidance for critical care staffing levels to ensure sufficient trained critical care staff care for critically ill patients safely and effectively. These patients require complex care, and therefore staffing provision reflects these demands (Royal College of Nursing (RCN), 2017).

The critical care environment

Critical care units range in size, design, and structure and a typical bedspace can be seen in Figure 1.1. In the UK, Department for Health and Social Care (2013) guidelines specify the recommended design and layout, to ensure each critical care unit has sufficient space to provide appropriate bedside care and treatment. Consequently, there is tendency for critical care units to be larger, more technological, and highly clinical environments in comparison to other hospital wards.

Sufficient staff are needed to safely care for critically ill patients, and the complexity of patient treatment reflects the severity of their illness, which is often compounded by

Box 1.1   The four levels of patient care (*Source:* FICM & ICS, 2019).

Level 0	Patients whose needs can be met through normal ward care in an acute hospital
Level 1	Patients at risk of their condition deteriorating, or those recently relocated from higher levels of care, whose needs can be met on an acute ward with additional advice and support from the critical care team
Level 2	Patients requiring more detailed observation or intervention including support for a single failing organ system or post-operative care and those 'stepping down' from higher levels of care
Level 3	Patients requiring advanced respiratory support alone, or basic respiratory support together with support of at least two organ systems. This level includes all complex patients requiring support for multi-organ failure.

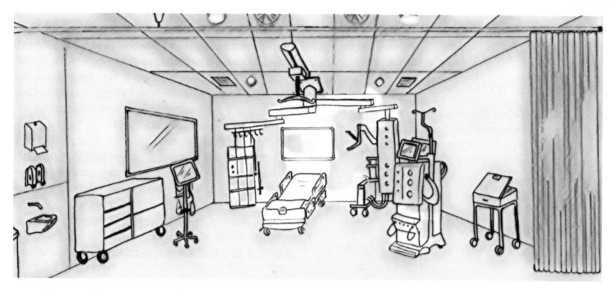

Figure 1.1   Layout of a critical care bed space (Illustrated by Vikki Park 2021 ©).

comorbidities. Therefore, the critical care unit can quickly become crowded with members of the interprofessional team, with machinery and equipment. Consequently, patients can experience sensory overload with elevated and prolonged periods of excessive light, noise, and activity. Critical care teams are hindered, and their collaboration is deterred in units that have poorly positioned equipment, irregular lighting and near constant alarms (Ervin et al., 2018). FICM and ICS (2019) guidelines emphasise that critical care unit design needs to consider environmental factors such as natural light levels, noise reduction and sufficient storage space, and they advocate access to outdoor space. Furthermore, critically ill patients can experience sleep deprivation. Richardson et al. (2013) identify numerous factors that can disturb patient sleep cycles, including mechanical ventilation, noise, light, and critical illness factors such as pain, clinical interventions and medication.

Critical care can be overwhelming for patients, families and all staff, particularly for new workers, students or redeployed colleagues. For patients specifically, this can lead to memories that are upsetting and like nightmares (Bienvenu and Gerstenblith, 2017) and these experiences are often associated with delirium. Tait and White (2019) claim that lack of awareness and knowledge of the adverse effects of delirium can lead to traumatic stress for patients and post-traumatic stress disorder (PTSD). Patients that overcome critical care illness and are discharged from the critical care unit often experience long-term effects as 'survivors' (Connolly et al., 2014). One fifth of 'critical illness survivors' experience PTSD-related symptoms in the first year of discharge from critical care (Bienvenu and Gerstenblith, 2017). Therefore, the need to holistically support patients with psychological recovery from critical illness is apparent, and guidelines from the National Institute for Health and Clinical Excellence (NICE, 2009) outline ways that multidisciplinary critical care rehabilitation can be given to patients.

Orange Flag

Patients admitted to critical care can experience sensory overload, sleep deprivation and can develop delirium and PTSD during their recovery. Rehabilitation support for critical care survivors is advocated, including the utilisation of outside spaces to promote critical care patient recovery. Increased evidence is needed to support critical care patient recovery, such as consideration of the role of psychologists in critical care.

Critical care patients

Whilst patients of all ages can develop critical illness, statistics show that on average patients admitted are older and have comorbidities (Intensive Care National Audit and Research Centre (ICNARC), 2020) and older patients with comorbidities are being increasingly admitted to critical care units (FICM & ICS, 2019). Jones et al. (2020) add to this demographic trend, stating in the last two decades more older patients have been admitted to critical care than can be explained by the demographic shift of the ageing population, but outcomes for critical patients continue to improve and they claim most patients return home following critical care admission. The COVID-19 pandemic has affected the demographics of patients admitted to critical care, and in the UK, early admission data indicated that demographics such as being male or having a body mass index of 30 or higher were commonly associated with critical care patients with COVID-19 (ICNARC, 2021).

Critically ill patients require continuous monitoring, often using invasive medical devices such as central venous catheters (CVC) to monitor central venous pressure (CVP) and to administer multiple intravenous infusions (IVI), and arterial lines to continuously measure

Box 1.2   Examples of patient conditions at Levels 1, 2 and 3.

Level 1   Post-operative observation for a complex patient with extensive previous medical history or comorbidities. Care transitioning down from Level 2 or up from Level 0.

Level 2   One organ failure e.g., respiratory failure. Care transitioning down from Level 3 or up from Level 1.

Level 3   Patient with sepsis and multi-organ failure. Care has transitioned up from Level 2 due to deterioration.

blood pressure and obtain arterial blood samples. Critically ill patients may require clinical interventions to support respiratory, cardiovascular, genitourinary, and gastrointestinal function. Interventions can include invasive or non-invasive ventilation, urinary catheterisation, or parenteral nutrition. Examples of patients that are categorised across Levels 1–3 are provided in Box 1.2.

Level 1 care

Level 1 category patients have the potential to deteriorate, warranting regular vital observations to ensure haemodynamic stability. For example, a Level 1 patient with a NEWS2 score of 4, which is low-risk and requires a ward-based response, needs 4–6 hourly observations, unless one parameter scores 3 and then hourly observations are required (RCP, 2012). This group of patients may include people with a critical care bed booked post-operatively for close observation and monitoring, or patients who have a previous medical history or comorbidities that increase risk of complications or mortality. Level 1 patients may be transitioning their care down from Level 2 and could be ready for transfer to a ward setting, or they could be at risk of deterioration and may therefore require support from the Critical Care Outreach Team (CCOT).

Level 2 care

Patients at Level 2 are historically referred to as 'high dependency patients', and they require support for one failed organ. An example of a Level 2 condition would be a patient with respiratory failure due to Chronic Obstructive Pulmonary Disorder (COPD). Level 2 care is recommended to adopt a nursing care ratio of one nurse to two patients (RCN, 2017; FCM & ICS, 2019). Patients require frequent assessment and close monitoring, are usually conscious and conditions tend to be more stable.

Level 3 care

People who develop multi-organ failure from illnesses such as sepsis require one-to-one nursing care (RCN, 2017; FCM & ICS, 2019) and have severe and life-threatening conditions that need intensive treatment. Patients receiving Level 3 care will probably be intubated and ventilated, often invasively with an endo-tracheal tube (ETT) or tracheostomy tube, rather than non-invasively via a mask. Nutrition and hydration need to be maintained, and sedated ventilated patients are dependent upon the interprofessional critical care team to provide all care, from personal hygiene and positional changes, to organ support. Patients with kidney failure require haemofiltration and cardiovascular support with inotropic medication or vasopressor drugs commonly used in critical care to maintain vascular pressure and perfusion.

Medications management – inotropic and vasopressor medication

Critical care patients with organ failure, decreased vascular resistance, vasodilation, reduced circulating volume or reduced cardiac output may require inotropic or vasopressor medication to improve the blood flow around the body to perfuse tissues and organs.

Inotropes are used to support the cardiovascular system, improving cardiac muscle function, thereby supporting blood pressure, and increasing cardiac output. Inotropes work by affecting heart rate and contractility. Dopamine and dopexamine are examples of inotrope drugs.

Vasopressors increase the vascular tone of the circulation through vasoconstriction, thereby increasing blood pressure, perfusion, and organ function. Vasopressors constrict blood vessels, reducing their diameter, increasing vascular resistance, and raising blood pressure. Noradrenaline and vasopressin are examples of vasopressors.

Inotropes and vasopressors are given intravenously in small volumes with syringe pumps, usually via central venous catheters. Administration of inotropes and vasopressors require close monitoring and careful titration, and caution must be exercised with management of such medication to avoid side effects, to ensure safe administration and to maintain the haemodynamic stability of patients receiving these potent medications.

See Chapters 11 and 13 for a further discussion of medications used in the critical care environment.

The snapshot (a patient referred to CCOT) gives an example of a deteriorating patient that requires admission to the critical care unit.

Snapshot

An example of a patient referral to the Critical Care Outreach Team (CCOT)

The CCOT nurse receives a referral from a surgical ward nurse for an urgent review of a patient who is 2 days post-operative following a hemi-colectomy (bowel surgery). The patient is John, a 67-year-old man who had a bowel resection for cancer. The nurse reports concern about his vital observations and reports he has new-onset confusion and agitation. The nurse is concerned John has sepsis, so has completed an infection screen. John's latest observations are:

Airway (A): Airway is patent and speaking in full sentences.

Breathing (B): Oxygen saturations 93% (NEWS2 = 2), on room air (NEWS2 =0), respiratory rate (RR) 28 breaths per minute (NEWS2 = 3).

Cardiovascular System (C): Blood Pressure (BP) is 90/58 (NEWS2 = 3), Heart Rate (HR) is 112 beats per minute (NEWS2 = 2), capillary refill time (CRT) is 4 seconds.

Disability (D): New-onset confusion is noted (NEWS2 = 3), John is assessed as 'C' on the ACVPU scale (see Chapter 14), Body Temperature (T) is 38.6°C (NEWS2 = 1).

Exposure (E): Wound dressing intact. No abnormalities detected (NAD).

Total NEWS2 score: 14

Nursing actions

- The CCOT nurse attends the ward within 30 minutes to perform an urgent review in line with NEWS2 guidelines (Royal College of Physicians (RCP), 2020).
- John gives consent to be assessed and is updated about his condition.
- Vital observations are repeated and a thorough ABCDE assessment is conducted, with a head-to-toe assessment.
- The medical team is informed of the assessment findings for senior clinical review within 60 minutes (RCP, 2020).
- The patient is categorised as Level 2 – a bed is arranged on critical care to move the patient to an 'environment with monitoring facilities' (RCP, 2020).
- The CCOT nurse liaises with critical care and transfers John to the unit.
- The ward staff contact the patient's family.

Diagnosis

- John is diagnosed with sepsis.
- The Sepsis 6 protocol is initiated.
- The source of the infection is unknown, pending culture and sensitivity results from the infection screen. A broad-spectrum antibiotic is commenced after blood cultures have been obtained.
- 30-minute observations are commenced initially on the ward.
- Oxygen and intravenous (IV) fluids are commenced.

Red Flag

New-onset confusion is an indicator of acute illness and requires urgent clinical assessment. Acutely altered consciousness and cognition can be caused by sepsis, hypoxia, hypotension, or metabolic disturbances.

RCP (2020)

Critical care competence

Critical care requires 'specific knowledge and skills' (ICS, 2020), and to holistically care for critically ill patients, a range of professions are required. The professional boundaries between staff often blur and overlap, and scope of professional practice is influenced by professional jurisdiction based upon profession-specific knowledge (D'Amour and Oandasan, 2005). This means that every profession works within their individual and professional levels of competence and within the remit of their professional field, which is often regulated by professional regulatory bodies such as the Nursing and Midwifery Council (NMC), the Health and Care Professions Council (HCPC) and the General Medical Council (GMC).

6Cs: Competence

To provide high-quality, safe and effective care, healthcare professionals must recognise and work within the limits of their competence for their professional field.

Professionals are perceived as accountable by professional regulatory bodies to effectively apply their knowledge to inform practice-based decisions (Scholes et al., 2013). Healthcare staff registered with a professional regulatory body must possess a minimum level of competence to be entered onto their profession-specific register as a qualified healthcare practitioner, and to maintain registration they must maintain competence through regular learning, skill development and appraisal.

For nurses, the adult critical care nursing role is recognised as highly skilled. However, in the UK, to counter concerns about nurses' competence and post-registration education (Deacon et al., 2017), a national critical care

Box 1.3   Step 1 competency example.

Step 1 Competencies
National Competency Framework for Critical Care Nurses (CC3N, 2015b)

1.1.1 Promoting Psychosocial Wellbeing
You must be able to demonstrate through discussion essential knowledge of (and its application to your supervised practice):

Concept of holistic care and how it can be incorporated into your practice:

- Physical
- Psychological
- Social and family
- Spiritual and cultural

Box 1.4   Some of the healthcare professions working in the critical care unit.

Healthcare professions common to critical care units
Nurses, medical staff, physiotherapists, healthcare support workers, pharmacists, microbiologists, dieticians, speech and language therapists, psychologists, rehabilitation teams, health scientists, critical care outreach teams, advanced critical care practitioners, occupational therapists, infection control teams and students.

competency framework was developed to standardise knowledge and skills, and to develop insight into the critical care nurse role (Critical Care Network National Nurse Leads (CC3N), 2015a). The framework aims to promote safe, effective, transferable levels of care to patients and their families. Nurses new to critical care are expected to complete Step 1 competencies within 12 months, and newly registered nurses need a minimum of 6 weeks supernumerary status. The first element in the Step 1 competencies identified as a priority to achieve relates to promoting psychosocial wellbeing (see Box 1.3). Step 2 and Step 3 competencies are completed alongside academic programmes to develop expertise and competence (CC3N, 2015b).

The interprofessional team

Different professions are involved in providing complex patient care and the number of professionals involved reflects the trajectory patient treatment takes. Box 1.4 illustrates key healthcare professions that may provide critical care.

Critical care nurses are described as the one constant professional presence who advocate for patients and liaise with other professions (Park, 2019), nurses must develop rich knowledge and many skills to provide critical care safely and effectively. Nurses require technical skills, such as operating ventilators or haemofiltration equipment, and they need highly developed assessment skills and interpersonal skills to communicate effectively with patients, families, and colleagues.

Whilst critical care nurses provide 24-hour patient care, often on a one-to-one nurse to patient basis, they are supported by healthcare support workers such as healthcare assistants. Healthcare assistants and nursing support workers are essential members of the critical care unit team, and their role involves supporting healthcare professions

and providing direct care to patients. As a staff group that is not registered with a professional regulatory body, their training and career pathways are supported by organisations such as the RCN (2021), and a code of conduct has been produced by Skills for Care & Skills for Health (2013) to guide training, outlining role expectations and promoting consistent standards for practice.

Teams of doctors from different specialities plan and oversee the patient's treatment. Medical teams present in the critical care unit can include intensivists (critical care consultants), anaesthetists, junior doctors, advanced critical care practitioners (ACCPs), and visiting specialists such as surgeons or gastroenterologists. In the UK, doctors are registered and regulated by the General Medical Council (GMC) and have clearly defined training programmes, career pathways and appraisal processes.

Critically ill patients will often be cared for by physiotherapists. This independent body of practitioners, whose professional focus is on the optimisation of muscularskeletal and respiratory function, are registered with the Health and Care Professions Council (HCPC) in the UK. Physiotherapists are vital in the recovery and rehabilitation of critically ill patients, and they can assist with breathing, ventilation, and mobility.

The intensity and complexity of patient care has resulted in extended roles in the interprofessional team. Several roles now exist, such as advanced critical care practitioners, nursing associates, physiotherapy assistants and critical care assistants. Extended roles in the critical care team have been associated with increased interprofessional learning and holistic care provision (Park, 2019).

To meet the needs of patients and to provide expert care, other professions common to critical care include dieticians to optimise nutritional status, pharmacists to oversee pharmacological management and speech and language therapists to ensure patients can safely swallow, additionally supporting patient communication.

Patients outside of the critical care unit receiving care at Level 1 or above may be cared for by the CCOT, emergency response teams or rehabilitation teams. These external teams are resourced with experienced critical care practitioners and their goal is to stabilise and support patients at specific stages of their critical illness to promote recovery and prevent deterioration.

Communication

Effective communication occurs when staff understand professional roles and share collaborative goals, and Hawryluck et al. (2002) link a lack of understanding with increased tension. Whilst critical care teams have low temporal stability because the team membership frequently changes (Ervin et al., 2018), Alexanian et al. (2015) note that teams continue to work effectively when they communicate shared knowledge and when they have shared expectations of professional roles. Therefore, effective communication between interprofessional team members is fundamental to the success of the collaborative critical care team (Van den Bulcke et al., 2016).

6Cs: Communication
To provide high-quality, safe care, healthcare professionals must communicate clearly and effectively to meet the complex needs of critically ill patients.

Ways of working

The critical care team develops routines and ways of working in the culture of their daily practice. The definitive starting and end point of a shift for most professionals is demarcated by the practice of handover. At the point of a shift change, healthcare staff such as doctors and nurses conduct handovers to update colleagues about the care given to patients and the events that have occurred. Handovers have also been associated with culture and rituals which have shared meanings within teams (Philpin, 2006). Whilst handovers tend to be profession-specific, they can be interprofessional, and interprofessional handovers are advocated within critical care standards to promote engagement in interprofessional activities (FICM & ICS, 2019). In the critical care unit, handover shapes the way professions work.

Each profession works in their own way to meet the remit of their professional focus and has its own goals for patient care, viewing patients through a different professional lens (Park, 2019). Staff are professionally socialised into their roles and Stephens et al. (2011) indicate it takes time for different professions to become professionally socialised in the critical care unit. Socialisation in healthcare happens when profession-specific frameworks shape staff based upon a shared disciplinary worldview with firmly defined professional jurisdictions (D'Amour and Oandasan, 2005). As a multidisciplinary environment, critical care staff share the same goal to care for critically ill patients, but they have different outlooks, professional standards, and regulations (Gagan and Tait, 2019). Therefore, different professions share similar beliefs and values when caring for patients, but their professional perspectives differ.

A core goal shared by the interprofessional critical care team is to promote the provision of safe, effective, high-quality care that is patient-centred and holistic in nature (Park, 2019). This commonality between professions unite staff and forge a community of critical care practice which has shared values and shared purpose.

6Cs: Commitment
All critical care professions are committed to the shared goal of providing safe, holistic, patient-centred care.

Healthcare professions should raise concerns, identify safeguarding issues, and ask questions to learn and promote a safe working environment. The term 'psychological safety' refers to the feeling that staff are free from detrimental consequences if they speak up in the workplace. Ervin et al. (2018) claim that critical care functioning improves when psychological safety enables team members to contribute to problem solving and collaborative decision making. Avoiding 'authoritative decision making' approaches further promotes interprofessional decision making, enabling professions to highlight problems and challenges as they arise (Van den Bulcke et al., 2016).

6Cs: Courage
Healthcare professions require courage to ask questions, to raise concerns and to contribute to collaborative interprofessional decision making and care provision.

Red Flag
Most mistakes and clinical errors can be linked to communication. The extensiveness and low temporal stability of the critical care team means that communication must be exemplary between all interprofessional colleagues to always ensure the safety of critically ill patients.

Understanding philosophies of care

Care given to critically ill patients can become subsumed by the pragmatics of using technology and urgently treating the patient's physical presentation with the aim of monitoring haemodynamic stability and therefore prioritising the treatment of life-threatening conditions. One of the challenges in the critical care unit is to ensure that care remains patient-centred and holistic. It is imperative that the health care team do not lose focus of the patient amidst all the care interventions and invasive treatments, and that care is humanised and based on compassion.

6Cs: Compassion

Compassion in critical care is needed to ensure that the critically ill patient remains the focus of care provided.

The term 'philosophy of care' refers to the philosophical perspectives that individuals position themselves from in the pursuit of providing care to others. Philosophies of care are therefore theoretical belief systems that staff adopt to guide and underpin patient care. The provision of healthcare is based upon the ethical concepts of beneficence and non-maleficence. In simple terms, these are the acts of 'doing good' (Kozier et al., 2012) and 'to do no harm' (Gagan and Tait, 2019).

An example of a philosophy of care advocated in current healthcare practice is holism. Holistic approaches to care are concerned with the whole person, addressing their complex needs, considering the environment and following a bio-psycho-social care model (Kozier et al., 2012). The ICS (2020) caution that 'task-based approaches' to practice create barriers to holistic care. When care is fragmented into discrete tasks, the focus on the patient as a whole person becomes obscured and patients' complex holistic needs cannot be fulfilled. However, White and Tait (2019) recognise that for critically ill patients, critical care nurses may focus on the 'immediacy of sustaining life' rather than providing holistic care.

Patient-centred care as a concept centralises the patient as the focal point of care. Derived from theorist Carl Rogers' interest in client-centred therapy, it has a long history in nursing practice, and is recognised as a core philosophy in healthcare which is associated with quality improvement, adopting a holistic viewpoint (White and Tait, 2019).

Family-centred care is a philosophy that recognises family members need support when relatives become critical care patients, and healthcare professions need to involve families in patient care in person or remotely where possible. Brannay and Brannay (2019) discuss the importance of family access to the critical care unit and associate 'well managed' family visits with improvements

in patient recovery. However, it is known that families experience distress with uncertainty over their relative's recovery and as they adapt to the intimidating unfamiliar critical care environment, therefore staff must care for family in addition to patients (Tait and White, 2019). Family presence in the critical care unit is affected by visiting hours, hospital policies, patient acuity and culture. The COVID-19 pandemic influenced family access to the critical care unit, where prevention measures to reduce infection rates created an absence of families within hospitals. Montauk and Kuhl (2020) explain that increased family separation in critical care during the pandemic is likely to exacerbate psychological dysfunction experienced by families leading to increasingly complex decision making and exclusion from patient care, which prevents information processing, grief and closure.

Humanising critical care

Being human in such an intense clinical environment promotes care that is personable and kind. In such a highly technologically driven environment, with medical crises and invasive treatments, the challenge for those providing critical care is to remain patient-focused and person-centred. White and Tait (2019) propose that as healthcare becomes increasingly technical, the need for humanisation becomes increasingly essential. Humanising care is fundamental to the patient and family experience, and philosophically underpins the approach to critical care.

Humanisation as a philosophical concept can be traced back to key authors such as Carl Rogers and is rooted in the Renaissance and Enlightenment movements (Létourneau et al., 2017). When applied to healthcare, this philosophy perceives patients as people rather than the conditions they have or as a subset of biological systems. Critical care involves the complex balance of caring for patients physically, psychologically, socially, and emotionally, whilst primarily meeting the physiological needs of the body. One of the greatest risks in the critical care unit is for the acute environment to overshadow the human aspects of care, and when this happens, care becomes dehumanised (Todres et al., 2009) and holistic care becomes unachievable. An example of humanised care is patient diaries that capture the lived experience of being in critical care.

Adopting a humanised approach can enhance the therapeutic relationship with patients and their families, building trust and collaboratively working towards shared care goals. Humanising care extends to health professional colleagues as well. Additionally, trust and respect between colleagues can enable open interprofessional communication (Van den Bulcke et al., 2016) and affects interprofessional decision making (Alexanian et al., 2015), Humanising approaches between staff have been linked to improved staff morale, effective teamwork, and open environments where staff can ask questions, use professionally apt humour, share emotions and learn interprofessionally (Park, 2019).

Surviving critical care

Patient and family recovery after critical illness extends beyond admission to critical care. Rehabilitation teams, psychologists and use of outdoor spaces recognise and respect the person experiencing the critical illness with the goal of promoting healing and recovery. Effective patient care is built on a foundation of trust, and rapport developed between patients and the interprofessional team are associated with higher levels of morale and improved patient and family experiences. Survivors of critical care require rehabilitation support after discharge from the unit (NICE, 2009), and rehabilitation teams and voluntary organisations like ICU Steps can offer emotional and social support to patients and families once they have left the critical care unit.

Death in critical care

Whilst many people are discharged, they often experience long-term health conditions and may be readmitted for further treatment. Due to the fragility of patients' health, and the extent of critical illness, many patients do not survive and will die in the critical care unit. Mortality rates in the critical care unit can be high. Chapter 32 discusses dying and death. For staff, ensuring a dignified death that protects patient and family wishes is paramount. Measures taken to promote a humanised and dignified death can include:

- agreeing 'ceilings' of treatment to limit the invasiveness of interventions, where early decisions are made between staff, patients and families to predetermine the limit and 'highest level of intervention' that the medical team consider to be contextually appropriate to promote quality care (Walzl et al., 2019)
- implementing DNACPR orders (Do Not Attempt Cardiopulmonary Resuscitation) and
- initiatives such as ReSPECT (Recommended Summary Plan for Emergency Care and Treatment), endorsed by the Resuscitation Council (UK), which is a document which can capture patients' wishes about ceilings of treatment and CPR, to inform and guide decision making within clinical practice (Hawkes et al., 2020).

Resilience

Critical care staff are repeatedly exposed to stressful and emotional circumstances. Burnout, emotional labour, and moral distress are all associated with staff in the critical care unit, and the workforce is challenged to manage these stressors in a way that promotes health and well-being.

Work in the critical care unit can be emotionally challenging (Highfield, 2019). Critical care provision is complicated, consuming emotional energy (Lindahl and Norberg, 2002), and can evoke intense emotions (Brindley and Reynolds, 2011) which can be culturally stigmatised in relation to coping (Jackson et al., 2018). The process of emotional investment that people make in their daily working lives is often referred to as 'emotional labour' (Hochschild, 2003). Stayt (2009) acknowledges that caring for critically ill patients and their families in the critical care unit expends significant amounts of emotional labour. Further psychological distress can arise for staff in situations where clinical decisions or situations conflict with their personal or professional morals, and this term is referred to as moral distress (Jameton, 2017). Exposure to moral distress in the workplace can lead to burnout and staff attrition as nurses leave the profession (Gutierrez, 2005).

Resilience is often referred to as a means of managing stressful circumstances, although there is no universal definition within research literature (Aburn et al., 2016). Resilience enables nurses to adapt positively to stressors and adversity in the workplace and is recognised as a dynamic and complex process (Cooper et al., 2020) and from these challenging experiences, individuals can learn and gain strength (Grant and Kinman, 2013). In critical care, resilience explains how staff can 'bounce back' from exposure to traumatic situations (Arrogante and Aparicio-Zaldivar, 2017). Resilience is associated with enhanced performance (Hartwig et al., 2020), staff retention, increased job satisfaction, increased quality of care, successful coping, and protection from psychopathology (Cooper et al., 2020). As a complex process, the concept of resilience in nurses is outlined in Figure 1.2, and resilience can be viewed from the perspective of individuals, teams, and organisations.

Personal resilience

From a personal perspective, resilience reduces the effect of workplace stress on critical care professionals' mental health (Arrogante and Aparicio-Zaldivar, 2017) and reflects a nurse's personal response to stressors. Research has indicated multiple factors that can influence resilience for individuals. Key factors include achieving work-life balance and self-care, being realistic and having social support (Cooper et al., 2020), having flexibility (Thomas and Revell, 2016), and having optimism, a sense of humour and self-efficacy (Thomas and Revell, 2016, Cooper et al., 2020). Critical care nurses experience different levels of workplace adversity and awareness of adversity shapes the nurse response (Jackson et al., 2018).

Team resilience

Nurses need resilience to respond to different adverse situations (Arrogante and Aparicio-Zaldivar, 2017), but having a group of individuals with high levels of resilience does not always produce a resilient team. Hartwig et al. (2020) consider a team's ability to face adversity as a collective response that is facilitated through effective collaboration, communication, and coordination, and they refute the aggregation of individual resilience as a representation of a team's overall resilience. Being in a resilient team can reduce workplace stressors for individuals because teams with strongly developed shared identities experience less stress and have higher well-being (van Dick et al., 2018). Shared identities can create commonalities and a community of critical care practice (Park, 2019) and can reduce workloads and increase capacity for team

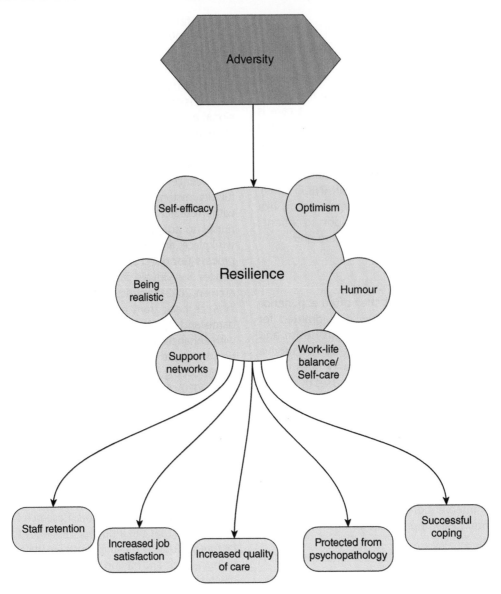

Figure 1.2   The concept of resilience in nurses.
Source: Cooper et al., 2020.

resilience (Hartwig et al., 2020). Team resilience is critical for situations where failure to collaborate as a team at work would jeopardise people's lives (Hartwig et al., 2020), which applies to the critical care unit.

Organisational resilience

Supportive clinical environments are needed to address workplace adversity, to promote retention of staff in critical care units and to promote well-being (Jackson et al., 2018). Therefore, organisational resilience can be viewed as the collective response of multiple teams when facing challenges and threats. Sustaining resilience requires individuals and organisations to engage and take action (Cooper et al., 2020). Overcoming stress in healthcare organisations is the focus of publications such as the 2015 RCN guide *Healthy Workplace, Healthy You. Stress and You: A Guide for Nursing Staff* and the DH 2009 paper *NHS Health and Well-being Final Report*.

Whilst resilience definitions are broad and research remains limited, the links between workplace adversity, burnout and resilience are clear within the acute environment of critical care and several mechanisms have been associated with improved management of workplace stressors, as illustrated in Figure 1.3.

Learning event: reflections

Consider the COVID-19 pandemic and reflect on an experience related to this where you or someone else may have become overwhelmed or required support in the workplace. Consider the coping strategies adopted, mechanisms of support available and ways to promote well-being and resilience.

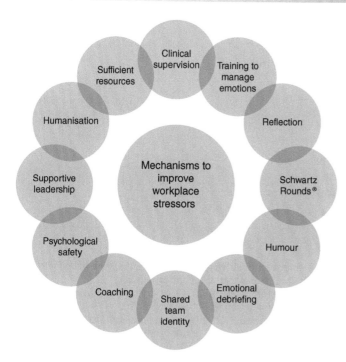

Figure 1.3 Examples of mechanisms to improve workplace stressors.

NMC (2018) Prioritising People

3. Make sure that people's physical, social, and psychological needs are assessed and responded to.

To achieve this, you must:

3.1 pay special attention to promoting wellbeing, preventing ill health, and meeting the changing health and care needs of people during all life stages,

3.2 recognise and respond compassionately to the needs of those who are in the last few days and hours of life,

3.3 act in partnership with those receiving care, helping them to access relevant health and social care, information, and support when they need it,

3.4 act as an advocate for the vulnerable, challenging poor practice and discriminatory attitudes and behaviour relating to their care.

Nursing considerations and recommendations for practice

Nurses must prioritise people, as indicated in the code of professional conduct (NMC, 2018). As indicated in Box 1.5, nurses must assess and respond to patients' holistic needs promoting their health, well-being and preventing illness during all life stages. Partnership working with patients provides information and support, giving access to relevant health and social care. Nurses must act as patient advocates, and upon recognising the patient at the end of their life must provide compassionate care. Complex care must be thoroughly and accurately assessed, and care plans must meet patient's individual needs.

Future challenges

Critical care in the 21st century faces many challenges. The increasingly ageing population presents global challenges of treating more people with increasingly complex needs (Jones et al., 2020). However, the unexpectedness of the COVID pandemic and the rapidity with which the virus spread across the world is a stark reminder that the role of the critical care team has never been more intrinsic to global health and demands persist for increased numbers of highly skilled knowledgeable staff to meet these increasing health demands of the population. Technology is ever-evolving, and clinical practice advances at pace, underpinned by research and evidence as the face of healthcare adapts. Future critical care units need to be flexible to adapt to healthcare challenges, to respond to global health needs, and to maintain a humanised approach to care. The shared goal of providing safe holistic person-centred care is the driver that will ensure the future critical care workforce is versatile and resilient to rise to future challenges.

Conclusion

As a specialised area, the critical care unit often cares for the most critically ill patients in hospital. The large technological units are frequented by many different professions with their own professional perspectives, but all staff work towards the shared goal of providing safe, effective, holistic care to critically ill patients. Therefore, communication within the interprofessional critical care team must be exemplary. Due to the complexity of care provision, those working in critical care units need to become highly skilled and knowledgeable, and sufficient staffing levels are essential to safely provide specialist care. Critical care is emotionally demanding, affecting patients, families and the workforce, and is associated with emotional labour, moral distress and burnout. Individuals, teams and organisations develop resilience to overcome workplace adversities. Adopting a humanising approach to critical care supports patients, families and staff, and this can be challenging in such an acute environment. The critical care team must collaboratively work together to assess and respond to the physical, psychological and social needs of critically ill patients (NMC, 2018).

12

Take home points

1. The critical care unit tends to be large, fast-paced and highly technological.
2. Critically ill patients have complex needs.
3. It takes many different professions to provide holistic critical care.
4. It is important to understand professional roles in critical care.
5. Clear effective communication is needed.
6. Care must be humanised and holistic in approach.
7. The critical care unit can be an emotionally demanding environment.
8. The critical care team must find ways to develop resilience.
9. Critical care patients may require rehabilitation after critical illness.
10. Families require information and support.

References

Aburn, G., Gott, M., and Hoare, K. (2016). What is resilience? An integrative review of the empirical literature. *Journal of Advanced Nursing* 72(5): 980–1000. doi: 10.1111/jan.12888.

Albarran, J.W. and Richardson, A. (2013). Scope and delivery of evidence-based care. In: *Critical Care Manual of Clinical Procedures and Competencies* (ed. J. Mallett, J. Albarran, and R. Richardson), 1–10. Singapore: John Wiley & Sons, Ltd.

Alexanian, J.A., Kitto, S., Rak, K.J., and Reeves, S. (2015). Beyond the team: Understanding interprofessional work in two North American ICUs. *Critical Care Medicine* 43(9): 1880–1886.

Arrogante, O. and Aparicio-Zaldivar, E. (2017). Burnout and health among critical care professionals: The mediational role of resilience. *Intensive and Critical Care Nursing* 42: 110–115. doi: 10.1016/j.iccn.2017.04.010.

Bienvenu, O.J., and Gerstenblith, T.A. (2017). Posttraumatic stress disorder phenomena after critical illness. *Critical Care Clinics* 33(3): 649–658. doi: 10.1016/j.ccc.2017.03.006.

Brannay, J. and Brannay, D. (2019). Haemodynamic instability. In: *Critical Care Nursing: The Humanised Approach* (ed. S.J. White and D. Tait), 99–114. London: Sage.

Brindley, P.G. and Reynolds, S.F. (2011). Improving verbal communication in critical care medicine. *Journal of Critical Care* 26(2): 155–159.

Connolly, B., Douiri, A., Steier, J. et al. (2014). A UK survey of rehabilitation following critical illness: implementation of NICE Clinical Guidance 83 (CG83) following hospital discharge. *British Medical Journal Open* 4(5) e004963. doi: 10.1136/bmjopen-2014-004963.

Cooper, A.L., Brown, J.A., Res, C.S., and Leslie, G.D. (2020). Nurse resilience: A concept analysis. *International Journal of Mental Health Nursing* 29: 553–575. doi: 10.1111/inm.12721.

Critical Care Network National Nurse Leads (2015a). *National Competency Framework for adult critical care nurses: Version two*. Birmingham: Critical Care Network National Nurse Leads (CC3N) – Critical Care Nurse Education Review Forum.

Critical Care Network National Nurse Leads (2015b). *National Competency Framework for Registered Nurses in Adult Critical Care: Step 1 Competencies*. Critical Care Network National Nurse Leads (CC3N) – Critical Care Nurse Education Review Forum.

D'Amour, D. and Oandasan, I. (2005). Interprofessionality as the field of interprofessional practice and interprofessional education: An emerging concept. *Journal of Interprofessional Care* 19(sup 1): 8–20.

Deacon, K.S., Baldwin, A., Donnelly, K.A. et al. (2017). The national competency framework for registered nurses in adult critical care: an overview. *Journal of Intensive Care Medicine* 18(2): 149–156. doi: 10.1177/1751143717691985.

Department for Health and Social Care (2013). *Health Building Note 04-02 Critical care units*. London: HMSO.

Department of Health (2009). *NHS Health and Well-being Final Report November 2009*. London: HMSO.

Department of Health (2000). *Comprehensive Critical Care: A Review of Adult Critical Care*. London: HMSO.

Department of Health (1996). *Guidelines on Admission to and Discharge From Intensive Care and High Dependency Units*. London: HMSO.

Ervin, J.N., Kahn, J.M., Cohen, T.R., and Weingart, L.R. (2018). Teamwork in the intensive care unit. *The American Psychologist* 73(4): 468–477. doi: 10.1037/amp0000247.

Faculty of Intensive Care Medicine and Intensive Care Society (2019). Guidelines for the Provision of Intensive Care Services, 2e. https://www.ficm.ac.uk/sites/default/files/gpics_v2_-_version_for_release_-_final2019.pdf (accessed 18 January 2021).

Gagan M.and Tait, D. (2019). Legal and ethical issues in critical care. In: *Critical Care Nursing: The Humanised Approach* (ed. S.J. White and D. Tait), 223–242. London: Sage.

Grant, L. and Kinman, G. (2013). *The Importance of Emotional Resilience for Staff and Students in the 'Helping' Professions: Developing an Emotional Curriculum*. London: American Psychological Association.

Gutierrez, K.M. (2005). Critical care nurses' perceptions of and responses to moral distress. *Dimensions of Critical Care Nursing* 24(5): 229–241.

Hartwig, A., Clarke, S., Johnson, S., and Willis, S. (2020). Workplace team resilience: A systematic review and conceptual development. *Organizational Psychology Review* 10(3–4): 169–200. doi: 10.1177/2041386620919476.

Hawkes, C.A., Fritz, Z., Deas, G. et al. (2020). Development of the Recommended Summary Plan for Emergency Care and Treatment (ReSPECT) *Resuscitation* 148: 98–107. doi: 10.1016/j.resuscitation.2020.01.003.

Hawryluck, L.A., Espin, S.L., Garwood, K.C. et al. (2002). Pulling together and pushing apart: tides of tension in the ICU team. *Academic Medicine* 77(10): S73–S76.

Highfield, J.A. (2019). The sustainability of the critical care workforce. *Nursing in Critical Care* 24(1): 6–8.

Hochschild, A.R. (2003). *The Managed Heart: Commercialization of Human Feeling*. University of California Press.

Intensive Care National Audit and Research Centre (2021). *ICNARC report on COVID-19 in critical care: England, Wales and Northern Ireland 15 January 2021*. https://www.icnarc.org/Our-Audit/Audits/Cmp/Reports (accessed 19 January 2021).

Intensive Care National Audit and Research Centre (2020). *Key statistics from the Case Mix Programme – adult, general critical care units 1 April 2019 to 31 March 2020*. https://www.icnarc.org/Our-Audit/Audits/Cmp/Reports/Summary-Statistics (accessed 19 January 2021).

Intensive Care Society (2020). *Intensive Care 2020 and Beyond: Co-developing the Future*. London: ICS.

Jackson, J., Vandall-Walker, V., Vanderspank-Wright, B. et al. (2018). Burnout and resilience in critical care nurses: A grounded theory of Managing Exposure. *Intensive and Critical Care Nursing* 48: 28–35.

Jameton, A. (2017). What moral distress in nursing history could suggest about the future of health care. *AMA Journal of Ethics* 19(6): 617–628.

Jones, A., Toft-Petersen, A.P., Shankar-Hari, M. Harrison, D.A., and Rowan, K.M. (2020). Demographic shifts, case mix, activity, and outcome for elderly patients admitted to adult general ICUs in England, Wales, and Northern Ireland. *Critical Care Medicine* 48(4): 466–474. doi: 10.1097/CCM.0000000000004211.

Kozier, B., Erb, G., Berman, A., Snyder, S., Harvey, S., Morgan-Samuel, H. (2012). *Fundamentals of Nursing: Concepts, Process and Practice*, 2e. Harlow: Pearson.

Leon-Villapalos, C., Wells, M., and Brett, S. (2020). Exploratory study of staff perceptions of shift safety in the critical care unit and routinely available data on workforce, patient and organisational factors. *BMJ Open* 10 (e034101). doi: 10.1136/bmjopen-2019-034101.

Létourneau, D., Cara, C., and Goudreau, J. (2017). Humanizing nursing care: An analysis of caring theories through the lens of Humanism *International Journal for Human Caring* 21(1): 32–40.

Lindahl, B. and Norberg, A. (2002). Clinical group supervision in an intensive care unit: a space for relief, and for sharing emotions and experiences of care. *Journal of Clinical Nursing* 11(6): 809–818.

Montauk, T.R., and Kuhl, E.A. (2020). COVID-related family separation and trauma in the intensive care unit. *Psychological trauma: theory, research, practice and policy* 12 (S1) S96–S97. doi: 10.1037/tra0000839.

National Institute for Health and Clinical Excellence (2009). *Rehabilitation after critical illness NICE Clinical Guideline 83*. London: NICE.

Nursing and Midwifery Council (2018). *The Code. Professional Standards of Practice and Behaviour for Nurses, Midwives and Nursing Associates*. https://www.nmc.org.uk/globalassets/sitedocuments/nmc-publications/nmc-code.pdf (accessed 23 May 2020).

Paradis, E., Leslie, M., Gropper, M.A. et al. (2013). Interprofessional care in intensive care settings and the factors that impact it: Results from a scoping review of ethnographic studies. *Journal of Critical Care* 28(6): 1062–1067.

Park, V. (2019). Learning in Critical Care: A Focused Ethnography of Interprofessional Learning Culture. Doctoral thesis. Northumbria University.

Philpin, S. (2006). 'Handing over': Transmission of information between nurses in an intensive therapy unit. *Nursing in Critical Care* 11(2): 86–93.

Richardson, A., Allsop, M., and Coghill, E. (2013). Assessment of sleep and sleep promotion. In: *Critical Care Manual of Clinical Procedures and Competencies* (ed. J. Mallett, J. Albarran, and R. Richardson), 421–434. Singapore: John Wiley & Sons, Ltd.

Rothschild, J.M., Landrigan, C.P., Cronin, J.W. et al. (2005). The Critical Care Safety Study: The incidence and nature of adverse events and serious medical errors in intensive care. *Critical Care Medicine* 33(8): 1694–1700.

Royal College of Nursing (RCN) (2021). *Careers resources for Nursing Support Workers: Resources for Healthcare Assistants, Support Workers, Assistant Practitioners and Nursing Associates*. https://www.rcn.org.uk/professional-development/your-career/hca (accessed 22 January 2021).

Royal College of Nursing (2017). *Safe and Effective Staffing: Nursing Against the Odds*. London: RCN.

Royal College of Nursing (2015). *Healthy Workplace, Healthy You. Stress and You: A Guide for Nursing Staff*. London: RCN.

Royal College of Physicians (2020). *National Early Warning Score (NEWS) 2 Standardising the assessment of acute-illness severity in the NHS Additional implementation guidance*. London: RCP.

Royal College of Physicians (2012). *National Early Warning Score (NEWS) 2 Standardising the assessment of acute-illness severity in the NHS*. London: RCP.

Scholes, J., Richmond, J., and Mallett, J. (2013). Competency-based practice. In: *Critical Care Manual of Clinical Procedures and Competencies*, 11–26. Singapore: John Wiley & Sons, Ltd.

Skills for Care & Skills for Health (2013). *Code of Conduct for Healthcare Support Workers and Adult Social Care Workers in England*. Leeds: SfC/SfH.

Stayt, L.C. (2009). Death, empathy and self preservation: the emotional labour of caring for families of the critically ill in adult intensive care. *Journal of Clinical Nursing* 18(9): 1267–1275.

Stephens, J., Abbott-Brailey, H., and Platt, A. (2011). 'Appearing the team': from practice to simulation. *International Journal of Therapy & Rehabilitation* 18(12): 672–682.

Tait, D. and White, S.J (2019). The impact of critical illness on recovery and rehabilitation. In: *Critical Care Nursing: The Humanised Approach* (ed. S.J. White and D. Tait), 243–258. London: Sage.

Thomas, L.T. and Revell, S.H. (2016). Resilience in nursing students: An integrative review. *Nurse Education Today* 36: 457–462. doi: 10.1016/j.nedt.2015.10.016.

Todres, L., Galvin, K.T., and Holloway, I. (2009). The humanization of healthcare: A value framework for qualitative *research International Journal of Qualitative Studies on Health and Well-being* 4(2): 68–77.

Van den Bulcke, B., Vyt, A., Vanheule, S., Hoste, E., Decruyenaere, J., and Benoit, D. (2016). The perceived quality of interprofessional teamwork in an intensive care unit: A single centre intervention study. *Journal of Interprofessional Care* 30(3): 301–308.

van Dick, R., Ciampa, V., and Liang, S. (2018). Shared identity in organizational stress and change. *Current Opinion in Psychology* 23: 20–25 http://dx.doi.org/10.1016/j.copsyc.2017.11.005

Walzl, N., Jameson, J., Kinsella, J., and Lowe, D.J. (2019). Ceilings of treatment: a qualitative study in the emergency department. *BMC Emergency Medicine* 19(9): 1–8. doi: 10.1186/s12873-019-0225-6.

White, S.J. and Tait, D. (2019). Humanised care and clinical decision making in critical care. In: *Critical Care Nursing: The Humanised Approach* (ed. S.J. White and D. Tait), 5–34. London: Sage.

Chapter 2

Organisational influences

Vikki Park

Aim

This chapter discusses the organisational influences that affect critical care provision in the United Kingdom (UK). The critical care unit is affected by legislation, in addition to local, national, and international influences. These will be explored with consideration of the changing landscape of critical care with advances in evidence-based practice and current UK legislative review.

Learning outcomes

After reading this chapter the reader will be able to:

- Have an awareness of organisational influences that affect critical care.
- Appreciate legislation affecting critical care.
- Understand the role of Professional Regulatory Statutory Bodies.
- Consider national and international influences on critical care.
- Recognise the influence of local policies and voluntary agencies.

Test your prior knowledge

- Name three Professional Statutory Regulatory Bodies (PSRBs) in the UK.
- What is the name of the UK law that focuses on capacity for decision making?
- Which international organisation advocates using 5 moments of hand hygiene?
- Identify what types of patient information are personal data.
- Based upon current evidence, critically discuss published standards and guidelines that influence critical care practices.

Fundamentals of Critical Care: A Textbook for Nursing and Healthcare Students, First Edition. Edited by Ian Peate and Barry Hill.
© 2023 John Wiley & Sons Ltd. Published 2023 by John Wiley & Sons Ltd.
Companion website: www.wiley.com/go/peate/criticalcare

Introduction

Chapter 2 explores wider organisational influences that affect the provision of critical care in the UK. Legislation, guidelines and professional organisations shape the standards of care, the infrastructure and critical care practices. The way the critical care unit is organised and operates reflects the standards and requirements outlined by local, national and international governments and organisations.

The four UK nations

In Great Britain (GB), health and social care provision is managed differently, and the roles, remit and power of England, Scotland and Wales health and social care regulators differ. Northern Ireland (NI) additionally has different healthcare provision and forms the UK in combination with the three GB nations.

England

In England, the Department of Health and Social Care (DHSC), previously known as the Department of Health (DH), is the government department responsible for health and adult social care policy. DHSC policies primarily relate to England, where other matters are devolved to the Scottish Government, Welsh Government or Northern Ireland Executive. The DHSC oversees the English National Health Service (NHS), and works with 29 agencies and public bodies. These include the executive agency Public Health England, and executive non-departmental public bodies such as NHS England, Health Education England and the Care Quality Commission (CQC) which regulates the quality and safety of all health and social care services in England (UK Government, 2021a).

Scotland

The Scotland Act 1998 is a UK General Public Act which devolved healthcare to the Scottish Parliament from the UK Parliament (UK Legislation, 1998). In Scotland, the NHS is therefore managed by Scottish Government, and most of the care provision is paid for through taxation. NHS Scotland comprises 14 regional NHS Boards, 1 Public Health Body and 7 Special NHS Boards. Regional NHS Boards provide healthcare services responsible for the protection and improvement of health in each board population. The NHS Scotland Public Health Body is Public Health Scotland, which is Scotland's 'lead national agency' responsible for the improvement and protection of health and well-being (Public Health Scotland, 2020). Seven Special NHS Boards are part of NHS Scotland, and they include Healthcare Improvement Scotland (HIS), which evaluates the quality and safety of Scottish healthcare, further outlined within their 5-year strategy (Healthcare Improvement Scotland, 2017).

Wales

Previously, the Wales health system was administered through the UK Governments Welsh Office, but from 1999 responsibility for most health policy was devolved to Wales (Longley et al., 2012). NHS Wales is a publicly funded healthcare system, which is part of the UK National Health Service. Welsh healthcare is delivered using various providers, including seven Local Health Boards which cover geographical areas in Wales and three NHS Trusts, including Public Health Wales. The independent inspectorate and regulator of healthcare quality in Wales is the Healthcare Inspectorate Wales (Healthcare Inspectorate Wales, 2019).

Northern Ireland

Northern Ireland (NI) is part of the UK, and health and social care is government-funded and free at the point of delivery. The NI Department of Health have responsibility for health and social care, including health workforce policy and management, governance in health and social care, and safety and quality standards. The Health and Social Care Board, Public Health Agency and other Health and Social Care (HSC) bodies are accountable to the NI Department of Health for the commissioning and provision of effective health and social care services (Northern Health and Social Care Trust, 2020). The quality of health and social care in NI is regulated by the Regulation and Quality Improvement Authority (Regulation and Quality Improvement Authority, 2021).

6Cs: Competence

To be competent, nurses need to have awareness of legislation and guidelines to understand their relevance to clinical practice and to appropriately apply them.

Legislation

Critical care practice is shaped by legislation with regards to patient treatment, professional conduct, and care provision

Professional Statutory Regulatory Bodies (PSRBs)

In the UK, the following Professional Statutory Regulatory Bodies (PSRBs) determine and regulate the professional knowledge, competence and conduct of registered health professionals: Nursing and Midwifery Council (NMC), General Medical Council (GMC) and Health and Care Professions Council (HCPC). The PSRB standards of practice are based upon legislation such as the Health Professions Order (2001), and practising professionals must be registered with their respective PSRB to lawfully practise in the UK. It is unlawful to practise as a nurse without being a registrant with the NMC in the UK (NMC, 2018).

16

With the ultimate purpose of protecting the public, registered health professionals have a legal duty of care. Within their 2021–2026 Corporate Strategy, the HCPC (2021) emphasise that the core of their PSRB work is to promote protection of the public. The NMC (2020) similarly position patient protection as a core principle within their 5-year strategy *NMC Strategy: Regulate, Support, Influence, 2020–2025*, whereas the GMC (2020) emphasise that patients need to trust medical staff with their lives and must maintain standards of practice across four domains: knowledge, skills and performance; safety and quality; communication, partnership and teamwork; and maintaining trust. Therefore, the legal duty of care is central to the professional standards outlined by PSRBs for health professionals working within UK critical care.

Red Flag

To maintain a legal and professional duty of care to patients, critical care professionals need to protect patients from harm, often making decisions on their behalf.

Shared decision making

Ethical and legal principles advocate that where possible patients should plan care with health professionals. NHS England (2020) state that it is a statutory duty from the National Health Service Act 2006 (as amended by the Health and Social Care Act 2012) for Clinical Commissioning Groups and NHS England, to involve people in their care and to make shared decisions with individuals about any health services provided. Shared decision making is noted by all UK PSRBs and underpins the philosophy of patient-centred care (NMC, 2018; GMC, 2019; HCPC, 2016).

For critically ill patients potentially unable to make informed independent decisions about their care during their admission to the critical care unit, the NMC requires that nurses must safeguard the privacy and dignity of patients and must act as an advocate to promote the patient's best interests (NMC, 2018). Consent for treatment becomes challenging to obtain in the critical care environment, and the complexity of this process is compounded when patients are unconscious, critically unwell or medicated for example. Chapter 3 discusses legal and ethical issues in more detail.

Gagan and Tait (2019) emphasise that, legally, any treatment risks to patients need to be disclosed and alternative strategies or treatments need to be discussed to ensure informed consent can be obtained. Whilst care decisions should always involve the patient wherever possible, in the acute environment of critical care decisions may need to be made with urgency, requiring compassion, consultation with others, and decisions must be based on principles of non-maleficence and beneficence to respect ethical and legal frameworks. Beneficence is indicated by Bester (2020) as the means of providing benefit to patients to promote and protect wellbeing, and non-maleficence is ensuring that care provided does not cause harm (Gagan and Tait, 2019).

6Cs: Care

The primary goal of health care is to benefit patients by restoring or maintaining their health as far as possible, thereby maximising benefit and minimising harm. If treatment fails, leads to more harm or burden than benefit (from the patient's perspective), ceases to benefit the patient, or if an adult with capacity has refused treatment, that treatment is no longer justified.

British Medical Association, Resuscitation Council (UK), Royal College of Nursing (2016)

Capacity for shared decision making

The urgent nature of critical care can require action, without delay, to support and protect patients from harm, and this indicates that treatment is needed to sustain life (Mental Capacity Act (MCA), 2005). Such urgency in treatment can prevent time to seek informed consent from patients and alternative measures or associated risks from alternative treatments may not be possible to discuss in advance with patients receiving life-saving treatment. The NMC (2018) requires nurses to act in the best interests of patients without delay, and therefore, emergency situations in critical care are recognised as presenting ethical and legal challenges for healthcare professionals.

For a person to provide consent, they require mental capacity to make independent decisions and capacity is presumed until proven otherwise (Mental Capacity Act (MCA), 2005). The Mental Capacity Act (2005) outlines four elements required to enable people to have capacity to provide consent (see Box 2.1).

Box 2.1 Determinants of mental capacity to make decisions. *Source:* MCA, 2005.

A person has capacity if they can:

1. Understand any information relevant to the decision in question.
2. Retain that information.
3. Use the information to make their decision.
4. Communicate their decision MCA (2005)

The capacity of critically ill patients to make decisions is often detrimentally affected when a patient's cognitive functioning is affected. Cognition is discussed further in Chapter 15.

Confidentiality

Confidentiality is key in critical care and numerous legislations govern management of personal data and information. UK GDPR (United Kingdom General Data Protection Regulation) is a regulation that outlines legal management of personal data and therefore determines the context within which patient information, personal data, or other confidential information can be shared with others in critical care. The General Data Protection Regulation (GDPR, 2016) is European Union (EU) legislation that has been amended, incorporated into UK law as UK GDPR, and updated following the end of the agreed transition period leaving the EU. The Data Protection Act (DPA, 2018) is legislation which sits alongside GDPR and provides a framework for data protection in the UK. The Freedom of Information Act (FOIA, 2000) is another regulation which gives members of the public a means of requesting information from organisations. FOIA is a UK General Public Act which outlines the disclosure of information permitted by public authorities or people providing public services (UK Legislation, 2000).

6Cs: Communication

Legislation regulates the lawful retention and exchange of personal information and nurses must be aware of the law and its relation to data protection when communicating with others.

Personal data is defined as information which relates to an 'identified or identifiable natural person' referred to as the 'data subject' and this includes any information which if provided could make an individual identifiable (Information Commissioner's Office (ICO), 2020). The ICO statutory Data Sharing Code of Practice (ICO, 2020) indicates that exemptions include sharing data in an emergency, as is necessary and proportionate, for example if there is risk of serious harm to individuals. In critical care, this has implications for the patient information that nurses may consider sharing with others, particularly with family members, or during emergency situations if a patient's condition deteriorates. Box 2.2 outlines the seven key principles of UK GDPR which are central to the approach taken to processing personal data (ICO, 2021).

Box 2.2 Key principles of personal data processing with UK GDPR. *Source:* ICO, 2021.

Seven key principles of UK GDPR:

1. Lawfulness, fairness, and transparency
2. Purpose limitation
3. Data minimisation
4. Accuracy
5. Storage limitation
6. Integrity and confidentiality (security)
7. Accountability

6Cs: Commitment

Nurses and health professionals must commit to upholding legislation principles to ensure that patient confidentiality and privacy is lawfully protected for critically ill patients who cannot provide consent to share personal or sensitive information.

Decisions relating to end-of-life care

Decisions and treatment provided for patients at the end of their life are often influenced by legislation. Healthcare professionals must have awareness of their legal and ethical responsibilities relating to refusal of treatment and when making decisions about end-of-life care (Gagan and Tait, 2019). Patients with capacity have a right to refuse consent to treatment (MCA, 2005). Patients with capacity may also have made advance directives or decisions to be used in any future event where they lose capacity but still wish to refuse specific nursing or medical treatments (Gagan and Tait, 2019). Pattison (2013) states that withdrawing and withholding treatment from a critically ill patient will cause patient death and notes the ethical implications and complexities of making end-of-life care decisions in critical care.

Do not attempt cardiopulmonary resuscitation (DNACPR) orders may be obtained for patients, and these would be considered for patients who for example would not benefit from CPR if their prognosis were considered poor or their condition deemed irreversible (Pattison, 2013). A joint guideline about making cardiopulmonary resuscitation decisions has been published by the British Medical Association (BMA), the Resuscitation Council UK (RCUK), and the Royal College of Nursing (RCN) (2016). These guidelines provide healthcare professionals with a framework to make decisions about CPR which comply with the Human Rights Act (1998).

6Cs: Compassion

To care for patients at the end of their life, nurses must uphold the ethical and legal principles that frame care provision and must care with compassion, respecting the privacy and dignity of patients and their families.

Risk management

Effective risk management is essential in critical care. The Health and Safety Executive (HSE) is the government agency responsible for maintaining workplace safety in GB, and they are therefore pivotal to healthcare organisations to ensure safe operational practices. Within critical care for example, the HSE regulate clinical waste management, and policies and practices such as disposal of sharps and clinical waste are regulated by legislation and standards that are outlined by this government agency. Fire safety, evacuation procedures, safe use of medical devices, radiological protection, and moving and handling practices are all underpinned by HSE legislation and the Health and Safety at Work Act etc. UK Legislation (1974). Nurses are responsible for ensuring safe and effective practice, and nurses must be competent with risk management and courageous enough to raise concerns and challenge unsafe practice (NMC, 2018).

6Cs: Courage

In the 2021–2026 Strategy the NMC outline their vision for safe, effective, and kind nursing and midwifery, to improve everyone's health and wellbeing. Nurses must use courage to challenge behaviours or practices which may be unsafe.

International influences

The current UK legal system is experiencing a period of historical significance as the nation adapts to its transition out of its partnership with the European Union. The UK exited from the EU on the of 31 January 2020, and 11 months later, the transition period ended on the 31 December 2020. Legislation such as the EU Working Time Directive, embedded into UK law with The Working Time (Amendment) Regulations 2003 and enforced by the HSE (UK Legislation, 2003), may be subject to review. The NMC entered a period of consultation to review the EU Recognition of Professional Qualifications regulations (UK Legislation, 2015) which stipulates a minimum completion of 2300 hours of clinical

Box 2.3   Examples of international critical care nursing organisations.

International organisations for critical care nurses:

- World Federation of Intensive and Critical Care
- World Federation of Critical Care Nurses
- World Federation of Societies of Intensive and Critical Care Medicine
- European Federation of Critical Care Nursing Associations
- European Society of Intensive Care Medicine

placement required for professional nurse registration. Future working practices of UK critical care units may be shaped by these legislative changes.

The World Health Organization (WHO) is an influential international organisation within the United Nations' system with the role of promoting international health and leading responses to global health issues. The organisation produces reports, guidelines and launches global campaigns such as *Save Lives: Clean Your Hands* which advocated 5 moments for hand hygiene (WHO, 2009). These evidence-based campaigns and guidelines continue to influence the care provided within critical care units across the world. There are numerous international organisations for critical care nurses and examples of these are provided in Box 2.3.

National influences

In the UK, critical care is influenced by government organisations, professional organisations, operational delivery networks, guidelines, independent quality assurance agencies, and evidence-based research.

UK government organisations

England, Scotland, Wales and Northern Ireland governments shape the provision of healthcare in the UK. For critical care services in England, the Department of Health (2000) publication *Comprehensive Critical Care: A Review of Adult Critical Care Services* transformed the operationalisation of critical care. The review advocated integration of services, it extended critical care provision based on patient need rather than location within a critical care unit and advocated roles such as critical care outreach teams. This publication changed the landscape of critical care provision in England and illustrates how government publications can influence critical care practice.

The design of critical care units in the NHS is outlined by the Department for Health and Social Care (2013), who published building guidelines which influence the physical and practical design of critical care units within hospitals. Critical care units are 'highly technological' environments, treating the hospitals most critically ill patients, within large bedspaces using a wide range of equipment which enables constant monitoring and treatment of patients (Park, 2020). Building guidelines are therefore required to ensure sufficient space is provided for safe and effective working, compliant with the Safety at Work Act legislation, to safeguard critical care patients, families and staff.

NHS England is an organisation that is an executive non-departmental public body, sponsored by the Department of Health and Social Care (UK Government, 2021b). The operationalisation of the critical care unit is influenced by NHS England Service Specifications. Service Specifications define the standards of care required by NHS England funded organisations and describe core standards which should be demonstrable by these organisations and developmental service standards which include those requiring adaptation and improvement over time (NHS England and NHS Improvement, 2021b). The Service Specification for Adult Critical Care (NHS England, 2019) outlines care pathways, outcomes and quality standards, and service standards which underpin the infrastructure and organisation of critical care units. For example, the Service Specification for Adult Critical Care states that half of nursing staff need to have a post-registration award in critical care nursing and there must be a training strategy to achieve this. Therefore, these specifications influence the function of critical care units regarding staff activity, service structure and development.

In 2019, NHS England and NHS Improvement combined to work as one organisation to support the NHS delivery of care in England. They have made a recommendation to parliament for legislative change that would ensure that place-based partnerships within Integrated Care Systems are supported by a statutory NHS Integrated Care System body that would comprise wider health and care organisations and in partnership they would develop plans for health, social care, and public health (NHS England and NHS Improvement, 2021a). For critical care, Integrated Care Systems and the potential for a statutory NHS Integrated Care System body offer potential to improve further streamlining of services and increased collaborative working with sectors of health, social care and public health that have historically been operationalised within fragmented systems separate to the work of critical care. This is of particular significance in view of recent statistics which indicate that in 2018/2019, 10,431 patients, which equates to 5.3% of the critical care discharge destination data received, were transferred home from the critical care department (NHS Digital, 2019); streamlined working with primary health and social care services within Integrated Care Systems will therefore influence the care and services given to critical care patients and families.

Networks

The Critical Care Service Specification additionally recognises the relationship with operational delivery networks. Currently there are 18 critical care operational delivery networks in England, Wales and Northern Ireland (Association of Chartered Physiotherapists in Respiratory Care, 2021). These were developed after the DH (2000) review of critical care services, with the purpose of coordinating regional and local resources to ensure optimal efficiency, standardised equipment use, protocols and training, and to facilitate safe patient transfers between regional hospitals (Baker and Whitley, 2013).

Critical Care Network National Nurse Leads (CC3N) comprises nurse leads from critical care operational delivery networks across England, Wales and Northern Ireland and they meet quarterly with other critical care forums such as the UK Critical Care Nursing Alliance (UKCCNA) and the Critical Care Leadership Forum to improve the safety, quality and experience of critical care service users (CC3N, 2018). The CC3N Communication Strategy illustrates the large number of organisations and networks which influence UK critical care, and some of these are listed in Box 2.4 and include the BACCN (British Association for Critical Care Nurses), the ICS (Intensive Care Society) and the FICM (Faculty of Intensive Care Medicine). These organisations support and develop the knowledge of critical care staff, they contribute to the development of policy, guidelines and standards, and promote high-quality provision of critical care to patients and families.

Box 2.4 Critical care networks in UK.

Examples of UK networks which influence critical care units:

- British Association for Critical Care Nurses
- UK Critical Care Nursing Alliance
- Royal College of Nursing
- National Outreach Forum
- Intensive Care Society
- National Critical Care Network Forum
- Advanced Critical Care Practitioner Forum
- Faculty of Intensive Care Medicine

Orange Flag

Voluntary organisations, such as ICU Steps, are important organisations which influence critical care. They promote the holistic recovery of patients and families, and all critical care patients need access to a follow-up clinic for psychological support.

National guidelines

Many UK organisations produce national guidelines which are applicable to critical care provision. Publication of the Core Standards for Intensive Care Units (FICM and ICS, 2013) preceded Guidelines for the Provision of Intensive Care Services (GPICS) first published in 2015. The second version of the GPICS guidelines, published in 2019, affects planning, commissioning, and delivery of critical care in the UK (FICM and ICS, 2019). Epic3 guidelines for preventing healthcare-associated infections in NHS hospitals in England (Loveday et al., 2014) are an example of research commissioned by the Department of Health and the evidence-based guidelines are advocated to promote patient safety by the NHS Improvement organisation.

Evidence-based guidelines are also produced for NHS organisations to promote the safety and well-being of patients and staff. In England and Wales (subject to Welsh legislation), guidelines are produced by the National Institute for Health and Care Excellence (NICE) to guide practice and to find new cost-effective treatments and interventions to implement into the NHS (Walsh and Dark, 2019). In Northern Ireland, the NI Department of Health has adopted a process whereby the transferability of NICE guidelines produced for England and Wales are endorsed, implemented, monitored and reviewed. During the COVID-19 pandemic, such guidelines included the NICE COVID-19 rapid guidelines for critical care NG159 (NICE, 2020) developed to promote the safety of staff and patients and to promote the 'best use' of NHS resources. This guideline was updated and replaced by NG191 NICE (2021) COVID-19 rapid guideline: managing COVID-19, to apply to all patients, children, young people and adults, across all care settings, and included new recommendations on treatment, alongside previous guidelines for managing symptoms with conditions such as reducing the risk of venous thromboembolism in over-16s with COVID-19 and antibiotics for pneumonia in adults in hospital.

In Scotland, evidence-based guidelines are produced by the Scottish Intercollegiate Guidelines Network (SIGN). SIGN is from the Evidence Directorate of Healthcare Improvement Scotland but maintains editorial independence from the Scottish Government-funded organisation (Scottish Intercollegiate Guidelines Network, 2020a). The goal of SIGN is to improve the quality of care for patients in Scotland, promoting standardisation of practice, by disseminating national clinical evidence-based guidelines. Recent SIGN guidelines relating to the COVID-19 pandemic include Assessment of COVID-19 in primary care (SIGN, 2021) and Managing the long-term effects of COVID-19 (SIGN, 2020b).

Examples of other national guidelines that have influenced critical care provision include Rehabilitation after Critical Illness guidelines (NICE, 2009), Difficult Airway Society ICU intubation guidelines (Higgs et al., 2018), and the Royal College of Anaesthetists (2018) Care of the critically ill woman in childbirth; enhanced maternal care guidelines.

Such national guidelines shape the provision of critical care services as the evidence base evolves.

Quality assurance

To ensure high standards of care provision within critical care, several quality assurance processes have been established. For example, critical care units in England need to have surveillance systems for nosocomial infections, structured clinical audit programmes to compare practice to published standards and must participate in a national audit programme such as ICNARC (Intensive Care National Audit & Research Centre) to monitor quality and improvement (Rooney and Mathieu, 2019). Macnaughton and Webb (2019) note that the GPICS guidelines have been used in critical care as the benchmark to peer review and have been used to base assessment upon by the England healthcare regulator the Care Quality Commission (CQC).

To assess the quality of critical care services, each UK nation has quality review processes. In England, the CQC use the *Inspection framework: Critical Care (Acute and independent healthcare)* (CQC 2019) to review critical care provision. This document outlines the standards, services, and practices with respect to evidence and guidelines to benchmark critical care services against as indicators of quality.

In Scotland, Healthcare Improvement Scotland (HIS) is responsible for evaluating the quality and safety of Scottish healthcare. Their five-year strategy outlines five strategic priorities which includes providing objective assessments of the quality and sustainability of care, to meet the priority of offering and embedding quality assurance to give people confidence in the sustainability and quality of services in Scotland (Healthcare Improvement Scotland, 2017).

Quality assurance of healthcare in Wales is provided by the Healthcare Inspectorate Wales (Healthcare Inspectorate Wales, 2019). Healthcare Inspectorate Wales regulates and inspects NHS and independent healthcare organisations in Wales against standards, guidance, policies and regulations with the aim of highlighting areas for improvement.

In Northern Ireland, the quality of health and social care is regulated by the Regulation and Quality Improvement Authority (RQIA) which is an independent body that inspects the quality of care and leadership, highlighting good practice and areas of concern to drive improvements (Regulation and Quality Improvement Authority, 2021).

In addition to quality assurance organisations, critical care has also been influenced by benchmarking practice as illustrated with Essence of Care benchmarking (DH, 2010), and research influences critical care with the use of care bundles such as Sepsis 6 from the UK Sepsis Trust. Daniels et al. (2011) researched the Surviving Sepsis Care resuscitation bundle, and their findings indicated an association with reduced mortality, demonstrating that simplified treatment pathways such as Sepsis 6, used with education programmes such as Survive Sepsis, can improve the delivery of life-saving interventions for critically ill patients.

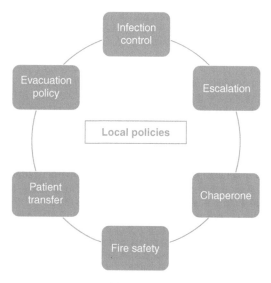

Figure 2.1   Examples of local policies in critical care.

Local policies

Policies used within hospitals and within critical are units are based upon legislation, organisations, PSRBs, research and evidence-based guidelines. Examples of local policies are indicated in Figure 2.1 and they affect the daily practice of critical care experienced by patients, families, and critical care staff.

Nursing considerations and recommendations for practice

Nurses must act in the best interests of patients, as indicated in Box 2.5, and nurses must respect the right to privacy and confidentiality (NMC, 2018). Professional, ethical and legal factors impact on caring for critically ill patients and decision-making processes about provision or withdrawal of critical care treatment should involve all professions, patients and families wherever possible to meet professional, ethical and legal requirements (Pattison, 2013). Nurses must be competent to balance the best interests of patients, complying with legislation, and have a 'duty of confidentiality' based upon respect, dignity, effective communication, and appropriate information sharing (NMC, 2018).

Box 2.5   Ethically and legally acting in best interests. *Source:* NMC, 2018.

NMC (2018) Prioritising People

4.   Act in the best interests of people at all times.

To achieve this, you must:

4.1   balance the need to act in the best interests of people at all times with the requirement to respect a person's right to accept or refuse treatment

4.2   make sure that you get properly informed consent and document it before carrying out any action

4.3   keep to all relevant laws about mental capacity that apply in the country in which you are practising, and make sure that the rights and best interests of those who lack capacity are still at the centre of the decision-making process

4.4   tell colleagues, your manager and the person receiving care if you have a conscientious objection to a particular procedure and arrange for a suitably qualified colleague to take over responsibility for that person's care.

Conclusion

Critical care nurses must have awareness of organisational influences on the provision of critical care to ensure that safe high-quality patient-centred care is provided to patients. Albarran and Richardson (2013) emphasise that the delivery of high-quality critical care that reflects national standards is within the remit of all healthcare professionals irrespective of their grade or status within the organisation. Nurses working within critical care must have an awareness of legislation, evidence, national guidelines, and standards to continue to care for critically ill patients and families within professional, ethical, and legal frameworks.

Take home points

1. Critical care is influenced by local, national and international factors.
2. Legislation underpins the provision of critical care services.
3. The United Kingdom is experiencing an extensive period of legislative review with the exit from the European Union.
4. Consent is complex in critical care and shared decision making is the goal.
5. Critically ill patients often lack mental capacity to consent for treatment.
6. Nurses must be advocates and act in the patient's best interests.
7. Ethically and legally, patient confidentiality must be maintained.
8. The infrastructure of UK critical care services is affected by guidelines and standards produced by many different national organisations.
9. Evidence-based guidelines are integrated into critical care practice.
10. Voluntary organisations, such as ICU Steps, influence critical care services.

References

Albarran, J.W. and Richardson, A. (2013). Scope and delivery of evidence-based care. In: *Critical Care Manual of Clinical Procedures and Competencies* (ed. J. Mallett, J. Albarran, and R. Richardson), 1–10. Singapore: John Wiley & Sons.

Association of Chartered Physiotherapists in Respiratory Care (2021). *Critical care network: Index of UK Critical Care Networks (or Operational Delivery Networks)*. https://www.acprc.org.uk/resources/critical-care/critical-care-networks/ (accessed 2 April 2021).

Baker, A., and Whitley, S.M. (2013). Transfer of the critically ill patient. In: *Critical Care Manual of Clinical Procedures and Competencies* (ed. J. Mallett, J. Albarran, and R. Richardson), 469–488. Singapore: John Wiley & Sons.

Bester, J.C. (2020). Beneficence, Interests, and Wellbeing in Medicine: What It Means to Provide Benefit to Patients. *The American Journal of Bioethics* 20(3): 53–62. doi: 10.1080/15265161.2020.1714793.

British Medical Association, Resuscitation Council (UK), Royal College of Nursing (2016). *Decisions relating to cardiopulmonary resuscitation: Guidance from the British Medical Association, the Resuscitation Council (UK), and the Royal College of Nursing (previously known as the 'Joint Statement')*, 3e. https://www.resus.org.uk/library/publications/publication-decisions-relating-cardiopulmonary (accessed 2 April 2021).

Care Quality Commission (2019). *Inspection framework: Critical Care (Acute and independent healthcare)*. https://www.cqc.org.uk/sites/default/files/20191218_Core_service_framework_for_critical_care_for_NHS_and_IH_providers_v8.pdf (accessed 3 April 2021).

Critical Care Network National Nurse Leads (CC3N) (2018). *About CC3N*. https://www.cc3n.org.uk/about-us.html (accessed 2 April 2021).

Daniels, R., Nutbeam, T., McNamara, G., and Galvin, C. (2011). The sepsis six and the severe sepsis resuscitation bundle: a prospective observational cohort study. *Emergency Medicine Journal* 28: 507–512.

Department of Health (2010). *Essence of Care 2010: Benchmarks for the Fundamental Aspects of Care*. London: HMSO.

Department of Health (2000). *Comprehensive Critical Care: A Review of Adult Critical Care*. London: HMSO.

Department for Health and Social Care (2013). *Health Building Note 04-02 Critical Care Units*. London: HMSO.

Faculty of Intensive Care Medicine and Intensive Care Society (2019). Guidelines for the Provision of Intensive Care Services, 2e. https://www.ficm.ac.uk/sites/default/files/gpics_v2_-_version_for_release_-_final2019.pdf (accessed 18 January 2021).

Faculty of Intensive Care Medicine and Intensive Care Society (2013). *Core Standards for Intensive Care Units* https://www.ics.ac.uk/ICU/Guidance/PDFs/Archive-Core_Standards_for_ICU (accessed 2 April 2021).

Gagan M.and Tait, D. (2019). Legal and ethical issues in critical care. In: *Critical Care Nursing: The Humanised Approach* (ed. S.J. White and D. Tait), 223–242. London: Sage.

General Medical Council (2020). *Guidance on Professional Standards and Ethics for Doctors: Decision Making and Consent*. https://www.gmc-uk.org/-/media/documents/gmc-guidance-for-doctors---decision-making-and-consent-english_pdf-84191055.pdf?la=en&hash=BE327A1C584627D12BC51F66E790443F0E0651DA (accessed 1 April 2021).

General Medical Council (2019). *Good Medical Practice*. https://www.gmc-uk.org/-/media/documents/good-medical-practice---english-20200128_pdf-51527435.pdf?la=en&hash=DA1263358CCA88F298785FE2BD7610EB4EE9A530 (accessed 1 April 2021).

Health and Care Professions Council (2021). *HCPC Corporate Strategy 2021–2026*. https://www.hcpc-uk.org/about-us/what-we-do/corporate-strategy/ (accessed 30 March 2021).

Health and Care Professions Council (2016). *Standards of conduct, performance and ethics*. https://www.hcpc-uk.org/globalassets/resources/standards/standards-of-conduct-performance-and-ethics.pdf?v=637171211260000000 (accessed 1 April 2021).

Healthcare Improvement Scotland (2017). *Making Care Better – Better Quality Health and Social Care for Everyone in Scotland: A strategy for supporting better care in Scotland 2017–2022*. http://www.healthcareimprovementscotland.org/previous_resources/policy_and_strategy/strategy_2017-2022.aspx (accessed 5 April 2021).

Healthcare Inspectorate Wales (2019). *Inspect Healthcare*. https://hiw.org.uk/ (accessed 5 April 2021).

Higgs, A., McGrath, B.A., Goddard, C. et al. (2018). Guidelines for the management of tracheal intubation in critically ill adults. *British Journal of Anaesthesia* 120(2): 323–352.

Information Commissioner's Office (2021). *Guide to the Data Protection Regulation*. https://ico.org.uk/media/for-organisations/guide-to-data-protection/guide-to-the-general-data-protection-regulation-gdpr-1-1.pdf (accessed 2 April 2021).

Information Commissioner's Office (2020). *Data Sharing Code of Practice*. https://ico.org.uk/media/for-organisations/data-sharing-a-code-of-practice-1-0.pdf (accessed 2 April 2021).

Intensive Care Society (2020). *Intensive Care 2020 and Beyond: Co-developing the Future*. London: ICS.

Longley, M., Riley, N., Davies, P., and Hernandez-Quevedo, C. (2012). United Kingdom (Wales): Health system review. *Health Systems in Transition* 14(11): xiii–84.

Loveday, H.P., Wilson, J.A., Pratt, R.J. et al. (2014). epic3: National evidence-based guidelines for preventing healthcare-associated infections in NHS hospitals. *England Journal of Hospital Infection* 86(S1): S1–S70.

Macnaughton, P. and Webb, S. (2019). Foreword. In: Faculty of Intensive Care Medicine and Intensive Care Society (2019). Guidelines for the Provision of Intensive Care Services, 2e. https://www.ficm.ac.uk/sites/default/files/gpics_v2_-_version_for_release_-_final2019.pdf (accessed 18 January 2021).

National Institute for Health and Care Excellence (2021). *COVID-19 Rapid Guideline: Managing COVID-19: NICE Guideline [NG191]*. London: NICE.

National Institute for Health and Care Excellence (2020). *COVID-19 Rapid Guideline: Critical Care in Adults: NICE Guideline [NG159]*. London: NICE.

National Institute for Health and Care Excellence (2009). *Rehabilitation After Critical Illness in Adults: Clinical Guideline [CG83]*. London: NICE.

NHS Digital (2019). *Hospital Adult Critical Care Activity – 2018–19 Data Tables*. https://digital.nhs.uk/data-and-information/publications/statistical/hospital-admitted-patient-care-activity/2018-19 (accessed 2 April 2021).

NHS England and NHS Improvement (2021a). *Legislating for Integrated Care Systems: Five Recommendations to Government and Parliament*. https://www.england.nhs.uk/publication/legislating-for-integrated-care-systems-five-recommendations-to-government-and-parliament/ (accessed 2 April 2021).

NHS England and NHS Improvement (2021b). *Service Specifications*. https://www.england.nhs.uk/specialised-commissioning-document-library/service-specifications/ (accessed 2 April 2021).

NHS England (2020). *Shared Decision Making to Comply with National Legislation and Policy*. https://www.england.nhs.uk/shared-decision-making/why-is-shared-decision-making-important/shared-decision-making-to-comply-with-national-legislation-and-policy/ (accessed 1 April 2021).

NHS England (2019). *Adult Critical Care Service Specification*. https://www.england.nhs.uk/publication/adult-critical-care-services/ (accessed 2 April 2021).

Northern Health and Social Care Trust (2020). *Health and Social Care in Northern Ireland*. http://www.northerntrust.hscni.net/

about-the-trust/trust-overview-2/health-and-social-care-in-northern-ireland/ (accessed 5 April 2021).

Nursing and Midwifery Council (2020). *NMC Regulate, Support, Influence: Strategy 2020–2025*. https://www.nmc.org.uk/globalassets/sitedocuments/strategy/nmc-strategy-2020-2025.pdf (accessed 30 March 2021).

Nursing and Midwifery Council (2018). *The Code. Professional Standards of Practice and Behaviour for Nurses, Midwives and Nursing Associates*. https://www.nmc.org.uk/globalassets/sitedocuments/nmc-publications/nmc-code.pdf (accessed 23 May 2020).

Park, V. (2020). COVID 19: What to expect if you are deployed to a critical care setting. *Nursing Standard*. https://rcni.com/nursingstandard/careers/career-advice/covid-19-what-to-expect-if-you-are-deployed-to-a-critical-care-setting159646 (accessed 31 March 2021).

Pattison, N.A. (2013). Withdrawal of treatment and end of life care for the critically ill patient. In: *Critical Care Manual of Clinical Procedures and Competencies* (ed. J. Mallett, J. Albarran, and R. Richardson), 499–530. Singapore: John Wiley & Sons, Ltd.

Public Health Scotland (2020). *Our vision and values*. https://publichealthscotland.scot/our-organisation/about-public-health-scotland/our-vision-and-values/ (accessed 5 April 2021).

Regulation and Quality Improvement Authority (2021). Hospitals. https://www.rqia.org.uk/what-we-do/inspect/hospitals/ (accessed 5 April 2021).

Rooney, K.D. and Mathieu, S. (2019). Audit and quality improvement. In: Faculty of Intensive Care Medicine and Intensive Care Society (2019). Guidelines for the Provision of Intensive Care Services, 2e. https://www.ficm.ac.uk/sites/default/files/gpics_v2_-_version_for_release_-_final2019.pdf (accessed 18 January 2021).

Royal College of Anaesthetists (2018). *Care of the Critically Ill Woman in Childbirth; Enhanced Maternal Care Guidelines*. https://www.rcoa.ac.uk/sites/default/files/documents/2020-06/EMC-Guidelines2018.pdf (accessed 3 April 2021).

Scottish Intercollegiate Guidelines Network (2021). *Assessment of COVID-19 in Primary Care*. https://www.sign.ac.uk/media/1824/assessment-covid-primary-care-update-feb-21.pdf (accessed 5 April 2021).

Scottish Intercollegiate Guidelines Network (2020a). About us. https://www.sign.ac.uk/about-us/ (accessed 5 April 2021).

Scottish Intercollegiate Guidelines Network (2020b). *Managing the Long-term Effects of COVID-19*. https://www.sign.ac.uk/media/1833/sign161-long-term-effects-of-covid19-11.pdf (accessed 5 April 2021).

UK Government (2021a). Departments, agencies and public bodies. https://www.gov.uk/government/organisations#department-of-health-and-social-care) (accessed 5 April 2021).

UK Government (2021b). Organisations: NHS England. https://www.gov.uk/government/organisations/nhs-commissioning-board (accessed 1 April 2021).

UK Legislation (2015). The European Union (Recognition of Professional Qualifications) Regulations 2015. https://www.legislation.gov.uk/uksi/2015/2059/contents/made (accessed 1 April 2021).

UK Legislation (2003). The Working Time (Amendment) Regulations 2003. https://www.legislation.gov.uk/uksi/2003/1684/contents/made (accessed 1 April 2021).

UK Legislation (2000). Freedom of Information Act. https://www.legislation.gov.uk/ukpga/2000/36/introduction (accessed 2 April 2021).

UK Legislation (1998). Scotland Act 1998. https://www.legislation.gov.uk/ukpga/1998/46/contents (accessed 5 April 2021).

UK Legislation (1974). Health and Safety at Work etc. Act 1974. https://www.legislation.gov.uk/ukpga/1974/37/contents (accessed 1 April 2021).

Walsh, T. and Dark, P. (2019). Research and development. In: Faculty of Intensive Care Medicine and Intensive Care Society (2019). Guidelines for the Provision of Intensive Care Services, 2e. https://www.ficm.ac.uk/sites/default/files/gpics_v2_-_version_for_release_-_final2019.pdf (accessed 18 January 2021).

World Health Organization (2009). *WHO Guidelines on Hand Hygiene in Health Care: First Global Patient Safety Challenge Clean Care is Safer Care*. https://www.who.int/publications/i/item/9789241597906 (accessed 1 April 21).

Chapter 3

Legal and ethical issues

Leonie Armstrong, Tracey Carrott, and Jacqueline Newby

Aim

This chapter aims to focus on end-of-life care ethics including confidentiality, withdrawal of life-sustaining treatments and organ donation after death.

Learning outcomes

After reading this chapter the reader will be able to:

- Review ethical principles.
- Recognise ethical issues at the end of life.
- Provide an overview of key ethical and legal issues related to organ donation.
- Develop an understanding of the role of consent in the organ donation process.
- Describe the two types of cadaveric organ donation in the UK.

Test your prior knowledge

- Name the four ethical principles.
- When was the Mental Capacity Act written?
- What are the two types of organ donation after death?
- How do the types of organ donation differ?
- Recognise the changes introduced in the UK relating to deemed consent for organ donation.

Fundamentals of Critical Care: A Textbook for Nursing and Healthcare Students, First Edition. Edited by Ian Peate and Barry Hill.
© 2023 John Wiley & Sons Ltd. Published 2023 by John Wiley & Sons Ltd.
Companion website: www.wiley.com/go/peate/criticalcare

Introduction

Ethics, legal requirements and professional conduct shapes all decisions within healthcare. They help us to question what is good, what is right and how that will impact on patient care (Ogstan-Tuck, 2017). The critical care environment provides more frequent ethical and legal situations than other health care settings. The advances in medical technology, including life support and sustaining interventions, can lead to many questions of what is right and what is good for the patient. Just because we can, does not mean we always should.

There are many ethical theories that can be considered in relation to end-of-life care and organ donation. The authors will refer to utilitarianism and deontology but the chapter will focus on the ethical framework Principles of Biomedical Ethics' (Beauchamp and Childress, 2001; see Box 3.1).

The Nursing and Midwifery Council (NMC) Code of Conduct 2018 provides an ethical framework for nurses, midwives and nursing associates. The code sets out principles to prioritise people, practise effectively, preserve safety and promote professionalism and trust. It provides the nursing and midwifery professions with standards of conduct and behaviour to uphold and serves to protect its service users.

Nurses and other healthcare professionals will use a blended mix of professional ethical frameworks, ethical theory, personal moral beliefs and principles to reflect on their clinical practice and experiences. Law and policy provide a governance structure as to how individuals and professionals should and should not act in certain situations. These will provide 'absolute' rules to follow, with an accepted societal understanding that consequences will result if rules are broken or not followed. On occasions, an individual's belief and views may well be challenged when looking after patients. A nurse may not agree with termination of pregnancy on religious or personal beliefs, and therefore if faced with that situation in the clinical setting could result in difficult decisions, whether to compromise their own beliefs or to compromise their duty of care. The NMC (Code of Conduct 2018a, NMC Standards 2018b) recognises this particular situation and permits the nurse the statutory right of conscientious objection, the nurse must inform their manager and identify another individual to care for the patient. All other situations will require the nurse to balance their own beliefs whilst adhering to the code and maintaining the standards set out, ensuring patient care is not compromised.

In order to maintain the principles of the code, nurses should develop the essential skills and knowledge to provide effective care in their designated area of practice. The care needs of patients in the critical care setting are highly specialised and require specific training. The National Competency Framework (2015) for registered nurse in critical care has many domains, including end-of-life care and organ donation. Undertaking such training and meeting the competency requirements promotes critical thinking and reflection which should lead to improved patient care and experience.

Confidentiality

All aspects of nursing care demand explicit attention to issues of patient confidentiality. Ethical issues can often place us in a position of question or clarification in relation to sharing of information and maintaining confidentiality. The code demands that we share confidential information with other professionals at the lowest level as possible (on a need to know basis only) and that patient confidentiality is maintained at all times, even after death.

Box 3.1 The four principles (*Source*: Beauchamp and Childress, 2001).

Autonomy	Respect for the autonomy of the patient 'What is important to the patient?'
Beneficence	Acting for their beneficence. To promote the well-being of patients.
Non-maleficence	Avoiding harm. 'Do no harm'
Justice	Being fair to others in how we use resources

Snapshot

Bill is a 72-year-old gentleman with severe left-sided heart failure. He has been admitted to the critical care unit for renal support as he has developed an acute kidney injury. Bill is detained in the local prison. He has two prison officers with him at all times and is restrained with handcuffs.

How do you feel looking after a prisoner? Does it feel different to any other patient?

It could be perceived that Bill does not deserve to have the intensive support that critical care provides, as he has previously committed a crime. This consideration may be viewed from a position of justice. If there are limited critical care resources, would an individual who has committed a crime be less worthy of treatment than an individual who had had not committed a crime? The NMC Code would override this position, stating that all individuals are treated with respect, that their rights are upheld and any discriminatory attitudes towards them challenged. This results in all individuals being treated equally, irrespective of social background or criminal behaviour.

You may wonder what offence Bill has committed. This is of no concern to healthcare staff. It is good practice to avoid any speculation to ensure that no bias arises. We cannot judge how another person chose to act or understand their actions. Bill's rights have been restricted in terms of freedom and independence but his human rights remain, therefore he should not be excluded from receiving the same care as any other patient.

Snapshot – continued

Bill's condition has been deteriorating during his admission to critical care and the consultant has spoken to Bill and discussed putting a DNACPR (do not attempt cardio-pulmonary resuscitation) form in place, as they feel that his heart failure and renal failure are now at a point where they will not recover.

One of the prison officers asks what is Bill's prognosis. Should they be asking for personal information about Bill? Does Bill have different rights relating to confidential information because he is a prisoner?

The prison officer should not be told clinical information about Bill. The prison officer is there in relation to custody and security issues. Bill's health information is confidential and therefore should not be shared with anyone unless Bill gives consent.

In this situation, the prison officer has known Bill for a number of years and his question regarding prognosis comes from a place of care and concern. He knows that if Bill has a prognosis of less than three months then he could be considered for early release from prison on compassionate grounds. The information regarding Bill's prognosis should only be discussed with the prison healthcare team or the prison governor. The governor can then consider Bill's case for early release by weighing up his offence, time left on his sentence, the risk that he poses to others and Bill's health needs in light of the poor prognosis. The information can be considered in relation to the Dying Well in Custody Charter (DWiCC) 2018. The debate or decision regarding early release from custody is not within health care staff's scope of practice, although they may be approached to provide information regarding diagnosis and prognosis. The decision maker in the first instance will be the prison governor and then HMPPS Public Protection Group. The most common reasons for refusing early release is an unclear diagnosis, or that death is not expected within three months (Independent Advisory Panel on Deaths in Custody, 2020). To consider compassionate release from a custodial sentence can be argued to be supporting the ethical principle of autonomy and human rights. This is encouraging

that Bill could be considered and his preferences taken into consideration despite his sentence. However, the number of successful applications for early release remains low and therefore there continues to be high number of prisoners who die expected deaths in custody.

If Bill is not considered to be an appropriate case for early release, the health professionals will consider an appropriate place for his end-of-life care. When Bill dies, his death will be reviewed and investigated as a death in custody, the same process as if he had died in prison. All of the medical notes are retained and reviewed by the police and the HMS coroner.

End-of-life care and best interest decisions

End-of-life care poses many challenging decisions that patients and clinicians need to navigate. The key areas that will be explored in relation to ethics and the law will be:

- Withdrawal of life-sustaining treatment
- Best interest decisions
- Right to life and right to die

Decisions to withdraw life-sustaining treatment can be complex; there is potential for differences in opinion between professionals and patients' relatives. The patients in critical care are often unconscious, and unable to express their own thoughts or wishes, thus best interest decisions are likely to made for them. The Mental Capacity Act (MCA) 2005 advises that all reasonable measures must be taken to support the patient to regain capacity to be involved in decision making, in times of temporary lack of capacity. In the situation of a patient who has been sedated and ventilated, it could be suggested that the sedation is impacting on their capacity and ability to engage in in decisions about their care.

To reduce or remove sedation to improve mental capacity and engagement may increase harm to the patient, with an increased risk of dying without the level 3 support, e.g. inotropic support, intubation and ventilation (level 2 and 3 support, discussed in Chapter 2). It would therefore be unethical to cause more harm to the patient to establish if they could be included in the decision-making process.

The decision maker when a patient lacks capacity can be a previously appointed person; for example, a lasting power of attorney (LPA) (health and welfare or finance) or court appointed deputy. These individuals can make decisions for the patient who lacks capacity, even in a withdrawal of life-sustaining treatment decision, but like any situation the LPA and court appointed deputy would require the necessary facts and information to be able to weigh up the decision appropriately. It would therefore be the role of the senior clinician to set out the facts of the case. Often there is no attorney or appointed deputy and at this point the most suitably informed professional will become the decision maker. The decision maker should consider a range of factors and opinions including; the clinical situation, the professional opinion of the MDT (multidisciplinary team) members, any previously expressed wishes of the patient and the views of the relatives of what the patient would have wanted if they were able to be part of the discussion. The process requires careful navigation and accurate documentation. Some critical care units will use mental capacity assessments to document best interest decisions such MCA 1 (Record of mental capacity assessment) and MCA 2 (Record of actions taken to make a best interest decision) forms. The decision-making process can be time-consuming and in the event of an emergency it may not be possible to take the time required. The principle to consult those closest to the patient to establish the patients' views and preferences should always be maintained. It is good practice to understand the local policies and guidelines of the clinical area you are working in, in advance of a best interest decision or a withdrawal of life-sustaining treatment situation.

In the event of disagreement or conflict between parties regarding a withdrawal of life-sustaining treatment, then the local ethics committee or organisational solicitor could be involved. If a patient has no identified family or significant others to act on their behalf or a situation conflict arises, then the MCA advises that an independent mental capacity advocate (IMCA) should be allocated to act as the patient's advocate. In some high-profile cases of disagreement, court action may be taken utilising processes from the court of protection through to the Supreme and European Court to act on behalf of the patients' rights (Faculty of Intensive Care Medicine (FICM), 2019).

The Mental Capacity Act provides a legal framework for decision making and decision making on behalf of the patient. The framework should be adhered to at all times.

Ethical themes

Belief systems surrounding words can bring about very different views between health care professionals and patients/families. For example, withdrawal of care and withdrawal of treatment could mean the same thing to some groups or individuals. However, a focus on the word 'care' and the withdrawal of it could be viewed negatively. This could be seen as causing harm, negligent, lacking compassion and an infringement of human rights. Therefore, it is imperative to consider the words and terminology used in any sensitive conversations, so as not to cause any confusion or misunderstanding.

Consideration of withdrawal of life-sustaining treatments should only take place when there is no chance of meaningful recovery from the underlying diagnosis and problems. In the situation of neurological death or vegetative state, then to continue with life-sustaining interventions could be argued to be cruel and prolonging death.

Life-sustaining treatments need to be considered within the context that they are being used (MCA 2007). In some

situations, intravenous antibiotics could be deemed to be life-sustaining but, in another situation, the same treatment may not be life-sustaining and merely treating infection. The decision to stop intravenous antibiotics is likely to feel less controversial than a decision regarding withdrawal of ventilation. Does this reflect the impact of the intervention? There are observations and diagnostic tests that identify those patients who cannot breathe for themselves and investigations that establish those who will not recover from their clinical situation. The factual information can help to guide the decision-making process from a scientific basis.

The time from withdrawal of intervention to death can play a part in how the situation is reflected upon. If dying occurs quickly after withdrawal of ventilation, then the decision to withdraw ventilation could be argued to be right from a position of non-maleficence; the patient died quickly and therefore any further harm was prevented. However, if we consider withdrawal of artificial nutrition, this can be a more complex and emotive situation. Dying following withdrawal of nutrition and hydration is likely to take days or weeks. At a simplistic level this could appear cruel or even negligent to a nurse, some could say that the patient is being starved to death. Food and nutrition are seen as fundamental care needs by the code that nurses have a duty to provide such care. Thus, to withdraw artificial nutrition and hydration could be argued to deny a patient of a fundamental care need and a failure to deliver nursing standards.

Some high-profile cases of withdrawal of nutrition and hydration include *Airedale v Bland* (1993), and the House of Lords judgment provides some clarity to these concerns. The judgment states that artificially administered hydration and nutrition can be lawfully withdrawn if it is no longer serving a therapeutic purpose and is not in the best interests of the patient. It also concludes that the patient will die of their underlying condition, not the lack of nutrition or hydration (Szawarski and Kakar, 2012). There is a natural reduction from appetite and thirst that occurs in the dying phase of illness. To continue with artificial nutrition or hydration when a patient is diagnosed to be dying could be seen as burdensome and lead to prolonged death. This could be argued to be maleficent and therefore unethical. This clearly demonstrates the different ethical positions that can be worked through if you look at a situation from duty, outcome or belief.

Mental Capacity Act

The Mental Capacity Act supports individuals with capacity the right to refuse treatments but not to demand treatments. An Advance Decision to Refuse Treatment (ADRT) is a legally binding document that allows an individual to consider treatments that they may want to refuse in the future and if they lacked capacity their wishes would be documented and could be applied. Some individuals with neurological conditions, for example motor neuron disease,

28

may document in advance any treatments that they may want to refuse in the future, e.g. mechanical ventilation or artificial nutrition. An advance decision to refuse treatment has serious consequences for the individual, therefore they should be written correctly and shared appropriately with the patient's family and healthcare professionals. Before applying an ADRT the healthcare professional must have evidence that the ADRT exists, is valid and applies to the current circumstances (Mental Capacity Act Code of Practice 2007).

Further terminology and phrases that can provide focus for end-of-life ethical discussion and debate are examined below.

Euthanasia

Euthanasia versus 'allowing to die' can be considered under the principles of maleficence and autonomy. Some will describe the 'act' of withdrawal of life-sustaining treatments such as mechanical ventilation or artificial nutrition as euthanasia, in a passive sense or 'backdoor euthanasia'. This is not a strong ethical position, Rachels (1999) argues that that there is no moral difference between active and passive euthanasia. However, there is a legal difference; the law and professional conduct codes will support withdrawal of such treatments if the patient has no chance of recovery and death is expected. The use of the term 'euthanasia' even when paired with 'passive' can cause controversy. Healthcare professionals will not want their practice being tarnished by being described in such ways, it could have a significant impact on their professional reputation. Euthanasia and assisted dying are illegal within the United Kingdom, but remain areas of high public interest and debate. Clarity as to what the patient is dying from is vital when considering withdrawal of life-sustaining treatments. This should be clearly communicated with the patient's family or significant others to prevent misunderstanding and to support acceptance of the situation. It can be argued ethically that prolonged life support interventions cause harm to that patient from a position of maleficence. Painful and distressing interventions such as insertion of cannulas, nasogastric feeding and endotracheal tubes go against the fundamental principle of healthcare and medicine to 'do no harm', when there is no prospect of recovery for the patient. Conversely, allowing the patient to die could be argued to be supporting that patient's autonomy, when they have previously expressed a wish not to live a life of prolonged life support, which lacks quality. Such complex situations require time and expertise to navigate the ethical concerns. Many tools are available to aid the moral balance dynamic of weighing up the burden benefit ratio of a clinical situation; such as MORAL balance (Nottingham University Hospitals); this is an applied medical ethics technique grounded in principle-based bioethics (see Box 3.2).

Abandonment

Abandonment can be considered under the principles of maleficence and justice. In some cases, withdrawal of

Box 3.2   The MORAL Balance (*Source:* Harvey and Gardiner, 2019).

- Make sure of the facts surrounding the clinical situation.
- Establish Outcomes Relevant to the Agents involved.
- Level up options by balancing likely outcomes with and without critical care support.

Orange Flag

Make yourself aware of the formal and informal systems that your clinical unit use to support ethical and legal dilemma's. Remember to acknowledge specific situations that stay with you and have challenged your own moral beliefs. Reflection and de-brief are essential skills that all nurses need to develop and master.

life-sustaining treatments may be viewed by patients' relatives as a sense of abandonment, 'giving up' or needing the critical care bed for someone else. The critical care team may see the situation from an opposing position in that there are scarce resources (limited critical beds) and a patient who is expected to survive would benefit more than the patient who is dying but being kept alive by the interventions. Such situations require time and gradually developed conversations, setting out the situation and expectations with the patients' relatives to enable them to adjust to the change in focus and direction of care for their loved one. We may well run the risk of causing the relatives harm in their grief by allowing them to feel abandoned, but we must also ensure that false hope is not given. Ensuring appropriate allocation of resources is fulfilled is a daily requirement of critical care teams, reviewing patient needs, escalation and de-escalation of treatment levels requires a high level of clinical knowledge, excellent teamwork, organisation, trust and communication to ensure that the patients who are the most needy, have access to the required interventions. FICM (2019) provide a simple but effective flow chart to consider end-of-life dilemmas within a critical care setting (see Box 3.3).

6Cs: Commitment

Being aware of your own values, beliefs and morals is an important starting position. To then be able to consider others views and beliefs around a situation. We will not all agree all of the time therefore it is important to have mechanisms to work through difficulties and differences when they arise.

Box 3.3   Dealing with dilemma at end of life (*Source:* FICM, 2019).

DEALING WITH DILEMMA AT END OF LIFE

Severe acute illness and critical care admission
(uncertain prognosis)

Be honest and clear about uncertainty. **AVOID FIRM PREDICTIONS**
(absolute predictions create misunderstanding and fuel conflict)

Are there any advance statements outlining patients' values or wishes?
(verbal or written)

Do proposed treatments offer a minimum quality of life acceptable
to the patient, and can they achieve their goals for a good life?

Preservation of life as a physiological entity is not necessarily paramount.
Preservation of a patient's preferences and values can enable a good death.

Organ donation

Ethical and legal issues related to organ donation in the UK

At the time when the critical care team recognise that the patient is dying and the level 2 and 3 interventions as discussed in Chapter 2 are prolonging death rather than extending life, then a decision about the direction of that patient's care should be made. This will likely result in doctors testing a patient's brain function in order to diagnose neurological death, or doctors making a plan regarding withdrawing life-sustaining treatment and allowing the patient to die. Once a plan for further care is made, these plans should include a consideration regarding possible organ donation, making donation a usual part of end-of-life care for patients on the critical care unit.

Organ donation is 'the gift of life' where organs are offered freely and without financial or other recompense to those in need; and this is recognised as a true act of altruism. The direction of care may change in order to facilitate organ donation; however, the overall aim of care will always be the comfort of the patient, and providing care for patients before their death remains the responsibility of the lead consultant and the critical care team.

The act of donation itself fulfils a broad utilitarian perspective as organs and tissue are provided from one person for the good of the many. One donor can go on to help nine people through organ donation, and up to 50 people can have their lives improved through eye and tissue donation. However, less than 1% of the deceased population die in circumstances where organ donation can be facilitated, with only patients dying within critical care areas being able to donate, and not everyone in a position to donate does so. The current UK consent rate for organ donation is around 68% (NHSBT, 2020) and a utilitarian proposal to increase donation would be that organ donation should become a duty rather than a gift in order to help more people (Veatch, 2002). As this would override autonomy and personal choice, there are no plans to introduce such a duty in the UK.

Organ donation in the UK and other democratic countries is more aligned to a deontological perspective where the decision of the person is of the highest concern and should be followed. The recent changes in donation consent law in the UK states that the last known decision of the individual is of the highest importance in gaining consent to donate – more on this area later in this chapter. However, not everyone's decision to donate is respected, and 11% of families override a loved one's decision to donate (Morgan et al., 2017). While it is legal to proceed to donation on a documented decision such as an opt-in registration on the UK organ donation register, there is currently no example of recourse to the courts to ensure donation proceeds.

When donation is opposed and very much against the wishes of the family, potentially causing distress and mental ill health to family members, it would be difficult and un-empathetic to pursue organ donation therefore strategies to increase donation rates remain focused on increasing consent through communication and education.

Organ and tissue donation and transplant in the UK is tightly regulated. The management of donated organs and tissue for transplant is undertaken solely by NHS Blood and Transplant (NHSBT), who work in close association with the UK government regulator the Human Tissue Authority (HTA). Together NHSBT and the HTA ensure that all donation and transplant meets legal requirements regarding removal, use, storage and disposal of human tissue, as set out by two acts of parliament, the Human Tissue Act (2004) and the Human Tissue (Scotland) Act (2006).

The HTA (2020) has four guiding principles for organ and tissue donation:

- Consent – appropriate and valid consent is the fundamental principle
- Dignity – in the treatment of human bodies and their organs and tissue
- Quality – underpinning the management of bodies and their organs and tissue
- Honesty and openness – should be a foundation for communication

The donation process

Organ donation is a complicated process taking time and necessitating further patient tests to ensure organs are safe and suitable to transplant. Most people are unable to donate due to medical contraindications or clinical instability and it would be unethical to offer donation in either circumstance. Therefore, the National Institute for Health and Care Excellence guidelines 135 (NICE 2011) request that all patients having neurological tests, or patients with a plan to withdraw life-sustaining treatment, are referred for consideration for organ donation by a specialist nurse who will confirm if the patient is suitable to donate organs. Referral before any discussions with the patient or family is preferable to ensure clinicians have accurate information and families are not approached unnecessarily. For those patients who are in a position to donate, the responsible team and the Specialist Nurse Organ Donation will approach the patient or their family to establish consent.

Red Flag

Absolute contraindications to organ donation

Patients may have conditions which prevent them donating organs after their death; there are absolute contraindications where no organ donation is possible or organ specific contraindications where certain organs can be donated safely.

Some examples of absolute contraindications include:

- Current haematological cancers and most solid organ cancers with metastasis
- Creutzfeldt–Jakob disease (CJD)
- Current infections such as Severe Acute Respiratory Syndrome (SARS), Coronavirus, Middle East Respiratory Syndrome (MERS), viral haemorrhagic fevers, rabies, yellow fever.

Consent (authorisation in Scotland) for organ donation

Consent is required for any procedure within healthcare, whether it be a physical examination, surgical hip replacement or organ donation after death. Informed consent is a fundamental aspect of medical ethics and international human rights law and the requirement of consent in the medical setting is grounded in respect for autonomy (Parsons and Moorlock, 2020).

Individuals also have a right to determine what happens to their organs and tissue following their death and acknowledging and acting in accordance with a person's wishes regarding treatment of their body signals respect for their autonomy. However, organ donation usually occurs at a point in life where the person can no longer exercise their autonomy or object in any way to what is done to their body. The UK Organ Donor Register operated by NHS Blood and Transplant provides a system whereby people can register their organ donation decisions.

The Human Tissue Authority are responsible for providing advice and guidance on what counts as lawful consent (HTA 2020). Lawful consent can be viewed as a hierarchy of 4 steps of decreasing importance

1. First person consent – by documenting a decision on the organ donor register or making you decision known to others.

2. Nominated or appointed representative – someone you choose to make decisions on your behalf (not Scotland)
3. Deemed consent – where you have made no decisions about donation and it is presumed that you would have wanted to donate.
4. Consent on your behalf – from the person highest in a hierarchy of relationships.

It is vital that each of these steps are understood and are followed in order to ensure that consent conforms to legal and ethical requirements.

First person consent

A person can make a decision to donate after their death or alternatively they can also make a decision not to donate after their death. Having their decision documented through either 'opt in or opt out' on the UK organ donation register, or making others aware of their decisions by witnessed communication is regarded as first person consent regardless of the actual decision.

First person opt-in

Opt-in exists when the patient in some form has given or expressed consent, whether they have joined the NHS Organ Donor Register (ODR) or made known their decision. When a decision to donate is registered on the ODR, details of whether a person wants to donate some or all of their organs when they die can be specified. This expressed statement of intention to donate is the most important form of consent as it comes direct from the individual and states that donation is consistent with their views on what should be done to their body after their death. An individual can access the ODR at any time and can amend or rescind their consent.

First person opt-out

People can also record their decisions not to donate any or all of their organs or tissues after their death by registering an opt-out decision on the ODR.

When someone dies in circumstances where organ donation is possible an NHS Specialist Nurse will check the NHS Organ Donor Register (ODR) to see if a decision regarding organ donation has been recorded. Where a decision has been made this will be shared with the patient's family to ensure it was the last known decision of that person. If the family state the person had actually changed their decision after the initial decision then this new decision should be followed wherever possible (HTA 2020).

Appointed/nominated representative (not Scotland)

If a person does not wish to make a decision about their health care which includes organ and tissue donation, then they can appoint someone to make the decision for them and this person is known as an appointed or nominated representative. This may be a formally nominated person known as having lasting power of attorney (LPA) or an informally nominated person recognised and acknowledged as being that person's representative (HTA 2020). A decision made by a recognised representative will override those of anyone else where no first person decisions have been made with the exception of Scotland where a nominated representative is not recognised in law.

Deemed consent

Many countries have looked to improve consent rates for organ donation. Countries including Spain, Belgium, Austria and Singapore have moved to a system of 'deemed consent' whereby in the absence of an organ donation decision made by the patient in their lifetime, and where no objection to donation recorded, then consent to organ donation can be presumed (Abadie et al., 2006). In this scenario. where no decision or objections have been made, then it is assumed that a person would have wanted to donate their organs for transplantation after their death.

Many families are unable to make a decision regarding organ or tissue donation on behalf of their loved one if they have not previously discussed donation. In this scenario families may feel more comfortable agreeing to deemed consent which assumes that donation was the option the person would have chosen.

Wales became the first nation in the United Kingdom to move to a deemed consent system, enshrining in law the Human Transplantation (Wales) Act 2013. The majority of UK countries have since followed this example, with Scotland becoming the latest country to move to a deemed authorisation system in March 2021 with the implementation of the Human Tissue (Authorisation) (Scotland) Act 2019.

The various deemed consent laws all have similar guidelines and in the situation where there is no first person consent although there are nuances in each legislation or no nominated representative, then a patient can be deemed to have consented/authorised to donation if they meet the following criteria.

- Are an adult aged over 18 (aged over 16 in Scotland)
- Have lived voluntarily in the country deeming consent for 12 months

- Have mental capacity for a significant period of time before their death
- Have died in the country deeming consent

Snapshot

Can consent to organ donation be deemed?

A 37-year-old man has moved from Scotland 14 months ago to live with his partner in England. He is currently in Critical Care Unit following an intracranial haemorrhage and has been neurologically declared dead. He has been referred for potential organ donation and his partner and family have been approached for consent to organ donation.

They reveal that they are not aware of any prior decisions made regarding organ donation as they had never spoken about it.

Consent can be deemed as he meets the criteria and in agreement with his partner and family organ donation could proceed.

The new laws have not changed regarding children. If anyone under the age of 18 dies in a way that makes donation possible (under 16 in Scotland), then their parents would be approached about organ donation and they would be given the opportunity to consent on their child's behalf.

Orange Flag

It is common for laws to be named after campaigners in recognition of their efforts to bring important issues to the attention of the public. The English Organ Donation (Deemed Consent) Act 2019 has also been termed Max and Keira's Law to recognise two children who have raised awareness and understanding about donation and transplant.

Whilst these legislative changes provide a legal basis for deeming (presuming) consent, the patient's family are still closely involved and they are asked for their support in deeming consent for their loved one. Families have the opportunity to provide any additional or more recent information about any prior decisions made, and these decisions would be respected.

In 2018 a faith and beliefs declaration was added to the NHS Organ Donor Register, allowing a person to register if they want their religion to be consulted prior to any organ donation decisions being made.

The ethics of deemed consent

Much has been written on the ethics of deemed consent, with opponents stating that a lack of objection to donation does not equate to consent. A presumed consent framework puts a utilitarian and a rights and justice approach into conflict. Concerns are grounded on whether presumed consent accurately reflects the patient's wishes, with the potential to violate a donor's autonomy if they did not want to donate but omitted to register an opt-out decision. Arguably the taking of organs is no longer a gift or donation in the true sense of the word. In this way deemed consent may represent a breach of the right of autonomy (Horvat, 2010) in that the individual's body becomes public property unless claimed otherwise.

Concern also exists around whether the potential donor was fully informed of the process of organ donation at the time of consent. It can be argued that consent such as an ODR or deemed consent is not true informed consent as there may be newer procedures associated with organ retrieval that were not envisioned by the patient at the time the intent was expressed (Simonsson et al., 2019).

Current practice within the UK is that a family can oppose and override both first person and deemed consent, preventing donation from proceeding. If a family objects to organ donation even when permission has been expressed either by joining the NHS ODR, carrying a donor card or by telling relatives or friends, then healthcare professionals will discuss this matter sensitively with the patient's family members. Families are encouraged to accept the patient's decision. In law a family does not have the legal right to overrule a consent decision, however this 'hard' form of consent for organ donation which would force donation to proceed irrespective of the views of the family members is not currently in consideration in the UK. Indeed, consent to organ donation may be considered by some as inaccurate and misleading and the HTA (2020) state that consent permits an activity to take place but does not mandate it, which does mean consent can be overturned.

Learning event: reflection

How do you think you would feel regarding deemed consent if you or a member of your family required an organ transplant?

Consent from a person in the highest-ranking relationship

In cases where there is no first person consent, no nominated representative and where consent can't be deemed, then the family or friends will be asked to give their consent to organ donation. There is a hierarchy of relationships set out in the Human Tissue Act 2004 (see Box 3.4) providing guidance regarding who should be approached to give consent.

Box 3.4   Hierarchy of qualifying relationships.

1. Spouse or partner (including civil or same sex partner). A person is another person's partner if the two of them (whether of different sexes or the same sex) live as partners in an enduring family relationship
2. Parent or child (in this context a child biological or adopted may be of any age, but must be competent in accordance with MCA (2005)
3. Brother or sister
4. Grandparent or grandchild
5. Niece or nephew
6. Stepfather or stepmother
7. Half-brother or half-sister
8. Friend of long standing.

Relationships listed together are accorded equal ranking; it is sufficient to obtain consent from just one of them for donation to proceed provided they are ranked equal highest.

6Cs: Communication

Having effective communication skills is vital in the complex discussions that take place around organ donation. Verbal and written communication are equally important and great skill is required to effectively communicate verbally and document accurately what has been said.

Organ donation and ethical issues require defensible documentation of all communication situations.

Cadaveric organ donation

As there are two ways of dying in the UK – you can be certified neurologically dead or you can be certified circulatory or cardiac dead – then it follows that there are also two different forms of donating organs after death. Please see Chapter 32 for further discussion on the diagnosis of death in the UK. The Human Rights Act (1998) states that a fundamental human right is not to be killed, therefore surgeons must not remove organs that will lead to the death of the individual and this 'dead donor' rule governs all cadaveric donation.

With neurological death, organ donation is usually discussed with the family after the person has been certified dead and death has been diagnosed following clinical testing by two senior doctors following strict guidelines.

The UK currently diagnose neurological death using the Code of Practice issued by the Academy of Medical Royal Colleges (2008) updated in 2019 (AoMRC, 2008). Neurological death tests must be carried out by doctors qualified for over 5 years and the tests must be carried out twice in order to diagnose and then confirm death.

Red Flag

Diagnosing neurological death is a 3-step process:

1. There must be evidence of irreversible brain damage of known aetiology.
2. Doctors performing the tests must make sure there are no other causes for the coma, namely drugs (sedatives or neuromuscular blocking agents), hypothermia, metabolic or endocrine disorders.
3. Doctors performing the tests must test for the absence of brainstem function using six separate cranial nerve tests and one apnoea test.

The process of testing must be repeated in full to confirm the results of the first test.

(AoMRC, 2008)

With circulatory death, the discussion around organ donation must be made while the person is still alive, though they are usually unresponsive and in a coma. The approach is based on a decision by the caring team that the withdrawal of life-sustaining therapies are in the best interests of the individual, and the patient is expected to die once these life-sustaining therapies are removed.

This significant difference, between a diagnosis of death or a decision to withdraw life-sustaining treatment, can lead clinical staff to feel that donation in a neurological death situation is somewhat easier because the clinical situation has been established.

Orange Flag

Health care workers may experience psychological stress when caring for organ donors, especially looking after those who donate following circulatory death (Zelweger et al., 2017). There can be a perceived conflict of duty away from the patient and towards the organ recipients and there can be discomfort from the uncertainty involved in this type of donation. It is important to discuss these issues and seek clarity and support from the donation nurse involved.

The organ donation process

As stated earlier, quality is a guiding principle of organ donation and this necessitates further investigations by donation nurses to ensure safety of organs offered for transplant.

All potential organ donors have pre-donation blood tests in order to detect transmissible infections such as hepatitis B, C and E, Human Immunodeficiency Virus (HIV) and Coronavirus. A positive test may have implications for the health of family members as they may have been unknowingly exposed to an infection, therefore it is necessary to gain consent from the family to undertake these tests. Other tests such as blood tests, X-ray or echocardiography may also be requested to assist with the donor to recipient matching process. If a person has made a decision to help others after their death then it is expected that they would want to provide the best opportunity for recovery for the recipient, and in this way requesting further testing can be viewed as ethical when it does not harm the individual.

Past medical history and the current clinical picture are scrutinised and documented. There is then a period of time before organ retrieval surgery can proceed to allow transplant surgeons time to review the donor characteristics and to discuss potential organ transplants with both their medical colleagues the intended organ recipients. Organs are not taken without there being an intended recipient.

All organ donation will require the donor to remain on the ITU for a period of time to facilitate donation, and its important that the organ function is preserved by maintaining or optimising the cardiovascular status of the donor.

Snapshot

Jo is 62-year-old and has been admitted to the Critical Care Unit overnight with a cerebrovascular accident. Jo is currently ventilated and has an arterial line and 2 peripheral cannulas. Following discussion between the stroke and critical care teams, both agree that Jo cannot survive this event, and a decision is made to withdraw ventilation. The family have been contacted and have been asked to attend hospital to discuss the clinical situation. Following the phone call a DNACPR (do not attempt cardiopulmonary resuscitation) order is documented.

Before the family arrive to discuss withdrawal of life-sustaining treatment Jo becomes unstable, the blood pressure drops and the heart rate rises to 146 beats per minute. Should doctors start medications in order to stabilise? is it ethical to start new therapies when clinical staff have already documented a plan to withdraw ventilation as she cannot survive this event?

Both NICE 135 (2016) and DOH (2009) state that measures should be taken in order to stabilise a patient in order to establish any organ donation decisions made by the patient. Clinicians need to balance the risks of harm from any possible treatments and interventions, against the wishes of the donor to be altruistic.

In this scenario intravenous fluids and peripheral metaraminol are started as doctors felt this would not harm their patient. Jo's known decision to donate was established with the family and Jo remained clinically stable until organ donation could proceed.

Only when organs are matched and an organ retrieval surgical team are in the hospital ready to perform the surgery can the withdrawal of life-sustaining therapy occur. The intensive care team decide where and how the withdrawal of life-sustaining treatment will take place, and the intensive care team will carry out the planned withdrawal of these therapies,

ensuring that the patients comfort and dignity is their main priority. The intensive care team will stay with their patient until asystole and following certification of death the patient is immediately taken to theatre for the organ retrieval surgery.

Those patients who have been certified neurologically dead are taken directly into theatres where ventilation is discontinued and organs are retrieved.

6Cs: Care

In a situation where life is prolonged for the purpose of organ donation it is vital to ensure that care of the patient remains the utmost priority.

Post organ retrieval

Another of the guiding principles of organ donation is dignity. For all cadaveric organ donation, the body is surgically closed after the organs have been retrieved with dressings applied to incision line. Formal care after death procedures are performed by the specialist nurse with help from theatre or intensive care staff, and often this care is individualised such as washing and styling hair, shaving or placing the donor in clothes important to them before they are taken to the mortuary.

6Cs: Compassion

It is vitally important to treat the person who is donating organs with dignity and compassion throughout the retrieval operation and once surgery is complete in care after death.

Organ allocation

In any situation where supply does not meet demand, such as that seen in organ donation and transplant, the ethical decisions behind resource allocation are vital to ensure equity and justice.

NHS Blood and Transplant are responsible for matching and allocating organs nationally in accordance with guidelines decided by each UK organ advisory groups, with allocations schemes comprising of recipient clinical need, immunological and blood group compatibility, expected benefit from the transplant, waiting times and geographical location.

Over recent years as the storage and transport of organs has improved, organ allocation has moved away from a mix of local and national allocation, to predominantly national allocation. These national allocation schemes ensure equity in opportunity for all people waiting for a transplant and they are only deviated from in cases where time pressures for transplant may result in an organ not being utilised.

Conditional donation where donors or their family specify who can receive an organ from their loved one, is not permitted in accordance with the Equality Act 2010 which regulates against any bias within healthcare.

One situation does exist where directed donation is possible. A family can ask that one kidney be given to a named person on the waiting list as long as other organs are also being donated, and provided the intended recipient is already on the waiting list and is a suitable match for the kidney.

Snapshot

Paul is 21 and has a suffered hypoxic brain damage due to a prolonged asthma attack. He has been certified neurologically dead and the family have agreed to donation with the stipulation that his organs are not given to an alcoholic.

Can his family make this request?

Following donation, in accordance with the final guiding donation principle of honesty and openness the family are informed of the donation outcome. Some basic information will be given about who received the organs or tissue, and families often receive letters from the recipients who have benefitted from the donation.

Conclusion

The ethical and legal issues surrounding end-of-life care and organ donation are numerous and complex. The legal frameworks and law are there to protect the individual and professionals in such difficult situations. It can often be difficult to separate the emotions from the facts in such situations; this highlights the importance of effective communication, teamwork and opportunities to reflect and debrief following such cases.

Take home points

1. If a patient is able to be involved in end-of-life discussions, always involve them. The NMC 2018 Code of Conduct directs nurses to prioritise people and treat them as individuals, in part to recognise patients' individual preferences and advocate for them when needed.
2. In a best interest decision, remember that individuals speaking on behalf of the patient must present what the patient's view would be should they be able to speak for themselves, not what the relatives would want for the patient.
3. Open and honest conversations are imperative to support all ethical dilemmas. It is essential when caring for patients in a WLST and organ donation situation that all documentation is accurate, clear and defensible.
4. Plans to withdraw life-sustaining treatments or to perform neurological tests to ascertain brain function must always be made before, and independent of, any consideration for organ donation.
5. The Human Tissue Authority is a statutory body responsible for regulating and monitoring organ and tissue donation and transplant guidelines in accordance with UK law.
6. Families of patients can overrule an NHS Organ Donation Resister registration if they are aware of a recent decision change.
7. Cadaveric organ donation can only go ahead after legal certification of death by a competent individual.
8. Patients and families cannot ask that organs are withheld from individuals or groups of people.

References

Abadie, A. and Gay, S. (2006). The impact of presumed consent on cadaveric organ donation: A cross country study. *Journal of Health Economics* 25(4): 155–166.

Airedale Hospital Trustees v Bland (1993). AC 789. www.bailii.org/uk/cases/UKHL/17.pdf (accessed November 2020).

Academy of Medical Royal Colleges (2008). *A Code of Practice for the Diagnosis and Diagnosis of Death*. PPG Design and Print.

Beauchamp, T. and Childress, J. (2001). *Principles of Biomedical Ethics*, 5e. Oxford: Oxford University Press.

Organ Donation (Deemed Consent) Act (2019). www.legislation.gov.uk/ukpga/2019/7/pdfs/ukpga_20190007_en.pdf (accessed 20 November 2020).

Department of Health (2009). Legal issues relevant to non – heart beating donation. https://www.dh.gov.uk/en/Publicationsandstatistics/Publications/PublicationsPolicyAndGuidance/DH.082122 (accessed 15 November 2020).

Equality Act (2010). https://www.equalityhumanrights.com/en/equality-act-2010 (accessed 1 December 2020).

Faculty of Intensive Care Medicine (2019). *Care at the End of Life: A guide to best practice, discussion and decision making in and around critical care*. https://www.ficm.ac.uk/sites/default/files/ficm_care_end_of_life.pdf (accessed October 2020).

Harvey, D.J.R. and Gardiner, D. (2019). MORAL balance – decision making in critical care. *BJA Education* 19(3): 68–73.

Horvat, L.D., Cuerden, M.S., Kim, S.J. et al. (2010). Informing the debate: Rates of kidney transplantation in nations with presumed consent. *Annals of International Medicine* 10: 641–649.

Human Tissue Act (2004). http://www.legislation.gov.uk/ukpga/2004/30/pdfs/ukpga_20040030_en.pdf (accessed 12 November 2020).

Human Tissue (Scotland) Act 2006. http://www.opsi.gov.uk/legislation/scotland/about/htm. (accessed 12 December 2020).

Human Transplantation (Wales) Act 2013. https://www.hta.gov.uk/sites/default/files/HTA_CoP_on_Human_Transplantation_

(Wales)_Act_2-13_- Final - May_2014.pdf (accessed 6 November 2020).

Human Rights Act (1998). https://www.legislation.gov.uk/ukpga/1998/42/contents (accessed 1 December 2020).

Human Tissue (Authorisation) (Scotland) Act 2019 https://www.legislation.gov.uk/ssi/2020/80/contents/made (accessed 1 December 2020).

Human Tissue Authority 2020: Guiding principles and the fundamental principle of consent. https://www.hta.gov.uk/sites/default/files/HTA%20Code%20of%20Practice%20A%20-%20Guiding%20principles%20and%20the%20fundamental%20principle%20of%20consent%201.pdf (accessed March 2021).

Independent Advisory Panel on Deaths in Custody and RCN (2020). *Avoidable Natural Deaths in Prison Custody: Putting Things Right.* https://www.iapondeathsincustody.org/news/iap-rcn-preventing-natural-deaths-prison (accessed 21 December 2020).

Mental Capacity Act (2005). Great Britain: HMSO. https://www.legislation.gov.uk/ukpga/2005/9/contents (accessed 6 November 2020).

Morgan, J., Hopkinson, C., Hudson, C. et al. (2017). The rule of threes: three factors that triple the likelihood of families overriding first person consent for organ donation in the UK. *Journal of Intensive Care Society* 19, Issue 2 101–106.

National Competency Framework for Registered Nurses in Adult Critical Care (2015). https://www.cc3n.org.uk/uploads/9/8/4/2/98425184/02_new_step_2_final.pdf (accessed November 2020).

National Competency Framework for Registered Nurses in Adult Critical Care (2015). https://www.cc3n.org.uk/uploads/9/8/4/2/98425184/03_new_step_3_final.pdf (accessed November 2020).

National Institute for Health and Care Excellence (2011). Organ Donation and Transplantation: improving donor identification and consent rates for deceased donation. https://www.nice.org.uk/guidance/cg135 (accessed 1 December 2020).

NHS Blood and Transplant (2020). National Potential Donor Audit https://nhsbtdbe.blob.core.windows.net/umbraco-assets-corp/19199/section-13-national-potential-donor-audit.pdf (accessed 1 December 2020).

Nursing and Midwifery Council (2018a). *The Code. Professional Standards of Practice and Behaviour for Nurses, Midwives and Nursing Associates.* https://www.nmc.org.uk/globalassets/sitedocuments/nmc-publications/nmc-code.pdf (accessed 23 May 2020).

Nursing and Midwifery Council (2018b). *Standards of Proficiency for registered Nurses.* https://www.nmc.org.uk (accessed November 2020).

Ogstan-Tuck, S. (2017). Ethical issues in palliative and end of life care. In: *Palliative and End of Life Care in Nursing*, 2e (ed. J. Nicol and B. Nyatanga), 99–199. London. Sage.

Parsons, J.A. and Moorlock, G. (2020). A global pandemic is not a good time to introduce 'opt-out' for organ donation. *Medical Law International* 20(2): 155–166. doi: 10.1177/0968533220950002.

Rachels, J. (1999). Active and passive euthanasia. In *Bioethics* (ed. H. Kuhse and P. Singer), 227–230. Malden: Blackwell Publishing Ltd.

Simonsson, J., Keijzer, K., Sodereld, T., and Forsberg, A. (2009). Intensive critical care nurses with limited experience: Experiences of caring for an organ donor during the donation process. *Journal of Clinical Nursing.* 29: 1614–1622.

Szawarski, P. and Kakar, V. (2012). Classic cases revisited: Anthony Bland and withdrawal of artificial nutrition and hydration in the UK. *Intensive Care Society* 13(2): 126–129.

Veatch, R.M. (2002). *Transplantation Ethics.* Georgetown University Press.

Zelweger, A., Gasche, Y., Moretti, D. et al. (2017). A qualitative pilot study on donation after cardiac death: feelings experienced by the nursing and medical staff in the adult intensive care unit of the Geneva hospitals. *Transplantation* 101: S22.

Chapter 4

Professional issues in critical care

Aurora Medonica

Aim

The aim of the chapter is to provide an overview of a range of professional issues that may be encountered in the critical care setting and to support those students who are approaching the critical care environment for the first time.

Learning outcomes

After reading this chapter the reader will be able to:

- Have an understanding of the values that underpin professional performance in the critical care setting.
- Understand the importance of critical thinking in healthcare.
- Have an initial understanding of the prioritising process that operates in a critical care setting.
- Be familiar with the UK national competencies framework.
- Be able to make use of the many opportunities for learning and professional growth available in the critical care setting.

Test your prior knowledge

- In relation to the critical care environment, describe how the Code of Professional Conduct (NMC, 2018a) relates to this care environment
- Explain why prioritising actions is crucial in critical care and the importance of critical thinking
- When commencing a placement in the critical care unit, what are the ideal characteristics of a practice assessor/supervisor and what is an ideal learning environment?

Fundamentals of Critical Care: A Textbook for Nursing and Healthcare Students, First Edition. Edited by Ian Peate and Barry Hill.
© 2023 John Wiley & Sons Ltd. Published 2023 by John Wiley & Sons Ltd.
Companion website: www.wiley.com/go/peate/criticalcare

Introduction

This chapter explores professional issues in critical care units (CCUs) with a particular focus on healthcare students allocated to this care environment. The chapter will include an overview of the values and standards advocated by the Nursing and Midwifery Council (NMC) Code (2018a), discussions related to being a student in a charged environment, leadership in healthcare and the United Kingdom's (UKs) national Competencies Framework for critical care.

The critical care environment is a unique environment, with many opportunities for learning and professional growth. Each patient brings with them their own personality, needs and aspirations, each shift is an adventure. They are filled with complex issues that require the critical care nurse to engage in critical thinking on a number of levels whilst maintaining a professional and patient-centred approach at all times.

Opportunities for learning

For many students an opportunity to undertake a clinical placement in a critical care environment brings feelings of elation and trepidation. The critical care environment is a highly charged area of care provision. CCUs and CCU nurses provide care to the most severely ill hospitalised patients. When entering the CCU you will experience new dynamics and a range of unknown expectations (remember, this is the same for the patient and their family).

Orange Flag

There are a number of emotional constraints that you will experience when in the critical care setting such as, death and dying as a daily occurrence.

Those working in the critical care environment are working in a highly charged emotional environment that is characterised by persistent grieving and moral distress. This is why it is important to access the support that is available to you, to help you talk through issues and to manage your own health and wellbeing.

The goal of intensive care nursing is to stabilise, monitor and manage, intervene and evaluate, transfer the patient to other care areas (for example a medical or surgical ward) when stable and safe to do so or to transfer to another health care facility (for example a regional tertiary care centre). Critical care nursing concerns the acute management of critically ill people and their families.

When starting on your learning journey, the learning process can be very frightening. Try not to let this overwhelm you. You are expected to know a minimal amount of information regarding common concepts, it is understood that you will not walk on to the CCU knowing all the answers. You are

a student; your learning outcomes, the level of your training and the requirements of the programme will be tailored to meet your needs as you discuss these with your practice supervisor. As you progress, you will hone your nursing skills and those important critical thinking processes.

There will be groups of patients (patient populations) that you will never have come across previously, there will be diseases and conditions that you are unfamiliar with, and this is all expected. You must remain open to any learning opportunities and remain positive. Set realistic weekly goals for yourself; this will keep you focused and positive throughout the experience. Acknowledge there will be challenges.

Take your time to settle in and make use of the resources that are available to you such as managers, practice supervisors, peers and patients. Always seek advice if you are unsure, know your limits. You are bringing something to the CCU setting, it is just different to what those nurses who are already working in the CCU bring.

Visit the care area before the placement commences, this gives you the chance to meet staff and to ascertain if there is anything specific that they would like you to study before arriving for duty. When in the CCU, making your initial visit, have look around the unit if you can, look at the equipment in use and listen to the various sounds, they may all be new to you.

Snapshot

Mark is a nursing student attending his second year of university and has recently discovered his allocation for the next placement.

Mark is allocated to the Critical Care Unit of a large teaching hospital and he is worried as it is his first time working in a critical care area. What should Mark do at this point? What are your ideas?

Here are few suggestions:

- Visit the unit and find out the daily dynamics (shifts timing, Nurse in charge, building specifics).
- Meet with the staff and ask if there are basic concepts that they want the student to know before the placement.
- Identify the Practice Supervisors/Assessor and the Clinical Educators Team for guidance and support whenever needed.

NMC Code in critical care units: journey to independent, safe practice

The role and function of the NMC is to protect the public. The NMC does this by maintaining the register of nurses, nursing associates and midwives as well as setting standards of education, training, conduct and performance.

Through the revalidation process the NMC ensure that nurses, nursing associates and midwives keep their skills and knowledge up to date.

Students are enrolled on an educational programme that is preparing them to enter the profession. This brings great privilege and responsibility with it. It is expected that as a nursing student, you should uphold the values and standards that all registered nurses must maintain. You must, even as a student, conduct yourself professionally at all times so as to justify the trust that the public places in the nursing profession. These sentiments apply to other healthcare students undertaking a programme of study that leads to registration with a statutory and regulatory body, for example the Health and Care Professions Council or the General Medical Council. Support mechanisms are in place to help you to aspire to and achieve the high standards that the regulatory bodies lay down.

Throughout your placement in CCU you will continue to learn about the behaviours and conduct that the public expects from a registered nurse. As you develop, you will continue to be assessed in relation to the knowledge, skills and behaviours you need to demonstrate in order to perform safely and effectively in the critical care setting. You will also need to evidence these qualities so to be entered on to the professional register.

The NMC's various regulations, standards and guidance outline common principles of practice and behaviour by those who are on the register. This enables patients, employers and colleagues to understand what to expect from a registered nurse. By using the principles within the Code, students, and those supporting them in practice (for example, clinical educators), can use it to help making sense of what it means to be a registered professional and what standards are required for practice. The key core principles of the NMC code of conduct are detailed in the Box 4.1 (NMC, 2018a)

Box 4.1   NMC Code of Conduct principles (NMC, 2018a).

- **Prioritise people:** The registered professional puts the interests of people first using or needing nursing or midwifery services.
- **Practise effectively:** The registered professional assesses needs and delivers treatments or gives help to the best of his/her abilities, on the basis of best available evidence.
- **Preserve safety:** The registered professional makes sure that patient and public safety is not affected.
- **Promote professionalism and trust:** The registered professional should display a personal commitment to the standards of practice and behaviour set out in the Code.

The core principles

A nursing student's conduct is based on the four core principles that have been set out in the Code. Adhering to the standards and responsibilities presented in the Code, will help to ensure safe, fair and ethical treatment of patients and their families. You should never undermine the values associated with the core four principles, these are essential for good practice and professional accountability.

Prioritise people

You must make the care of people your first concern, treating them as individuals as well as respecting their dignity. Prioritising people is key, this requires you to put the interests of service users first. A fundamental component of the care process is treating patients with respect. You must uphold the rights of patients.

Always be polite, kind, caring and compassionate to patients and, if appropriate, their families. The nurse must not be discriminatory, judgemental or disrespectful to patients, irrespective of personal views or patient behaviour. Do not discriminate in any way against those for whom you offer care and support. Acknowledge diversity, respect cultural differences and the values and beliefs that others hold. This will include the people you care for and other members of staff.

Respect a person's right to confidentiality. You must not disclose information to anyone who is not entitled to have that information. If you are concerned about this, then seek advice from your practice supervisor/assessor or academic supervisor prior to disclosing any information. Ensure you are aware of and follow any guidelines or policy concerning confidentiality (refer to your higher education provider or a clinical placement provider policies), refer to the guidance on confidentiality within the Code (NMC, 2018a).

Make every effort to collaborate with those in your care, listening to people and responding to their concerns and preferences. Offer support to people in caring for themselves, to improve and maintain their health. Provide people with information and advice, in a way they are able to understand, this can help them to make choices and decisions concerning their care.

You must ensure that you gain consent prior to providing care. Ensure that people know that you are a student. It is important to respect the right for people to ask if care could be provided by a registered professional only.

Maintain clear professional boundaries concerning the relationships that you have with others. Maintain clear sexual boundaries at all times with those whom you provide care, their families and carers.

Learning event

On different occasions nursing assessment and care in CCU will involve unconscious patient exposure or hygiene manoeuvres. Dignity and respect for the patient, always needs to be paramount even in emergency situations.

Few useful tips are:

- Make sure you close the room door or pull the curtains around the bed space when assessing chest movement or genitourinary tract.
- When performing hygiene care, keep genitals and chest covered by a towel, once the area is cleaned.

Reflect on the preservation of dignity and respect for the patient and think about how emergency situations could affect both.

Practise effectively

You must always practise under supervision as you offer people care and support and within your scope of practice. You will be supported in the critical care setting to enable you to meet proficiencies and programme outcomes (NMC, 2018a, 2018b, 2018c).

It is acknowledged that registered nurses are required to assess the needs of patients, interpret the results of tests, or offer advice on treatment regimens while adhering to the best available evidence. Student nurses will be aspiring to achieve these requirements. Nurses must be able to deliver the standards of care within a timeframe, and, at the same time, clearly communicating with patients and maintaining professional standards of record keeping or knowledge sharing. Within a busy CCU this can be daunting and challenging, but support mechanisms are in place to help to achieve the various programme requirements so you can become a safe and effective nurse.

Learning event

Critical Care can often be a fast-paced unit to work in. Especially during emergencies, healthcare staff must work cohesively and quickly to save people's lives.

Students, as well as novice CCU staff, can feel overwhelmed or inadequate during such scenarios:

- It is important to take a step back and discuss the situation with your Practice Supervisor/Assessor or with the senior member of the team.
- A revision of what went well and what did not go well is often useful to focus on what the student needs to improve on and what the Practice Supervisor/Assessor needs to do to be more supportive.

Try to explore the use of reflective cycles and think about how you might address the topic with your Practice Supervisor/Assessor.

Preserve safety

At the core of all nurse decision-making processes there is patient safety. While working with your practice supervisor/assessor, you have to recognise and work within your sphere of proficiency, monitoring the quality of your work and maintaining the safety of people for whom you provide care.

Red Flag

Practising outside your scope of practice refers to anyone who attempts to perform a task that is outside of their qualifying skill set. Doing this can put patients' and staff's lives at risk. You must let people know and express concerns if you are asked to act outside of your scope of practice.

All nurses have to be aware of their limitations and skill set, they have to know when they are out of their depth and seek help. If you lack the necessary skills or knowledge when attempting to offer care and support to people, or if you are doubtful, then this is not safe. Be aware also of the care processes of others (how others are practising) and potential lapses in the provision of care. If you are concerned or you identify unsafe practice, report this and address any safety concerns in a timely manner.

Learning event

Mark recently started his placement in CCU and assisted one of his practice supervisors with a telephone call in relation to the patient they are both looking after. Mark noticed that his practice supervisor did not confirm if the person he was talking to was effectively the patient's next of kin.

Mark, considering that is placement had only just started, decided not to ask questions and finished the shift without mentioning his doubts.

- What would you do in the same situations? Who would you contact to seek support?

Promote professionalism and trust

The promotion of professionalism and trust is the fourth underpinning principle of the Code. Nurses have to act with integrity and be trusted to use the powers they have in a responsible manner. All nurses and student nurses are required to uphold the values of the profession, ensuring that nurses remain respected members of the healthcare team. This can be achieved by adopting all of the necessary behaviours and attitudes outlined in the Code. Ensuring professionalism in everyday practice means that patients are more likely to trust you and as such they will be more confident in your abilities.

UK National Competency Framework: critical care

Many chapters in this text will refer to competency frameworks. Competency frameworks are often described as the core abilities that are required in order to fulfil a specific role, as such, critical care nurses have a structured competency framework including the abilities required to practise as a critical care nurse. These competencies have to be dynamic, reflecting the changing needs of those who use health services and health care provision. Chapters 1 and 2 provide an insight to the broader frameworks that underpin service provision.

The student or newly qualified health care practitioner allocated to work in critical care settings may be assessed against the competency levels described in the National Standards for Adult Critical Care Nurse Education (Critical Care Network, 2016). The student may also have to ensure that competencies laid down by their education provider (in the form of a practice assessment document) are also achieved during their clinical placement.

Critical Care Network (2016) explains how the Competency Framework will guide the novice practitioner from the initial stage (Step 1) to more independent and safe practice (steps 2–3) within the CCU environment. The goals expected to be achieved for each phase are outlined as follows (Critical Care Network, 2016).

Step 1

During Step 1 competencies, the novice will work mainly under direct supervision, student nurses must always work under supervision. Therefore, this first step will be performed as a supernumerary team member. Step 1 focuses on novice nurses who are new to the CCU with no previous critical care experience. This step is the step that healthcare students will be working at. The Critical Care Network (2016) suggest that the Step 1 competencies should be completed before any postgraduate academic qualifications and within a year from the starting date. Whilst this may not apply to student health care professionals this could be an aspirational landmark.

Step 2

In relation to the Step 2 competencies (it is not anticipated that students would be working to achieve the competencies in Step 2), the aims change to linking the theoretical knowledge, acquired in Step 1, to clinical practice. During this phase, specific skilled practice could be discussed with a clear rationale. Moreover, the person undertaking Step 2 competencies should understand and apply relevant policies, procedures and guidelines used within the critical care environment. The advice in this case is to complete the

competencies before or alongside an academic qualification. Another goal of the Step 2 phase is to involve the healthcare professional in problem solving of more complex cases, assessing the way in which critical analysis is used to achieve a specific goal. During this phase supervision should be minimal, allowing the candidate to improve their professional independence (Critical Care Network, 2016).

Step 3

As with Step 2 competencies, Step 3 competencies should be completed as part of an academic qualification. At this stage the supervision should take place for complex situations where the problem-solving ability of the candidate might need to be supported. The aim is to increase the number of hours without direct supervision and to develop solid critical analysis and problem-solving skills. The candidate may undertake the supervision with a range of activities related to the candidate's role and responsibilities. Another focus will include the in-depth knowledge of policies, procedures and guidelines commonly used in the CCU environment (Critical Care Network, 2016).

The full competency framework is available on the Critical Care Network website at https://www.cc3n.org.uk. The website also contains useful recommendations related to the assessment process.

Competency assessment is described as teamwork, driven by the learner. It is the responsibility of the learner to collaborate with the practice supervisor/assessor and clinical educators in order to establish and agree achievable goals and clarify specific developmental needs. A useful guide to establish achievable goals is the SMART acronym shown in Box 4.2.

Suggestions are made to help the novice nurse transitioning in the new CCU environment and settle in with the various competency requirements. The Critical Care Network suggest scheduling regular meetings, on a minimum three-month basis, to check the progression of knowledge, to express any concerns by both parties and to establish new learning goals. In relation to the establishment of new goals, the suggestion is to start with achievable and realistic goals according to the learner's skills and needs. The student allocated to the critical care setting will also be required to undergo initial, mid-point and final interviews so as to discuss development needs and to celebrate achievements.

Box 4.2   SMART goals (Williams, 2012).

1. **Specific:** Define exactly what is being pursued.
2. **Measurable**: Is there a number to track completion?
3. **Attainable**: Can the goal be achieved?
4. **Realistic**: Is it doable from a clinical perspective?
5. **Timely**: Can it be completed in a reasonable amount of time?

If the student raises any concerns, this should be discussed, and support provided. If this support is perceived as not adequate or minimal then a tripartite discussion is needed (see Figure 4.1).

If needed, a development plan or action plan may need to be devised or changed to ensure that the students receive the support required to help them achieve the competencies and proficiencies required. The plan should be agreed by all involved in the discussion (see Figure 4.1).

The relationship of the Code and the competency framework is not only linked to safe standards of practice and the knowledge level of the student, but also from a logistical point of view the two are connected. The layout and the assessment documentation presented by the competency framework has been designed to facilitate the candidates to support, with evidence, their progressive learning. The practice assessment document will also follow similar lines. As per the NMC description, reflection in practice and receiving practice-related feedback, will constitute progression and also provide evidence of achievement (NMC, 2018a).

Moreover, through the competency framework, the learning provided could be participatory (learning while on clinical practice) or non-participatory (self-independent study) (Critical Care Network, 2016). The amount of learning hours will be directed by the educational institution as well as the commitment and willingness to complete all the steps within the practice assessment document and the competency framework (if this is being used to assess a student's progression) in an appropriate time frame.

The steps of competence identified within the National Competency Framework aim to provide support for educational teams and to structure the content of critical care education and training programmes. However, it is important to remember that, if the student is being assessed against a set of criteria provided by the educational institution, then these requirements must also be met.

Development of critical thinking in healthcare

Critical thinking is a fundamental skill in healthcare. Hajrezayi et al. (2015) defined critical thinking as self-regulatory judgment that leads to interpretation, analysis and evaluation of specific knowledge, situations and scenarios. During an initial placement in critical care, the healthcare student should aim to develop their own clinical judgement and learn how to prioritise patient needs, under supervision. The interpretation of clinical findings by healthcare professionals allows the focus on relevant signs and symptoms shown by the patient (Smeltzer et al., 2010), whilst ensuring appropriate care provision.

Critical thinking includes two major components: cognitive and metacognitive (Vaghar et al., 2009). While the cognitive component is mainly related to the acquisition of knowledge and reasoning, the metacognitive one is related to the control of the learning process and therefore entails self-awareness, self-evaluative and self-reflective skills (Josephsen et al., 2014). Nursing and healthcare students should work on developing both cognitive and metacognitive components of critical thinking. Gholami et al. (2016) state that the introduction of problem-based learning in teaching methods could help the improvement of such skills. This method is particularly suitable for healthcare students as it focuses on the active role taken by students on their own learning. Problem-based learning is described as inquiry learning, where a small group of students direct their way of learning through the process of solving an open-ended problem (Tang et al., 2020).

Healthcare students should aim to achieve most of the critical thinking component by the end of their academic course. Observing and reflecting on practice within the CCU can help to achieve this aim. Some key qualities of a critical thinker include gathering and seeking information, questioning and investigating, analysing, evaluating, problem solving and the application of theory to practice (Chan, 2013). Therefore, students need to be able to assess a situation from different perspectives and consider all aspects before converting the assessment into action.

Consequently, a thorough analysis has to be performed before determining the solution to a clinical problem. Familiarity with the process of understanding and discriminating data (Chan, 2013) makes this a reality. Problem-based learning together with clinical experience will help to link theoretical data and clinical practice in order to elaborate a patient-centred approach. See Box 4.3 for an overview of issues related to critical thinking in action.

The prioritising process

This section considers the ways in which care is prioritised in the critical care setting. There are a number of skills required to be able to prioritise effectively. Prioritisation is reliant on discretionary judgement and ongoing

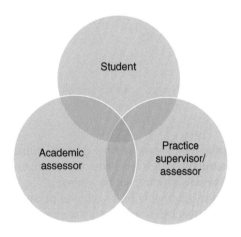

Figure 4.1 The tripartite model.

Box 4.3 General inquiries to facilitate critical thinking in action (*Source*: Adapted from Smeltzer et al., 2010).

- What relevant assessment information do I need? And how do I interpret them in relation to the clinical context?
- What problems identify the information gathered? Are there any other problems that need to be considered?
- Have I gathered all the information needed (think about your history-taking skills)?
- Is there anything that requires immediate priority? Do I need additional assistance?
- Have I considered potential and actual risk factors? What can I do to minimise them?
- Is there any complication that I can anticipate?
- Does the family and the patient perceive important problems in the same way? If not, what are the priorities given by both?
- Are relationships with relatives/families affecting the situation I am assessing in any way? Is my clinical plan going to be affected too?

assessment to manage complex and uncertain situations (Lake et al., 2009).

Whilst undertaking a clinical placement in a critical care setting, use this opportunity to experience what prioritising is about and how it is developed in this fast-paced critical setting. Continued exposure to the critical care routine will enable you to gain confidence in eventually making appropriate choices for action, developing competence and moving beyond the need to work with explicit rules to proficient nursing practice (Lake et al., 2009).

The components of the prioritising process have been researched using scientific research since the beginning of this millennium, there is no single notion of what the prioritising process entails. The literature review conducted by Lake et al. (2009) identified three main areas of nursing decision making and nursing prioritisation:

1. Time
2. Resource constraints
3. Multidisciplinary interactions

Time

Time impacts considerably on nursing/healthcare prioritisation, especially in the critical care environment where the number of tasks during an emergency are multiple and diverse. The general rule would be to prioritise all the interventions aimed at preserving the patient's life (e.g. airway manoeuvres, invasive haemodynamic procedures).

Resource Constraints

Resource constraints also play an important role during the prioritisation process as it influences the amount of human and technical resources available to perform an intervention. For example, from a nursing perspective, the seniority and the skills presented by staff, influence the decision making of the nurse coordinator whose role is to prioritise the allocation of senior members to the most complex patients.

Multidisciplinary interactions

Multidisciplinary interaction often impacts the prioritisation process in critical care as several specialists will cooperate with the CCU team and will integrate interventions in the daily clinical plan. Once again, the critical care healthcare professional will assess the situation and rearrange priorities according to the new clinical plan, such as suspending enteral nutrition before surgical procedures.

Exposure to the clinical environment will increase the ability of the healthcare student to recognise a situation previously experienced and to act/prioritise accordingly. This constant exposure will build the so called pattern recognition: a key component of the skills required to make a healthcare decision (Lake et al., 2009).

After considering the components of the prioritising process, it is useful to look at the method of prioritisation used by healthcare professionals. Patterson et al. (2011) aimed to investigate the method with which nurses prioritised their interventions in the clinical environment. The results demonstrated that there were different levels of nursing prioritisation (see Box 4.4).

Another interesting finding from Alspach (2000) also aimed to look at the prioritising methods used by healthcare practitioners. Results included what they referred to as the five Fs of prioritisation (see Box 4.5).

Box 4.4 Nursing prioritisation method (*Source*: Adapted from Patterson et al., 2011).

1. Imminent clinical concerns
2. High uncertainty activities
3. Core clinical care giving
4. Managing pain
5. Relationship management
6. Documenting
7. Helping others
8. Patient support
9. Cleaning/preparing supplies
10. Personal breaks and social interactions

Box 4.5 Nursing prioritisation method 2 (*Source*: Adapted from Alspach, 2000).

1. Fatal (could cause death or injury)
2. Fundamental (essential to nurse)
3. Frequent (must be conducted many times)
4. Fixed (must be done within certain times)
5. Facility (standard by the organization)

Learning event

As you commence your placement in the critical care setting, take note of the ways in which prioritisation occurs. Drawing on the information provided in Boxes 4.4 and 4.5. Can you identify any of the component parts?

Support systems: the student

The primary role of the student, who is undertaking a practice experience, is that of a learner. Pre-registration nursing students must be supernumerary when they are in clinical placement (the critical care setting). This means that students cannot be counted as part of the workforce while they are learning on placement in a clinical setting. The aim of supernumerary status is to give student nurses the opportunity to achieve their own learning needs as well as understanding their professional responsibilities, giving students the space and time to learn. Supernumerary status makes it clear to staff that students are primarily in the critical care area to learn, making it easier for students to articulate their learning needs in a more confident manner. Moreover, the supernumerary period enable them to access the appropriate clinical activities and experiences

that can help ensure they are safe and effective practitioners at the point of registration.

Every student should have access to adequately staffed settings that are characterised by high-quality patient care, delivered by skilled, up-to-date, enthusiastic and supportive health care staff. These are the key components of an excellent practice learning environment, ensuring that student and staff learning is maximised in the workplace.

Students are allocated a negotiated workload that is within their scope of practice, meeting their learning needs. This means that the experience gained during practice experiences should be guided by educational needs. Students do not need to be purely observers so as to develop their required skills and to achieve the identified learning outcomes. Students are required to take part in supervised clinical activities, and they should discuss with their practice assessor/supervisor the best ways of achieving their learning outcomes. The student may be required to experience the 7 day a week, 24 hours per day provision of the critical care environment or following a variety of working patterns.

Red Flag

Supernumerary status means that the critical area where the student has been allocated would continue to be able to deliver care without the student's presence.

Student nurses are usually allocated a practice assessor/supervisor who oversees progress and achievements, playing a crucial role in the development of healthcare students. The Critical Care Network (2016) outlines specific practice assessor/supervisor responsibilities such as the promotion of a positive learning environment, the ability of setting realistic, achievable goals and consequent action plans to fulfil them.

Conclusion

The journey of healthcare students in CCUs is complex, challenging and exciting, all at the same time. Having an insight into the professional requirements and responsibilities, the opportunities available for learning and the support mechanisms in place will help you settle into this highly charged care environment.

Take home points

1. There are many learning opportunities available to you in the critical care setting.
2. The exposure to the clinical environment will increase your ability to act/prioritise accordingly.
3. The supernumerary period aims to allow adequate time for you to develop skills and competence to care safely for the critically ill patient.
4. There are number of support systems in place, including practice supervisors, and you should aim to make use of the various systems.
5. The Competency Framework can also be a guide to help you during the clinical placement.

References

Alspach G., (2000). *From Staff Nurse to Preceptor: A Preceptor Development Program Instructor's Manual*, 2e. Aliso Viejo, CA: American Association of Critical Care Nurses.

Chan Z. (2013). A systematic review of critical thinking in nursing education. *Nurse Education Today* 33(3): 236–240.

Critical Care Networks – National Nurse Leads Forum (2016). *National Standards for Adult Critical Care Nurse Education*. www.cc3n.org.uk (accessed November 2020).

Gholami M., Moghadam P., Mohammadipoor F. et al. (2016). Comparing the effects of problem-based learning and the traditional lecture method on critical thinking skills and metacognitive awareness in nursing students in a critical care nursing course. *Nurse Education Today* 45: 16–21.

Hajrezayi, B., Roshani alibinasi, H., Shahalizade, M. et al. (2015). Effectiveness of blended learning on critical thinking skills of nursing students. *J. Nurs. Educ.* 4 1): 49–59.

Josephsen, J., 2014. *Critically reflexive theory: a proposal for nursing education*. Adv. Nurs. 1–7.

Lake S., Moss C., and Duke J., (2009). Nursing prioritization of the patient need of for care: A tacit knowledge embedded in the clinical decision-making literature. *International Journal of Nursing Practice* 15: 376–388.

Nursing & Midwifery Council (2018a). *The NMC Code*. https://www.nmc.org.uk/globalassets/sitedocuments/nmc-publications/nmc-code.pdf (accessed November 2020).

Nursing & Midwifery Council (2018b). *Standards of Proficiency for Registered Nursing Associates*. London: Nursing & Midwifery Council.

Nursing & Midwifery Council. (2018c). *Standards for Student Supervision and Assessment*. London: Nursing & Midwifery Council.

Patterson, E., Ebright, P., and Saleem, J. (2011). Investigating stacking: How do registered nurses prioritize their activities in real-time? *International Journal of Industrial Ergonomics* 41: 389–393.

Smeltzer S., Bare B., Hinkle J., and Cheever K. (2010). *Brunner & Suddarth's Textbook of Medical-Surgical Nursing*. Lippincott Williams & Wilkins.

Tang M. (2020). Interdisciplinarity creativity. In: *Encyclopaedia of Creativity* (ed. S. Pritzker and M. Runco).

Vaghar Seyyedin, A., Vanaki, Z., Taghi, S., and Molazem, Z. (2009). The effect of guided reciprocal peer questioning (GRPQ) on nursing students' critical thinking and metacognition skills. *Iran. J. Med. Educ* 8(2): 333–339.

Williams, C. (2012). *MGMT*, 5e. USA: South-Western College Publishing.

Chapter 5

Using an evidence-based approach

Sadie Diamond-Fox and Alexandra Gatehouse

Aim

The aim of this chapter is to provide the reader with an introduction to the principles of evidence-based practice (EBP) and the implications these have upon critical care practice.

Learning outcomes

After reading this chapter the reader will be able to:

- Understand the historical context of the development of EBP.
- Gain an appreciation of the development of the hierarchy of evidence.
- Understand how the hierarchy of evidence has since been translated in to a practical approach by the Centre for Evidence-Based Medicine (CEBM).
- Apply the principles of evidence-based frameworks to your own practice within critical care.
- Gain an understanding of the underpinning principles of critical appraisal and begin to apply these within your own practice.

Test your prior knowledge

- Can you define the term 'evidence-based practice' and what it means?
- List the components of the hierarchy of evidence
- List the four elements of the PICO method used to formulate a clinical research question
- Can you define the term 'critical appraisal' and what it means?
- Can you list the five stages of the clinical audit cycle?

Fundamentals of Critical Care: A Textbook for Nursing and Healthcare Students, First Edition. Edited by Ian Peate and Barry Hill.
© 2023 John Wiley & Sons Ltd. Published 2023 by John Wiley & Sons Ltd.
Companion website: www.wiley.com/go/peate/criticalcare

Introduction

Evidence-Based Practice (EBP) forms the basis of healthcare theory and practice and has become the language of patients, clinicians, policymakers, managers and researchers. Recognition of wide variations in clinical practice, the continued use of ineffective interventions, in addition to the underuse of effective therapies, led to the concept of EBP. It is beyond the scope of this chapter to explore all aspects of EBP; however, further information can be found in Glasper and Rees (2017). This chapter begins to explore the areas that are pertinent to nursing and healthcare students who have an interest in critical care and the process used to search for high-quality evidence and implementation into clinical practice.

Step 2 competencies

The following CC3N competencies will be covered in this chapter:

2:9.1:   Enhancing professionalism – ability to be a motivated self-directed learner

2:10.1:   Actively seek opportunities and challenges for personal learning and development

2:10.2:   Working with others – promote the sharing of information and resources

2:10.3:   Ensuring patient safety – understand your role in influencing the quality of safe and effective critical care services

2:10.4:   Improving services – question existing practices and challenge present performance/culture, contribute to quality improvement projects being undertaken in your unit

What is evidence-based practice (EBP)?

Since 1992 the major policy drivers and key strategies for implementing EBP within the NHS have focused upon integrating robust research from the laboratory setting into patient care (Department of Health, 1992), a process since termed 'from bench to bedside'. As illustrated in Figure 5.1, EBP focuses upon a triad of integrating clinical expertise, best internal/external evidence and individual patients' values and expectations, with the ultimate aim being to provide improved patient outcomes in a safe and cost-effective manner (Hamer and Collinson, 2005; Sacket et al., 1996) (see Figure 5.1).

Despite there being a long-standing movement towards EBP there are counter-arguments that exist, as EBP is not restricted to evidence with a particular grade of methodological rigour and therefore requires caution when implementing recommendations into practice (Greenhalgh, 2020). Other salient viewpoints include that of the reliance of the practitioner using EBP to be able to formulate the appropriate question to enable them to find the appropriate evidence, often working with limited information concerning the patient and within a fast-paced and stressful environment. These are particularly important factors for critical and emergency care departments. However, all clinically based NHS employees have a contractual duty to provide evidence-based care as part of the Knowledge and Skills Framework's (KSF) (NHS Employers, 2020) core dimension 'Quality'. This also underpins all other dimensions within this framework with a need to ensure that a conscious effort to embrace EBP occurs within one's daily practice. According to the NMC code and the Standards of Proficiency, the provision, leading and co-ordinating of care should always

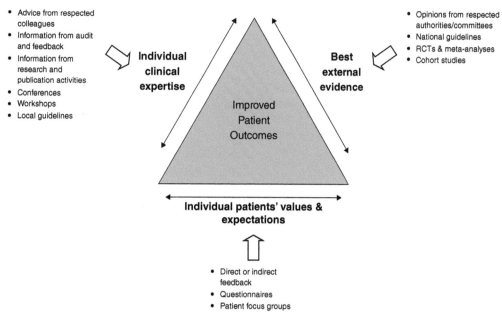

Figure 5.1   Evidence-based practice: a triad of factors aiming to improve patient outcomes.
Source: Adapted from Sacket et al. (1996) and Hamer and Collinson (2005).

be evidence-based (NMC, 2018a; NMC, 2018b). Petrie and Sabin (2020) advocate that in order to practise EBM, the clinician needs to be able to:

1. Formulate a relevant clinical question using the four main elements (PICO – explored further in this chapter)
2. Locate research/evidence relevant to their patient group (e.g. regarding diagnosis, prognosis or therapy)
3. Assess the strength of the findings of said research/evidence through the application of critical appraisal skills and recognise the varying levels of research/evidence
4. Extract the most relevant and useful results
5. Apply the results in to clinical practice.

6Cs: Commitment

Commitment to improving the care of patients and populations is the cornerstone of what we do as healthcare professionals. We need to build upon the commitment to practise EBP in our practice in order to improve the care and experience of patients.

The following sections of this chapter will explore the 5 steps in detail.

Step 1: formulating a clinical question – the PICO method

There are four main elements to consider when formulating a research question in order to provide meaningful information that can be used by the clinician to guide decision making. The mnemonic PICO is often used to remember them. Table 5.1 explores the PICO model in more detail.

Step 2: locating the evidence/research: performing a systematic literature review

Evidence may come from a variety of sources, but the primary search often begins by using an online database such as PubMed. It is important that the clinician can justify the chosen databases dependent on the type of information identified in the PICO model. There is vast coverage of medical, nursing and allied professional related literature with the aim of reducing bias towards one professional discipline. The National Institute for Health and Care Excellence (NICE), in association with Health Education England (HEE)

provide a useful platform entitled 'Healthcare Databases Advanced Search (HDAS)' (https://hdas.nice.org.uk/).

Bettany-Saltikov and McSherry (2016) advocate using a simple tabular format to detail the combination of the synonyms identified using the PICO model with Boolean operators (combination phrases) (see Table 5.2) to ensure a sensitive and specific literature search (Table 5.3). The use of quotation marks within a search also allows the phrase used to be considered as a single search term and not individual words which could lead to an inappropriate search. The InterTASC Information Specialists' Sub-Group Search Filter Resource database (https://sites.google.com/a/york.ac.uk/issg-search-filters-resource/home), a resource

Table 5.1 The PICO Model and a critical care example.

			Example
P	**P**atient, **P**opulation, **P**atient Location or **P**roblem	Describe the patient characteristics, population, patient location, or intervention you wish to study. This could include: · General population (e.g. adult patients) · Specific community types (e.g. rural or urban-dwelling) · Other population-based descriptors such as: · Age · Location	Adult patients with acute respiratory distress syndrome (ARDS).
I	Intervention	Describe the length, location and type	Low tidal volume ventilation (LTVV) at ≤8 mL/kg ideal body weight
C	**C**omparison	A different intervention, no intervention, or the location of the intervention	Standard therapy at >8 mL/kg ideal body weight
O	**O**utcome	A measurable effect	Mortality

Table 5.2 Boolean operators and their meaning. *Source:* Bettany-Saltikov and McSherry, 2016.

Boolean operator	Meaning
AND	Enhances specificity of the search by finding citations which contain all of the specific keywords
OR	Enhances sensitivity of the search by finding citations which contain either of the specific keywords
NOT	Disregards/excludes citations containing the specified keywords

Table 5.3   PICO model, synonyms and Boolean operators. *Source:* Bettany-Saltikov and McSherry, 2016.

Column terms combined with	Population/Patient condition AND	Intervention AND	Comparative intervention AND	Outcomes AND
	"......"	"......"	"......"	"......"
OR	"......"	"......"	"......"	"......"

endorsed by the National Institute for Health and Care Excellence, should also be used to aid in the identification and assessment of valid search filters where possible.

When performing a formalised systematic review of the literature, the search terms are usually developed after conducting a brief initial literature search and analysing common terminology used within various primary and secondary literature. This ensures that the search criteria for the review is consistent with the literature already in circulation.

The use of truncations when performing a database search enables variations of common words without having to state each of those variations separately. This is a technique advocated when conducting literature searches in order to ensure appropriate inclusion of studies within the search strategy, particularly those that may use American versus English spelling of certain words (Bettany-Saltikov and McSherry, 2016). Each database uses slightly different truncation symbols, but for the purpose of illustration a '*' has been used in Table 5.4, which details some of the truncations that may be used in the PICO example in Table 5.1.

The nature of literature reviews is such that many studies will inevitably be returned from initial searches. If undertaking a systematic review of the literature, it is recommended that the original search criteria may need to be refined to ensure that only studies that are relevant to the original research question are included. This process should include:

1. Title sifts whereby studies are excluded if their title does not relate to the research question. Reference lists of published meta-analyses identified during the initial search may also be interrogated and the same inclusion/exclusion criteria applied.
2. After this stage, the references of the remaining articles may be interrogated to ensure that articles that may have been missed in the original search strategy may be identified to locate further literature.
3. A subsequent abstract sift of the remaining articles' abstracts after the title sift stage.
4. The fourth stage should involve full text sifts, which by definition excludes any articles where full text access is not available. Duplicate articles are also excluded at this stage. All remaining studies are then examined against strict inclusion and exclusion criteria.

Being transparent about the search protocol used to conduct a systematic review is not only important in order

Table 5.4   Example truncations of chosen synonyms and Boolean operators applied to an example literature search.

Column terms combined with	Population/ Patient condition AND	Intervention AND	Outcomes AND
	1. "Acute respiratory failure"	9. "Artificial vent*"	17. Mortality
OR	2. "Acute respiratory distress syndrome"	10. "Tidal volume"	

for the review to potentially be reproduced in the future due to updating of the literature, but also to ensure that bias is not unintentionally introduced. There are eight areas for consideration, as detailed in Table 5.5, which have been applied to our example from the PICO model in Table 5.1.

Step 3: critical appraisal and the hierarchy of evidence

With the dawn of EBP so has come a plethora of resources that could be constituted as evidence with varying degrees of methodological quality and rigour behind their recommendations. In 1995 a key paper by Guyatt et al. (1995) was published which presented a new way of grading healthcare recommendations when using primary literature. The newly proposed framework suggested that there were three key elements to be considered when making a recommendation about a health care intervention:

1. The strength of the evidence, presented in the overview
2. The threshold or magnitude of intervention effect at which benefit exceeds the risks of therapy, including both adverse effects and costs
3. The relationships between the estimate of the magnitude of the intervention effect, the precision of that estimate, and the threshold.

Table 5.5   Rationale for inclusion and exclusion criteria.

Area for consideration	Inclusion criteria	Exclusion criteria	Rationale
1. Topic of study	Low Tidal Volume Ventilation (LTVV) versus Conventional Tidal Volume Ventilation (CTVV)	Studies not comparing LTVV to CTVV	This is the essential component of the primary research question and the subject of this review
2. Patient population	Patients with Acute Lung Injury (ALI)/Acute Respiratory Distress Syndrome (ARDS)/ hypoxaemic respiratory failure	All non-human studies Patients with alternative forms of respiratory failure	To ensure that the data can be extrapolated to the UK critical care population which includes both males and females
	Studies conducted within both male and female adult intensive care patients	Studies that only included single-sex participants	
3. Age group	Studies conducted within the adult intensive care population.	Studies including participants less than 18 years of age	NHS England's Standard contract for the provision of adult critical care calls for critically ill children and young (those <18 years) to be managed within paediatric units or lead centres, where possible. Only under exceptional circumstances would a child or young person be managed in an adult ICU within the UK. Therefore including studies that include a mixed adult and paediatric ICU population mean that data cannot be extrapolated to the UK population and therefore would not be useful in achieving the aim of this review; to improve evidence-based practice within the practitioners' current clinical environment.
4. Publication language	Studies published in English	Studies not available in English	The author's first language and the reliance on external sources for translation could possibly have introduced bias and/or the potential for mistakes in translating data.
5. Study design	Primary studies Randomised controlled trials Outcome data includes mortality rates (the primary outcome of this systematic review)	Secondary studies or any study that did not use a randomised, controlled design Outcome data does not include mortality rates	A systematic review of the available literature aims to summarise the highest quality of research relevant to the review question. By definition a systematic review aims to examine primary literature to eliminate bias through the adherence to a set of specific, rigorous methods (Bettany-Saltikov, 2016). A well-conducted systematic review of Randomised Controlled Trials (RCTs) is at the pinnacle of the hierarchy of evidence and as RCTs assess the impact of effectiveness of an intervention upon a well defined population group whilst aiming to eliminate bias through randomisation and blinding, it was therefore decided that this would provide the best quality evidence to answer the review question.
6. Publication dates	Studies published between 1996 and 2020	Studies published earlier than the year 1996	Although evidence-based literature recommends using search strategies that limit inclusion of studies from the previous 10 years, the initial literature search for this review revealed that seminal works had been performed in the late 1990s and that these works have often been referred to in subsequent literature. Therefore, the decision to exclude such works would not reflect the current literature in wider circulation at the present time.
7. Publication scrutiny	Peer-reviewed primary studies	Non peer-reviewed studies	To ensure that only evidence from high-quality, robust studies were appraised.
8. Availability of full text	Available	Not available	This is an essential criterion to ensure that the data within each of the studies sourced was able to be analysed.

Guyatt et al. (1995) suggested that if the strength and heterogeneity of the primary study are combined with the magnitude and precision of the treatment which directly relates to the number of patients that would need to be treated to prevent one additional bad outcome (number needed to treat (NNT)), the clinician can then make an analytical decision as to whether there is strength in the recommendation suggested, ultimately the deciding factor as to whether to treat or not to treat. The 'hierarchy of evidence' was produced based upon these key factors and is detailed in Figure 5.2. This new method of grading evidence has been widely adopted within the healthcare literature since its inception.

More recently the Centre for Evidence-Based Medicine (CEBM) has proposed an alternative framework which reflects clinical decision making. It has been 'designed so that it can be used as a short-cut for busy clinicians, researchers, or patients to find the likely best evidence' (CEBM, 2011).

In order to ensure methodological rigour of any systematic review, the evaluation of quality of the included studies is an essential component, with the central aim being to promote transparency and minimise bias. There are multiple tools available to aid the healthcare practitioner in critical appraisal of research and evidence, the use of which are also endorsed by the Centre for Reviews and Dissemination (CRD) (2009) guidance. One of the most common tools which is widely recommended across the NHS is the Critical Appraisal Skills Programme (CASP) (https://casp-uk.net/). There are eight critical appraisal tools which are designed to be used when reading and appraising research that has been identified as part of the systematic literature search. CASP has appraisal checklists designed for use with Systematic Reviews, Randomised Controlled Trials, Cohort Studies, Case Control Studies, Economic Evaluations, Diagnostic Studies, Qualitative studies and Clinical Prediction Rule.

Several seminal studies (Miller et al., 2007; Noyes and Popay, 2007; Schneider et al., 2014) have used the CASP tool to assess the quality of studies prior to inclusion in a subsequent systematic literature review, with an equivalent quality assessment agreement range of a minimum of 75%. Therefore, if the clinician performing the systematic review identifies studies with a percentage quality assessment score <75%, they may wish to consider discarding said studies at this stage.

6Cs: Competence

Competence in the principles of critical appraisal skills is vital in order to be able to practise EBP, and in turn, improve the care and experience of patients.

Learning event

Reflect upon how you may have previously used critical appraisal skills within your practice.

Step 4: extracting the most relevant and useful results

In order to ascertain the answer to any research questions/outcomes the most appropriate data included within each of the selected studies needs to be extracted following a transparent and rigorous process. The CRD (2009) and Greenhalgh (2020) advocate that a standardised extraction tool be used at this stage in order to aim to provide consistency, reduce bias and improve validity and reliability. An example tool can be found in Table 5.6.

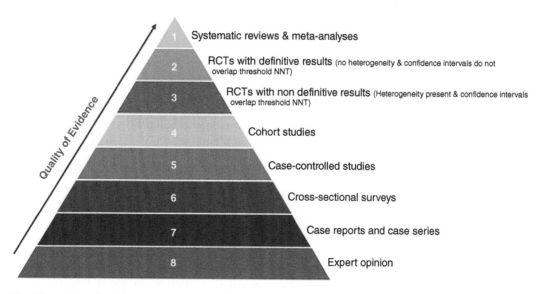

1 Systematic reviews & meta-analyses

2 RCTs with definitive results (no heterogeneity & confidence intervals do not overlap threshold NNT)

3 RCTs with non definitive results (Heterogeneity present & confidence intervals overlap threshold NNT)

4 Cohort studies

5 Case-controlled studies

6 Cross-sectional surveys

7 Case reports and case series

8 Expert opinion

Quality of Evidence

Figure 5.2 The hierarchy of evidence.

51

Table 5.6   Example data extraction tool. *Source:* based upon Centre for Research Dissemination, 2009; Greenhalgh, 2020.

Study Reference:						
Authors, date and country and focus of study	Study design	Participants, recruitment and sampling methodology	Intervention	Outcome measures	Results	Comments

Synthesis of data involves the collation and summarising of findings of the individual studies identified for the systematic review (Bettany-Saltikov and McSherry, 2016). There are two main forms of data synthesis classically used in systematic literature reviews; narrative and quantitative via the performance of a meta-analysis. In the case of therapeutic trails, such as those analysed in this review, meta-analyses of the data is considered to provide 'the best evidence' according to the hierarchy of evidence (Guyatt et al., 1995) due to its ability to aid in the control of bias which may confound the outcome of a RCT leading to an under- or over-estimation of the true effect of the intervention studied (Greenhalgh, 2020).

Step 5: implementing research into practice

Translational research is the application of knowledge derived in basic laboratory biology to clinical practice (Burnham and Moss, 2020; Davis UC, 2018). It is viewed as a spectrum or continuum and includes biomedical discovery, clinical efficacy research, clinical effectiveness research and implementation science (Weiss et al., 2016). The significance of translational research has increased considerably over recent years and is vital to the future of medicine to inform interventions, improve dissemination and implementation, bridging the 'bench to bedside' gap and reducing healthcare inequalities (Mensah et al., 2015). Nurses account for the majority of frontline health care workers and nurse-led research is critical to improving patient outcomes (World Health Organisation, 2012).

Worldwide healthcare is constantly changing and with the emerging wealth of reliable and robust evidence, evolution of clinical practice is essential. Despite these changes and increased understanding of the gap between healthcare research and clinical practice in critical care, the lack of translation of research to practice continues to be apparent, resulting in a lack of guideline-recommended therapy and preventable morbidity and mortality (Weiss et al., 2016). The aim of implementation science is to understand why healthcare interventions are adopted, or not, incorporating principles from research of health services, operations management, behavioural economics, epidemiology and organisational psychology (Khan, 2017). The subsequent development and testing of strategies aids patients, healthcare professionals and systems to overcome the research-practice gap, ensuring all suitable patients receive evidence-based care.

Implementation science acknowledges that interventions are complex and multi-component, target multilevels in a system and focus upon adaptive challenges to behaviour change (Weiss et al., 2016). There are many reasons as to why evidence-based practice has not been successfully adopted within critical care clinical practice. Conceptual frameworks have been developed within implementation science to impart common terms and definitions that are widely adopted, increase the understanding of research findings and allow investigation by multiple users, targeting factors that promote or prevent behavioural change. The overall aim of a framework is to explain the process of implementation, provide classification of implementation strategies and guide the evaluation of implementation, and over 100 frameworks have been developed (Powell et al., 2012; Proctor et al., 2009; Tabak et al., 2012; Weiss, 2017).

The consolidated framework for implementation research (CFIR) is based upon manifold of concepts and comprises of five domains:

- Intervention – characteristics of the evidence-based practice being implemented, including core and adaptable components
- Outer setting – general context (economic, political, social) of the organisation within which implementation occurs
- Inner setting –specific context (cultural, political, structural) through which implementation occurs such as networks and communication
- Individuals – the people (behaviour, characteristics) included within the implementation process
- Implementation process – the change required to effect implementation (Weiss et al., 2016)

Implementation is distinct from implementation science and is the process by which certain practices are adopted, incorporating audit, clinical guidelines, continuing professional education and financial incentives (Grimshaw et al., 2010). An evaluation framework, such as the Reach, Effectiveness, Adoption, Implementation, Maintenance (RE-AIM), may be used to assess the effectiveness of the implementation strategy in translating research into practice using clinical and process outcomes (Glasgow et al., 1999).

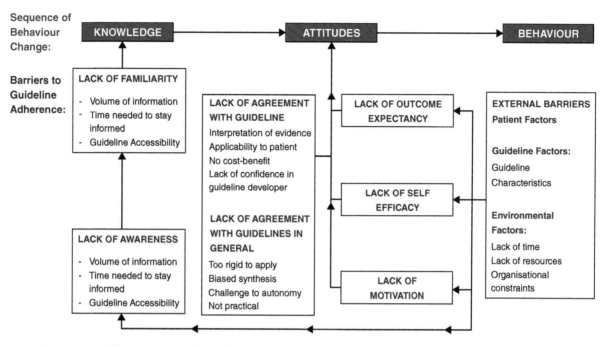

Figure 5.3 Barriers to adherence to evidence-based practice guidelines in relation to behaviour change.
Source: Adapted from Cabana et al. (1999).

Ideally these should be tested, allowing evaluation of impact and refinement prior to dissemination.

Seminal research identified that dissemination and implementation of research and evidence-based practice is more effective if active approaches are combined, rather than passive approaches (Grimshaw et al., 2001, 2004, 2006). Active approaches include the development of guidelines and protocols, active reminders, educational outreach, integration of decision-support systems and audit with feedback. Changing practice requires multilevel and systematic strategies which are dependent upon available resources, the perceived barriers to the adoption of EBP and the evidence relating to the effectiveness and efficiency of different strategies.

Behavioural strategies are critical in translating research into evidence-based guidelines and subsequently into clinical practice (Cabana et al., 1999; Cochrane et al., 2007). EBP is central to the NMC code and standards of proficiency and therefore it is important to have an understanding and appreciation of barriers to adherence and factors that influence implementation of evidence-based practice, recognition of which may facilitate change and improve clinical practice. These are outlined in Figure 5.3 and Table 5.7.

Quality healthcare in critical care

Quality assurance and clinical governance are frameworks employed within critical care to assure the quality of clinical services, improve patient safety and the performance of healthcare providers. In 2001, the Institute of Medicine defined quality healthcare as 'safe, effective, efficient, equitable, timely and patient-centred'. National standards and monitoring ensure quality of services within critical care and these include NICE, the Faculty of Intensive Care Medicine (FICM), the Intensive Care Society (ICS), the Care Quality Commission (CQC) and the National Confidential Enquiry into Patient Outcome and Death (NCEPOD). Clinical audit, quality improvement, guidelines, incident reporting, continuing professional development (CPD) and appraisal all contribute to the development and maintenance of the quality of healthcare provided.

Clinical audit and quality improvement

Clinical audit is a process in which healthcare provided is systematically reviewed against proven and agreed standards, allowing both patients and healthcare professionals to assess service performance and identify areas for development, with the aim to improve overall patient care and outcomes (FICM, 2019; NICE, 2002). Quality improvement (QI) involves the implementation of these changes with ongoing monitoring to verify enhanced healthcare delivery through better system performance, patient outcome and professional development (Batalden and Davidoff, 2007; NICE, 2002).

The guidelines for the provision of intensive care service (GPICS) (FICM, 2019) recommend that critical care units have planned and structured clinical audits programmes, participate in national audits such as the Intensive Care National Audit and Research Care (ICNARC) and the Scottish Intensive Care Society Audit Group (SICSAG), in addition to auditing and providing feedback nationally with regards to nosocomial infections via the Public Health England Infections in Critical Care Programme (ICCQIP) and the Scottish nosocomial infections in ICU audit (FICM, 2019).

54

Table 5.7   Factors influencing the implementation of evidence-based guidelines into practice. *Source:* based on Cochrane et al., 2007.

Barrier	Sub-types
Cognitive/behavioural	Knowledge/awareness Skills/expertise Critical appraisal skills
Attitudinal/rational-emotive barriers	Efficacy/perceived competence Perceived/outcome expectancy Confidence in abilities Authority Accurate self-assessment
Health care professional/physician barriers	Characteristics Age/maturity of practice Professional boundaries Legal issues Peer influence/models Gender Inertia
Clinical practice guidelines/evidence barriers	Utility Evidence/disagree content Access Structure Local applicability
Patient barriers	Patient characteristics/factors Patient adherence
Support/resource barriers	Time Support Costs/funding issues Resources
System/process barriers	Organisational System HR/workload/overload Team structure/work Referral process

There are several stages of the clinical audit, which is cyclical in nature and depicted in Figure 5.4.

The topic should be pertinent to critical care and the standard of best practice agreed, forming the basis of the audit criteria. Data is collected and analysed via comparison against the standards. Feedback of results with discussion regarding changes are subsequently agreed and implemented. Sufficient time should then be allowed for embedding of the changes prior to re-auditing to conclude if practice has improved.

Clinical audit and QI programmes are inextricably linked, enabling implementation of improvements in care, which can then be regularly measured in terms of structure, process and outcome. The process of improvement may be accelerated through the use of the Plan Do Study Act (PDSA) cycle which enables testing of changes on a small scale, in a structured way, prior to whole-scale implementation. The advantage of which is less disruption to patients and staff

with a safer process of change (NHS Improvement, 2018). The framework comprises three key questions with a process that allows testing of changes or full implementation. This is detailed in Figure 5.5. All measures should be specific, measurable, achievable, realistic and timely (SMART). QI is interdisciplinary with quality indicators

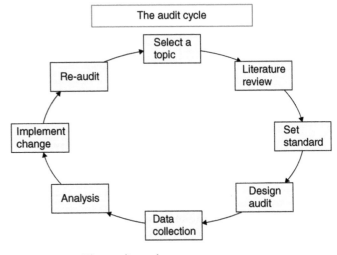

Figure 5.4   The audit cycle.

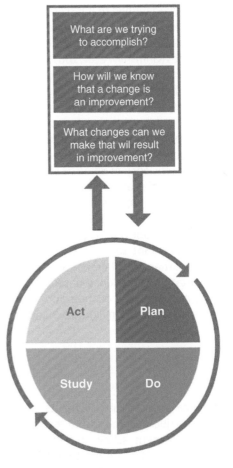

Figure 5.5   The PDSA cycle.
Source: NHS Improvement (2018).

ensuring high standards of clinical practice by individuals, units and organisations.

Clinical governance contributes to quality improvement and is a framework, through which health organisations are accountable for quality of services in addition to the safeguarding of high standards of care (FICM, 2019). Clinical effectiveness informs, changes and allows monitoring of practice and this, with clinical governance is supported by clinical audit.

Research and development in critical care

Research is concerned with discovering the right thing to do; audit with ensuring that it is done right.

Smith, 1992

Research uses clearly defined hypotheses to acquire innovative knowledge with regards to best practice, leading to the development of new treatments or services. If evidence is high-quality and demonstrates clinical and cost-effectiveness, widespread adoption may occur, ensuring patients benefit from state of the art treatment (FICM, 2019). Research is essential within critical care due to the high rates of morbidity and mortality associated with critical illness, in addition to patients' reduced quality of life and the significant cost associated with acute hospitals stays.

NICE collaborates with researchers, as well as charities, funders and organisations, to attain high-quality evidence, developing guidance and identifying gaps within the evidence base, making recommendations for further research. Alongside this in 2019 the NHS Long Term Plan was written stating that the NHS was committed to research and innovation to improve future patient outcomes.

The National Institute for Health Research (NIHR) funds health and care research, within the UK, and the NIHR Clinical Research Network (CRN) supported 104 studies within critical care, in 2018–2019. Within England there are 15 Local Clinical Research Networks (LCRNs), each of which has a critical care research lead, with government funding to support the delivery of research within healthcare organisations in the form of clinical research nurses, research support services and research time. The CRN supports a national portfolio which comprises of high-quality research studies relating to critical care specialities such as sepsis, ARDS, long-term implications of critical illness, brain injury and minimising risk and morbidity associated with major surgery. International critical care trails and experimental medicine in critical care studies are also included within the portfolio. These are easily accessible on the NIHR website.

Good Clinical Practice (GCP) is the international ethical, scientific and practical standard to which all clinical research is conducted. It protects the rights, safety and wellbeing of study participants and is a requirement stipulated by the UK Policy Framework for Health and Social Care Research (National Institute for Health Research, 2020). The completion of GCP is recommended for any clinician interested in

healthcare research as it provides a sound introduction to the multiple areas concerning clinical research, including ethical and safeguarding considerations.

The National Confidential Enquiry into Patient Outcome and Death (NCEPOD) aims to improve the quality of healthcare for adults and children, in the UK, through conducting confidential surveys and research of patient management. These reviews are then published within the public domain, are widely available, and make recommendations to clinicians and service providers. Essentially NCEPOD assesses and establishes levels of standards within multiple specialities with an overarching review programme of medical and surgical, as well as child health clinical outcomes. Specific topics are explored but there are several common themes that are relevant to the care related to patient's hospital admission. These include (NCEPOD, 2018):

- Timely consultant review
- Ongoing supervision of trainee doctors
- Improved multidisciplinary review
- Accuracy of documentation in case notes
- Frequency of monitoring and use of early warning scores
- Morbidity and mortality review attendance and occurrence
- Critical care review
- Use of networks of care
- Consent
- Greater existence and audit of policies, protocols, proformas, guidelines and standard operating procedures

Several NCEPOD reports have identified deficiencies in recognition and assessment of acutely unwell patients including poor management of simple aspects of acute care in addition to lack of knowledge and supervision, failure to seek advice leading to delayed response, poor communication and organisational failure (NCEPOD, 2018). This led to the publication of a NICE Clinical Guideline for recognition and response to acutely ill adults in hospital (NICE, 2007), following which a standardised approach to the management of these patients was developed, the National Early Warning Score (NEWS2) (Royal College of Physicians, 2017). This is a monitoring tool wherein scores are given to physiological measurements including respiratory rate, oxygen saturations, heart rate, blood pressure, level of consciousness and temperature. NCEPOD (2018) recommends that the NEWS2 tool should be used in all acute healthcare settings to ensure rapid identification of patients at high risk of acute deterioration, ensure an appropriate and timely response and improve communication between clinicians regarding deterioration of a patient. This is based upon 17 NCEPOD reports published since 2000 (NCEPOD, 2018). The use of early warning scores is also a key element of Critical Care Outreach services which should be available 24 hours a day, seven days a week. It is recommended that these services not only use a track and trigger system to identify at-risk patients but also rapid referral to experts, timely transfer to critical care and facilitation of discharge and rehabilitation of critical care patients (NCEPOD, 2018).

Conclusion

In conclusion, there are major policy drivers and a professional duty to implement and provide EBP within the clinical arena, otherwise there is a risk that certain practices may become outdated and sometimes highly questionable in their potential to cause patient harm. This chapter has explored some of processes by which the healthcare student may begin to address these issues, from the formulation of an appropriate clinical questioning using the PICO technique through to applying relevant implementation strategies.

Take home points

1. NHS professionals have a contractual duty to implement and provide EBP.
2. The traditional hierarchy of evidence has since been adapted via the CEBM and provides a more practical 'bedside' approach to grading relevant evidence for clinical practice.
3. There are several evidence-based frameworks available in order to guide you in the steps of implementing EBP in to your own practice, from identifying the 'problem' to developing and implementing clinical practice guidelines.

References

Batalden, P.B. and Davidoff, F. (2007). What is 'quality improvement' and how can it transform healthcare? https://www.ncbi.nlm.nih.gov/pmc/articles/PMC2464920/pdf/2.pdf (accessed December 2020).

Bettany-Saltikov, J. and McSherry, R. (2016). *How to Do a Systematic Literature Review in Nursing*, 2e. Open University Press.

Burnham, E.L. and Moss, M.(2020). Translational research: Basic concepts and the importance of heterogeneity. https://www.thoracic.org/professionals/clinical-resources/critical-care/critical-care-research/translational-research.php#1 (accessed December 2020).

Cabana, M.D., Rand, C.S., Powe, N.R. et al. (1999). Why don't physicians follow clinical practice guidelines? A framework for improvement. *Journal of the American Medical Association* 282: 1458–1465. http://jama.jamanetwork.com/article.aspx?articleid=192017 (accessed December 2020).

Centre for Evidence-Based Medicine (2011). OCEBM Levels of Evidence Working Group. The Oxford 2011 Levels of Evidence. https://www.cebm.ox.ac.uk/resources/levels-of-evidence/explanation-of-the-2011-ocebm-levels-of-evidence/resolveuid/78a5245777444c8ea440b734e30ca724 (accessed December 2020).

Centre for Reviews and Dissemination. (2009). Systematic Reviews: CRD's guidance for undertaking reviews in health care. https://www.york.ac.uk/media/crd/Systematic_Reviews.pdf (accessed December 2020).

Cochrane, L.J., Olson, C.A., Murray, S. et al. (2007). Gaps between knowing and doing: Understanding and assessing the barriers to optimal health care. *Journal of Continuing Education in the Health Professions* 27(2): 94–102.

Davis, U.C. (2018). What is translational research? https://www.ucdavis.edu/one-health/translational-research/ (accessed December 2020).

Department of Health (1992). *The Health of the Nation – A Strategy for Health in England*. London: Her Majesty's Stationary Office.

Faculty of Intensive Care Medicine (FICM) (2019). Guidelines for the Provision of Intensive Care Services, 2e. https://ficm.ac.uk/sites/default/files/gpics-v2-final2019.pdf (accessed December 2020).

Glasgow, R.E., Vogt, T.M. and Boles, S.M. (1999). Evaluating the Public Health impact of health promotion interventions: The RE-AIM framework. https://www.ncbi.nlm.nih.gov/pmc/articles/PMC1508772/pdf/amjph00009-0018.pdf (accessed December 2020).

Glasper, A. & Rees, C. (2017). Nursing and Healthcare Research at a Glance. Wiley Blackwell.

Greenhalgh, T. (2020). *How to Read a Paper: The Basics of Evidence-based Medicine and Healthcare*, 6e. Wiley Blackwell.

Grimshaw, J.M., Shirran, L., Thomas, R. et al. (2001). Changing Provider Behavior: An Overview of Systematic Reviews of Interventions. Medical Care. 39. 8. Supp 2.

Grimshaw, J.M., Eccles, M.P., Walker, A.E., and Thomas, R.E. (2002). Changing physicians' behavior: What works and thoughts on getting more things to work. *Journal of Continuing Education in the Health Professions* 22: 237–243. http://onlinelibrary.wiley.com/doi/10.1002/chp.1340220408/abstract (accessed 12 April 2014).

Grimshaw, J.M., Eccles, M.P., and Tetroe, J. (2004). Implementing clinical guidelines: current evidence and future implication. *The Journal of Continuing Education in the Health Professions* 24 ppS31–S37.

Grimshaw, J., Eccles, M., and Vale, L. (2006). Toward Evidence-Based Quality Improvement: Evidence (and its limitations) of the Effectiveness of Guideline Dissemination and Implementation Strategies 1966–1998. Journal of Internal Medicine. 21, supp2. http://www.ncbi.nlm.nih.gov/pmc/articles/PMC2557130/ (accessed 4 April 2014).

Grimshaw, J., McAuley, L.M., Bero, L.A. et al. (2010). Systematic reviews of the effectiveness of quality improvement strategies and programmes. https://qualitysafety.bmj.com/content/qhc/12/4/298.full.pdf (accessed December 2020).

Guyatt G.H., Sackett D.L., Sinclair J.C. et al. (1995). Users guide to the medical literature: IX. A method for grading healthcare recommendations. JAMA 274,1800–1804.

Hamer, S. and Collinson, G. (2005). *Achieving Evidence-based Practice. A handbook for Practitioners*, 2e London: Balliere Tindal.

Institute of Medicine (U.S.) (2001). *Crossing the Quality Chasm: A New Health System for the 21st Century*. Washington, D.C., National Academy Press.

Khan, J.M. (2017). Bringing implementation science to the intensive care unit. https://www.ncbi.nlm.nih.gov/pmc/articles/PMC6020843/pdf/nihms972031.pdf (accessed December 2020).

Lissauer, T., Fanaroff, A.V., Miall, L. et al. (2015). *Neonatology at a Glance*, 3e Wiley & Sons.

Mensah, G.A., Engelgau, M., Stoney, C. et al. (2015). News from NIH: a center for translation research and implementation science. https://europepmc.org/article/pmc/4444711 (accessed December 2020).

Miller, T., Bonas, S., Dixon, M. (2007). Qualitative research on breastfeeding in the UK: A narrative review and methodological reflection. *Evidence & Policy* 3: 197–230.

National Confidential Enquiry into Patient Outcome and Death (NCEPOD) (2018). Themes and recommendations common to all hospital specialities https://www.ncepod.org.uk/CommonThemes/Common Themes.pdf (accessed January 2021).

National Institute for Health and Care Excellence (2002). Principles for best practice in clinical audit. https://www.nice.org.uk/media/default/About/what-we-do/Into-practice/principles-for-best-practice-in-clinical-audit.pdf (accessed December 2020).

National Institute for Health and Care Excellence (2007). Acutely ill adults in hospital: recognising and responding to deterioration. Clinical Guideline (CG50). https://www.nice.org.uk/guidance/cg50 (accessed January 2021).

National Institute for Health Research (2020). http://www.nihr.ac.uk (accessed December 2020).

NHS Employers (2020). Simplified Knowledge and Skills Framework (KSF) https://www.nhsemployers.org/SimplifiedKSF (accessed December 2020).

NHS Health Research Authority (2020). UK Policy Framework for Health and Social Care Research. https://www.hra.nhs.uk/planning-and-improving-research/policies-standards-legislation/uk-policy-framework-health-social-care-research/uk-policy-framework-health-and-social-care-research/ (accessed December 2020).

National Health Service Improvement (2018). Online library of Quality, Service Improvement and Redesign tools: Plan, Do, Study, Act (PDSA) cycles and the model for improvement. https://improvement.nhs.uk/documents/2142/plan-do-study-act.pdf (accessed December 2020).

Noyes, J. and Popay, J. (2007). Directly observed therapy and tuberculosis: how can a systematic review of qualitative research contribute to improving services? A qualitative meta-synthesis. *Journal of Advanced Nursing* 57(3): 227–243.

Nursing and Midwifery Council (NMC) (2018a). The Code. Professional standards of practice and behaviour for nurses, midwives and nursing associates. https://www.nmc.org.uk/globalassets/sitedocuments/nmc-publications/nmc-code.pdf (accessed January 2021).

Nursing and Midwifery Council (NMC) (2018b). Future nurse: Standards of proficiency for registered nurses. https://www.nmc.org.uk/globalassets/sitedocuments/education-

standards/future-nurse-proficiencies.pdf (accessed January 2021).

Petrie, A. & Sabin, C. (2020). *Medical Statistics at a Glance*, 4e Wiley-Blackwell.

Powell, B.J., McMillen, J.C., Proctor, E.K. et al. (2012). A compilation of strategies for implementing clinical innovations in health and mental health. https://www.ncbi.nlm.nih.gov/pmc/articles/PMC3524416/ (accessed December 2020).

Proctor, E.K., Landsverk, J., Aarons, G. et al. (2009). Implementation research in mental health services: an emerging science with conceptual, methodological, and training challenges. https://www.ncbi.nlm.nih.gov/pmc/articles/PMC3808121/ (accessed December 2020).

Sacket, D.L. et al. (1996). Evidence based medicine: what it is and what it isn't. *BMJ*. 312. doi: 10.1136/bmj.312.7023.71.

Schneider, C., Mohsenpour, A., Joos, S., and Bozorgmehr, K. (2014). Health status of and health-care provision to asylum seekers in Germany: protocol for a systematic review and evidence mapping of empirical studies. *Systematic Reviews*. 3. 139.

Smith, R. (1992). Audit and research: Research is concerned with discovering the right thing to do; audit with ensuring that it is done right. *BMJ* 305(6859): 905–906.

Tabak, R.G., Khoong, E.C., Chambers, D.A. et al. (2012). Bridging research and practice: models for dissemination and implementation research. https://www.ncbi.nlm.nih.gov/pmc/articles/PMC3592983/pdf/nihms-396032.pdf (accessed December 2020).

The National Health Service (2019). *The Long Term Plan*. https://www.longtermplan.nhs.uk/wp-content/uploads/2019/08/nhs-long-term-plan-version-1.2.pdf (accessed December 2020).

Weiss, C.H. (2017). Why do we fail to deliver evidence-based practice in critical care medicine? https://www.ncbi.nlm.nih.gov/pmc/articles/PMC5784774/pdf/nihms935847.pdf (accessed December 2020).

Weiss, C.H., Krishnan, J.A., Au, D.H. et al. (2016). An official American Thoracic Society Research Statement: Implementation science in pulmonary, critical care and sleep medicine. https://www.atsjournals.org/doi/pdf/10.1164/rccm.201608-1690ST (accessed December 2020).

World Health Organization (2012) *Enhancing Nursing and Midwifery Capacity to Contribute to the Prevention, Treatment and Management of Noncommunicable Diseases in Practice*. Human Resources for Health Observer, No. 12. https://www.who.int/hrh/resources/observer12.pdf (accessed December 2020).

Chapter 6

Nursing care

Sarah Crowe and Fiona McLeod

Aim

The aim of this chapter is to provide the reader with evidence-based understanding of the nursing care provided to patients in critical care settings.

Learning outcomes

After reading this chapter the reader will be able to:

- Gain an appreciation of the complexities of care provided to critical care patients.
- Understand the common complications associated with critical care and the role nursing care plays in prevention of these.
- Describe how to care for a critically ill patient, under supervision.

Test your prior knowledge

- Can you name six common complications that critically ill patients may experience?
- Can you identify the preventive measures for delirium?
- Can you describe how to safely mobilise a critically ill patient?
- Do you know how often a critically ill patient should be assessed?

Fundamentals of Critical Care: A Textbook for Nursing and Healthcare Students, First Edition. Edited by Ian Peate and Barry Hill.
© 2023 John Wiley & Sons Ltd. Published 2023 by John Wiley & Sons Ltd.
Companion website: www.wiley.com/go/peate/criticalcare

Introduction

This chapter explores the nursing care provided to patients admitted to critical care units. The aim of nursing care in critical care is to support patients who are faced with actual or potential life-threatening events. The care provided in critical care settings includes advanced knowledge, monitoring, and technology; and generally includes a lower nurse to patient ratio than on other general hospital units.

Critically ill patients face numerous difficulties during their critical care stay, and beyond; and it is the care provided by Critical Care Registered Nurses (CCRNs) that optimises comfort and promotes a return to quality of life when possible (Canadian Association Critical Care Nurses, 2017). The majority of the care provided by CCRNs is focused on providing therapeutic treatment and support, monitoring the patient's response to therapy, and minimising the risk of complications. Patients can experience a high burden of physiological and psychological burden while in critical care, and many of these effects are continued beyond critical care. The term Post Intensive Care Unit Syndrome or PICS has been coined to describe the constellation of symptoms and sequelae associated with critical care (Kiernan, 2017; Rawal et al., 2017). Common complications of critical care include delirium, muscle wasting, pressure injuries, depression/anxiety, and nosocomial infections. Cognitive impairment associated with critical care is often related to critical care delirium, acute brain dysfunction (e.g. stroke), hypoxia, hypotension, glucose dysregulation, prolonged ventilation and prior poor cognitive function, which can all contribute to PICS (Harvey and Davidson, 2016). Many of the physical symptoms associated with PICS, often referred to as critical care unit (CCU) acquired weakness, are due to prolonged ventilation, sepsis, multiorgan dysfunction and the use of medications such as high dose analgesia, sedation, and neuromuscular blocking agents (Ferguson et al., 2018). Nursing care, while often thought of as a basic function of nursing, when caring for critically ill patients focuses on mitigating potential complications to optimise a patient's potential for recovery and comfort; and to minimise PICS.

6Cs: Commitment

A commitment to patients to improve their care and experience.

Standards of care

Standards of care are guidelines that are used to define the minimum expected safe care to be provided to patients in a designated area. In critical care it will be important to determine the unit or hospital's specific level of acuity and expectations in order to create guidelines to guide the CCRNs' practice. Components that are important to consider when developing standards include expectations during

---

6Cs: Care

Caring for patients defines the work we do as critical care nurses.

---

preadmission, admission and ongoing daily care.

At all times the nurse is required to ensure that they up hold the tenets associated with Nursing and Midwifery Council's (NMC) Code (NMC, 2018). The Code provides the professional standards that those on the professional register must uphold in order to be registered to practise in the UK. It is arranged around four themes – prioritise people, practise effectively, preserve safety and promote professionalism and trust (see also Chapter 4).

Preadmission

During the preadmission phase, standards of care should focus on preparing the patient room or space for readiness to admit a critically ill patient. This will include checking to ensure all relevant equipment is present, clean and functional. This includes items such as the bed, intravenous pumps, suction devices, mechanical lifts, cardiac monitors, ventilators and safety equipment. Examples of safety equipment include a bag-mask-valve for manual breath delivery, oral and/or nasal airways, suction catheters, and oxygen masks. Another important phase during the preadmission check is to consider possible isolation needs of the potential patient, and ensuring all necessary personal protective equipment (PPE) is available.

Admission

Standards of care for the admission process should provide criteria about the expectations for not only the components of physical assessment, but also the timing and documentation requirements. In general, a newly admitted critical care patient should have a full comprehensive assessment completed within 30 minutes or less of arriving to the critical care unit. Aspects of the initial comprehensive assessment include verifying the patient's identification, working diagnosis, and any special consideration such as allergies, infectious disease precautions, and goals of care or cardiopulmonary resuscitation (CPR) wishes. Documentation of the initial patient assessment should include a review of systems or head-to-toe account of the patient status on arrival to the unit. The patient's vital signs including, blood pressure (BP), mean arterial pressure (MAP), heart rate and rhythm (including a rhythm strip with analysis), respiratory rate, temperature, oxygen saturation and the amount of supplemental oxygen (if any), invasive or non-invasive mechanical ventilation support (if any), and level of consciousness should all be documented on arrival (Royal College of Physicians, 2017). Any patient-specific parameters should also be assessed, such as neurological or neurovascular function. Medication infusions should be documented, including the rate and dose being delivered. All physician orders should be reviewed and verified during the initial admission. This should include reviewing and providing any prescribed medications, intravenous (IV) fluids, and diagnostic tests that may be outstanding. The full comprehensive assessment should be documented as soon as possible.

Comprehensive assessments

CCRNs are required to assess the patient's status each shift, and should involve a comprehensive overall assessment as well as focused reassessments throughout their shift. The comprehensive assessment is important to provide the CCRN with an in-depth understanding the of the patient's current acuity and status. This will help the CCRN plan care throughout the day and also allow the CCRN to anticipate potential deterioration or improvement. It is also an important part of developing a relationship with the patient.

The comprehensive assessment can be divided into two sections, the initial quick safety survey and the secondary in-depth assessment. The initial quick safety survey of the patient should involve a fast assessment of the 'ABCDEs' (airway, breathing, circulation, disability and exposure). It involves assessing to ensure the patient has a secure and patent airway, is breathing effectively, has appropriate circulation, assesses the neurological status of the patient and identifies any immediate threats or exposures to patient and nurse safety. Once the 'ABCDEs' have been determined to be stable, it is safe to continue on with an in-depth secondary aspect of the assessment (Urden et al., 2018). If there is any concern over the stability of the 'ABCDEs' the CCRN should immediately intervene as required and call for help. The CCRN should not proceed with the secondary assessment until it is safe to do so.

The comprehensive assessment involves performing an overall head-to-toe or systems assessment of the patient. Some hospitals or units will start at the head of the patient and work down the body, assessing all aspects; others will use a systems approach (e.g. neurological, cardiovascular, and so on). Either style of assessment is acceptable (Morton and Fontaine, 2013). The purpose of this assessment is to be thorough and to gain a full understanding of the patient's status as soon as care is assumed (e.g. at admission or start of shift). It is important to use inspection, palpation, auscultation and percussion where applicable.

Table 6.1   Glasgow Coma Scale.

Best eye-opening response	Score
Spontaneously	4
To speech	3
To pain	2
No response	1

Best verbal response	Score
Orientated	5
Confused conversation	4
Inappropriate words	3
Garbled Sounds	2
No response	1
Not testable	NT

Best motor response	Score
Obeys Commands	6
Localises stimuli	5
Withdrawal from stimulus	4
Abnormal flexion (decorticate)	3
Abnormal extension (decerebrate)	2
No response	1

Other chapters in this text will provide detail on system specific assessment details.

There are several important assessment scales that may be incorporated into the comprehensive assessment process depending on local policy and procedure that assess a patient's neurological status. These assessments are important regardless of why a patient is admitted, as many patients are at risk for neurological impairment in the critical care unit related to disease process, cardiac output, and hypoxaemia. A few examples of important scales include the Glasgow Coma Scale (GCS), Richmond Agitation-Sedation Scale (RASS), Riker Sedation-Agitation Scale (SAS), and the Confusion, Assessment Method-ICU (CAM-ICU) Delirium Scale. The GCS is comprised of three assessment parameters of neurological function, eye opening, verbal responses, and motor responses (see Table 6.1) (Nik et al., 2018). It is used to determine the neurological functioning of a patient, in particular those with or potential of neurological injury; and has been helpful in predicting outcomes (Nik et al., 2018). A benefit of the GCS is that it is quick, standardised and can be conducted and scored by a CCRN. A score of 3 to 8 suggests severe neurological impairment, 9 to 12 suggests moderate neurological impairment, and 13 to 15 suggest minor or minimal impairment (Morton and Fontaine, 2013).

The RASS and SAS are scales used to assess sedation and agitation in critical care (Sessler et al., 2002). It is important to assess both sedation and agitation levels of critical care patients, both to manage and titrate medications (e.g. sedatives, analgesics) and to help monitor for delirium and changing patient status (Khan et al., 2012).

Table 6.2 Richmond Agitation-Sedation Scale (RASS).
Source: Khan et al., 2012 with permission of Elsevier.

Score	Term	Description
+4	Combative	Overtly combative, violent, danger to staff
+3	Very agitated	Pulls or removes tubes or catheters; aggressive
+2	Agitated	Frequent non-purposeful movement, fights ventilator
+1	Restless	Anxious, but movements not aggressive or vigorous
0	Alert and calm	
−1	Drowsy	Not fully alert, but has sustained wakening (eye opening/eye contact) to voice (>10 seconds)
−2	Light sedation	Briefly awakens with eye contact to voice (<10 seconds)
−3	Moderate sedation	Movement or eye opening to voice (but no eye contact)
−4	Deep sedation	No response to voice, but movement or eye opening to physical stimulation
−5	Unable to rouse	No response to voice or physical stimulus

The RASS scores patients on a continuum from +4 (combative) to −5 (no response to voice or physical stimulus) (Khan et al., 2012). A score of zero is optimal in most circumstances and is indicative of alert and calm (See Table 6.2). The SAS scores patients on a scale ranging from 1 (unable to rouse) to 7 (dangerous agitation) (Khan et al., 2012).

Delirium is a common problem in the critical care unit therefore assessment of and prevention of delirium is an important part of critical care nursing (Ely et al., 2001). The lasting effects of delirium can be significant on patient outcomes and experiences, and contribute to the development of post-ICU care syndrome. All critical care patients are at risk for developing delirium and therefore must be assessed regularly for it (Haenggi et al., 2013). Chapter 15 will provide a more in-depth explanation of delirium, its assessment and management. Two common delirium assessment tools used in critical care are the CAM – ICU and the Intensive Care Delirium Screening Checklist (ICDSC) (Khan et al., 2017). Both have been validated within the critical care population and provide a positive (the patient is delirious) or negative (the patient does not have delirium) finding (Ely et al., 2001). Much of the nursing care provided in critical care is aimed at preventing delirium and optimising patient recovery.

Snapshot

A 63-year-old patient with chronic obstructive pulmonary disease (COPD) was admitted seven days ago with an exacerbation complicated with pneumonia. The patient required intubation. The patient was initially on high doses of propofol and fentanyl, but has since been weaned to low doses of fentanyl for pain control and minimal propofol.

During the nurse's initial assessment the patient opens his eyes to voice, is able to follow commands. He cannot speak as he is still intubated. During the assessment he falls asleep quickly and the nurse must speak loudly or gently touch him to wake him.

Other assessment findings are as follows:

Airway (A): airway is secured and patent, he has an oral endotracheal tube in place.
Breathing (B): Oxygen saturations are 95% on FiO_2 30% (NEWS2 score 2), respiratory rate 16 on pressure support ventilation (NEWS2 score 0).
Cardiovascular (C): Blood pressure (BP) is 110/50 (NEWS2 score 0), heart rate 80 (NEWS2 score 0).
Disability (D): patient is drowsy (NEWS2 score 2) and is normothermic (36.8°C).
Exposure (E): no abnormal findings.

Nursing Action:
- The nurse scores the patient's GCS 9NT, he receives an NT as he is not able to verbalise any words due to his endotracheal tube.
- The nurse scores the patient's RASS -2 as he is falling asleep quickly and needs stimulation to awaken.
- What was the NEWS2 score?

Diagnosis:
- The patient appears alert with moderate impairment likely due to the analgesia and sedation he is receiving.
- He should be assessed for the need for ongoing sedation and weaned off with a RASS goal of 0.

Ongoing care
Ongoing standards of care once a patient is admitted to a critical care unit, should include expectations surrounding timing of start of shift comprehensive assessments (e.g. within 15 to 30 minutes of arriving on shift), focused reassessments throughout the shift (e.g. a full head-to-toe assessment every four hours), hourly monitoring parameters, expected care practices, and documentation expectations. Evaluation of the patient status regularly is important to help guide therapies, to identify when patients are stable and ready for transition out of the critical care area, and also to identify those at risk for deterioration beyond the capacity of a particular unit or hospital, and which may require transfer to a higher level of care unit or hospital. Some sites may be using early warning systems, such as the National Early Warning System 2 (NEWS2) to help provide early identification of a patient deterioration (Royal College of Physicians, 2017).

Orange Flag

Asking patients and families if the patient likes music and bringing in music players for those that would benefit from music therapy. Music can be used in critical care to help manage complications from delirium, as well as reducing anxiety and the stress response (Bamikole et al., 2018).

Focused assessments

The focused assessment is an assessment that is purposeful and is related to the patient's main area(s) of concern. It is a more concise evaluation and is intended to be completed regularly throughout the shift in order to re-evaluate the patient's status and response to treatments (Urden et al., 2018). An example of a focused assessment is performing only a neurological and respiratory assessment on a patient who is admitted with a traumatic brain injury and is mechanically ventilated, versus a comprehensive assessment that would see all systems evaluated.

6Cs: Competence

A competent critical care nurse has insight and knowledge of the key issues enabling them to conduct meaningful assessments and provide appropriate patient care.

Safety assessments

Other standards that are important to consider are safety assessments each shift and appropriate shift-to-shift handover. The safety assessment should include reviewing and ensuring all relevant safety equipment is present and functional at the beginning of each shift. Patient-specific safety equipment needs should also be reviewed; this may include tracheostomy supplies, wire cutters, traction weights, temporary pacing pads, restraints. All medication infusions should be rechecked for the correct dosage and concentration at the beginning of each shift as well.

Snapshot: Safety Check

A 54-year-old male admitted two days ago to CCU post overdose. The patient is intubated and on vasopressors for hemodynamic instability. During the nurse's initial safety check they discover the norepinephrine infusion dose written on the mediation bag is different to the dose programmed into the intravenous (IV) pump.

Other assessment findings are as follows:

Airway (A): airway is secured and patent, he has an oral endotracheal tube in place.

Breathing (B): Oxygen saturations are 98% on FiO_2 30% (NEWS2 score 0), respiratory rate 24/24 on a control mode of ventilation (NEWS2 score 2).
Cardiovascular (C): Blood pressure (BP) is 105/48 (NEWS2 score 1), heart rate 65 (NEWS2 score 0).
Disability (D): patient is a RASS of -4(NEWS2 score 3) and has a temperature of 38.3°C (NEWS2 score 1).
Exposure (E): no abnormal findings.

Nursing action
A new bag of norepinephrine is mixed including priming a new IV line to ensure the patient is getting the appropriate dose.

Other considerations
All infusions should be checked from the insertion site at the patient to the IV bag including the rate and dose programmed into the pump to ensure they are labelled, dated and timed correctly per hospital guidelines).

Handover

Shift-to-shift and inter-department handover is a key component of patient safety and ensuring a methodical standardised approach is key to ensuring continuity of care (Malekzadeh et al., 2013). Handover of patient care information promotes continuity and quality of care of the patient and helps to prevent errors (Leenstra et al., 2018). A standardised approach to information handover facilitates this process (Kowitlawakul et al., 2015). The gold standard for information handover is a person to person verbal handover, providing the receiving nurse with the opportunity to ask questions and seek clarification from the outgoing CCRN (Kowitlawakul et al., 2015). Standardised checklists or templates that help guide the information exchange to ensure all relevant and necessary information is shared can help mitigate and prevent communication errors (Kowitlawakul et al., 2015).

Alarm settings

Another standard of care that is important to consider is personalising the monitoring alarm settings. The monitoring parameters must be individualised to the patient's current status to allow for reasonable alarms to alert the CCRN of potential deterioration. For example if a normal heart rate is 60–100 beats per minute (BPM) and the patient has a heart rate of 45 BPM, the alarm limit should be lowered to 40 to 70 to alert the nurse when there is a big change in heart rate. Standardised alarm settings are not best practice as this will not adequately capture potential changes in a patient's condition and will create an abundance of potential nuisance alarms leading to alarm fatigue. There are simple practices that CCRNs can employ to prevent alarm fatigue. Proper skin cleansing and drying of the skin in preparation to securing electrocardiogram electrodes to the skin can ensure a better fixation (AACN, 2018). Daily routine changing of electrocardiogram electrodes can also ensure proper placement and fixation. Daily assessment of the patient's status and subsequent personalising the alarms based on their current status can help prevent excessive alarms as well (AACN, 2018).

Learning event

Reflect on what you know about alarm settings. How will you ensure your patient's alarms are customised and will still alert you to significant events?

Step 2 competencies: National Standards

2:10.3 Ensuring Patient Safety

- Understand your role in influencing the quality of safe and effective critical care services
- Identify actual or potential risks or incidents and take required actions
- Promote a safe culture that learns from and responds to risk
- Instigate immediate response to safe guard patients
- Report adverse or potential risks through internal clinical incident reporting system

---

Physical care

Providing physical care to the critically ill patient is an important part of the CCRN's role. Providing physical care offers an opportunity to assess the patient, provide physical comfort and prevent many complications that are associated with a critical care stay.

Patient hygiene

Patients admitted to critical care areas are often acutely ill and unable to perform self-care. The act of providing physical hygiene care to a critically ill patient is a very important and intimate act. Not only does providing personal hygiene promote comfort, but it also helps to reduce the risk of colonisation of bacteria and potentially prevent nosocomial infections, as well as promoting skin integrity.

Patients should be approached and encouraged to perform as much of their own care as possible, and when help is needed CCRNs should seek permission before proving care. Always take into consideration any personal preferences that the patient may have or that you may be aware of when providing care that is associated with hygiene needs. Many patients are often so acutely ill that they require assistance with all aspects of care, and care

should be planned and prioritised based on the patient's status. Communication of what is happening should be done throughout, even if the patient is sedated or appears to be unaware. During hygiene care the CCRN has the opportunity to assess the status of the patient's skin and tissues, and also other aspects of their status such as level of consciousness, pain, agitation, haemodynamic stability and oxygen stability.

6Cs: Communication

Effective communication is a key requisite when undertaking assessment of patient needs.

Providing the patient with a bed bath daily is considered the standard of care. This is usually coupled with regular intermittent care provided to the face and hands, mouth, eyes, and perineum as required. It is important to remember that some patient may require more or less care depending on their individual needs. The diaphoretic patient, for example, may require a complete bed bath and linen change several times a day in order to protect the skin from excessive moisture which could lead to skin breakdown. In other cases of extreme instability the patient may not tolerate a bed bath, but this should be reassessed frequently. Personal hygiene should be timed to protect the normal sleep – wake – cycle to prevent unnecessary disruptions which could lead to delirium (Morton and Fontaine, 2013). Consideration should also be given to patients who are febrile or hypothermic, as exposure of the skin surfaces with moisture can lead to shivering and further vasoconstriction and increased oxygen consumption (Morton and Fontaine, 2013).

There are a wide variety of cleansing solutions and soaps available for providing patient hygiene, and often different solutions for different aspects of care (e.g. general body versus face and perineum). Being aware of what is available in your unit and what is recommended by the Tissue Viability Nurse is important.

Skin care

The critically ill patient can be haemodynamically unstable with altered blood flow to their skin and extremities, and have altered nutritional intake placing them at a higher risk for skin breakdown (Kim et al., 2009). Critically ill patients are often at the greatest risk for skin breakdown caused by pressure injuries or shear injuries. Skin breakdown and injuries may occur from routine care such as prepositioning, transferring or from excessive moisture (including incontinence and diaphoresis). Specific patient populations may be at a greater risk if they are frail, on long-term steroids, or have excessive oedema. Use of adhesives, such as tape, can also promote skin injuries.

Skin injuries can be prevented or minimised by careful handling of patients to mitigate shear or friction through the use of lifting and/or turning devices, such as overhead lifts and slings. Careful positioning of sheets or slings to ensure no additional creases or foreign objects are caught in the bed can also promote healthy skin. Regular assessment of the patient's skin using a validated assessment tool is important. Examples of assessment tools include the Braden Scale, the Song and Choi Scale, the Cubbin and Jackson Scale and the International Skin Tear Advisory assessment pathway (Cox, 2012; LeBlanc et al., 2013). There are challenges with many of the pressure injury scales and often critical care patients are deemed high risk despite which scale is utilised reducing their use in critical care areas, however careful assessment, intervention and documentation to promote healthy skin is important regardless scale used.

Red Flag

Monitor the patient's skin regularly including bruised areas and areas under dressings for skin tears.

Eye care

Eye care is important part of care provided to critically ill patients. The fluid produced by the tear ducts to lubricate the eyes in combination with the eyelids and lashes provide an immune defence to the eye to protect it from injury and infection (Alansari et al., 2015). Unnecessary harm can occur when the eyes are not cared for properly, leading to potentially permanent injuries that can alter a patient's quality of life far beyond their critical care stay.

Critical care patients who are unable to fully close their eyes or who have an impaired blink response are at risk for corneal dryness or abrasions. Patients with neurological conditions (e.g. Guillain–Barré Syndrome, stroke) or those receiving large amounts of sedative or neuromuscular blocking agents may be at increased risk of eye injuries. Patients with a large amount of medical equipment near their head or face may also be at risk for an unintentional mechanical injury (e.g. intravenous lines inadvertently hitting the eyes). Assessment of the patient's eyes should be done routinely every shift. The eyelid position, inspection of the external eyelid, lashes and closure using a penlight is key, in addition to the routine checking of the pupillary responses. Specific at-risk patients may require more frequent assessment and eye care including those who cannot properly close their eyelids, and also those who are receiving positive pressure ventilation who are at risk for developing conjunctival oedema, also known as chemosis, and those receiving high flow oxygen (e.g. via continuous positive airway pressure (CPAP) masks) and may develop excessive dryness (Ajibawo et al., 2020). Regular eye lubrication should be applied throughout the shift, and consideration for taping the eyelid closed in those unable to fully close their eyelids should be considered. Simple eye care protocols guiding assessments, product application (e.g. every 2–4 hours), and cleansing can prevent permanent injury (Alansari et al., 2015).

Oral care

Oral hygiene serves both to promote patient comfort and to promote health and wellness. Providing a patient with oral hygiene can be challenging, especially if the patient is intubated, requiring continuous non-invasive ventilation or is delirious; but it is important for not only the patient's oral health, but also their overall health (Prendergast et al., 2012). Without adequate oral care the naturally occurring bacteria in the mouth can flourish, putting the patient at risk for infection (Prendergast et al., 2012). Patients with pre-existing poor oral hygiene are at an increased risk. In addition to being at risk for increased bio-burden related to flourishing bacteria, critical care patients are also at risk for excessive drying of their mouths due to all the equipment (e.g. endotracheal tube) in their mouths and inability to properly close their lips. This can lead to a breakdown of the mucosal lining, which increases the risk of infection. The added equipment in their mouths can also place them at risk for oral pressure injuries related to the equipment pressing on their tongues and lips.

Without adequate oral hygiene critical care patients are at risk for infection, and in particular ventilator-associated pneumonia related to the bacteria-laden oral secretions that have the potential to be aspirated (AACN, 2017a). Oral hygiene should include: regular oral assessments, brushing the teeth, gums and tongue a minimum of once a shift (or twice in 24 hours), application of oral moisturiser every two to four hours to oral mucosa and tongue, and use of an approved oral cleansing solution such as oral chlorhexidine gluconate (0.12%) rinse twice a day will help promote oral health and reduce the risk of ventilator-associated pneumonia (Munro et al., 2009). Oral assessment should include visualisation of the inside of the patient's mouth, examining the teeth, tongue, gums and inside cheeks for any dryness, plaque build-up, excoriation or breakdown, and examining for pressure injuries related to any equipment in the mouth. This can be done every two to four hours during application of oral moisturiser. Although cleaning the oral cavity can be challenging, there are a variety of products available to assist the CCRN, including oral cleansing sponges, toothbrushes with built-in suction and endotracheal tubes with subglottic suction to help prevent aspiration of any excessive oral secretions that accumulate between cleansing to reduce the risk of ventilator-associated pneumonia (Mahmoodpoor et al., 2017). In addition to regular cleansing, regular rotation of oral devices to change the position in the mouth should be done as well (e.g. moving the endotracheal tube from the left side of the mouth, centre, to the right side).

Medication management: chlorhexidine gluconate mouthwash

Chlorhexidine gluconate mouthwash is an antiseptic solution used to prevent accumulation and proliferation of oral bacteria in the intubated patient. Generally chlorhexidine gluconate is used twice in 24 hours, applied throughout the oral cavity (teeth, gums, tongue, cheek mucosa) with an oral sponge. In combination with mouth care every 2–4 hours, this practice has demonstrated a reduction in ventilator-acquired pneumonia (Synders et al., 2011). Common side effects include mucosa drying.

There are many different products available for cleansing a patient's mouth, including toothpaste, mouthwash, impregnated oral sponges. Determining the right product to use will depend on the patient's status (intubated, extubated, tracheostomy), and available supplies and policies. Patients that are awake and able to should be encouraged to participate in their care, even if it is a simple as controlling the oral suction catheter to help remove excessive secretions.

Perineum and elimination care

Many critically ill patients require assistance with body waste elimination (urinary and faecal), and care of their perineum areas. Critical care patients' skin is often exposed to excessive moisture, and stool and urine incontinence which can lead to perineal dermatitis (Pather and Hines, 2016). Patients at higher risk for perineal dermatitis include those with advanced age, diabetes, smokers, liquid stool, febrile and low oxygen saturation (Van Damme et al., 2018). Perineal dermatitis may be asymptomatic or can be quite distressing and involve pruritis and pain (Driver, 2007). Regular cleansing with a product created specifically for the perineum is preferred over regular soap and water to help prevent excessive drying often associated with soap which can lead to further breakdown (Driver, 2007). Use of barrier creams to protect the integrity of skin is valuable in minimising the impact of moisture on the skin. It is very important when providing perineum care to fully explain to the patient and ask permission to proceed prior to beginning. Cleaning a patient's perineum area is a very delicate and intimate act, and many patients may find it very invasive and distressing. Be aware of the patient's past histories and any trauma that may be present and proceed with kindness and caution.

6Cs: Compassion

Compassion is how care is given through relationships based on empathy, respect and dignity.

Urinary incontinence

Many patients in the critical care area will initially have a urinary catheter for urine measurement and collection as a part of the monitoring required for the renal system and response to therapies. It is important to provide regular care to the catheter and perineum, especially if the patient has faecal incontinence to prevent a catheter-associated urinary tract infection (CAUTI). Catheters interfere with the body's natural defence mechanism, the urethral length and micturition that normally prevent migration of pathogens into the bladder (Chenoweth and Saint, 2013). The presence of the catheter promotes bacterial growth and transfer to the bladder, leading to a CAUTI.

To prevent CAUTI, regular re-assessment of the need for a catheter should be undertaken, and the catheter should be removed as soon as possible (AACN, 2017b). Evidence-based sterile insertion technique, maintenance of a closed drainage system, and prohibition of flushing or bladder washouts can also help prevent infections (Rahimi et al., 2019). Flushing of catheters that do not appear to be draining well can actually introduce bacteria into the bladder and cause an infection (Rahimi et al., 2019). If catheter drainage is an issue, a bedside bladder scan can be conducted to determine if the patient is indeed retaining urine, and if so exchanging the catheter for a new one if still required is preferred over flushing. If catheter removal is possible, a plan for urination should be in place. This may include either toileting if possible, a bedpan, or, if needed, an absorbent pad or properly fitted incontinence product. If using an incontinence pad or brief, adherence to the manufacturers' recommendation and fit guidelines is important to prevent incontinence dermatitis. Once a catheter has been removed, if the patient is incontinent and urine output is still important to measure, patient daily weights or incontinence product weights can be used.

Bowel care

Regular bowel movements are an important part of health and wellbeing. In the critical care setting there are many different factors that interfere with regular bowel routines. Medications and treatments required in critical care can contribute to both constipation and diarrhoea (Hay et al., 2019). Constipation can be related to the use of opioids, vasoactive drugs, sepsis, bed rest or decreased mobility, inflammatory mediators, electrolyte disorders, dehydration and more (de Souza Guerra et al., 2013). Whereas diarrhoea in critical care is often related to changes in nutrition (e.g. tube feed formulas), antibiotics, infectious aetiologies, electrolyte imbalances, and other medications, including those used to treat constipation (Dionne et al., 2019).

Many bowel protocols use a stepwise approach, increasing in intensity each day the patient does not have a bowel movement. Unfortunately the use of bowel protocols is inconsistent, and can also lead to the new onset of diarrhoea (Knowles et al., 2015; Hay et al., 2019). Routine use of

65

laxatives such as senna, bisocodyl, polyethylene glycol, and lactulose are used in many critical care bowel protocols (Vazquez-Sandoval et al., 2017).

Medication management: bisacodyl

Bisacodyl is a laxative/stimulant that can be administered orally or rectally. Oral doses range from 5–15 mg once daily and rectally it can be administered as an enema or suppository as a 10 mg dose, once daily. Bicosadyl is typically used for temporary relief of constipation and irregularity. In the critical care setting there is a high frequency of constipation with opioid therapy being a significant risk factor Routine administration of laxatives/ stimulants can help to reduce the prevalence of constipation and irregularity (Patanwala et al., 2006).

Diarrhoea also plays a critical role in patient outcomes as it can cause hypovolaemia, electrolyte and acid-base imbalances, and skin breakdown of the perineum. Incontinence dermatitis from liquid stool can cause significant discomfort and harm to the patient. Faecal incontinence-associated dermatitis can occur rapidly, and is often associated with sensory impairment, friction/shear from movement and the use of vasoactive drugs (Ma et al., 2017). Removing the stool from skin and preventing contamination of any urinary catheters or wounds is important to prevent infection and further skin breakdown. Timely cleaning of stool with appropriate cleansers specific for the perineum is important. Application of a barrier cream after cleansing can help in prevent further skin breakdown.

Some critical care units utilise faecal collection systems. These systems can be external or internal, and are designed to collect faecal matter to aid in the protection of the perineal skin, aid in cleaning (in particular for patients who are haemodynamically unstable and do not tolerate frequent movement), and to help measure output.

Mobility

Many complications associated with critical care that contribute to post-ICU care syndrome are related to patient immobility (Crowe et al., 2019). Many critical care units have multidisciplinary teams to help provide holistic care, including physiotherapist, rehabilitation specialists/assistants and respiratory therapists; however, patient mobilisation should not be delayed due to lack of their availability. A team of CCRNs can safely and effectively mobilise critical care patients (Schallom et al., 2020). Critically ill patients who are mobilised earlier experience improved outcomes and have an increased chance of returning to their pre-hospital baseline (Hall and Clark, 2016; Vollman, 2010).

Early mobilisation can help promote retention of muscle strength, functional mobility, and prevent delirium; all leading to improve patient outcomes (Schallom et al., 2020). Early mobility can also help reduce haemodynamic instability. Bed rest promotes immobility of muscle fibres leading to shortening of the collagen which can produce contractures and reduced functioning of a limb in as little as two weeks (Truong et al., 2009; Vollman 2013). Immobility also has a significant impact on the cardiovascular system, including an 8–10% reduction in plasma volumes within the first three days leading to increased cardiac workload from elevated heart rate and decreased stroke volume (Truong et al., 2009). Immobility can also decrease the responsiveness of the carotid-cardiac baroreflex responsiveness which can lead to worsening postural hypotension and tachycardia (Vollman, 2013).

There are often many barriers to mobilising critically ill patients. Critical care patients are often haemodynamically unstable and may have a lot of equipment (intravenous lines, catheters, ventilators) attached (Jolley et al., 2014). The idea that the patient is too sick to mobilise, or is receiving a therapy such as continuous renal replacement therapy and is not able to be mobilised is a barrier (Crowe et al., 2019). Another barrier often encountered is the assumption that mobility means getting out of bed and either sitting in a chair or going for a walk; whereas in reality there are a number of different ways a patient can be mobilised (Crowe et al., 2019). In-bed mobility is a key first step to mobilising a patient. This involves turning the patient from side to side and elevating the head of the bed throughout the day. It is recommended to turn and reposition the patient every two hours (Vollman, 2013). It also includes passive and active range of motion exercises. Passive range of motion (PROM) is the act of moving and bending the patient's limbs and joints for them when there are unable to complete this on their own. Active range of motion (ROM) occurs when the patient is able to conduct the movements on their own. During this phase of mobility involvement of the family may be possible to assist with PROM exercises (Crowe et al., 2019). Assessing the patient for tolerance of these exercises is key prior to advancing the mobility plan. Once the patient has been assessed as ready to progress bedside sitting and dangling the legs at the edge of the bed can be done, then progressing to transferring to a chair and finally walking (Schallom et al., 2020).

Red Flag

Families can be encouraged to participate in PROM. This will not only promote PROM but also give families the opportunity to participate in patient care.

6Cs: Courage

Courage enables us to do the right thing for the patients we care for. It means having personal strength and vision to innovate and to embrace new ways of working.

Mobility should be considered on a continuum, and a stepwise approach to safe, slow mobility should be implemented (Dammeyer et al., 2013; Talley et al., 2013). A mobility pathway or protocol can help safely guide the process (Schallom et al., 2020). Frequent reassessment of a patient's status is important to ensure patient safety. Another key point to remember in mobility is if the patient is unable to mobilise or to progress to the next level of mobility they should still be reassessed for readiness frequently (Crowe et al., 2019).

Snapshot: early mobilisation in critical care

An 82-year-old female was admitted post-operatively from a laparotomy for a bowel obstruction. The patient is requiring ongoing ventilation and pain control following surgery. She is on post-operative day 8, and has a RASS of 0.

During the nurse's initial assessment the patient is awake, alert and orientated and is following commands. The patient has been able to complete ROM exercised while in bed and has been transferred to a chair daily for the last 3 days using a ceiling lift.

Other assessment findings are as follows:

Airway (A): airway is secured and patent, he has an oral endotracheal tube in place.
Breathing (B): Oxygen saturations are 95% on FiO_2 40% (NEWS2 score 1), respiratory rate 22 on pressure support ventilation (NEWS2 score 2).
Cardiovascular (C): Blood pressure (BP) is 115/78 (NEWS2 score 0), heart rate 70 (NEWS2 score 0).
Disability (D): patient is alert and orientated with a RASS score of 0 (NEWS2 score 0) and is normothermic (36.9°C) (NEWS2 score 0).
Exposure (E): no abnormal findings.

Nursing action
In collaboration with the physiotherapy team the patient will attempt to stand at the bedside prior to being transferred to the chair. The team ensures all safety measures are in place and there is clear communication prior to ambulation as well as during the process. The nurse ensures the patient's pain level has been assessed and that analgesia is given prior to ambulation if required.

Considerations for mobilisation in CCU
- Time requirements and adequate nursing
- Staff training
- Need for teamwork and coordination
- Sedation levels
- Devices that have the potential to become dislodged (central venous catheters, endotracheal tubes, feeding tubes, catheters)
- Haemodynamic stability
- Pain
- Patient cognition

Critical care bundles

Much of the physical care provided to critically ill patients is focused on preventing PICS, and some is delivered in an evidence-based bundle approach. Care bundles are a series of evidence-based practices grouped together in a single protocol used to enhance patient outcomes (Fulbrook and Mooney, 2003). Care bundles provide both a succinct approach to patient care, and also serve to increase quality across a system by standardising care delivery. The key bundles of care provided in critical care include:

- ventilator-associated pneumonia (VAP) bundle
- preventing venous thromboembolism (VTE) bundle
- central line-associated bloodstream infection (CLABSI) bundle.

Other important bundles are dedicated to delirium prevention and management. They include the pain, agitation, delirium, interrupted sleep (PADIS) bundle, and the delirium ABCDEF bundle; however, these will be discussed in a later chapter.

Conclusion

The care provided by CCRNs is extremely important for the wellbeing and recovery of the critically ill patient. Critically ill patients have many obstacles to overcome in their recovery to wellness, and preventing and minimising complications through excellent nursing care is important. Many of the complications commonly associated with PICS can be prevented through CCRN-instigated care.

Take home points
1. Nursing care is vital to critical care patient outcomes.
2. CCRNs have a direct role in preventing post-ICU care syndrome (PICS) and other complications of critical care.
3. A bundled approach to nursing care in critical care allows for evidence-based practices to be implemented and evaluated to prevent complications.

References

Abu-Ssaydeh, D.A., Rechnitzer, T.W., Knowles, B.P., and Richmond, T.S. (2018). Major haemorrhage associated with the Flexi-Seal (R) Fecal Management System. *Anaesth Intensive Care* 46(1): 140.

Ajibawo, T., Zahid, E., and Leykind, Y. (2020). An unusual case of bilateral hemorrhagic chemosis in the intensive care unit. *Cureus* 12(8). doi: 10.7759/cureus.9679.

Alansari, M.A., Hajazi, M.H., and Maghrabi, K.A. (2015). Making a difference in eye care of the critically ill patients. *Journal of Intensive Care Medicine* 30(6): 311–317. doi: 10.1177/0885066613510674.

American Association of Critical-Care Nurses (AACN). (2017a). Oral care for acutely and critically ill patients. *Critical Care Nurse* 37(3), e19–21. doi: 10.4037/ccn2017179.

American Association of Critical-Care Nurses (AACN). (2017b). Prevention of catheter-associated urinary tract infection in adults. *Critical Care Nurse* 1–3. https://www.aacn.org/~/media/aacn-website/clincial-resources/practice-alerts/adultcauti2017practicealert.pdf (accessed March 2022).

American Association of Critical-Care Nurses (AACN). (2018). Managing alarms in acute care across the lifespan: electrocardiography and pulse oximetry. *Critical Care Nurse* 38(2), e16–e20. doi: doi: 10.4037/ccn2018468

Bamikole, P.O., Theriault, B., Caldwell, S., and Schlesinger, J.J. (2018). Patient-directed music therapy in the ICU. *Critical Care Medicine* 46(11). doi: 10.1097/CCM.0000000000003365.

Canadian Association of Critical Care Nurses (CACCN). (2017). *Standards for Critical Care Nursing Practice*. London, Ontario. https://caccn.ca/wp-content/uploads/2019/05/STCACCN-2017-Standards-5th-Ed.pdf (accessed March 2022).

Chenoweth, C. and Saint, S. (2013). Preventing catheter-associated urinary tract infections in the intensive care unit. *Critical Care Clinics* 29(1): 19–32. doi: 10.1016/j.ccc.2012.10.005.

Cox, J. (2012). Predictive power of the Braden scale for pressure sore risk in adult critical care patients: a comprehensive review. *Journal of Wound, Ostomy and Continence Nursing* 39(6): 613–621. doi: 10.1097/WON.Ob013e31826a4d83.

Crowe, S., Brook, A., and Haljan, G. (2019). Continuous renal replacement therapy and mobilization: yes, it is possible. *Canadian Journal of Critical Care Nursing* 30(1): 12–16.

Dammeyer, J., Dickinson, S., Packard, D. et al. (2013). Building a protocol to guide mobility in the ICU. *Critical Care Nursing Quarterly*, 6: 37–49.

de Souza Guerra, T.L., Mendonca, S.S., and Marshall, N.G. (2013). Incidence of constipation in an intensive care unit. *Rev Bras Ter Intensiva* 25(2): 82–92. doi: 10.5935/0103-507X.20130018.

Dionne, J.C., Sullivan, K., Mbuagbaw, L. et al. (2019). Diarrhoea: interventions, consequences and epidemiology in the intensive care unit (DICE-ICU): a protocol for a prospective multicentre cohort study. *BMJ Open* 9(6). doi: 10.1136/bmjopen-2018-028237.

Driver, D.S. (2007). Perineal dermatitis in critical care patients. *Critical Care Nurse* 27(4): 42–46. doi: 10.4037/ccn2007.27.4.42.

Ely, E.W., Inouye, S.K., Bernard, G.R. et al. (2001). Delirium in mechanically ventilated patients: validity and reliability of the confusion assessment method for the intensive care unit (CAM – ICU). *JAMA* 286(21): 2703–2710. doi: 10.1001/jama.286.21.2703.

Ferguson, A., Uldall, K., Dunn, J. et al. (2018). Effectiveness of a multifaceted delirium screening, prevention, and treatment initiative on the rate of delirium falls in the acute care setting. *Journal of Nursing Care Quality* 33(3): 213–220.

Fulbrook, P. and Mooney, S. (2003). Care bundles in critical care: a practical approach to evidence-based practice. *Nursing in Critical Care* 8(6): 249–255.

Haenggi, M., Blum, S., Brechbuehl, R. et al. (2013). Effect of sedation level on the prevalence of delirium when assessed with CAM-ICU and ICDSC. *Intensive Care Medicine* 39: 2171–2179. doi: 10.1007/s00134-013-3034-5.

Harvey, M.A. and Davidson, J.E. (2016). Postintensive care syndrome: right care, right now . . . and later. *Critical Care Medicine* 44(2): 381–385. doi: 10.1097/CCM.0000000000001531.

Hall, K.D. and Clark, R.C. (2016). A prospective, descriptive, quality improvement study to investigate the impact of a turn and position device on the incidence of hospital acquired sacral pressure ulcers and nursing staff time needed to reposition patients. *Ostomy Wound Management* 62(11): 40–44.

Hay, T., Bellomo, R., Rechnitzer, T. et al. (2019). Constipation, diarrhea, and prophylactic laxative bowel regimens in the critically ill: a systematic review and meta-analysis. *Journal of Critical Care* 52: 242–250. doi: 10.1016/j.jcrc.2019.01.004.

Jolley, S.E., Regan-Baggs, J., Dickson, R.P., and Hough, C.L. (2014). Medical intensive care unit clinician attitudes and perceived barriers towards early mobilization of critically ill patients: a cross-sectional survey study. *BMC Anaesthesiology* 14(84): 1–9.

Kiernan, F. (2017). Care of ICU survivors in the community: A guide for GPs. *British Journal of General Practice* 67(663): 477–478.

Khan, B.A., Guzman, O., Campbell, N.L. et al. (2012). Comparison and agreement between the Richmond Agitation-Sedation Scale and the Riker Sedation-Agitation Scale in evaluating patients' eligibility for delirium assessment in the ICU. *Chest* 142(1): 48–54. doi: 10.1378/chest.11-2100.

Khan, B.A., Perkins, A.J., Gao, S. et al. (2017). The CAM-ICU-7 delirium severity scale: a novel delirium severity instrument for use in the intensive care unit. *Critical Care Medicine* 45(5): 851–857. doi: 10.1097/CCM.0000000000002368.

Kim, E., Lee, S., Lee, E., and Eom, M. (2009). Comparison of the predictive validity among pressure ulcer risk assessment scales for surgical ICU patients. *Australian Journal of Advanced Nursing* 28(4): 87–94.

Knowles, S., Lam, L.T., McInnes, E. et al. (2015). Knowledge, attitudes, beliefs and behaviour intentions for three bowel management practices in intensive care: effects of a targeted protocol implementation for nursing and medical staff. *BMC Nursing* 14(6). doi: 10.1186/s12912-015-0056-z.

Kowitlawakul, Y., Leong, B.S., Lua, A. et al. (2015). Observation of handover process in an intensive care unit (ICU): barriers and quality improvement strategy. *International Journal for Quality in Health Care* 27(2): 99–104. doi: 10.1093/intqhc/mzv002.

LeBlanc, K., Baranoski, S., Christensen, D. et al. (2013). International skin tear advisory panel: a tool kit to aid in the prevention, assessment, and treatment of skin tears using a simplified classification system. *Advances in Skin & Wound Care* 26(10): 459–476. doi: 10.1097/01.ASW.0000434056.04071.68.

Leenstra, N.F., Johnson, A., Jung, O.C. et al. (2018). Challenges for conducting and teaching handovers as collaborative conversations: an interview study at teaching ICUs. *Perspectives on Medical Education* 7: 302–310. doi: 10.1007/s40037-018-0448-3.

Ma, Z., Song, J., and Wang, M. (2017). Investigation and analysis on occurrence of incontinence-associated dermatitis of ICU patients with fecal incontinence. *Int J Clin Exp Med* 10(5): 7443–7449.

Mahmoodpoor, A., Hamishehkar, H., Hamidi, M. et al. (2017). A prospective randomized trial of tapered-cuff endotracheal tubes with intermittent subglottic suctioning in preventing ventilator-associated pneumonia in critically ill patients. *Journal of Critical Care* 38: 152–156. doi: 10.1016/j.jcrc.2016.11.007.

Malekzadeh, J., Mazluom, S.R., Etezadi, T., and Tasseri, A. (2013). A standardized shift handover protocol: improving nurses' safe practice in intensive care units. *Journal of Caring Science* 2(3): 177–185. doi: 10.5681/jcs.2013.022.

Morton, P.G. and Fontaine, D.K. (2013). *Critical Care Nursing: A Holistic Approach*, 10e. Philadelphia, PA: Lippincott Williams & Wilkins.

Munro, C.L., Grap, M.J., Jones, D.J. et al. (2009). Chlorhexidine, toothbrushing, and preventing ventilator-associated pneumonia in critically ill adults. *American Journal of Critical Care* 18(5): 428–437. doi: 10.437/ajcc2009792.

Nik, A., Andalibi, M.S.S., Ehsaei, M.R. et al. (2018). The efficacy of Glasgow Coma Scale (CGS) score and Acute and Chronic Health Evaluation (APACHE) II for predicting hospital mortality of ICU patients with acute traumatic brain injury. *Bull Emerg Trauma* 6(2): 141–145. doi: 10.29252/beat-060208.

Nursing and Midwifery Council (2018). *The Code: Professional Standards of Practice and Behaviour for Nurses, Midwives and Nursing Associates*. https://www.nmc.org.uk/standards/code/ (accessed November 2020).

Patanwala, A.E. Abarca, J., and Huckleberry, Y. (2006). Pharmacological management of constipation in the critically ill patient. *Pharmacotherapy* 26(7): 896–902. doi: 10.1592/phco.26.7.896.

Pather, P. and Hines, S. (2016). Best practice nursing care for ICU patients with incontinence-associated dermatitis and skin complications resulting from faecal incontinence and diarrhoea. *International Journal of Evidence-Based Healthcare* 14(1): 15–23. doi: 10.1097/XEB.000000000000067.

Prendergast, V., Jakobsson, U., Renvert, S., and Hallberg, I.R. (2012). Effects of a standard versus comprehensive oral care protocol among intubated neuroscience ICU patients: results of a randomized control trial. *Journal of Neuroscience Nursing* 44(3): 134–146. doi: 10.1097/JNN.Ob013e3182510688.

Rahimi, M., Farhadi, K., Babaei, H., and Soleymani, F. (2019). Prevention and management catheter-associated urinary tract infection in intensive care unit. *Journal of Nursing and Midwifery Sciences* 6(2): 98–103. doi: 10.4103/JNMS.JNMS_47_18.

Rawal, G., Yadav, S., and Kumar, R. (2017). Post-intensive care syndrome: an overview. *Journal of Translational Internal Medicine* 5(2). doi: 0.1515/jtim-2016-0016.

Royal College of Physicians. (2017). *National Early Warning Score (NEWS2) 2: Standardising the Assessment of Acute-Illness Severity in the NHS*. London: RCP. https://www.rcplondon.ac.uk/projects/outputs/national-early-warning-score-NEWS-2 (accessed March 2022).

Schallom, M., Tymkew, H., Vyers, K. et al. (2020). Implementation of an interdisciplinary AACN early mobility protocol. *Critical Care Nurse* 40(4), e7–e17. doi: 10.4037/ccn2020632.

Sessler, C.N., Gosnell, M.S., Grap, M.J. et al. (2002). The Richmond Agitation-Sedation Scale: validity and reliability in adult intensive care unit patients. *American Journal of Respiratory Critical Care Medicine* 166(10): 1338–1344. doi: 10.1164/rccm.2107138.

Synders, O., Khondowe, O., and Bell, J. (2011). Oral chlorhexidine in the prevention of ventilator-associated pneumonia in critically ill adults in the ICU: a systematic review. *SAJCC* 27(2): 48–55.

Talley, C.L., Wonnacott, R.O., Schuette, J.K. et al. (2013). Extending the benefits of early mobility to critically ill patients undergoing continuous renal replacement therapy: the Michigan experience. *Critical Care Nursing Quarterly* 36: 89–100.

Truong, A.D., Fan, E., Brower, R.G., and Needham, D.M. (2009). Bench-to-bench review: mobilizing patients in the intensive care unit – from pathophysiology toclinical trials. *Critical Care* 13(216). doi: 10.1186/cc7885.

Urden, L.D., Stacy, K.M., and Lough, M.E. (2018). *Critical Care Nursing: Diagnosis and Management*, 8e. St. Louis, Missouri: Mosby.

Van Damme, N., Clays, E., Verhaeghe, S. et al. (2018). Independent risk factors for the development of incontinence-associated dermatitis (category 2) in critically ill patients with fecal incontinence: a cross-sectional observation study in 48 ICU units. *International Journal of Nursing Studies* 81: 30–39. doi: 10.1016/j.ijnurstu.2018.01.014.

Vazquez-Sandoval, A., Ghamande, S., and Surani, S. (2017). Critically ill patients and gut motility: are we addressing it? *World Journal of Gastrointestinal Pharmacology and Therapeutics* 8(3): 174–179. doi: 10.4292/wjgpt.v8.i3.174.

Vollman, K.M. (2010). Progressive mobility in the critically ill: introduction to progressive mobility. *Critical Care Nurse* 30: S3–S6. doi: http://hx.doi.org/10.4037/ccn2010803.

Vollman, K.M. (2013). Understanding critically ill patients hemodynamic response to mobilization: using the evidence to make it safe and feasible. *Critical Care Nursing Quarterly* 36(1): 17–27.

Chapter 7

Skin integrity

Victoria Clemett

Aim

The aim of this chapter is to provide the reader with an evidence-based understanding of the appropriate assessment and management of skin integrity in the critical care environment.

Learning outcomes

After reading this chapter the reader will be able to:

- Understand the pathophysiology of the skin and its functions.
- Understand the factors that contribute to the development of pressure ulcers.
- Describe how to assess, prevent and manage pressure ulcers.
- Understand the principles of undertaking a holistic wound assessment and understand the factors that delay wound healing.
- Understand the principles of basic wound management and develop an appreciation on the reassessment of wounds that are harder to heal, including when to escalate care.

Test your prior knowledge

- What are the functions of the skin?
- What changes happen to the skin as people age?
- What are the two pathways that occur during pressure ulcer development?
- What are the four stages of wound healing?
- What signs indicate that a wound infection is spreading?

Fundamentals of Critical Care: A Textbook for Nursing and Healthcare Students, First Edition. Edited by Ian Peate and Barry Hill.
© 2023 John Wiley & Sons Ltd. Published 2023 by John Wiley & Sons Ltd.
Companion website: www.wiley.com/go/peate/criticalcare

Introduction

This chapter will examine skin integrity and some of the problems in skin integrity and wound healing that may be encountered in the critical care and acute nursing environment. This chapter will focus on requirements relevant to tissue integrity and wound care set out in the Critical Care National Network of Nurses (CC3N) competencies and the Nursing and Midwifery Council (NMC) standards of proficiency.

CC3N Competencies: Step 1

1:7.1 Anatomy and physiology of skin and its functions.

1:7.2 Aetiology of damage to skin integrity, including risk assessment and prevention of pressure ulcers.

NMC Standards of proficiency for registered nurses: Nursing procedures

3.3 Use appropriate positioning and pressure-relieving techniques.

4.1 Observe, assess and optimise skin and hygiene status and determine the need for support and intervention.

4.2 Use contemporary approaches to the assessment of skin integrity and use appropriate products to prevent or manage skin breakdown.

4.6 Use aseptic techniques when undertaking wound care.

4.7 Use aseptic techniques when managing wound and drainage processes.

9.1 Observe, assess and respond rapidly to potential infection risks using best practice guidelines.

Anatomy and physiology of the skin

The skin's main functions are: providing a barrier between the assaults of the external environment (such as protection from microbials, mechanical injury, UV radiation, irritants and allergens), protecting the internal environment (by acting as a barrier to water loss and maintaining body temperature), and as an interface between external influences and internal responses (such as pressure and temperature receptors, or the synthesis of vitamin D from sunlight).

Fundamentally the skin consists of the epidermis, dermis and a subcutaneous fat layer (sometimes called the hypodermis) (Figure 7.1), although the thickness of these layers and the distribution of their appendages (sweat glands, sebaceous glands, hair follicles and nails) differs throughout the body.

The epidermis consists of five layers with new skin cells (keratinocytes) forming in the basal layer (bottom layer, known as stratum germinativum). As new skin cells form, older cells are pushed upwards towards the skin surface and flattened to form dead cells on the skin surface to be removed. In adults it usually takes 3–4 weeks for the epidermis to replicate. The dermis has two layers, the papillary region and reticular region (Figure 7.1). The smaller papillary region is covered with conical projections known as dermal papillae, thought to maximise the adhesion of the dermis to the epidermis. The reticular layer is thicker characterised by dense collagen bundles and interconnecting elastic fibres. The skin also contains an number of specialised cells and appendages that assist the skin's functions (Table 7.1). The subcutaneous fat layer provides insulation and protects the body from injury.

Impact of ageing on skin and tissue integrity

When people age, there is a reduction of epidermal and dermal thickness, regression of sebaceous glands and fat loss (Figure 7.2). These age-related changes in strength and elasticity mean the skin becomes more vulnerable as people age and they become at increased risk of compromised skin integrity (Wounds UK, 2018). Epidermal turnover also decreases leading to a reduced ability to repair the epidermis, and there is a reduction in the number of melanocytes and Langerhans cells which has a negative effect on the skin's ability to protect itself from UV light and infections.

Pressure ulcers

Pressure ulcers (previously known as decubitus ulcers or pressure sores) occur because of pressure, or pressure in combination with shear – usually over a body prominence (National Pressure Ulcer Advisory Panel & European Pressure Ulcer Advisory Panel, 2014). There are two pathways to pressure ulcer development: pressure damage progressing from Grade 1 to Grade 4 pressure ulcers (Figure 7.3) where superficial damage becomes deeper. And pressure damage starting in the deeper tissues (deep tissue injury, Figure 7.3) before resulting in damage to the skin's surface (Kottner et al., 2020).

The sites susceptible to pressure damage are associated with patient positioning (Figure 7.4). However, certain positions are at higher risk of pressure ulcer occurrence such as lying in the prone position for extended periods (National Pressure Ulcer Advisory Panel, European Pressure Ulcer Advisory Panel, Pan-Pacific Pressure Injury

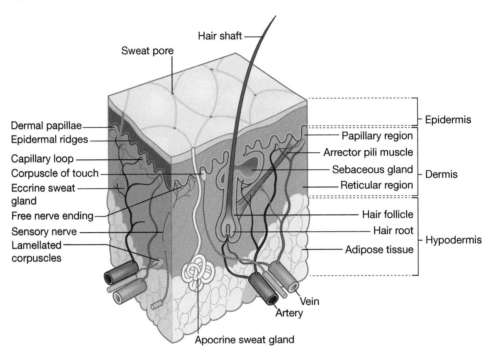

Sweat pore

Hair shaft

Dermal papillae
Epidermal ridges
Capillary loop
Corpuscle of touch
Eccrine sweat gland
Free nerve ending
Sensory nerve
Lamellated corpuscles

Epidermis
Papillary region
Arrector pili muscle
Sebaceous gland
Reticular region

Dermis

Hair follicle
Hair root
Adipose tissue

Hypodermis

Vein
Artery
Apocrine sweat gland

Figure 7.1   Anatomy of the skin. *Source:* Dutton & Finch (2018) with permission from John Wiley & Sons.

Table 7.1   Specialised cells and appendages involved in the skin's functions. *Source:* Peate and Stephens, 2020; Stephens, 2018.

Name	Location	Role
Melanocytes	Basal layer of the epidermis (stratum germinativum)	Produces the pigment (melanin) which is responsible for people's skin colour and protection from UV light
Langerhans cells	A middle layer of the epidermis (stratum spinosum)	Involved in immunity by phagocytosis and by presenting foreign antigens to the T-lymphocytes, as well as being involved in hypersensitivity reactions such as contact dermatitis
Merkel cells	A middle layer of the epidermis (stratum germinativum).	Involved in the detection of sensation
Sebaceous glands	Originate in the dermis and open on the skin surface through a hair follicle.	Secretion of sebum (a waxy/oily substance) which provides lubrication preventing moisture evaporation and conserving body heat.
Sweat glands	Originate in the dermis and open directly to the skin surface	Transport sweat to the skin surface to help regulate body temperature.
Hair follicle and hair muscle (arrector pili)	Originate in the dermis and open directly to the skin surface	Assist with thermoregulation through the formation of goose pimples and hair movement.
Free nerve endings	Detectors stimuli towards the top of the dermis	Detect pressure (nociceptors) and temperature (thermoreceptors)

Alliance, 2019). Individuals who are unable to detect the need to reposition themselves due to sensory impairment are also at more risk (National Pressure Ulcer Advisory Panel, European Pressure Ulcer Advisory Panel, Pan-Pacific Pressure Injury Alliance, 2019). Patients in the critical care environment are at added risk of pressure ulcer development due to factors such as the use of vasopressors and mechanical ventilation (National Pressure Ulcer Advisory Panel, European Pressure Ulcer Advisory Panel, Pan-Pacific Pressure Injury Alliance, 2019). Vasopressors cause peripheral vasoconstriction to increase mean arterial pressure (MAP) thus reducing blood flow to the tissues. This results in

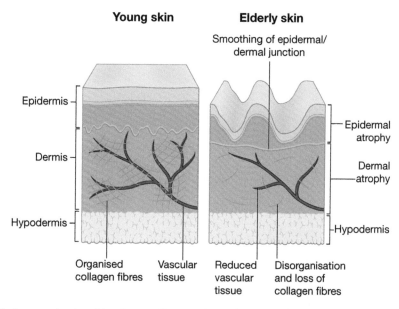

Figure 7.2 Age-related changes in the skin. *Source:* Dutton & Finch (2018) with permission from John Wiley & Son.

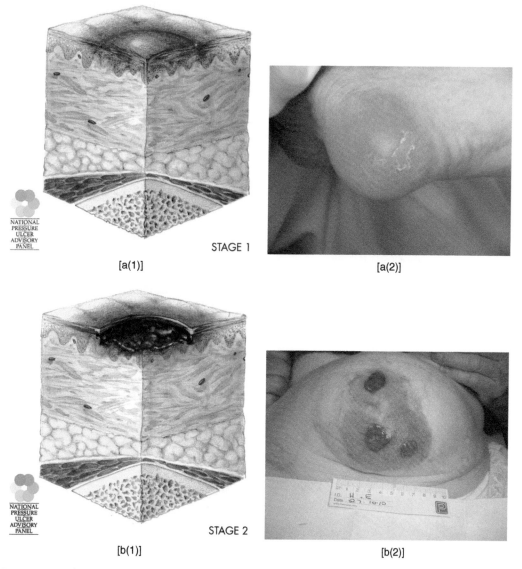

Figure 7.3 Categorises of pressure ulcers. *Source:* Flanagan et al. (2013) with permission from John Wiley & Sons.

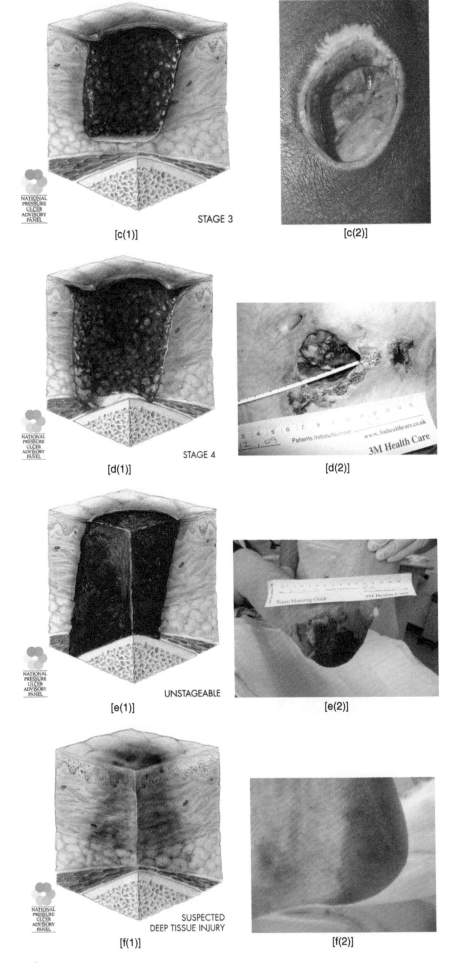

[c(1)]   STAGE 3   [c(2)]

[d(1)]   STAGE 4   [d(2)]

[e(1)]   UNSTAGEABLE   [e(2)]

[f(1)]   SUSPECTED DEEP TISSUE INJURY   [f(2)]

Figure 7.3   (Continued)

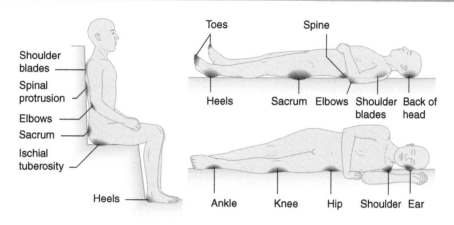

Figure 7.4 Common sites for pressure ulcers. *Source:* Peate and Stephens (2019) with permission from John Wiley & Sons.

vasopressors being an independent risk factor of pressure ulcer development (Alderden et al., 2017). Whereas the use of mechanical ventilation may indicate the severity of the illness meaning these individuals are more at risk of pressure ulcers (Alderden et al., 2017) or the use of oxygen delivery devices may lead to device related pressure ulcers (Gefen et al., 2020).

The use of medical devices is also an additional concern within the critical care environment where incidence of device-related pressure ulcers ranges from 0.9–41.2% (Baraket-Johnson et al., 2019). These occur at the interface between a device or object and the skin, resulting in a pressure ulcer conforming to the shape of the device (Gefen et al., 2020). Device-related pressure ulcers are often associated with respiratory devices including masks, endotracheal tubes, and oxygen tubing (Barakat-Johnson et al., 2017). However, they may result from any device with a medical purpose such as immobilisation devices or prosthetics, urinary catheters, feeding tubes, access devices or patient monitoring equipment, and objects without a medical purpose that may be left or dropped in the patient's bedspace such as mobile phones, hearing aids or pens (Gefen et al., 2020).

> # Learning event: reflection
> When undertaking personal care on a patient attached to numerous medical devices, consider what devices or objects may cause device-related pressures ulcers and reflect on how the patient and these devices are positioned to prevent pressure damage.

Where pressure damage has occurred it is important to be open with the patient and, where appropriate, their family to fully explain what has happened (NMC, 2018). Where this has occurred as a result of human factors such as environmental and organisational factors, work with colleagues to minimise the risk of this occurring in the future (NMC, 2018)

Nursing assessment

All patients must have a documented risk assessment on admission to hospital carried out using a validating tool (such as the Waterlow Score, PURPOSE-T or Braden Scale), which needs to be reassessed if there is a change in clinical condition (NICE, 2014) (see also Chapter 6). Pressure ulcer risk assessments consider several factors relating to the patient's underlying characteristics and comorbidities such as perfusion and circulation deficits, age or diabetes mellitus. Factors that may be related to their current condition such as impaired oxygen levels, and increased body temperature are also important (National Pressure Ulcer Advisory Panel, European Pressure Ulcer Advisory Panel, Pan-Pacific Pressure Injury Alliance, 2019). It is also important consider that all patients who have a medical device in situ are at risk of device-related pressure ulcers regardless of the outcomes of the rest of the risk assessment (Gefen et al., 2020).

All patients at risk of developing pressure ulcers should have their skin integrity assessed by visual inspection and, palpation by a trained and competent healthcare professional (National Institute for health and Care Excellence, 2014). To provide a structured approach to the exposure (E) component of assessment, begin at the patient's head and progress to the toes. Challenges may occur when inspecting and palpating the skin underneath medical devices where it is not possible to move the medical device due to clinical need. In such cases the healthcare professional may consider unusual sensation or discomfort beneath the device (Gefen et al., 2020). In all patients where it is possible, the skin underneath the medical device should be inspected at least twice a day to monitor for pressure damage (Gefen et al., 2020).

Scenario: assessing pressure damage in people with dark skin tones

Assessing pressure damage requires the nurse to inspect the skin and document findings reporting the surface area of pressure damage and record its depth using a validated tool, such as the NPUAP, EPUAP, PPPIA Classification shown in figure 7.3 (NICE, 2014). However, the recognition of category 1 pressure ulcers and deep tissue injury may be more challenging in people with darker skin tones.

Recognition of category 1 pressure ulcers: Darkly pigmented skin may not have visible blanching; its colour may differ from the surrounding area. But also assess for pain, and whether the area is firm, soft, warmer or cooler as compared to adjacent tissue (Figure 7.5a).

Recognition on deep tissue injury: Darkly pigmented skin tones may not have signs of discolouration, area may be painful, firm, mushy, boggy, warmer or cooler than adjacent tissues (Figure 7.5b).

Dark-coloured, thick, braided or beaded hair may also cause an additional challenge in assessment of pressure damage on the occiput region or under medical devices around the head. Therefore, additional care may be required to assess this area.

(a)

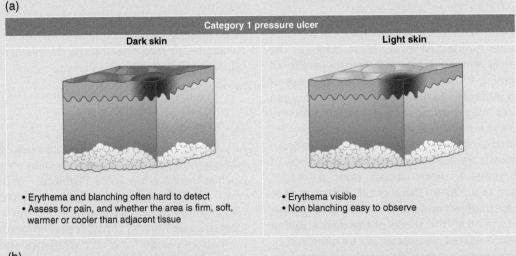

(b)

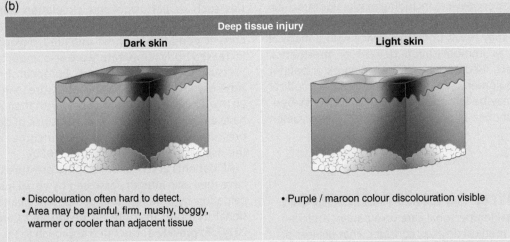

Figure 7.5 Presentation of pressure ulcers in different skin tones. *Source:* Modified from NPUAP, EPUAP, PPPIA 2009.

6Cs: Competence

Having the expertise to assess a patient is essential to deliver effective care. This competence is required when caring for patients who may have atypical presentation

Prevention of pressure ulcers

Encourage people (if able) who are at risk of pressure damage to change their position frequently, at least every four to six hours (NICE, 2014), with the frequency based on their individual risk, medical condition, treatment objectives and current levels of comfort and pain (NPAUP, EPAUP, PPPIA,

76

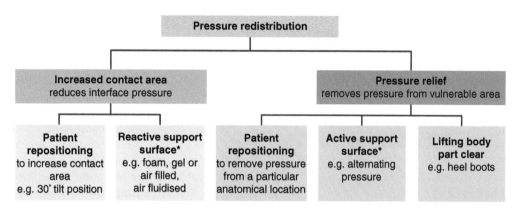

*A **reactive** support surface has the capability to change its load distribution properties only in response to applied load; an **active** support surface is able to change its load distribution properties with or without applied load.

Figure 7.6   Pressure redistribution. *Source:* Madeleine Flanagan (2013) with permission from John Wiley & Sons.

2019). This should be undertaken to relieve pressure from specific region and also increase contact area with the support surface where possible (Figure 7.6, Wounds International, 2010). However, within the critical care environment, it may not be possible to have regular repositioning between Left/Supine/Right lying, therefore in these cases it is considered best practice to frequently undertake small shifts in body positions using slow gradual turns to relieve pressure and also enable stabilisation of the patient's oxygenation and haemodynamic status (NPAUP, EPAUP, PPPIA, 2019).

Consider pressure redistribution surfaces to reduce pressure and friction (Figure 7.6). This may include choosing a support surface that enables the patient to sink into it or moulds itself to the patient, resulting in the patient's weight being spread over a larger area, thus reducing the pressure, or providing pressure relief by providing an alternating support surface or lifting the body part to relieve pressure on an affected area (Wounds International, 2010).

Snapshot: Liu

Presenting complaint: Liu is a 20-year-old female of mixed Chinese/White British heritage who was discharged from critical care 10 days ago and is being cared for on the high dependency unit for further rehabilitation and medical input.

History of presenting complaint: Liu was a passenger in a car that was involved in a road traffic collision. She sustained a traumatic brain injury as a result of contusion with associated cerebral oedema, rib fractures and haemothorax. All injuries were managed in the critical care unit with no complications. All drains were removed.

Past medical history: Known asthmatic. Underweight (BMI=18 kg/m²)

Social history: Lives in a shared house.

Drug history/drug allergies: No known drug allergies. Drinks 'moderate' amounts of alcohol (10 units/week).

Smoker (8–10 cigarettes/day). No known recreational drug use or over the counter medications.

Airway (A): Airway is patent, patient is speaking

Breathing (B): Respiratory rate:16 breaths per minute, chest movement: equal and bilateral, (Chest drain no longer in situ), Maintaining target saturations on room air (SpO$_2$ = 98%)

Circulation (C): Urine output within target 32–64 mL/hr, Blood pressure (BP): 109/68 mm/Hg, Heart rate (HR): 52 beats per minute. Capillary refill (CRT): 1.5 seconds, Temperature (T): 37.1°C

Disability (D): She is alert with some mild confusion and forgetfulness is noted. She is disoriented to time. Her Glasgow Coma Scale (GCS) has improved since admission and is currently 14/15.

Exposure (E): Anti-embolic stockings removed today and it is noted Liu has purple discolouration on both heels which is boggy to touch. No further pressure damage noted.

Total NEW2 Score: 4

Nursing actions:
- Confusion onset is not new and known to the team therefore, continue on observations as directed and inform medical team if GCS decreases.
- New observation relates to pressure damage on heels. Obtain heel offloading device to suspend heels off the bed.
- Ensure Liu is nursed on appropriate pressure-relieving equipment.
- Follow trust policy and complete Datex/incident report of pressure damage (it is suspected that a deep tissue injury has occurred on the posterior surface of the heel, where no muscle provides cushioning over the bone when in a supine position for a long period of time, and this has been unnoticed under anti-embolic stockings).

- Inform patient of the development of the pressure ulcer and discuss with her plan of care. Gain consent to discuss the development of this pressure ulcer with her family and involve both the patient and next of kin with the progress and plan of care as appropriate.
- Document care clearly and accurately in secure patient records

6Cs: Courage

Speak up when you have concerns about care or the care a patient has received. The development of this deep tissue injury may have been avoided and learning can take place as result of this mistake.

Red Flag: cautions when using heel offloading devices

The posterior heel contains no muscle and minimal subcutaneous fat, therefore cushioning over the bone is limited. When patients spend prolonged periods in the supine or semi-recumbent positions the heels are at risk of pressure damage. Therefore, heel off-loading devices can be used to elevate heels using a specific heel suspension device or a foam cushion.

The device should be placed to distribute the weight along the calf, avoiding pressure on the Achilles tendon or popliteal vein.

The heel offloading device changes where the contact between the support surface and patients' underlying tissue are, therefore may pose a risk of pressure damage in other areas.

A heel offloading device should be considered as a medical device and therefore the skin surface underneath the off-loading device needs to be inspected at least twice a day to ensure pressure ulcers are not developing under the device.

When medical devices are in use healthcare professionals can reduce the risk of skin breakdown by ensuring that the patient is not placed on the medical device and, where the medical condition allows, making effort to reposition the patient or device to redistribute the pressure (Gefen et al., 2020). The device chosen should also be sized and fit appropriately, secured without causing additional pressure and removed as soon as it is medically feasible (Gefen et al., 2020). Changes in the microclimate beneath the device, such as increases in humidity and temperature, also have a negative impact on pressure ulcer development therefore the area beneath the device should be clean and dry (Gefen et al., 2020).

Snapshot: Wilson

Presenting complaint: Wilson is a 72-year-old male of British Nigerian heritage currently in hospital receiving oxygen therapy via noninvasive ventilation (NIV) using CPAP (continuous positive airway pressure) device and corticosteroid as part of his treatment of COVID-19.

History of presenting compliant: Wilson developed a cough and loss of taste and smell four weeks ago. He received a positive COVID-19 test so was isolating at home, but his condition declined, and he was admitted to hospital with hypoxaemia.

Past medical history: Wilson is overweight (Weight = 101Kg, BMI 26 kg/m^2) and has diabetes (type 2 diabetes).

Social history: Widow. Wilson lives with his partner. He has 2 children and 1 grandchild.

Drug history/drug allergies: Metformin. No known allergies. Moderate drinker (18 units/week). Does not take illegal or over the counter drugs.

Airway (A): Patent

Breathing (B): Respiratory rate (RR): 18 breaths per minute, chest movement: equal and bilateral, Requiring CPAP (NIV), Maintaining target saturations with oxygen (SpO2 = 95%)

Circulation (C): Urine output within target 50.5–101 mL/hr, Blood pressure (BP): 130/78 mmHg, Heart rate (HR): 75. Capillary refill (CRT): 1.5 seconds, Temperature (T): 38.1°C

Disability (D): Alert, capillary blood glucose = 7.4 mmol/L, tenderness around face and discomfort from NIV mask

Exposure (E): No visible pressure ulcers but tissue appears firmer underneath where mask has been positioned.

Total NEW2 Score: 4

Nursing actions:
- Ensure the CPAP (NIV) device has been sized properly and secured properly without creating additional pressure using local policy and procedure.
- Maintain clean and dry surface under the device.
- Consider use of prophylactic dressing, following manufacturer's instructions.
- Plan to remove the device when medically feasible.
- Continue to inspect under the device at least twice a day.
- Follow trust policy and complete Datex/incident report of pressure damage (it is suspected that pressure damage has occurred undermark due to tenderness, discomfort and tissue firmness under NIV mask).
- Inform patient of the development of the suspected pressure ulcer and discuss with him plan of care. Gain consent to discuss the development of this suspected pressure ulcer with his family.
- Document care clearly and accurately in secure patient records.

6Cs: Commitment

The nurses' commitment to patients is essential when multiple reassessments are required of the same patient per shift.

Management of pressure ulcers

Ensure pressure redistribution and friction reduction continue alongside usual wound management practices (NICE, 2014).

Wound healing

Haemostasis occurs at the start of wound healing. This is initial vasoconstriction to prevent excessive blood loss but results in a coagulation cascade that results in the formation of a blood clot and also results in triggering the inflammation phase.

Inflammation phase

All wounds undergo a short period of inflammation (usually lasting less than 6 days), during this time chemical mediators cause capillary vasodilation, capillary permeability and attract leukocytes (white blood cells) to the site of injury. These changes cause localised swelling, heat, redness and minimal pain. During the inflammation phase phagocytosis commences removing debris.

Proliferation phase

The next phase is the proliferation phase, this includes the processes of granulation and epithelisation, this usually begins within 2–3 days of injury. During the granulation phase, macrophages release epidermal growth factor (EGF) which stimulates proliferation and migration of cells. The mix of budding blood vessels and collagen form granulation tissue. During epithelialisation keratinocytes (skin cells) at the wound margins and around hair follicles synthesise a temporary fibronectin matrix. Epidermal cells migrate over the surface of the wound using this temporary matrix to move over the wound surface under the influence of a range of growth factors.

The maturation, (also known as the remodelling or scarring phase) is where collagen bundles thicken, and scar tissue is formed. It is important to remember that this scar tissue does not retain the strength of skin that has not been wounded even after healing is completed.

Orange Flag: Body image and psychological wellbeing

Scars form when wounds heal during the maturation phase. However, different scarring may be more noticeable for some individuals.

Hypertrophic scarring is a raised scar along that is the same size as the original injury.

Keloid scarring is raised and larger than the original injury. It spreads beyond the original damaged area.

People with darker skin tones may also take some time for their original skin pigmentation to return so their scar is more noticeable.

These can have a negative impact on a patient's body image and therefore the impact of the wound on their quality of life should be assessed.

6Cs: Communication

Listening to patients' concerns is essential to determine the impact a wound is having on their quality of life and psychosocial wellbeing.

Learning event: reflection

Reflect on how and when psychological wellbeing and the impact of the wound on quality of life is assessed in the critical care setting. Does this capture the patient's concerns? What tools are available to assist in your assessment?

Patient factors that affect wound healing

A patient wound assessment includes the patient's general health information, wound baseline information and assessment parameters, wound symptoms and any specialist wound assessments (Coleman et al., 2017). This holistic assessment enables the nurse to determine how best to manage the patient's wound by considering the underlying patient factors, current wound factors and underlying patient and social variables (Atkin et al., 2019; Coleman et al., 2017). Several inpatient factors relate to poor healing and are associated with wounds becoming hard to heal (Atkin et al., 2019, Table 7.2). Some of these may be modifiable, but many of them are related to the patient's underlying health history and personal attributes.

Nursing assessment

Appropriate analgesia is likely to be required before undertaking a wound assessment or change of dressing. This is related to several wound-related factors such as nociceptors being excited during the haemostasis and inflammation phase, the presents of wound infection or bioburden causing further inflammation and pain by exciting nociceptors,

Table 7.2 Patient factors associated with hard-to-heal and non-healing wounds. *Source:* Atkin et al., 2019.

In-patient factors	Comorbidities	Psychosocial factors
Obesity Older age Poor nutrition Genetics Smoking Anaemia Hypoxia	Arterial disease Cancer Chronic inflammation Diabetes mellitus Immune suppression Lymphatic insufficiency Neuropathy Oedema Radiation Systemic medications Venous disease	Behavioural factors Demographic factors Economic status Patient adherence Patient choice Patient education

Table 7.3 Wound assessment should include this information. *Source:* Coleman et al., 2017.

Patient's general health information:	Risk factors that delay healing, skin sensitivities and allergies, impact of wound on quality of life.
Baseline wound information:	Number of wounds, location, type, duration, treatment aim, planned reassessment date.
Wound assessment parameters:	Wound size, undermining/tunnelling, category (for pressure ulcers only), wound bed type, wound bed amount, description of wound edges, colour/condition of peri-wound skin, has wound healed?
Wound symptoms:	Pain (frequency/severity), exudate (amount, consistency, type, colour), odour, systemic and local signs of infections, if wound swab taken
Specialists:	Investigations of the lower limb (i.e. ankle brachial pressure index), referrals (tissue viability nurse, vascular consultant, plastics consultant etc.).

and partial thickness wounds being more painful due to more nociceptors being exposed (Gardner et al., 2017). Although the perception of pain is also exacerbated by a patient's anxiety and anticipation of pain (Gardner et al., 2017) and therefore other techniques to manage pain at dressing changes should also be used.

Medication management: morphine for acute pain

Dose: 10 mg (5 mg in elderly), adjusting dose according to response.

Contraindications: Acute respiratory depression, head injuries (as effects reliability of neurological assessments), risk of paralytic ileus.

Route of administration: Oral solution, injections (intramuscular or intravenous),

Side effects: Respiratory depression, constipation, confusion, nausea, palpitations, may make the person sleepy/drowsy

Additional considerations: Use the STOPP/START criteria to review the use of this medication in elderly patients (patients over 65 years).

To provide a structured approach to the exposure (E) aspect of assessment, begin at the patient's head and progress to the toes. When undertaking a wound assessment, there is an agreed minimum data set for the information that should be documented (Coleman et al., 2017), detailed in Table 7.3. The general health information and wound baseline information is recorded when the patient develops a wound but the other parameters are recorded

when the wound is reassessed. This should occur at each dressing change but where trained auxiliary nursing staff (i.e.: a health care assistant) or nurses inexperienced in wound care undertake the dressing, there should be a formalised date when reassessment is undertaken by an appropriately trained and competent registered nurse (Coleman et al., 2017).

Wound photography is also considered good practice and may assist in the documentation of the patient's wound assessment (Coleman et al., 2017). When wound photography is taken from a consistent position and with a width and length measurement device shown in the photograph, it can quickly and easily show the progression or regression of the wound (Estocado and Black, 2019). However, wound photography was not included in the criteria of what must be included in a wound assessment due to current variations in access to high-quality and secure, digital cameras (Coleman et al., 2017).

Orange Flag: wound photography

Wound photography needs to comply with local policy and guidelines on consent and confidentiality, and be taken on appropriate devices and stored appropriately.

You must not take wound photographs on a personal phone.

Examination scenario: description of the wound bed

The base of the wound (known as the wound bed) needs to be inspected to determine how the wound is healing.

If the normal process of healing is occurring the wound bed will consist of granulation tissue (red, bumpy tissue) and/or epithelisation tissue (pale or pink in colour and may appear delicate).

However, other types of tissue may also exist on the wound bed and require removing so the wound can follow the normal process of healing.

Sloughy tissue: Devitalised tissue that is adherent, viscous and may be slimy or stringy. Often seen as yellow tough tissue that is usually wet but may look grey/dark if anaerobic bacteria is present or brown if it contains high levels of haemoglobin. May be thick, obscuring the wound bed, but may be patchy or present with some buds of granulation tissue showing through. Care should be taken that sloughy tissue is not confused with tendons or ligaments.

Necrotic tissue: Devitalised tissue that is usually black and hard with a leathery texture but necrosis that is starting to liquefy (by autolytic debridement) may appear yellow.

Assessment of the wound bed requires the nurse to decide the nature of the wound bed and what proportion of the wound bed is made up of each component. The nurse should also note any area that has tunnelling or undermining and where these are located.

6Cs: Compassion

Delivering care that respects the dignity of the patient demonstrates how compassionate care is given. Being aware of issues of consent and confidentiality enables the nurse to deliver dignified care.

Recognising wound infection

All wounds have some degree of inflammation; however, this generally resolves within 6 days. If signs of inflammation continue for longer and/or are accompanied by other signs of local or spreading infection (Figure 7.7) then this needs to be managed. Subtle signs of local wound infection, such as increasing exudate, may be present prior to the onset of the classic signs of local wound infection (International Wound Infection Institute, 2022), However, are often masked in those who are immunocompromised or have poor vascular perfusion (International Wound Infection Institute, 2022).

A patient's vital signs should also be assessed and considered alongside the local wound assessment to determine whether the infection has become systemic (Figure 7.7). Within the critical care environment c-reactive protein (CRP) and white blood cell counts (WBC) may be taken regularly and can also be reviewed alongside other assessments to determine whether the infection is systemic.

Red Flag: sepsis

Sepsis can occur as part of a systemic response to infection and may result in organ failure or death.

After an infection has been recognised there may be a clinical decision to commence a patient on antibiotics if this infection is spreading. It is best practice to take microbial samples before prescribing antibiotics and review the prescription when the results are available to ensure the antibiotic that has been prescribed is appropriate (NICE, 2015).

Clinical investigations: taking a wound swab

When undertaking a wound swab, local policy and procedure must be adhered to in relation to infection control, patient identification and consent. Once the dressing has been removed and there is a requirement to undertake a wound swab the following procedure should be followed.

Irrigate the wound with water or normal saline. This is to remove any transient bacteria as it is the microbials that have colonised the wound, formed a biofilm or causing a wound infection that are of interest.

Then undertake a wound swab using the Levine technique (Figure 7.8).

This involves rotating the wound swab over the area of greatest concern (including, if present, taking the sample from where any pus is present) covering at least a 1 cm² area.

The Levine technique is considered the most accurate way of taking a wound swab. Assessment of bacterial number and diversity, using this method is considered accurate compared to sampling using more invasive tissue culture punch biopsy.

Acute Wounds
e.g. surgical or traumatic wounds or burns

Localised infection	Spreading infection

• Classical signs and symptoms
    – New or increasing pain
    – Erythema
    – Local warmth
    – Swelling
    – Purulent discharge
• Pyrexia – in surgical wounds, typically five to seven days post-surgery
• Delayed (or stalled) healing
• Abscess
• Malodour
	As for localised infection PLUS:
	• Further extension or erythema
	• Lymphangitis
	• Crepitus in soft tissues
	• Wound breakdown/dehiscence

Notes
- Burns – also skin graft rejection; pain is not always a feature of infection in full thickness burns
- Deep wounds – induration, extension of the wound unexplained increased white cell count or signs of sepsis may be signs of deep wound infection
- Immunocompromised patients – signs and symptoms may be modified and less obvious

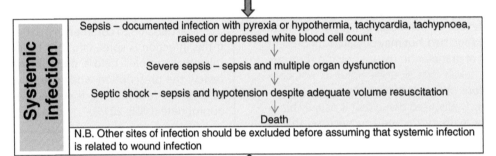

Systemic infection

Sepsis – documented infection with pyrexia or hypothermia, tachycardia, tachypnoea, raised or depressed white blood cell count
↓
Severe sepsis – sepsis and multiple organ dysfunction
↓
Septic shock – sepsis and hypotension despite adequate volume resuscitation
↓
Death

N.B. Other sites of infection should be excluded before assuming that systemic infection is related to wound infection

Chronic Wounds
e.g. diabetic foot ulcers, venous leg ulcers, arterial leg/foot ulcers or pressure ulcers

Localised infection	Spreading infection
• New increased or altered pain* • Delayed (or stalled) healing • Peri wound oedema • Bleeding or friable (easily damaged) granulation tissue • Distinctive malodour or change in odour • Wound bed discolouration • Increase or altered/purulent exudate • Induration • Pocketing • Bridging	As for localised infection PLUS: • Wound breakdown • Erythema extending from wound edge • Crepitus, warmth, induration or discolouration spreading into peri wound area • Lymphangitis • Malaise or other non-specific deterioration in patient's general condition

Notes
- In patients who are immunocompromised and/or who have motor or sensory neuropathies, symptoms may be modified and less obvious. For example, in a diabetic patient with an infected foot ulcer and peripheral neuropathy, pain may not be a prominent feature
- Arterial ulcers – previously dry ulcers may become wet when infected
- Clinicians should also be aware that in the diabetic foot, inflammation is not necessarily indicative of infection. For example inflammation may be associated with Charcot's arthropathy

*Individually highly indicative of infection. Infection is also highly likely in the presence of two or more of the other signs listed

Figure 7.7   Recognising infection. *Source:* Flanagan et al. (2013) with permission from John Wiley & Sons.

Clinical investigations: blood test for inflammatory markers

Blood tests are taken for tracking changes in inflammation makers (c-reactive protein, white blood cell count). These are usually taken alongside urea and electrolytes and full blood counts as they use the same collection bottles.

Snapshot: Arthur

Presenting complaint: Arthur has been readmitted to hospital via his GP due to dehisced and infected surgical wound.

History of presenting complaint: Arthur is a 68-year-old post-operative male patient who underwent total hip replacement for a hip fracture 4 weeks ago.

Past medical history: Has type 2 diabetes with uncontrolled blood glucose. Long-term tracheostomy following laryngectomy due to tumour in the larynx.

Social history: Arthur lives with his wife. He has 3 grown-up children.

Drug history/drug allergies: Metformin 500 mg three times daily. Was taking paracetamol to manage wound pain prior to admission.

Airway (A): Patient, talking in sentences.

Breathing (B): Respiratory rate (RR) 22 breaths per minute, chest moving equally and bilaterally, Long-term tracheostomy insitu (wearing Buchannan bib for humidification), oxygen saturations (SpO$_2$) 97%.

Circulation (C): Blood pressure (BP) 125/75 mm/Hg, heart rate (HR) 98 per minute, capillary refill (CRT) 1.5 seconds, urine output 40 mL/hr (target 34–68 mL/hr). Temperature (T): 38.1°C.

Disability (D): Alert and orientated. Capillary blood glucose = 6.4 mmol/L, Pain: moderate (localised to surgical site).

Exposure (E): Category 1 pressure ulcer on left hip, dehisced surgical wound (red/inflamed/hot to touch).

Total NEW2 Score: 4.

Nursing Actions:
- Complete sepsis screen, has several amber flags (RR 21–24 breaths per minute), surgery last 6 weeks, signs of clinical wound infection. Therefore, requires escalation and bloods being sent.
- Take wound swab, inform medical team of results so antibiotic regimen can be amended based on culture sensitivity.
- Consider appropriate antimicrobial dressing to manage wound.
- Inform patient of the development of wound infection and discuss with him plan of care. Gain consent to discuss the development of the wound infection with his family.

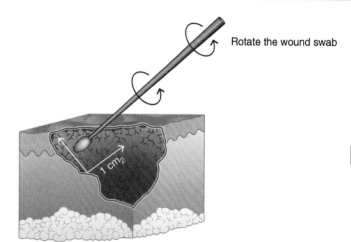

Rotate the wound swab

Figure 7.8 The Levine technique.

6Cs: Communication

Communication when making a referral is key to the workplace and is central to effective team working. Effective communication can also lead to positive patient outcomes.

Management of non-healing wounds

The majority of wounds heal by addressing any underlying causes and basic wound management. However, if the wound does not heal within the anticipated timeframe or when devitalised tissue is observed on the wound bed this needs to be managed before healing can occur. For healing to occur several areas need to be addressed, which make up the TIMERS framework (Atkin et al., 2019) (Figure 7.9). Referral to tissue viability nurses may be required to help you manage these more complex, hard-to-heal wounds.

Conclusion

Management of a patient's skin integrity is a basic skill of all nurses. However, it is fundamental in critical care because of the additional risk factors these individuals have for developing pressure ulcers and the negative impact a wound infection has on patient recovery. It is therefore important that a risk assessment for pressure ulcers is undertaken promptly and skin and wound assessments are conducted regularly. Special consideration should be given to all those who are using medical devices and those with darker skin tones, where initial signs of skin damage may be harder to spot.

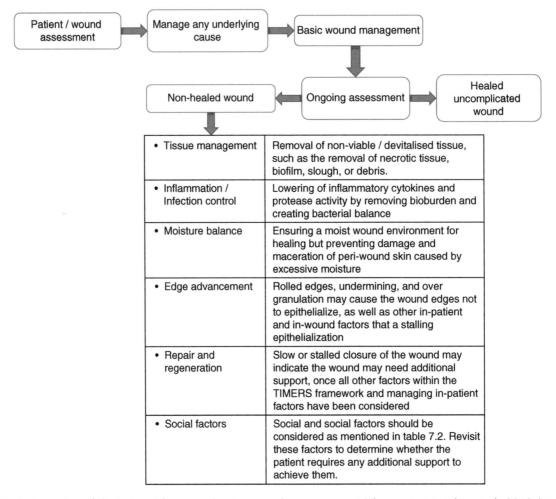

Figure 7.9 Integration of the TIMERS framework into wound management (Flanga, 2004; Atkin et al., 2019; Leaper et al., 2012).

Take home points

1. Pressure ulcer risk assessments must be completed on admission and reassessed if patient condition changes.
2. All patients are at risk of pressure ulcers from medical devices and objects left in the patient's bedspace.
3. Patients skin condition should be assessed head to toe, with special care taken of people with dark skin tones.
4. Wound assessments and re-assessment should be undertaken by a trained and competent registered nurse at agreed time points.
5. The patient's psychological wellbeing and quality of life should be considered when managing a patient with a wound.
6. In-patient factors and comorbidities impact risk of developing pressure ulcers and risk of poor healing.
7. Referral to a tissue viability nurse specialist may be required to manage complex and hard-to-heal wounds.

References

Alderden, J., Rondinelli, J., Pepper, G. et al. (2017). Risk factors for pressure injuries among critical care patients: A systematic review. *Int J Nurs Stud* 71: 97–114.

Atkin et al. (2019). Implementing TIMERS: the race against hard to heal wounds. *J Wound Care* 28(Suppl 3): S1–S49.

Barakat-Johnson, M., Lai, M., and Wand, T. (2019). The incidence and prevalence of medical device-related pressure ulcers in intensive care: a systematic review. *J Wound Care* 28(8): 512–521. doi: 10.12968/jowc.2019.28.8.512.

Barakat-Johnson, M., Barnett, C., Wand, T., and White K. (2017). Medical device-related pressure injuries: An exploratory descriptive study in an acute tertiary hospital in Australia. *J Tissue Viability* 26(4): 246–253. doi: 10.1016/j.jtv.2017.09.008.

Coleman, S., Nelson, E.A., Vowden, P. et al. (2017). Improving Wound Care Project Board, as part of NHS England's Leading Change Adding Value Framework. Development of a generic wound care assessment minimum data set. *J Tissue Viability* 26(4): 226–240.

Estocado, N. and Black, J. (2019). Ten top tips: Wound photo documentation. *Wounds International Journal* 10(3): 8–12.

Falanga (2004). Wound bed preparation: science applied to practice. http://ewma.org/fileadmin/user_upload/EWMA.org/Position_documents_2002-2008/pos_doc_English_final_04.pdf (accessed March 2022).

Gardner, S.E., Abbott, L.I., Fiala, C.A., and Rakel, B.A. (2017). Factors associated with high pain intensity during wound care procedures: A model. *Wound Repair and Regeneration* 25(4): 558–563. doi: 10.1111/wrr.12553.

Gefen, A., Alves, P., Ciprandi G. et al. (2020). Device related pressure ulcers: SECURE prevention. *J Wound Care* 29(Sup2a): S1–S52 doi: 10.12968/jowc.2020.29.Sup2a.S1.

International Wound Infection Institute (IWII) (2022). Wound Infection in Clinical Practice. *Wounds International*.

Kottner, J., Cuddigan, J., Carville, K. et al. (2020). Pressure ulcer/injury classification today: An international perspective. *J Tissue Viability* 29(3): 197–203. doi: 10.1016/j.jtv.2020.04.003.

Leaper, D.J., Schultz, G., Carville, K. et al. (2012). Extending the TIME concept: what have we learned in the past 10 years? *International Wound Journal* 9(6): 1–19.

NICE (2014). Pressure ulcers: prevention and management: NICE guideline CG179. https://pathways.nice.org.uk.

NICE (2015). Antimicrobial stewardship: systems and processes for effective antimicrobial medicine use: NICE guideline NG15. https://pathways.nice.org.uk.

NPUAP & EPUAP (2014). Prevention and treatment of pressure ulcers: quick reference guide. www.epuap.org.

NPUAP, EPUAP, and PPPIA (2019). Prevention and treatment of pressure ulcers/injuries: quick reference guide. www.epuap.org.

Peate, I. and Stephens, M. (2020). (2nd) *Wound Care at a Glance*. Oxford: Wiley.

Stephens, M. (2018). The principles of skin integrity. In: *Nursing Practice: Knowledge and Care*, 2e (ed. I. Peate and K. Wild), 350–375. Oxford: Wiley.

Wounds International (2010). Pressure ulcer prevention: pressure, shear, friction and microclimate in context. A consensus document. London: Wounds International, 2010. Available: https://www.woundsinternational.com/uploads/resources/5a517b64dacfb4fee06c221412f0b4e9.pdf.

Wounds UK (2018). Best Practice Statement Maintaining skin integrity. London: Wounds UK.

Chapter 8

Shock

Barry Hill

Aim

This aim of this chapter is to provide the reader with an evidence-based understanding of shock in the context of patients who are cared for in critical care settings.

Learning outcomes

After reading this chapter the reader will be able to:

- Be introduced to the different types of shock.
- Understand the underlying pathophysiology, risk factors and aetiology of shock.
- Gain knowledge of shock in the context of its effect on multiple organs.
- Explore the complications, investigations, and contemporary clinical management of shock.

Test your prior knowledge

- What are the clinical features of hypovolaemic shock?
- Can you explain the four stages of hypovolemic shock?
- What type of shock does severe left ventricular dysfunction usually trigger?
- What type of shock is caused by an inability to produce adequate cardiac output despite normal intravascular volume and myocardial function?
- What type of shock has the following three subtypes within it septic, anaphylactic/anaphylactoid, and neurogenic shock?

Fundamentals of Critical Care: A Textbook for Nursing and Healthcare Students, First Edition. Edited by Ian Peate and Barry Hill.
© 2023 John Wiley & Sons Ltd. Published 2023 by John Wiley & Sons Ltd.
Companion website: www.wiley.com/go/peate/criticalcare

Introduction

This chapter introduces the student to the different types of shock. It discusses the risk factors, aetiology, investigations, staging, complications, principles of management, education, and training.

Shock

Shock is generally classified according to its cause. There are four main pathological mechanisms that can result in a state of shock (Vincent and De Backer, 2013; Stratton, 2019):

- Hypovolaemia – loss of intravascular volume from internal or external fluid loss
- Cardiogenic – pump failure
- Obstructive barriers to cardiac filling or circulatory flow
- Distributive shock – due to vasoregulation and loss of vascular tone.

Shock is commonly defined as 'the life-threatening failure of adequate oxygen delivery to the tissues and may be due to decreased blood perfusion of tissues, inadequate blood oxygen saturation, or increased oxygen demand from the tissues that results in decreased end-organ oxygenation and dysfunction' (Stratton, 2019). If left untreated, shock results in sustained multiple organ dysfunction and end-organ damage with possible death. Tissue hypoperfusion may be present without systemic hypotension, but at the bedside shock is commonly diagnosed when both arterial hypotension and organ dysfunction are present (Stratton, 2019).

Step 3 competencies: National standards

3:2.3 Advanced Shock Management

You must be able to demonstrate the advanced knowledge and skills required to perform evidence-based practice safely and professionally in relation to the classifications, stages, pathophysiology, and treatment of:

1. Hypovolemic shock
2. Cardiogenic shock
3. Distributive:
   - Obstructive shock
   - Septic shock
   - Neurogenic shock
   - Anaphylactic shock

Hypovolaemic shock

Hypovolaemic shock (hypo=low, vol=volume and anaemic=blood) is characterised by a loss of intravascular volume of 15% or more, leading to inadequate perfusion of the tissues (Peate, 2020). Hypovolaemic shock occurs when the volume of the circulatory system is too depleted to allow adequate circulation to the tissues (Rull and Bonsall, 2017). Patients with hypovolaemic shock have severe hypovolaemia with decreased peripheral perfusion. If left untreated, ischaemic injury of vital organs can occur, leading to multisystem organ failure. The first factor to be considered is whether the hypovolaemic shock has resulted from haemorrhage or fluid losses as this will dictate treatment.

Pathophysiology and symptoms

Hypovolaemic shock results from depletion of intravascular volume, either by blood loss or extracellular fluid loss. The body compensates for this with increased sympathetic tone, resulting in increased heart rate and cardiac contractility, and peripheral vasoconstriction. Sympathetic tone is the condition of a muscle when the tone is maintained predominantly by impulses from the sympathetic nervous system. Changes in vital signs include an increase in diastolic blood pressure with narrowed pulse pressure. As volume status decreases, systolic blood pressure drops. Oxygen delivery to vital organs is unable to meet demand as a result and cells switch from aerobic to anaerobic metabolism, resulting in lactic acidosis. Blood flow is diverted from other organs to preserve the flow to the heart and brain as sympathetic drive increases. This propagates tissue ischaemia and exacerbates lactic acidosis. If this is not corrected, there will be worsening haemodynamic compromise and, eventually, death (Gayet-Ageron et al., 2018).

Symptoms of hypovolaemic shock can be related to volume depletion, electrolyte imbalances or acid-base disorders that accompany hypovolaemic shock. Patients with volume depletion may experience thirst, muscle cramps and/or orthostatic hypotension (decrease in systolic blood pressure of 20 mmHg or decrease in diastolic blood pressure of 10 mmHg within 3 minutes of standing compared to a sitting or supine blood pressure). In severe hypovolaemic shock, patients can experience abdominal, or chest pain caused by mesenteric and coronary ischaemia. Brain malperfusion can cause agitation, lethargy, or confusion.

Physical assessments because of volume depletion may find dry mucous membranes, decreased skin elasticity, reduced jugular venous pressure (JVP), tachycardia, hypotension and decreased urinary output. Patients may also appear cold, clammy and cyanotic (Annane et al., 2013).

Clinical assessment: cardiac output

Cardiac output (CO) is heart rate (HR) × stroke volume (SV). A reduction in CO causes reduced activity of arterial baroreceptors causing increased sympathetic and reduced parasympathetic activity. Heart rate increases and cardiac output is restored towards normal. An increase in heart rate is an early sign of compensation but its absence does not exclude significant compromise. While most patients with acute blood loss demonstrate the typical tachycardic response it is important to be aware that as many as 30–35% may present with an initial relative bradycardia (heart rate less than 60 beats/minute). This is in addition to patients taking beta-blockers who are pharmacologically prevented from mounting a tachycardia and those in whom a tachycardia may go unrecognised as their normal resting heart rate is lower than average (i.e., athletes). Bradycardia may of course be the cause of the shock state (e.g. complete heart block, beta-blocker or calcium antagonist overdose).

Risk factors

A healthy adult can withstand the loss of 0.5 litre of fluid from a circulation of about 5 litres without ill effect (Rull and Bonsall, 2017); however, larger volumes and rapid loss cause progressively greater problems. Risk of shock is related to the degree of hypovolaemia and the speed of correction. In children and young adults, tachycardia is one of the earliest signs of hypovolaemia as the circulatory system is better able to cope with the rigours of loss. The risk of morbidity and mortality is much greater as age increases because older people often do not tolerate having low blood volume (Rull and Bonsall, 2017). Abnormal pathology in the cardiovascular, respiratory and renal systems increases risk.

Aetiology

The annual incidence of shock of any aetiology is 0.3 to 0.7 per 1000, with haemorrhagic shock being most common in the critical care unit (Taghavi and Askari, 2019). Hypovolaemic shock is the most common type of shock in children and is frequently due to diarrhoeal illness in the developing world. Haemorrhagic shock is hypovolaemic shock from blood loss and is mostly caused by traumatic injury. Other causes of haemorrhagic shock include gastrointestinal (GI) bleed, bleeding from an ectopic pregnancy, bleeding from surgical intervention or vaginal bleeding (Taghavi and Askari, 2019).

Orange Flag

Patients who are actively bleeding may trigger the major haemorrhage protocol and procedure. It is imperative that the healthcare professional understands the patients wishes in relation to receiving blood components and is open and honest about what interventions they are performing.

Hypovolaemic shock because of extracellular fluid loss can be of the following aetiologies.

Gastrointestinal losses

GI losses can occur via many different aetiologies. The GI tract usually secretes between 3 to 6 litres of fluid per day. However, most of this fluid is reabsorbed as only 100–200 mL is lost in the stool. Volume depletion occurs when the fluid ordinarily secreted by the GI tract cannot be reabsorbed. This occurs when there is intractable vomiting diarrhoea, or external drainage via a stoma or fistulas (Taghavi and Askari, 2019).

Renal losses

Renal losses of salt and fluid can lead to hypovolaemic shock. The kidneys usually excrete sodium and water in a manner that matches intake. Diuretic therapy and osmotic diuresis from hyperglycaemia can lead to excessive renal sodium and volume loss. In addition, there are several tubular and interstitial diseases beyond the scope of this chapter that cause severe salt-wasting nephropathy (Taghavi and Askari, 2019).

Skin losses

Fluid loss also can occur from the skin. In a hot and dry climate, skin fluid losses can be as high as 1 to 2 litres/hour. Patients with a skin barrier interrupted by burns or other skin lesions can also experience large fluid losses that lead to hypovolaemic shock (Taghavi and Askari, 2019).

Third-space sequestration

Sequestration of fluid into a third-space (known as third spacing) can also lead to volume loss and hypovolaemic shock. Third spacing of fluid can occur in intestinal obstruction, pancreatitis, obstruction of a major venous system or any other pathological condition that results in a massive inflammatory response (Taghavi and Askari, 2019).

Blood analysis

Monitoring electrolytes and acid/base status in patients in hypovolaemic shock is of utmost importance. Biochemical analysis will identify any electrolyte and acid-base disturbances, for example contraction alkalosis, metabolic acidosis, which could affect choice of replacement fluid, and rate of repletion. In some cases, arterial blood gas is needed if mixed acid-base disturbance is suspected (Galvagno, 2014). More about Arterial Blood Gases (ABGs) can be seen in Chapter 16.

Orange Flag

When a patient is experiencing the symptoms of hypovolemic shock, it is imperative that the healthcare professional offers reassurance and acts as an advocate to alleviate any additional anxiety and fear.

Multiple organ dysfunction syndrome

The combination of direct and reperfusion injury may cause multiple organ dysfunction syndrome (MODS) – the progressive dysfunction of more than 2 organs consequent to life-threatening illness or injury (Procter, 2019). MODS can follow any type of shock but is most common when infection is involved; organ failure is one of the defining features of septic shock. MODS also occurs in more than 10% of patients with severe traumatic injury and is the primary cause of death in those surviving longer than 24 hours (Procter, 2019).

During MODS, the permeability of lung parenchyma leads to inflammation and oedema collection within the alveoli. Lactate production and metabolic acidosis produces abnormal levels of hydrogen ions. This decreases the pH in the blood and the level of bicarbonate. To compensate for this the respiratory rate is increased, resulting in hyperventilation (Galvagno, 2014). Progressive hypoxia may be resistant to supplemental oxygen therapy. This condition is termed acute lung injury or, if severe, acute respiratory distress syndrome (ARDS) (Procter, 2019).

The kidneys are injured when renal perfusion is critically reduced, leading to acute tubular necrosis and renal insufficiency manifested by oliguria and a progressive rise in serum creatinine (Procter, 2019).

In the heart, reduced coronary perfusion and increased mediators (including tumour necrosis factor and inter-leukin-1) may depress contractility, worsen myocardial compliance, and down-regulate beta-receptors. These factors decrease cardiac output, further worsening both myocardial and systemic perfusion and causing a vicious circle often culminating in death (Procter, 2019).

In the GI tract, ileus and submucosal haemorrhage can develop. Liver hypoperfusion can cause focal or extensive hepatocellular necrosis, transaminase and bilirubin elevation, and decreased production of clotting factors (Procter, 2019).

Coagulation can be impaired, including the most severe manifestation, disseminated intravascular coagulopathy (DIC) (Procter, 2019).

Examination scenario

Disseminated intravascular coagulation (DIC) may complicate hypovolemic shock secondary to trauma. Treatment with heparin in such cases is contraindicated because of the risk of bleeding at the site of trauma.

Staging of hypovolaemic shock

Lavoie (2018) recognises that there are four stages of hypovolaemic shock based on how much blood volume has been lost. All stages require early treatment, but it is helpful to recognise the stage of hypovolaemia to provide the appropriate treatment quickly due to the complications hypovolaemic shock presents (Table 8.1).

The clinical features of hypovolaemic shock can be seen in Table 8.2. A list of investigations and their rationales is shown in Table 8.3.

Stage 1

During the earliest stage of hypovolaemic shock, a person will have lost more than 15% (>750 mL) of their intravascular fluid volume. This stage can be difficult to diagnose. Blood pressure, urine output and breathing will still be normal. The most noticeable symptom at this stage is skin that appears pale. The person may also experience sudden anxiety.

Table 8.1 Complications. *Source:* Data from Rull and Bonsall, 2017.

Complication	Wider implication
Blood is directed away from the kidneys and gut	This can produce acute kidney injury and complications of gut ischaemia
Obstetric shock	Acute tubular necrosis can occur
Inadequate perfusion	This leads to hypoxia and metabolic acidosis
About 75% of the blood flow to the right ventricle and 100% to the left ventricle occurs in diastole	A fall in diastolic pressure Will predispose to cardiac arrhythmias and even arrest. Upset of acid-base balance, hypoxia and disturbance of electrolytes will aggravate the problem
In those who are susceptible, dehydration	This may lead to haemoconcentration and sludging of the circulation with such complications as venous sinus thrombosis

Table 8.2 Clinical features of hypovolaemic shock. *Source:* Data from AMBOSS, 2020.

- Weak pulse, tachycardia, tachypnoea
- Cold, clammy extremities, poor capillary refill
- Hypotension with narrow pulse pressure in the decompensated stage
- Specific symptoms corresponding to the cause (e.g., bleeding, melaena, haematemesis, diarrhoea)
- Elevated lactate

Table 8.3 Investigations table. *Source:* Data from Rull and Bonsall, 2017.

Investigation	Rationale
Check haemoglobin (Hb), urea and electrolytes (U&E), liver function test (LFT) and, in haemorrhage and burns, group and save and crossmatch	There is likely to be a significant drop in Hb in early stages of hypovolaemic shock. This is because, in the earliest stage of the condition, a person will have lost up to 15%, or 750 ml, of their blood volume. Prompt administration of blood is essential in instances of severe or ongoing blood loss.
Coagulation screen	The coagulation screen is a combination of tests designed to provide rapid information and allows an initial broad categorisation of haemostatic function. In hypovolaemic shock, the acute fall in clotting factors is likely due to increased haemostatic demands, plasma dilution from resuscitation, and extravascular relocation from shock-induced extravascular expansion.
Blood gases: arterial blood gas (ABG) or venous blood gas (VBG)	These may show a metabolic acidaemia from poor perfusion; lactate levels particularly reflect hypoperfusion. Note: in clinical practice, an AE3G is always preferred as the respiratory component is captured, and with patients who are in shock, it is inevitable that they will deteriorate.
Monitor urine output, which may require a catheter	Urine output should be used to guide administration of fluids.
Ultrasound	This can be useful for differentiating hypovolaemic from cardiogenic shock; the vena cava can be assessed for adequate filling and echocardiogram can show any pump failure.
Central venous pressure (CVP)	Monitoring CVP may be useful where there is evidence of shock.

Stage 2

In the second stage, the body will have lost up to 30% (1500 mL) of blood. The individual may experience increased heart and breathing rates. Blood pressure may still be within the normal range. However, the diastolic pressure may be high. The person may begin sweating and feeling more anxious and restless. At this stage, capillary refill is delayed, and urine output may be about 20–30 mL/hour.

Stage 3

By stage 3, a person with hypovolaemic shock will have lost 30–40% (1500–2000 mL) of blood. The systolic blood pressure will be 100 mmHg or lower. The patient's heart rate may increase to over 120 beats per minute. They will also have a rapid breathing rate of over 30 breaths per minute. The patient will begin to experience mental distress, including anxiety and agitation. Their skin will be pale and cold, and they will begin sweating. Urine output drops to 20 mL/hour.

Stage 4

A person with stage 4 hypovolaemia faces a critical situation. They will have experienced a loss of blood volume greater than 40% (2000 mL). They will have a weak pulse but extremely rapid heart rate. Breathing will become be very fast and difficult. Systolic blood pressure will be under 70 mmHg. They may experience the following symptoms:

- Drifting in and out of consciousness
- Sweating heavily
- Feeling cool to the touch
- Looking extremely pale or a lighter shade of natural skin tone
- Absent capillary refill
- Negligible urine output.

Principles of managing hypovolaemic shock

Management of hypovolaemia involves assessing and treating the underlying cause, identifying electrolyte and acid-base disturbances, and assessing and treating the volume deficit. This will influence the choice of fluid and rate at which it should be administered (Mandel and Palevsky, 2019). Clinicians should identify the aetiology (or aetiologies) contributing to hypovolaemia so that therapies can be directed at the underlying cause of volume loss. Therapies may include anti-emetics to treat vomiting, cessation of diuretics, or controlling haemorrhage. It is important to identify electrolyte and acid-base disturbances. Biochemical analysis will alert the clinician to electrolyte (e.g., hypo-or hypernatraemia, hypo- or hyperkalaemia) and acid-base disturbances (e.g., contraction alkalosis, metabolic acidosis), which may affect choice of replacement fluid and rate of repletion. In some cases, an arterial blood gas (ABG) may be needed if mixed acid-base disturbance is suspected.

Clinical investigation: ABG

An ABG allows assessment of two related physiological functions: pulmonary gas exchange and acid-base homeostasis.

Clinical investigation: metabolic acidosis

Reduced bicarbonate is the defining feature of all cases of metabolic acidosis and occurs for one of three reasons. Firstly, bicarbonate can be consumed in buffering an abnormally high acid load, so the primary problem here is increased production of metabolic acids. The second reason is increased loss of bicarbonate from the body and the third reason is failure of kidneys to regenerate bicarbonate. In a critical care setting metabolic acidosis is the most frequent acid-base disturbance and the most common cause is increased production of the metabolic acid, lactic acid. Lactic acid is produced in excess by tissue cells that are poorly oxygenated, so metabolic (lactic) acidosis can arise in any clinical condition in which oxygen delivery to tissues is compromised.

Fluid resuscitation

It is suggested that fluid resuscitation should be commenced immediately to restore circulating volume and improve cardiac output. The National Institute for Health and Care Excellence (NICE) (2017a) recommends the administration of intravenous (IV) crystalloids that contain sodium in the range 130–154 mmol/L, with a bolus of 500 mL over less than 15 minutes, unless the patient presents with active internal or external bleeding. In such cases, red blood cells should be transfused to support the transportation of haemoglobin around the body (Dutton and Finch, 2018). Hypovolaemia directly impacts circulating blood volume and therefore contributes to decreased oxygen carriage, increased lactate for anaerobic respiration, cell death, and potentially leads to pre-renal failure.

Clinical considerations

In patients with hypovolaemic shock due to extracellular fluid loss, the aetiology of fluid loss must be identified and treated (Taghavi and Askari, 2019):

- Monitoring electrolytes and acid/base status in patients in hypovolaemic shock is of utmost importance
- Trauma is the leading cause of haemorrhagic shock
- Haemorrhagic shock should be treated with balanced transfusion of packed red blood cells, plasma and platelets
- Determining whether patients will be responsive to volume resuscitation should not rely on a single modality such as ultrasound, pulse pressure wave variation, passive leg raises, or central venous pressure
- The decision on fluid administration should be based on a complete systematic assessment to help direct volume resuscitation
- For patients with hypovolaemic shock due to fluid loss, crystalloid solution is preferred over colloid.

Training and education for Registered Nurses

Hospitals should establish systems to ensure that all health professionals involved in prescribing and delivering IV fluid therapy are trained on the principles covered in the NICE (2017b) guideline, and are then formally assessed and reassessed at regular intervals. Health professionals need to be able to assess, identify and escalate care.

Competence must be demonstrated in:

- Understanding the physiology of fluid and electrolyte balance in patients with normal physiology and during illness
- Assessing patients' fluid and electrolyte needs (the 5 Rs: resuscitation, routine maintenance, replacement, redistribution and reassessment)
- Assessing the risks, benefits, and harms of IV fluids
- Prescribing and administering IV fluids
- Monitoring the patient response
- Evaluating and documenting changes
- Taking appropriate action as required.

Hospitals should have an IV fluids lead, responsible for training, clinical governance, audit, and review of IV fluid prescribing and patient outcomes.

Cardiogenic shock

Cardiogenic shock is sustained hypotension with inadequate tissue perfusion regardless of adequate left ventricular filling pressure. This is manifested with organ dysfunction such as oliguria, confusion, cool extremities and lactic acidosis.

Cardiogenic shock is defined as:

- a systolic BP of <90 mmHg for greater than 30 minutes
- a cardiac index of <2.2 L/min/m² in the presence of a pulmonary capillary wedge pressure of >15 mmHg.

Cardiogenic shock (CS) is the most severe form of acute heart failure, characterised by insufficient cardiac output, hypotension, and systemic hypoperfusion. CS is the leading cause of death in acute coronary syndrome (ACS), which accounts for about 80% of CS cases (Kataja and Harjola, 2017). CS has several causes (Tables 8.4 and 8.5). In addition to acute cardiac cause, the diagnostic criteria for CS include persistent hypotension (systolic blood pressure < 90 mmHg) and clinical signs of hypoperfusion. Mortality rates in CS remain as high as 35–50%. Severe left ventricular dysfunction usually triggers the shock and leads to the activation of systemic inflammatory response and hypothalamic-pituitary-adrenal axis. Immediately after detection of the

Table 8.4 Causes of cardiogenic shock.

Acute myocardial infarction	
Pump failure	**Mechanical complications**
• Large infarction • Smaller infarction with pre-existing disease • Right ventricular failure	• Papillary muscle rupture • Ventricular septal defect • Cardiac rupture • Cardiac tamponade

Table 8.5 Other causes of cardiogenic shock.

Other causes may include:	
• Septic shock with myocardial depression • End-stage cardiomyopathy • Myocarditis • Drugs – e.g., beta-blocker overdose	• Aortic dissection with acute aortic regurgitation • Myocardial contusion • Left ventricular outflow tract obstruction

shock, electrocardiography and echocardiography should be performed to determine the aetiology of CS and to rule out mechanical complications. Urgent revascularisation by percutaneous coronary intervention, or less often by coronary artery bypass graft, is the most important treatment in CS caused by ACS. In the case of mechanical complication, immediate surgical treatment is essential. Regardless of the aetiology, the fundamental treatment strategy includes fluid challenge that aims at obtaining euvolemia and relieving tissue hypoperfusion. Inotropes and vasopressors are often needed to improve cardiac performance and to maintain sufficient blood pressure. Ventilation is often supported mechanically, and CS patients are best treated in specialist cardiac critical care units. Continuous invasive blood pressure monitoring, electrocardiography, and repeated echocardiography are required. In CS refractory to other treatments, mechanical circulatory support may be considered to maintain adequate perfusion pressure and to prevent multi-organ failure.

Pathophysiology

The pathophysiology of CS is poorly understood owing to a paucity of high-quality clinical data. Even for the most common cause, ACS, significant heterogeneity (e.g., STEMI vs type I and type II non-STEMI with more specific variables such as postcardiac arrest or renal failure) exists that likely informs management and influences outcomes. Ideally, management of CS would integrate general supportive measures such as pharmacological circulatory support and mechanical circulatory support (MCS) titrated to interventions directed at treating specific mechanisms in increasingly granular detail such as interrupting the cellular, metabolic and inflammatory pathways. In the absence of robust multicentre cohort studies providing detailed patient-level phenotyping, current management of CS necessarily focuses on the quantifiable and modifiable parameters of CS as collected from invasive haemodynamic assessment.

In general, CS is characterised by an initial insult resulting in impaired CO followed by progressive injury culminating in inadequate and ultimately maladaptive compensatory mechanisms and rapid deterioration to end-organ hypoperfusion and complete cardiovascular collapse. This is conceptualised as a vicious cycle of cardiac injury, systemic deterioration and further cardiac impairment. Perhaps more than any single feature, this self-perpetuating feedback loop, encompassing the heart and the whole patient, is what underlies CS. Interrupting this 'shock spiral' and restoring cardiovascular homoeostasis is central to the overarching treatment paradigm of CS. Any cause of acute, severe impairment of CO can trigger this cascade and precipitate CS.

Communication

Cardiogenic shock causes rapid deterioration throughout the body systems. It is essential healthcare professionals establish patient-centred care and orientate them to the critical care environment.

Medications management: epinephrine (adrenaline)

Epinephrine is an agonist of alpha1, beta1 and beta2 receptors. It can increase the mean arterial pressure (MAP) by increasing the cardiac index and stroke volume, as well as systemic vascular resistance (SVR) and heart rate. Epinephrine decreases the splanchnic blood flow and may increase oxygen delivery and consumption. Administration of this agent may be associated with an increase in systemic and regional lactate concentrations. The use of epinephrine is recommended only in patients who are unresponsive to traditional agents. Other undesirable effects include an increase in lactate concentration, a potential to produce myocardial ischaemia, the development of arrhythmias, and a reduction in splanchnic flow.

Symptoms

The symptoms of cardiogenic shock occur as a reaction to the loss of oxygen-rich blood in the body. The symptoms that a person experiences may depend on how quickly the blood pressure drops and how low it gets. Some individuals may experience mild symptoms at first, whereas others may have no symptoms and then immediately lose consciousness.

Red Flag

Symptoms of cardiogenic shock

- Sudden drop in blood pressure
- Bradycardia
- Raised Jugular Venous Pressure (JVP)
- Swollen ankles
- Pale, blue hue to white skin tones, and chalky pale discolouration to dark skin tones
- Cold hands and feet
- Sweaty skin
- Confusion
- Decreased consciousness
- Tachypnoea

If a person does not receive treatment, cardiogenic shock can cause life-threatening complications, such as organ damage and complete organ failure. It can also be fatal in some cases.

Management

Cardiogenic shock is a medical emergency and requires immediate treatment. The aim of treatment is to restore blood flow to the brain and other organs as quickly as possible to protect them from damage. Treatment may include:

- intravenous fluids
- cardiac catheterisation for coronary angiography
- oxygen supplementation
- mechanical ventilation
- mechanical circulatory support (MCS) devices
- medicines, such as vasopressors, to contract blood vessels and raise blood pressure.
- other treatments may need to focus on preventing or treating damage to other organs.
- supporting patients and relieving any anxieties and concerns

For example, acute kidney injury (AKI) is prevalent in people with cardiogenic shock. These individuals may need additional treatments, fluid replacement, inotropic drugs, or renal replacement therapy (RRT).

6Cs: Compassion

Compassionate care must be provided to the patient, their family and friends especially during life-threatening events.

Medications management: norepinephrine (noradrenaline)

Norepinephrine is a potent alpha-adrenergic agonist with only minor beta1-adrenergic agonist effects. Norepinephrine can increase blood pressure successfully in patients who remain hypotensive following dopamine. The dosage of norepinephrine may vary from 0.2 to 1.5 mcg/kg/min, and high dosages (up to 3.3 mcg/kg/min) have been used because of the alpha-receptor down-regulation in persons with shock.

Clinical investigations: fluid resuscitation

Fluid resuscitation strategy is a clinical challenge in the early management of CS as it is often difficult to assess and can vary over time. In right-sided heart failure, right atrial pressures and pulmonary artery wedge pressures are poor predictors of fluid response. Echocardiography can assess right-sided heart volume status and rule out pericardial fluid collection. The definitive method of volume status assessment and adequacy of resuscitation is right heart catheterisation, which should be performed in conjunction with coronary angiography. If hypovolaemia is present, conservative boluses of crystalloids (250–500 mL) are reasonable while the patient is being stabilised for cardiac catheterisation (de Asua and Rosenberg, 2017).

Obstructive shock

Obstructive shock is caused by the inability to produce adequate cardiac output despite normal intravascular volume and myocardial function. Causative factors may be located within the pulmonary or systemic circulation or associated with the heart itself. Examples of obstructive shock include acute pericardial tamponade, tension pneumothorax, pulmonary or systemic hypertension, and congenital or acquired outflow obstructions. Recognition of the characteristic features of these syndromes is essential because most of the causes can be treated provided the diagnosis is made early.

Altered pathophysiology

The three most common obstructive shock pathologies and their management (ACLS, 2021) are listed below.

Tension pneumothorax

Tension pneumothorax is the accumulation of air within the pleural space. Causes of tension pneumothorax in children include trauma, asthma, cystic fibrosis, pneumonia and excessive positive pressure during manual or mechanical ventilation. Once a tension pneumothorax occurs air can continue to accumulate within the pleural space but cannot escape. This continued accumulation of air increases pressure and ultimately obstructs venous blood return to the heart. The obstruction results in decreased diastolic filling.

Signs and symptoms

The following list provides other signs and symptoms of tension pneumothorax using the primary assessment model (ABCDE).

- Airway: tracheal deviation toward the contralateral side
- Breathing: increased work of breathing, increased respiratory rate, respiratory distress, and diminished lung sounds on the affected side
- Circulation: neck vein distention, rapid and severe hypotension, tachycardia rapidly degrades into bradycardia, and Pulseless Electrical Activity (PEA)
- Disability: decreased level of consciousness
- Exposure: pale and cool extremities

Cardiac tamponade

Cardiac tamponade is the accumulation of fluid or blood within the pericardial sac. As fluid accumulates, the increased pressure decreases venous return to the heart and causes right ventricular compression which results in a progressive decline in right ventricular end-diastolic volume. The decreased end-diastolic volume compromises cardiac output which results in shock symptoms.

Signs and symptoms

The following list provides other signs and symptoms of cardiac tamponade using the primary assessment model (ABCDE).

- Airway: may have compromised airway if level of consciousness is decreased
- Breathing: increased work of breathing and respiratory rate; respiratory distress
- Circulation: tachycardia, decreased peripheral pulses, jugular vein distention, poor capillary refill, muffled heart sounds, narrow pulse pressure
- Disability: decreased level of consciousness
- Exposure: cool extremities

Pulmonary embolism (PE)

Pulmonary embolism occurs when the pulmonary artery or its branches become partially or totally occluded. Common causes of pulmonary embolism include blood clots (most prevalent), air and fat. Children who have existing risk factors are at higher risk for pulmonary embolism. Some risk factors include indwelling central venous catheters, sickle cell disorder, and coagulation disorders.

Signs and symptoms

The following list provides signs and symptoms of pulmonary embolism using the primary assessment model (ABCDE).

- Airway: may have compromised airway if level of consciousness is decreased
- Breathing: increased work of breathing and respiratory rate; respiratory distress
- Circulation: tachycardia, cyanosis, chest pain and hypotension. Venous congestion – right-sided (hepatomegaly, ascites, abdominal pain, pleural effusion, oedema, jugular venous distention)
- Disability: decreased level of consciousness
- Exposure: cool extremities

The management of obstructive shock can be seen in Table 8.6.

> # 6Cs: Competence
>
> Ensuring patients are safe from avoidable harm is a fundamental right. The nurse must be competent when assessing, implementing, and evaluating the care of a patient in obstructive shock

Table 8.6   Management of obstructive shock.

Management of tension pneumothorax:	The definitive treatment for obstructive shock caused by tension pneumothorax is needle decompression and chest tube placement to the affected area.
Management of cardiac tamponade:	The primary treatment for cardiac tamponade is pericardiocentesis. If cardiac tamponade is suspected and the patient is not in cardiac arrest, expert consultation should take place. If cardiac arrest is ongoing or impending and cardiac tamponade is suspected, emergency pericardiocentesis can be performed.
Management of pulmonary embolism:	Pulmonary embolism must be confirmed by CT scan with contrast, or echocardiography, or angiography. The primary treatment for pulmonary embolism is anticoagulant therapy, but since anticoagulant therapy does not act immediately, fibrinolytic therapy should be considered for severe cases of pulmonary embolism.

Distributive shock

Distributive shock is a state of relative hypovolaemia resulting from pathological redistribution of the absolute intravascular volume and is the most frequent form of shock (Standl et al., 2018). The cause is either a loss of regulation of vascular tone, with volume being shifted within the vascular system, and/or disordered permeability of the vascular system with shifting of intravascular volume into the interstitium. The three subtypes are septic, anaphylactic/anaphylactoid, and neurogenic shock.

Septic shock

Septic shock is the most common cause of distributive shock. Sepsis is defined as life-threatening organ dysfunction due to dysregulated host response to infection, and organ dysfunction is defined as an acute change in total Sequential Organ Failure Assessment (SOFA) score of 2 points or greater secondary to the infection cause (Singer at el, 2016). Septic shock occurs in a subset of patients with sepsis and comprises of an underlying circulatory and cellular/metabolic abnormality that is associated with increased mortality. Septic shock is defined by persisting hypotension requiring vasopressors to maintain a mean arterial pressure of 65 mm Hg or higher and a serum lactate level greater than 2 mmol/L (18 mg/dL) despite adequate volume resuscitation. The 2016 definition, also called Sepsis-3, eliminates the requirement for the presence of systemic inflammatory response syndrome (SIRS) to define sepsis, and it removed the severe sepsis definition. What was previously called severe sepsis is now the new definition of sepsis.

Lactate

Blood lactate in circulation can be used as a marker for systemic tissue hypoperfusion and it reflects cellular dysfunction in sepsis patients. It is now included in the clinical criteria for septic shock defined in the Third International Consensus Definition for Sepsis and Septic Shock (Sepsis-3). When measuring lactate in critically unwell patients, the results are complementary to other test results, such as PCT for determination of level of bacterial or fungal infection, and together they serve as an important help in assessing the severity of the illness. Lactate levels should be measured within 3 hours of admission and if elevated repeated within 6 hours, as recommended by the Surviving Sepsis Campaign guidelines (Dellingher et al., 2013). This allows for the implementation and evaluation of effective hemodynamic management of the septic patient as early as possible, increasing the chances of survival.

Snapshot

Mel is a 44-year-old female who has presented to the critical care outreach team with signs and symptoms of septic shock. As the nurse caring for Melanie, you have been instructed to begin the sepsis 6 bundle (UK Sepsis Trust, 2018). The following steps are taken, can you give a rationale as to why?

1. Administer oxygen aiming to keep saturations > 94% (88–92% if at risk of CO_2 retention e.g., COPD).
2. Take blood cultures and consider other sources of infection i.e., CSF, urine, sputum. Think source control! Call surgeon/ radiologist if needed chest x-ray and urinalysis for all adults.
3. Give IV antibiotics according to Trust protocol. Consider allergies prior to administration.
4. Give IV fluids. If the patient is hypotensive, lactate >2 mmol/L, 500 mL of IV fluid should be infused stat. This may be repeated if clinically indicated do not exceed 30 mL/kg.
5. Check serial lactates. Corroborate high venous blood gas lactate with arterial sample. If lactate >4 mmol/L, call Critical Care and recheck after each 10 mL/kg fluid challenge.
6. Measure urine output. This should be a minimum of 0.5 mL/kg/hour.

Anaphylactic shock

Anaphylaxis is a severe, life-threatening, generalised, or systemic hypersensitivity reaction (Resus.org.uk, 2020). Anaphylaxis is a severe and potentially life-threatening reaction which may be the result of hypersensitivity. The hypersensitive reaction may be generalised or systemic and tends to occur within minutes. It can be considered an allergic reaction, which may or may not have an immunological basis. The airway is often compromised because of pharyngeal or laryngeal oedema causing breathing difficulty. Increased respiratory rate or bronchospasm can cause these breathing difficulties. There might be evidence of circulatory compromise, such as hypotension and an increased heart rate. In most cases of anaphylaxis, skin and mucosal changes occur. Skin changes include flushing and urticaria. Symptoms can worsen rapidly.

The Resuscitation Council (UK) advises emergency treatment using the 'ABCDE' approach. Calling for further assistance is vital. The patient can be laid flat with their legs raised to aid venous return.

Examination may reveal the following findings:

- General appearance and vital signs: Vary according to the severity of the anaphylactic episode and the organ system(s) affected; patients are commonly restless and anxious
- Respiratory findings: Severe angioedema of the tongue and lips; tachypnoea; stridor or severe air hunger; loss of voice, hoarseness, and/or dysphonia; wheezing
- Cardiovascular: Tachycardia, hypotension; cardiovascular collapse and shock can occur immediately, without any other findings
- Neurological: cognitive disturbance, depressed level of consciousness or may be agitated and/or combative

- Dermatologic: Classic skin manifestation is urticaria (i.e., hives) anywhere on the body; angioedema (soft tissue swelling); generalised (whole-body) erythema (or flushing) without urticaria or angioedema
- Gastrointestinal: Vomiting, diarrhoea, and abdominal distention

If a drug is suspected of causing an anaphylactic reaction, this should be stopped if appropriate. The Resuscitation Council (UK) does not advise inducing vomiting in the case of food-related anaphylaxis. In the case of venom-induced anaphylaxis, the trigger should be removed if possible: for example, the stinger after a bee sting.

Medication management: epinephrine (adrenaline) use in anaphylactic reactions

Adrenaline is the mainstay of treatment for anaphylactic reactions. It has the effect of reversing peripheral vasodilation through its adrenergic activity. Its effect on beta-receptors includes dilation of bronchial airways, increased myocardial contraction and suppression of histamine and leukotriene release. This means that adrenaline can reduce the severity of an anaphylactic reaction if the reaction is immunologically mediated. Intramuscular administration of adrenaline is recommended, so the needle used to administer the drug needs to be long enough to achieve this. The Resuscitation Council (UK) advises administration of adrenaline intramuscularly into the anterolateral aspect of the middle third of the thigh.

Neurogenic shock

Neurogenic shock is a devastating consequence of spinal cord injury (SCI) (Dave and Cho, 2021). It manifests as hypotension, bradyarrhythmia and temperature dysregulation due to peripheral vasodilatation following an injury to the spinal cord. This occurs due to the sudden loss of sympathetic tone, with preserved parasympathetic function, leading to autonomic instability. Neurogenic shock is mostly associated with cervical and high thoracic spine injury. Neurogenic shock should be differentiated from hypovolemic shock; the latter is often associated with tachycardia.

Neurogenic shock is not to be confused with a spinal shock, which is the flaccidity of muscles and loss of reflexes seen following spinal cord injury. Early identification and aggressive management are vital in neurogenic shock to

prevent secondary spinal injury. This section of the chapter is a concise overview to further aid the care for those patients who develop neurogenic shock.

Neurogenic shock is the clinical state manifested from primary and secondary spinal cord injury. Haemodynamic changes are seen with an injury to the spinal cord above the level of T6. The descending sympathetic tracts are disrupted most from associated fracture or dislocation of vertebrae in the cervical or upper thoracic spine. Primary spinal cord injury occurs within minutes of the initial insult. Primary injury is direct damage to the axons and neural membranes in the intermediolateral nucleus, lateral grey mater and anterior root that lead to disrupted sympathetic tone. Secondary spinal cord injury occurs hours to days after the initial insult. Secondary injury results from vascular insult, electrolyte shifts and oedema that lead to progressive central haemorrhagic necrosis of grey matter at the injury site. There is excitotoxicity from N-methyl-D-aspartate (NMDA) accumulation at a cellular level, improper homeostasis of electrolytes, mitochondrial injury and reperfusion injury, which all lead to controlled and uncontrolled apoptosis. Neurogenic shock is a combination of both primary and secondary injuries that lead to loss of sympathetic tone and thus unopposed parasympathetic response driven by the vagus nerve. Consequently, patients experience instability in blood pressure, heart rate and temperature regulation.

Initial management of neurogenic shock is focused on haemodynamic stabilisation. Hypotension should be treated first to prevent secondary injury. The first-line treatment for hypotension is intravenous fluid resuscitation. This is to allow appropriate compensation for the vasogenic dilation that occurs. If hypotension persists despite euvolaemia, vasopressors and inotropes are the second lines. No single agent is recommended. Phenylephrine is commonly used as it is a pure alpha-1 agonist that causes peripheral vasoconstriction to counteract the loss of sympathetic tone. However, the lack of beta activity leads to reflex bradycardia, which augments the already unopposed vagal tone. Norepinephrine has both alpha and beta activity, aiding both hypotension and bradycardia, thus the preferred agent. Epinephrine has been cited for refractory cases of hypotension and is rarely needed. Recommend keeping the MAP at 85 to 90 mmHg for the first 7 days to improve spinal cord perfusion. Caution should be used when using vasopressors as there may be co-existing injuries exacerbated with vasoconstriction (Dave and Cho, 2021).

Conclusion

Shock causes an imbalance between oxygen supply and demand. If left untreated, patients can develop ischaemic injury of vital organs, which leads to multi-system organ failure. It is important for nurses and healthcare professionals to be able to assess, identify and escalate care to ensure patients receive correct and timely treatment.

96

Take home points

1. Shock is a life-threatening medical condition and is a medical emergency.
2. Shock is generally classified according to its cause.
3. There are four main pathological mechanisms that can result in a state of shock; hypovolaemia – loss of intravascular volume from internal or external fluid loss; cardiogenic – pump failure; obstructive barriers to cardiac filling or circulatory flow and distributive shock – due to vasoregulation and loss of vascular tone.
4. The main symptom of shock is hypotension. Other symptoms include rapid, shallow breathing; cold and clammy skin; tachycardia with a weak pulse; dizziness and fainting.
5. Treatment for shock depends on the cause. Investigations will determine the cause and severity. Usually in severe cases, IV fluids are administered in addition to medications such as vasopressors and inotropes to raise blood pressure.
6. Septic shock is treated using the sepsis 6 bundle. Initial treatment is antibiotics and fluids.
7. Anaphylactic shock is treated with diphenhydramine, epinephrine (an 'Epi-pen'), and steroid medications.
8. Cardiogenic shock is treated by identifying and treating the underlying cause.
9. Hypovolaemic shock is treated with IV fluids in minor cases, and blood transfusions in severe cases of haemorrhage.
10. Neurogenic shock is the most difficult to treat as spinal cord damage is often irreversible. Immobilisation, anti-inflammatories such as steroids and surgery are the main treatments.

References

ACLS (2021). Advanced Cardiac Life Support. https://acls-algorithms.com/pediatric-advanced-life-support/pediatric-shock-overview-part-1/pals-review-obstructive-shock/#:~:text=The%20definitive%20treatment%20for%20obstructive,placement%20to%20the%20affected%20area (accessed March 2022).

AMBOSS (2020) Shock. https://www.amboss.com/us/knowledge/Shock (accessed 1 April 2020).

Annane, D., Siami, S., Jaber, S. et al. (2013). CRISTAL Investigators. Effects of fluid resuscitation with colloids vs crystalloids on mortality in critically ill patients presenting with hypovolemic shock: the CRISTAL randomized trial. *JAMA* 310(17): 1809–1817.

Dave, S. and Cho J.J. (2021) Neurogenic shock. In: StatPearls. Treasure Island (FL): StatPearls Publishing. https://www.ncbi.nlm.nih.gov/books/NBK459361/ (accessed March 2022).

de Asua, I. and Rosenberg A. (2017). On the right side of the heart: medical and mechanical support of the failing right ventricle. *J Intensive Care Soc* 18:113–120.

Dellinger, R.P., Levy, M.M., Rhodes A. et al. (2013). Surviving sepsis campaign. International guidelines for management of severe sepsis and septic shock *Crit Care Med* 41: 580–637.

Dutton, H. and Finch J. (2018). *Acute and Critical Care Nursing at a Glance*. Chichester: Wiley Blackwell.

Galvagno, S. (2014). *Emergency Pathophysiology*. Hoboken (NJ): Teton NewMedia Inc.

Gayet-Ageron, A., Prieto-Merino, D., Ker K. et al. (2018). Antifibrinolytic Trials Collaboration. Effect of treatment delay on the effectiveness and safety of antifibrinolytics in acute severe haemorrhage: a meta-analysis of individual patient-level data from 40 138 bleeding patients. *Lancet* 391(10116): 125–132.

Lavoie, L. (2018). What to know about hypovolemic shock. *Medical News Today*. https://www.medicalnewstoday.com/articles/312348.php (accessed 1 April 2020).

Mandel, J. and Palevsky, P. (2019). Treatment of severe hypovolemia or hypovolemic shock in adults. *UpToDate*. https://tinyurl.com/y9jpfk9v (accessed 1 April 2020).

National Institute for Health and Care Excellence (2017a). Composition of commonly used crystalloids. In: *Intravenous Fluid Therapy in Adults in Hospital. Clinical Guideline 174*. https://tinyurl.com/y9pgrax9 (accessed 1 April 2020).

National Institute for Health and Care Excellence (2017b). Intravenous fluid therapy in adults in hospital. Clinical guideline 174. https://www.nice.org.uk/guidance/cg174 (accessed 1 April 2020).

Peate I. (2020). *Alexander's Nursing Practice: Hospital and Home*, 5e. London: Elsevier.

Procter L. *Shock. MSD Manual* (2019). https://tinyurl.com/yd7rvjn8 (accessed 1 April 2020).

Rull, G. and Bonsall A. (2017). Resuscitation in hypovolaemic shock. Emergency medicine and trauma. Patient. https://patient.info/doctor/resuscitation-in-hypovolaemic-shock (accessed 1 April 2020).

Singer, M., Deutschman, C.S., Seymour, C.W. et al. (2016). The Third International Consensus Definitions for Sepsis and Septic Shock (Sepsis-3). *JAMA* 315,8: 801–810.

Standl, T., Annecke, T., Cascorbi, I., Heller, A.R. et al. (2018). The Nomenclature, Definition and Distinction of Types of Shock. *Deutsches Arzteblatt International* 115(45): 757–768. doi: 10.3238/arztebl.2018.0757.

Stratton S. Shock. *BMJ Best Practice*. March 2019. https://bestpractice.bmj.com/topics/en-gb/1013#referencePop4 (accessed 1 April 2020).

Taghavi, S. and Askari R. (2019). Hypovolemic shock. https://www.ncbi.nlm.nih.gov/books/NBK513297/ (accessed 1 April 2020).

UK Sepsis Trust (2018). Sepsis Screening & Action Tool. https://sepsistrust.org/wp-content/uploads/2018/06/ED-adult-NICE-Final-1107.pdf (accessed March 2022).

Vincent, J.L. and De Backer, D. (2013). Circulatory shock. *N Engl J Med* 369(18): 1726–1734.

Chapter 9

Communication

Paul Jebb

Aim

The aim of this chapter is to explore and discuss communication within the critical care environment

Learning outcomes

After reading this chapter the reader will be able to:
- Gain an undersetting of the importance of communication.
- Describe different ways to enhance communication in critical care settings.
- Gain understanding of the role of the nurse in communicating with patients.
- Gain an understanding of the role of the nurse in communicating with families.
- Reflect on your own communication skills and plan ways to enhance these.

Test your prior knowledge

- Reflect on your communication. How have you fulfilled the Nursing and Midwifery Council (2018a) Code requirements? What were the challenges in meeting these within critical care and what were the successes?
- Think about the communication methods that you used for the last patient you cared for. How did they work? Could other methods of communication have been used?
- How have you adapted existing communication methods to ensure you delivered effective communication during the COVID-19 pandemic? What has the feedback been?
- How will you ensure the adaptations you have highlighted are sustained to enhance the patient and family experience of care within critical care?
- Thinking of the four areas highlighted by Adam et al. (2015). How are your communication skills? What barriers do you find in communicating effectively? How do you overcome these? What was the feedback from the patient, family, carer, healthcare team?

Fundamentals of Critical Care: A Textbook for Nursing and Healthcare Students, First Edition. Edited by Ian Peate and Barry Hill.
© 2023 John Wiley & Sons Ltd. Published 2023 by John Wiley & Sons Ltd.
Companion website: www.wiley.com/go/peate/criticalcare

Introduction

This chapter aims to explore the importance of communication within the critical care environment. Critical care is complex, not only for the delivery of personal care, but also in relation to the environment and the enhanced care that individuals need.

Health care is becoming an increasingly multi-professional service. Nursing and nurses are at the centre of that team and pivotal in the delivery and coordination of quality person-centred care. Communication is essential not only between the nurse and the patients, but also with families, carers, multidisciplinary team members and of course each other.

All patients receiving nursing care have the right to participate and communicate their needs, this includes those cared for in critical care environment, this could, according to Johnson et al. (2021), avoid adverse medical outcomes due to the severity of the illness, their responsiveness and the level of consciousness.

The Universal Declaration of Human Rights, Article 19, section 2 (United Nations, 1948) states that 'Everyone has the right to freedom of opinion and expression: this right includes freedom to hold opinions without interference and to seek, receive and impart information and ideas through any media and regardless of frontiers', as well as outlining the principle that all people, irrespective of age, status, ability or communicative capacity have the right to communicate. The importance of communication is also highlighted in the World Health Organization's (1996) Patients' Rights, stating that people have the right to be communicated with effectively. This is also a fundamental part of the registered nurses role.

The NHS constitution (NHS, 2021) emphasises that the patient will be at the heart of everything the NHS does and that patients, with their families and carers where appropriate, will be involved in and consulted on all decisions about their care and treatment. This can also lead to challenges in patient care especially when their capacity to understand is impaired. Critical care staff need to ensure they act in the patient's best interests and this could mean enhancing communication with carers and families to understand what the patient's wishes are and what they would want.

Communication is a consistent theme within complaints about care and hospital services. The nursing team and other health care professionals need to be able to communicate effectively and to use communication methods that are appropriate to meet individual patients' needs and their understanding.

Communication is complex. Phillips (2013) states that communication involves:

- A message – statements, questions, commands
- A language – words, symbols, gestures all make up the language
- A system – communication occurs through touch, silence, voice, gestures and writing.

Using a message, a language and a system enables communication to be effective, but as communicators we also need to think about how the message is delivered.

Phillips (2013) highlights other important aspects that play a part in communication;

- Timing and speed
- Body language – eye contact, facial expressions
- Word choice
- Tone of voice – this can highlight feelings and emotions
- Proxemics – the use of space around people

The complexity relating to communication in critical care is the process of checking for understanding, which brings further challenges when patients are mechanically ventilated and unable to communicate as they may have done were they not being cared for within a critical care setting. Recently, more patients who are admitted into a critical care environment are receiving a reduction in the amount of sedation being given to them, which in itself can create new challenges as they may struggle to understand due to their impaired communication when they are conscious (Wallender Karslen et al., 2018), which could remove the notion of feeling human in a very strange and often noisy environment.

Step 1 Competencies

1.13 Communication and Teamwork
Deliver effective communication processes with patients and relatives, during clinical practice. You must be able to demonstrate through discussion essential knowledge of (and its application to your supervised practice):
The importance of:

- Focusing on the individual
- Personal space and positioning when communicating
- Body language and eye contact when communicating
- Using the individual's preferred means of communication and language
- Checking that you and the individuals understand each other
- Adapting your communication skills to aid understanding
- Active listening
- Medications
- Past medical history
- Learning disability

National Competency Framework for Registered Nurses in Adult Critical Care (2015)

6Cs: Communication

To build a relationship with patients and families, nurses and health care staff, need to ensure effective communication, when giving and receiving messages. Communication is pivotal within a critical care setting to enable decisions to be made that are person-centred, informed and understood.

99

Communication is a fundamental aspect of nursing care and is highlighted in the Nursing and Midwifery Council (NMC) Code (2018a) section 7:

Communicate clearly

To achieve this, you must:

- use terms that people in your care, colleagues and the public can understand
- take reasonable steps to meet people's language and communication needs, providing, wherever possible, assistance to those who need help to communicate their own or other people's needs
- use a range of verbal and non-verbal communication methods, and consider cultural sensitivities, to better understand and respond to people's personal and health needs
- check people's understanding from time to time to keep misunderstanding or mistakes to a minimum
- be able to communicate clearly and effectively in English

The NMC (2018a) highlight communication within the Code, but also within the essential aspects of the *Future Nurse: Standards for Proficiency for Registered Nurses* (NMC, 2018b). Communication should not only be a priority in relation to caring for patients within the critical care environment, but also with other colleagues, families and carers, this will ensure person-centred care is delivered to all those who need it and care is consistent whilst the person is being cared for in the critical care environment.

Learning event

Reflect on your communication, how have you fulfilled the NMC Code requirements? What were the challenges in meeting these requirements within the critical care arena and what were the successes?

Communicating effectively with patients

Communication with patients is an essential part of the role of all the multidisciplinary team caring for people within the critical care environment. Communication can be challenging and those staff within the critical care environment have to work together to find ways to ensure communication is effective and understood by patients whose communication can be impaired. Health care professionals must ensure that effective communication methods are devised and used with individual patients, this includes communication that uses more than words to relay essential messages to people.

Body language, facial expressions and the use of hand gestures all have an impact on the messages that are trying to be relayed. Communication will impact the individuals' care, safety and patient and family experiences of care whilst they are being care for in the critical care environment.

Communicating during a pandemic

During the COVID-19 pandemic, communication has been more challenging. This has been due to restrictions on visiting, as health care professionals we are still required to follow the policy and guidance relating to social distancing when communicating with individuals. Furthermore, the faces of staff delivering care have been very much obscured by the use of personal protective equipment (PPE) to ensure patients and staff are safe, face masks can causing voices to be muffled, with facial expressions being hidden the inability to facilitate lip reading all have had an impact on communicating with people. Wearing masks, goggles and other PPE reduces the ability to communicate non-verbally, preventing the observation of facial expressions, lip movements and other non-verbal cues (Mitchell and Hill, 2020). The use of face masks cause challenges when there is a need for others to lip read, the use of clear face masks can be a challenge to access and this is having an effect on care delivery to some groups of people, for example, those with a learning disability and those who lip read.

6Cs: Care

Care is what nurses do, this must be person-centred, support the individuals' needs as well as supporting those around them.

People receiving care need it to safe and effective, enabling their needs to be met

Health care professionals strive to develop effective communication methods that are used between themselves and the critically ill person. These methods have gone beyond the use of voice and have included the use of photographs to ensure the patient knows what the person caring for them looks like under their PPE and also what their name is by writing this on their gown or aprons. This enables some barriers to be broken down and enables the patient or family member to build some form of relationship with the professional delivering the care. The use of digital solutions to communication challenges have been paramount during COVID-19, not only with regard to communicating with the patient, but as a result of restrictions in visiting; digital solutions allow the patient to have input from the world outside of the critical care unit, see familiar faces and engage in conversations with other people outside the health care team.

Snapshot

Life Lines was established in March 2020 to support virtual visiting, and prides itself in the partnership working across clinical care, academia and innovation. Take a look at the Life Lines website (https://www.kingshealthpartners.org/our-work/lifelines) and review your organisation's involvement and how this would impact on patients.

Life Lines uses secure, safe virtual visiting methods at the patient's bedside. This will also help to reduce a sense of isolation and separation due to visiting restrictions during the COVID-19 pandemic.

Virtual visits can also allow time with clinicians so they can communicate with families, report progress and plans moving forward in the care of their loved one.

There are other specific interventions that can facilitate the use of voice which can be used within critical care. Colleagues from the speech and language therapy team are essential partners in care to enable interactions to occur and enhance the individual's care with the aim of supporting their communication needs.

These interventions could include, if, for example, a person is neck breathing:

- above cuff vocalisation
- leak speech
- in-line speaking valves

All of these interventions could be used but extra precaution is needed when using aerosol-generating procedures. At all times local policy and procedure must be adhered to.

Alternative communication methods could be used which could be high and low technological solutions for example pen and paper, facial expressions, lip reading, use of speaking valves, picture boards and alphabet boards. Many other solutions can be found within other specialities across the health and social care sector which have been used for many years, for example, finger spelling and electronic voice communication aids. Often more than one method is required as no one single method can work alone and many working solutions rely on staff ensuring that communication is given the priority it deserves. Johnson et al. (2021) found that patients were more satisfied and less stressed about their care and treatment when alternative communication methods were used to ensure they were involved in their care, and aware of the future plans to aid their recovery.

Technology can also act as a barrier: the noise, the lights as well as a reliance on technology rather than on person-centred care. Alternative communication strategies can also create potential barriers, as teams may consider them a challenge to use, and they may take extra time to set up, prepare and use, which will slow the communication process – that is, if staff are aware of alternative tools that can be accessed and used within the critical care department (Carruthers

et al., 2017). Nurses are experts at overcoming barriers, and through their advocacy role can ensure that the patient receives the care they need as well as respecting the patient's choices and cultural beliefs (Beeby, 2000).

As professional registered nurses, we need to ensure that the initial assessment clarifies what the patient's first language is and what language they wish to receive communication in. A nurse (or other professional) that does not communicate in the patient's first language could have a detrimental effect on the patient's understanding. Across health care we also have our own language as well as nursing and medical jargon. In order to communicate effectively the nursing and health care team need to be aware of the language – including acronyms – they are using, ensuring that this can be easily understood by the patients, their family and other members of the health care team.

Education and an understanding of the various solutions to overcome communication barriers are needed. These challenges have to be overcome to ensure that communication, engagement and involvement in care is prioritised. At times families may be need to be shown and taught how to use some of the various communication tools as well to ensure engagement and effective communication to make certain that messages are delivered effectively to those who need them. This will take time, and health care professionals need to prioritise this to enable ongoing effective communication with individuals.

Orange Flag

When there are ineffective channels of communication this can have a negative impact on health and wellbeing (for all parties). It is essential to ensure as far as possible that all interactions with patients, families and other members of the health care team are focused and effective. Poor communication and inappropriate communication methods can lead to confusion, frustration, stress and unwanted tensions.

The use of digital communication methods has been essential during the COVID-19 pandemic. This has enabled families to gain reassurance, to be involved in care, as well as supporting the delivery of care. This has been shown to reduce episodes of delirium by giving the patient a familiar voice to hear in the unfamiliar and noisy world of critical care.

Learning event

Take some time to think about how have you adapted existing communication methods to ensure that you delivered effective communication during the COVID-19 pandemic. What has the feedback been? Is there anything that you might have done differently?

6Cs: Commitment

A commitment to care is an essential role of the nurse; indeed, it is espoused throughout the Code (NMC, 2018a). Nurses need to have commitment to always strive to deliver high-quality, safe and effective care for patients and their families in all care settings.

Communication with families

Having a family member requiring care within a critical care environment is worrying for all concerned and this may cause stress and a variety of emotional responses from families. Families can be terrified when they visit the critical care area: the noise, overhearing others talking, other families' emotional responses, seeing other patients. These can be amplified if their loved one's prognosis is poor (McAdam et al., 2010).

Learning event

Reflect on a difficult communication you had with a family member. How effective was your communication? What response did the family member have? How did you react to the emotional response? How can you develop even further your communication skills with families of those who are being cared for in a critical care setting?

A fundamental skill of nursing relates to the ability to be able to connect to others and their families. Emotional intelligence is essential to demonstrate trust and commitment (Morse, 1991). The nature of nurse–patient relationships is dependent on when and where nursing care is delivered, being able to build a professional relationship and build rapport. This will not only support families at this distressing time but also enable questions to be asked, enable them understand the care being delivered and the environment that it is delivered in, and enable and encourage families to be involved in care – this will include involvement in decision making and discussions about future care delivery and care planning. When nurses don't communicate effectively, this will affect the nurse–patient relationship as well as break down the relationship with family members, who will be anxious when their loved one is being cared for within the critical care environment, as well as not delivering person-centred care. It will also lead to an inability to ensure shared decision making is achieved. The need for patient-centred communication is essential to enable positive continuity of patient care, patient safety and health outcomes (Johnson et al., 2021).

If families feel that they are unable to be involved in care provision, or it is inappropriate for them to be involved, then the decision-making process or discussions relating to the care of their family member may add to their anxiety. Person-centred care delivery and multidisciplinary care should have family members and carers at the heart, alongside the patient themselves where this is appropriate.

In a literature review in 2015 Adam et al. found results relating to four major themes when communication with families, these were:

Nurses as information and communication facilitators

This relates to the nurse's role in giving families understanding of what is happening and what the future will bring and supporting families coming to terms with potential outcomes.

Nurses as family support providers

This was seen as essential in the development of the nurse: family relationship, gaining trust, supporting hopes, supporting spiritual needs and supporting those who wanted to be closer to the patient during the delivery of care.

Nurses' non-specific behaviours

The Adam et al. (2015) review found a theme relating to behaviours nurses showed, which had an impact in reducing the amount of time that they delivered active care they offered families and also showed how nurses perceived families. This included avoiding emotional overload as well as avoiding increasing anxiety and stress. To avoid this nurses, needed further development, time and space to learn and deliver messages to families, as well as support in doing this; it takes courage for nurses to say, 'Sorry I don't know the answer to that. . .' as well as saying 'Can I get back to you on that. . .'

Health care professionals can at times deprive patients of their right to communicate by not giving some patients the opportunity to be part of their care, and be involved in their own decision making, as part of a shared care process and shared decision making (Johnson et al., 2021)

Improving nurses' communication skills

Nurses feel they are good communicators. Communication is a fundamental subject within pre-registration nurse education regardless of the field of study the individual student is enrolled in. Nurses' communication skills have been developed through their initial pre-registration education, through their individual experiences, through observation of how other health care professionals communicate as well as through their own professional experiences. Individuals and their managers need to ensure their communication skills are updated and nurses are able to access funded professional development in relation to communication skills, training and upskilling.

6Cs: Courage

Nurses need courage to do the right thing for the people they offer care and support to. If things are not right, we need to say so. This is also known as a Duty of Candour. If we cannot communicate effectively, we need to say and look at how we need to develop to enable appropriate communication to occur.

Nurses are central to the health care team, and are the constant professional group who are delivering care 24/7. They need to bring the health care team together, with the patient at the centre, as well as ensuring their family are involved in care, and communication is shared across the whole of the team, ensuring continuity of care and decision making with the patient and family at the heart of care (Propp et al., 2010).

Learning event

Think of the four areas highlighted by Adam et al. (2015) and rate your communication skills. Can you identify any barriers when you are making all efforts to communicate effectively? How do you overcome these? What was the outcome for the patient, family, carer and team?

Conclusion

Effective communication with patients and families within critical care environments is essential to person-centred care delivery, but communication in such environments can be a challenge. There are many resources that the nurse can use to overcome these challenges; however, these can take time to implement and develop, they may need some personal development and may also require support from the wider health care team as well in order to get this very import activity right. People cared for within a critical care unit are often unable to make their own decisions, which means that family members need to take on this responsibility (Shaw et al., 2014), communication methods need to be assessed with the family members and care plans developed accordingly to ensure that the whole team providing care and offering support are aware of what methods are to be used to enhance communication and understanding for the patient and their family.

In order to deliver true person-centred care, effective communication along with strong nurse–patient relationships are essential. Nurses need to develop their communication skills; the use of the nurse's reflective skills will highlight areas to develop and potential further learning which they may need to undertake in order to continue to enhance their communication skills.

Take home points

1. Communication is a fundamental aspect of delivering holistic care within the critical care environment.
2. Effective communication can reduce anxiety and stress.
3. Families need to be involved with care if they feel able, even when visiting is restricted.
4. Communication across the whole multidisciplinary team enables continuation of care and patient/family involvement in decision making.
5. Nurses need support to develop their communication skills.
6. Communication needs to be reassessed at regular intervals to ensure the best methods are being used.
7. An essential part of communication is ensuring understanding.
8. Innovation and the use of digital resources can enhance and benefit communication with patients, families and across the whole multidisciplinary team.

References

Adams, A.M.N., Mannix, T., and Harrington, A. (2015). Nurses' communication with families in the intensive care unit – a literature review. *Nursing In Critical Care* 22(2): 70–80.

Beeby, J.P. (2000). Intensive care nurses' experiences of caring Part 2. *Intensive and Critical Care Nursing* 16: 151–163.

Carruthers, H., Astin, F., and Munro, W. (2017). Which alternative communication methods are effective for voiceless patients within intensive care units: A systemic review. *Intensive Crit Care Nurse* 42: 88–96.

Johnson, E., Heyns, T., and Nilsson, S. (2021). Nurses' perspectives on alternative communication strategies use in critical care units. *Nurs Crit Care* 27(1): 120–129.

McAdam, J.L., Dracup, K.A., White, D.B. et al. (2010). Symptom experiences of family members of intensive care patients at high risk of dying. *Critical Care Medicine* 38: 1078–1085.

Mitchell, A. and Hill, B. (2020). How to communicate effectively while wearing face masks. *Practice Nursing* 31(12): 508–510.

Morse, J.M. (1991). Negotiating commitment and involvement in the nurse-patient relationship. *Journal of Advanced Nursing* 17: 809–821.

National Competency Framework for Registered Nurses in Adult Critical Care (2015). https://www.cc3n.org.uk/uploads/9/8/4/2/98425184/02_new_step_2_final.pdf (accessed February 2021).

NHS. (2021). NHS Constitution. https://www.gov.uk/government/publications/the-nhs-constitution-for-england/the-nhs-constitution-for-england (accessed March 2022).

Nursing and Midwifery Council (2018a). The Code. Professional Standards of Practice and Behaviour for Nurses, Midwives and Nursing Associates. www.nmc.org.uk/globalassets/sitedocuments/nmc-publications/nmc-code.pdf (accessed March 2021).

Nursing and Midwifery Council (2018b). Future Nurse: Standards of Proficiency for Registered Nurses. https://www.nmc.org.uk/standards/standards-for-nurses/ (accessed March 2021).

Phillips, A. (2013). *Developing Leadership Skills for Health and Social Care Professionals*. London: Radcliffe Publishing.

Propp, K. Apker, J., Zabave Ford, W. et al. (2010). Meeting the complex needs of the health care team: identification of nurse – team communication practices perceived to enhance patient outcomes. *Qualitative Health Research* 20(1): 15–28.

Shaw, D., Davidson, J., Smilde, R. et al. (2014). Multidisciplinary team training to enhance family communication in the ICU. *Crit Care Med* 42(2): 265–271.

United Nations (1948). *Universal Declaration of Human Rights*. United Nations.

Wallender Karlsen, M. Alexandra Olnes, M., and Guntenberg Heyn, L. (2018). Communication with patients a scoping review. *British Association of Critical Care Nurses* 24(3): 115–131.

Chapter 10

Electronic health records

Timothy Kuhn

Aim

The aim of this chapter is to introduce the reader to the operational and professional elements related to the keeping of effective electronic health records (EHRs) within the critical care setting.

Learning outcomes

After reading this chapter the reader will be able to:

- Understand your responsibilities and the law in relation to the use of EHRs.
- Understand the different types of EHRs in critical care and how they are used.
- Know what patient data is available within the critical care unit and how this is recorded in an electronic health record.
- Understand how EHRs are used in critical care audit and research.
- Develop awareness of the benefits and barriers to EHRs.

Test your prior knowledge

- What legislation governs the way data is used and handled?
- Describe some of the barriers to effective use of EHRs.
- What is a Clinical Information System?
- How can EHRs improve quality care?

Fundamentals of Critical Care: A Textbook for Nursing and Healthcare Students, First Edition. Edited by Ian Peate and Barry Hill.
© 2023 John Wiley & Sons Ltd. Published 2023 by John Wiley & Sons Ltd.
Companion website: www.wiley.com/go/peate/criticalcare

Introduction

This chapter will highlight some of main EHR systems commonly used and give examples of how an EHR system can be utilised when caring for a critically unwell patient. It will also highlight considerations that need to be made when using an EHR system such as information governance and explore how EHR functionality is used not only by clinicians at the bedside but also for audit and research purposes.

Digitisation within healthcare

Digitisation within healthcare is not a new concept, computers first started to be used within healthcare back in the 1970s and were initially used for administrative and research purposes. However, uptake and development of technology has been slow. In 2013 the National Audit Office reported that the government's digital agenda had failed to meet its objectives. These included establishing an integrated electronic health record system across secondary care but they did recognise that some important national digital services and infrastructures had been created (National Audit Office, 2013).

Electronic health records (EHRs)

Electronic health records are defined as electronically maintained information about individuals' health status and healthcare stored in such a way that allows multiple legitimate users to access the record. The evidence base for EHR systems has evolved over recent years. The evolution of EHRs is documented as far back as 1999 (Shortliffe, 1999). At that time, it was noted that healthcare organisations were developing integrated clinical work stations that provided a single point of access to administrative and research information. The publication went on to note that having electronic records allows clinical information to be kept accessible, confidential and secure. It was also highlighted that the paper-based medical record was 'woefully inadequate'. Now that innovation in technology has allowed EHRs to be integrated with other digital systems, EHRs have been shown to improve efficiency and quality of healthcare provision.

The NHS Long Term Plan and technology

The National Health Service Long Term Plan (2019) recognises that healthcare continues to be radically reshaped by new innovation and technology. The plan describes how there had been a significant delivery of high-quality digital systems over the previous three years prior to publication of the plan and note as an example that electronic patient prescriptions were used in 93% of England's 7,300 GP practices. Amongst its 10 pledges relating to digitally enhanced care, the NHS Long Term Plan commits to ensuring that clinicians can:

- Access and interact with patient care records wherever they are
- Capture data for clinicians that will reduce the administrative burden
- Protect patient privacy
- Ensure the security of health record systems and
- Encourage software development and innovation.

The Health and Care Act 2022 sets out plans to reform the NHS in a move to deliver more joined-up care. The Act introduces the requirement for all of England to be covered by an integrated care system.

Data security

Guidelines for the Provision of Intensive Care Services (GPICS) (2nd edition), published by The Intensive Care Society (ICS) (2019), discusses Clinical Information Systems (CIS), a system used within critical care which encompasses various EHRs and other electronic data systems which collect patient data. The guidance document highlights that a CIS can lead to efficient working, reduction in errors and greater compliance with standards in relation to clinical records as well as improved data reporting. EHRs in the critical care setting can be utilised in a number of different ways, not simply a stand-alone mechanism for documenting a care intervention – for example EHRs can be used in a broader sense in the surveillance of bloodstream infections from central venous catheter insertion and in the monitoring of unit mortality rates. A retrospective study conducted by Flatow et al. (2015) evaluated the key quality measures within a surgical intensive care unit (SICU) following implementation of the Apollo EHR system in a tertiary hospital, and the study demonstrated that after the implementation of the EHR system, the rate of central line-associated blood stream infection (CLABSI) was 85% lower than prior to the implementation of the EHR system.

Barriers to further development of EHRs

Although EHR systems can be of significant benefit, it is important to note that there can be barriers to their effective use such as a lack of interoperability (where one record cannot transfer across different EHR systems), errors in medical information and lack of financial commitment required to accommodate the technology.

Errors and personal responsibility

It is also important not to ignore the fact that medical errors can still occur despite the increase in information being gathered about patients through the use of EHRs. A literature review conducted in 2010 by Chan et al. looked at the reliability and validity of EHRs and found that in all the studies they reviewed relating to electronic recording, significant errors were reported in relation to medication lists. These errors where mainly attributed to retention of medications on electronic drug charts that should have been discontinued and incorrect medication regimens. It is therefore important that clinicians not only receive sufficient training on electronic health record systems but also validate data entries themselves without relying on the system to be correct.

Understanding your responsibilities and the law in relation to record keeping

Professional responsibility for record keeping

All clinicians have a responsibility to look after and protect personal information relating to patients. This is not only a moral responsibility but also a legal and professional responsibility.

The Nursing and Midwifery Council (NMC) (2018) require registrants to ensure that they keep clear and accurate records. This includes EHRs. In February 2020 an NMC Fitness Practice Committee heard an example of where a registrant had not practised in line with The Code and amongst other charges had copied and pasted electronic notes from one patient's records to another, detailing clinical assessments which had not been undertaken. As part of the panel's conclusions, they deemed that the registrant had practised dishonestly, and was subsequently struck off the register.

It is not only professional regulators that outline the responsibility for accurate and safe record keeping, whether that be paper-based or electronic. The Royal College of Nursing, a union that represents nurses and other healthcare workers, explain that record keeping is a vital component of nursing as it aids effective communication as well as being an integral part of maintaining patient safety (RCN, 2019).

The responsibilities of record keeping do not apply only to the nursing profession. The Royal College of Anaesthetists' guidelines (RCOA, 2021) talks about the requirements of anaesthesia in the non-theatre environment and emphasises that accurate records of the anaesthetic must be maintained.

Red Flag being aware of your local systems

There are various EHR systems used within critical care. The systems used will vary from unit to unit and depend on which system an individual organisation adopts. Although there are set standards of what functionalities and guidance on how the EHR system should be implemented, there is not a standard system across the UK.

It is important therefore to receive training on the systems your unit uses to reduce the risk of error. The Nursing and Midwifery Council (NMC) (2018) require registrants to ensure that they keep clear and accurate records. This includes electronic records.

Intensive Care Society Guidelines

The Intensive Care Society (ICS), a charity which provides guidance, research and educational resources relating to intensive care, provides guidance on EHRs and CISs and how critical care units should implement and manage these systems. Within their Guidelines For the Provision of Intensive Care Services 2019 (GPICS 2), the ICS state that staff should receive adequate training to use a CIS and the CIS should have adequate security measures such as the functionality for smartcards to be used.

Data protection

The rules and standards set by professional regulations and other regulatory bodies is underpinned by law regarding data protection and record keeping. The European Union (EU) General Data Protection Regulations (GDPR) added extra responsibilities to the Data Protection Act 1998 on the 25 May, 2018. At the core of GDPR are key principles, which do not act as hard rules, but instead work as an overarching framework that is designed to lay out the broad purposes of GDPR. The principles are largely the same as those that existed under previous data protection laws:

1. Lawfulness fairness and transparency
2. Purpose limitation
3. Data minimisation
4. Accuracy
5. Storage limitation
6. Integrity and confidentiality (security)

All businesses that handle personal data had to ensure that they were aware of the new regulations and had to examine the processes they previously had in place to ensure they continued to comply with the law. GDPR can be considered the world's strongest set of data protection rules, detailing how people can access information about other individuals. In the context of a patient in a critical care setting, these rules set limits on what organisations can do with personal data.

6Cs: Competence

In order to provide effective care and ensure that EHRs are being used appropriately, clinicians should receive training to maintain their competence.

Data security

In relation to security techniques that protect EHRs and CISs, a systematic review conducted by Kruse et al. (2017) looked at the most common security techniques used by healthcare organisations for EHRs and the frequency of data breaches. The authors reviewed 25 articles and were able to identify three themes that aided the security of EHRs. These themes included:

- Administrative, which focused on system security and contingency planning
- Technical, which looked at issues around system virus protection and
- Audit trails and physical, which looked at workstation security and access control.

The authors concluded that privacy and security concerns present the largest and most important barrier to adopting EHRs. However, they identified a number of methods health organisations can use that have proved to be successful for ensuring privacy and security of EHRs. For example, within critical care units that use EHRs/CISs, clinicians will often be given a username and password that logs then into each system, or they may be issued with a 'smartcard' (Figure 10.1) which grants them access to the EHR/CIS.

In practice it is the individual practitioner's/clinician's responsibility to ensure that they are aware of their own employer's policies and guidelines in relation to record keeping and EHRs, including the security systems in place in relation to accessing a CIS as well the understanding of local policy. It is also important for clinicians to understand the principles of GDPR, this ensures that the clinician is practising in a way that keeps patient-sensitive information safe.

Red Flag are you data compliant?

Data breaches are serious as potentially sensitive information is shared. To reduce the risk of you being involved in a data breach, ensure that you are familiar with the principles of GDPR and local policies and procedures where you work.

Understanding the different types of EHRs in critical care and how they are used

There are a number of different companies that supply EHR systems to healthcare organisations. It is the decision of a specific organisation as to what system(s) they adopt and implement. The main EHR systems used by critical care clinicians can be divided into three main categories: imaging systems, tests and results, and clinical documentation.

Imaging systems

Radiology information systems (RISs) have been used since the 1970s. Historically, a picture archiving and communication systems (PACS), a RIS which allows clinicians to review radiological imaging, was used exclusively in large academic medical centres and was usually expensive, cumbersome and lacked the ability to integrate with a CIS. However, they paved the way for filmless medical imaging. Over the years the cost of PACS has reduced and computer power has increased, which makes this system a justifiable alternative (Arenson et al., 2000). In the critical care environment electronic imaging systems allow clinicians to rapidly review radiological images and reports, which can guide patient treatment and intervention.

Test and result systems

Electronic requesting of laboratory tests and radiological imaging within critical care is common as well as reviewing these results and reports via an EHR. Once the sample request has been made by either the nursing or medical team, the label for the specimen can be printed by inserting the patient's hospital number into the system or by scanning a bar code on the patient's hospital wrist band. This ensures that the correct label is printed, and the correct specimen is sent for the correct patient. Once the samples have been received by the laboratory, the staff use the laboratory information system (LIS) to process the samples. Once processed, the sample results can be reviewed within

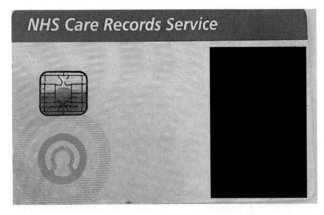
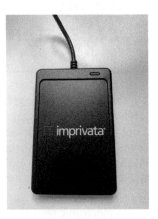

Figure 10.1   Smartcard and smartcard reader.

the system itself and often these systems are integrated into the CIS. In addition to laboratory tests, these systems can be used to request radiological tests such as ultrasounds, CT scans and X-rays. These electronic requests can usually be made by any trained member of the clinical team; however, it is important to note that some requests may be governed by other legislation, such as Ionising Radiation Medical Exposure Regulation (IRMER), which limits radiological requesting to those clinicians that have undertaken additional training covering the risk of radiation exposure (DHSC, 2018).

Clinical documentation

Electronic clinical documentation systems allow members of the multidisciplinary team such as the therapy teams and external visiting teams to document their assessment of a patient and progress made. A publication by Burton et al. (2004) highlighted the benefit of sharing of EHRs by the multidisciplinary team as clinicians treating people in a variety of settings are able to exchange and continuously update a patient's clinical record and then present the information in logical clinical groupings that other clinicians can access easily. When a team makes a clinical entry the electronic document falls into a relevant grouping. For example, if a member of the medical team makes an entry this will fall within the medical notes section and when a member of the therapy team documents an entry this will fall within the therapy grouping. Clinical documentation systems EHR will often be able to import data from other EHR systems such as test and result systems. This creates efficient working for clinicians as less time is spent manually copying data.

> # Learning event: Reflection
>
> Think about a critically unwell patient you have looked after recently. How could you utilise some of the EHR systems outlined above to provide more efficient care to that patient?

Despite there being a wide range of EHR platform suppliers, when these systems are categorised into their functions it can be appreciated that these systems have similar applications. Clinicians should ensure they have received appropriate training on the systems that their organisation use and should gain familiarity with the breadth of each of these systems in order to use them to their full potential.

> # 6Cs: Compassion
>
> When using an EHR, clinicians must still deliver care in a compassionate way by involving the patient in their care and decision making where possible.

Understanding what patient data is available within the critical care unit and how this is recorded in an electronic health record

The critical care bed space (Figure 10.2) can at first seem complex with a number of different machines, pumps and devices. However, as clinicians become more familiar with this environment, they can begin to appreciate the amount of data that is produced from these pieces of equipment and how this data can feed into the patient's EHR.

Monitoring a patient within the critical care unit differs from monitoring a patient on a ward as ward-based patients generally do not require the high-level monitoring carried out within the critical care unit and therefore less data is captured and entered into the EHR.

In the critical care setting patients are continuously monitored usually due to the severity of their condition and/or drugs that they are receiving which require specialised monitoring.

Most of the data within the critical care bedspace that comes from a machine such as the bedside monitor and ventilator automatically populates into the EHR. When the clinician wants to permanently record this data into the record they will be required to manually review the data on the EHR to ensure its accuracy and then, in order for the data to be permanently recorded, to validate the data by entering a password.

This system of machines integrating with the EHR is known as a Clinical Information System (CIS). Clinical Information Systems capture, store and process information and can display the data in graphs and tables for clinicians to then view. CISs are also often able to integrate with other hospital systems such as radiology and laboratory systems (Islam et al., 2018).

The Guidelines for the Provision of Intensive Care Services 2019 (GPICS 2) state that CISs should be part of an EHR and should include data capture from patient monitoring, infusion devices, ventilators, cardiac output devices, temperature management devices, intra-aortic balloon pumps, extracorporeal life support (ECLS) devices, blood gas analysers and renal replacement therapy (RRT) devices. But there is other data within the critical care bedspace which cannot be captured automatically by a CIS as it is not normally processed electronically. This data includes measurements such as drain and catheter outputs, if the patient has a pressure ulcer and devices that are being used to prevent deep vein thrombosis (DVT). The clinician has to manually enter this information into the EHR and again validate it by entering a password.

Hospitals are now moving towards greater use of EHR systems in all clinical areas and this means that even in a

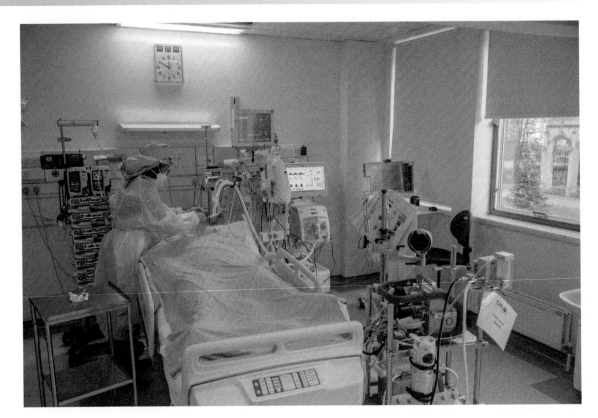

Figure 10.2   Critical care bedspace.

ward environment, where patients generally do not require continuous monitoring, a patient's vital signs data is either uploaded automatically or entered manually into an EHR instead of a paper chart.

This electronic recording of observations has linked in with the roll-out of the National Early Warning Score (NEWS) – a scoring system (now in revised version NEWS2) in ward-based environments, which acts as a method of detecting deteriorating patients. The published NEWS2 guidance from the Royal College of Physicians (RCP, 2017) notes that hospitals, at the time the guidance was published, were integrating the NEWS2 score into an EHR system. Subsequently mobile applications have been created whereby a NEWS2 score can be entered and calculated automatically. The advantage of this automated calculation of the NEWS2 score and subsequent automated alert system is that the system is not reliant on clinicians manually calculating scores and escalating a patient's care, which can result in errors due to inaccurate calculation and lack of verbal communication between teams. This technology has been utilised in other environments such as GP practices. Nevertheless is it vital to remember that importing the results electronically does not remove the risk of inaccurate recording. An observational study conducted in Denmark by Pederson et al. (2017) found that the NEWS2 score recorded manually and then transferred into an electronic form had an inaccuracy rate of 10%. The authors highlighted that the continual transferring of data was a limitation of the system not being fully automated.

6Cs: Courage

Clinicians must have the courage to speak up and alert the team if a mistake has been made in transferring data into an EHR.

Some clinical settings now have an integrated system in which observations are automatically uploaded to an EHR when monitored. This data is again validated by the clinician to ensure its accuracy and then the NEWS2 score is calculated automatically by algorithms within the system. This reduces the error of inaccurate data transfer as the clinician is not manually entering the data but still requires the clinician to validate the data that has been obtained by the system.

Understanding how EHRs are used in critical care audit and research

EHR use in research and audit

With the increased use of EHRs over recent years, these systems have played an important part in clinical audit and research by allowing clinicians to easily access clinical data and other clinical information such as imaging. Utilising EHRs for clinical audit and research not only allows researchers and auditors access to a large amount of data but has also been recognised as less resource-intense compared to traditional methods (Coorevits et al., 2013).

With the recent COVID-19 global pandemic, researchers have used EHRs as a means of obtaining a wealth of data to share with the international healthcare community, During the pandemic, EHRs have been used to collect demographic, clinical laboratory and radiological findings (Wang et al., 2020). Collecting data in this way enables researchers to share this information with the wider healthcare community. Rapidly obtaining data from EHRs and then sharing results allows clinicians to forward think and plan ahead. A recent single-centre randomised control trial (RCT) that looked at cytokine adsorption in patients with severe COVID-19 pneumonia requiring extracorporeal membrane oxygenation (ECMO) (Supady et al., 2021) used an EHR to obtain clinical data. The clinical data obtained in this trial was vast and included patient demographics, laboratory values, comorbidities, pre-ECMO treatments, ventilation parameters and blood gas values. The trial, which included 34 patients over a nine-month period, involved inserting a cytokine adsorption device into the ECMO circuit to establish if a cytokine adsorption device reduced serum cytokine (a protein released by the immune system) levels and had an effect on patient outcome. The trial found that early initiation of cytokine adsorption in patients with severe COVID-19 did not significantly reduce serum cytokine levels and had a negative effect on survival, This study not only provides an answer to the trial question but also demonstrates the range of data that can be obtained from an EHR for the purposes of research. Using EHRs in this way to share data with the wider medical community will no doubt become more common, especially as a result of the challenges caused by the latest pandemic.

6Cs: Communication

Communicating research to the global healthcare community enhances patient care.

In addition to research that answers specific clinical questions, there is also research underway that is investigating how EHRs can assist clinicians in their clinical practice and decision making. An RCT by Courtwright et al. commenced in 2018 (PONDER-ICU) is currently being conducted in which an EHR system will prompt clinicians to document a prognostic estimate of a patient's functional outcomes and document a justification if a clinician decides not to offer a patient the option of comfort orientated care. This trial aims to collect data on the rate of clinician adherence, response to intervention as well as challenges faced in implementing an EHR based trial. This demonstrates the versatility of EHRs and their use within clinical research.

EHR use in monitoring performance

In addition to research, EHRs have in recent years been used for monitoring of performance of critical care units and monitoring of quality outcomes. A literature review by DeMellow and Kim (2018) looked at how EHRs can be utilised for monitoring and providing feedback in relation to delivering quality care and improving patient outcomes through the use of evidence-based care bundles. From the literature reviewed, the study found that there had been a reported improvement in compliance following the implementation of an electronic-based monitoring and feedback system, compliance with care bundles rose from 3% to 60%.

Additionally, in the UK a collaboration of professional organisations representing adult, paediatric and neonatal intensive care, microbiology, and infection control which is supported by Public Health England (PHE), known as the Infection in Critical Care Quality Improvement Programme (ICCQIP), involves critical care units submitting data in relation to blood cultures that have a positive growth indicating a blood stream infection. The data submitted is obtained from laboratory EHR systems and allows microbiology and critical care teams to monitor the occurrence of blood stream infections (www.ficm.ac.uk/ICCQIP), this collection of data from EHRs and submission to a national database enables units to benchmark against each other and share good practice.

As well as aiding research and audit, EHRs have been used to create predictive models in order to improve patient outcomes, a study by Kaewprag et al. (2017) used data from an EHR in order to construct Bayesian networks from features of critical care patients in order to predict incidence of pressure ulcers. By obtaining data in this way the authors where able to develop predictive models that identified patients at risk of pressure ulcers, allowing clinicians to appropriately respond to patients with certain conditions associated with a higher incidence of pressure ulcers

It is evident that EHRs play a significant role in modern-day clinical research and audit. Using EHRs for these purposes not only allows clinicians access to a wide range of readily accessible data that can be shared with other clinicians globally but also allows critical care units to easily audit and improve their own clinical practices.

Learning event: reflection: using EHRs to improve patient care

Think of a quality improvement project you have been involved in. What functions of an EHR could you use to evaluate current performance and eventually improve patient outcomes?

Understanding the benefits and barriers to EHRs

EHRs have been shown to be of benefit in the clinical environment but they can also pose their own challenges. It is important therefore not only to appreciate the benefits but also to understand the challenges on EHRs. Table 10.1 summarises some of the benefits and barriers to EHRs.

Table 10.1   EHRs: benefits and barriers.

Benefits
Improved communication
Increased time efficiency
Reduction in prescribing errors
Ability to trigger a clinical response
Ability to automatically calculate clinical scores such as NEWS2

Barriers
Cost
Adoption by senior clinicians
Lack of training
Lack of interoperability of the EHR system
Integration of other electronic systems

Benefits of EHRs

The benefits an EHR provides in relation to clinical application, research and audit has previously been discussed and it has been reported that EHR users find that these systems improve clinical decision making, communication and their adoption can be related to a reduction in medication errors (Palabindala et al., 2016).

Regarding clinical decision making, non-adherence to evidence-based practice can be linked to not having sufficient access to a clinical guideline, not being aware a guideline is available and a lack of available time to find a particular guideline, EHRs have been linked with increased adherence to evidence-based practice through the linkage of clinical intervention and having evidence easily accessible via the EHR. A good example of this is the finding by researchers that computerised physician reminders increased the use of influenza and pneumococcal vaccinations from 0% to 35% for hospitalised patients (Dexter et al., 2001).

In the critical care setting, electronic prescribing is one aspect of EHRs that is widely used and has been shown to reduce medication errors. An observational study by Donyal et al. (2007) noted a 1.8% reduction in prescribing errors following the introduction of electronic prescribing.

Communication is an important factor when caring for the critically unwell patient but can be challenging in the fast-paced and complex environment of a critical care unit. Critical care research has shown poor communication between team members to be a common causal factor underlying adverse events (Wright et al., 1991). Recent studies have suggested that EHRs improve multidisciplinary team communication within the critical care team. A study by Bhise et al. (2018) looked at whether using data within an EHR to initiate a trigger system to flag patients that required escalation to critical care and/or needed a rapid response team review prevented patient harm. This observational study found that using EHR data to trigger a rapid response team review and/or escalation to critical care prevented adverse events and diagnostic errors.

Communication through EHRs is not limited to the acute phase of a patient's admission within critical care. EHRs have been shown to be of benefit during the rehabilitation phases of a patient's critical care journey. A cohort study (Anderson et al., 2018) looked at multidisciplinary communication within the critical care unit in relation to mobilisation of patients. The study was conducted in two phases – in phase one of the study staff members participated in an online learning module about a mobility protocol and mobility grading scale. Then in phase two a communication tool within the EHR was used to communicate mobility levels to all members of the MDT. The study demonstrated a statistically significant improvement in staff satisfaction with using the communication tool as well as a reduction in time for patients to reach a mobility goal, reduction in length of critical care stay and an average reduction in ventilation time of 27 hours.

6Cs: Care

Communicating to the wider team through an EHR is a component of care that benefits the patient and clinicians.

Barriers to implementation

Despite the documented benefits of EHRs there are some barriers to implementation and adoption of these systems.

The accuracy of EHR systems is heavily reliant on other electronic systems that feed into the EHR, for example if the CIS does not record accurate data into the EHR this could be missed or if noticed, the clinician would be required to manually change the data. This in turn would make using the EHR less time-efficient and would risk inaccurate records and potentially result in disengagement from clinicians.

Other barriers that can affect the implementation of EHRs include cost implications., The exact cost of implementing an EHR is difficult to ascertain but it is obvious from the scale of government investment that it comes at great cost. In 2015 the government announced it would invest £1 billion in new technology over the proceeding 5 years and

NHS England committed £100 million to support the delivery of comprehensive EHRs (Clarke et al., 2017). Although this might seem a generous level of funding, when spread across the entire National Health Service and taking into account others factors such as training and hardware one can see how implementation of these systems becomes very costly for individual hospitals.

Buy-in from clinicians

As discussed, two significant points to consider are the training of staff to use an EHR and the adoption of electronic systems by senior clinicians and managers. In order for an EHR system to be adopted by clinicians, consideration must be given to how these systems are implemented. A narrative review by Ajami and Arab-Chadegani (2013) examined 32 articles and reports with the aim of identifying the factors that limit the implementation of an EHR system. In the study the authors found that the main barriers to implementation of an EHR system were the disparity between the cost and the benefits of using an electronic system as well as technical issues, system interoperability and a lack of leadership for the implementation of such a system. This highlights the need for electronic systems to be implemented in a way that clearly demonstrates that their benefit outweighs the cost. To be successful, electronic systems need to be launched with the correct leadership and infrastructure in place. If EHRs are launched without this then adoption and engagement from clinicians is likely to fail (Atasoy et al., 2019).

6Cs: Commitment

For an EHR system to be effective and benefit patient care, clinicians must show commitment to the adoption and implementation of these systems.

Whilst there is a wealth of benefit to implementing and using EHRs, their success also relies on a number of factors which include how user-friendly the systems are, whether staff receive appropriate training and how these systems are adopted by senior clinicians. Significant barriers to EHRs remain the cost and how other systems integrate with the EHR.

Conclusion

EHRs have many uses both inside and outside the critical care unit. EHRs can aid more efficient working and can assist in decision making. Data collected within EHRs can be used retrospectively to share key clinical information and assist in designing models to improve patient care and outcomes. Whilst there is a wide range of benefits to EHRs, it is important to acknowledge some of the challenges with these systems such as the cost and training implications. Nevertheless, it is important to be aware of the improvements that can be put in place in order to overcome some of these barriers, such as sufficient infrastructure, support from senior clinicians and adequate training.

113

Take home points

1. Data protection laws as well as professional regulations and organisational policies should be adhered to when using EHRs.
2. The intensive care unit produces a vast amount of data that can be used to improve patient care and outcomes.
3. There is ongoing work to increase the digitalisation of healthcare.
4. EHRs can assist in audit and research activities.
5. EHR systems come with a significant cost implication.
6. There are a vast number of EHR platforms with different functionalities.
7. EHR users should ensure that they have received the appropriate training to use a particular system.

References

Ajami, S. and Arab-Chadegani (2013). Barriers to implement Electronic Health Records (EHRs) by physicians. *Acta Informatica Medica* 21(2): 129–134.

Anderson, R., Sparbel, K., Barr, R.,et al. (2018). Electronic Health Record Tool to Promote Team Communication and Early Patient Mobility in the Intensive Care Unit. *Critical Care Nurse* 38(6): 23–24.

Arenson, R., Andriole, K., Avrin, D., and Gould, R. (2000). Computers in Imaging and healthcare: Now and in the future. *Journal of Digital Imaging* 13: 145–156.

Atasoy, H., Greenwood, B., and McCullough, J. (2019). The digitization of patient care: A review of the effects of electronic health records on health care quality and utilization. *Annual Review of Public Health* 40: 487–500.

Bhise, V., Sittig, D., Vaghani, V., Wei, L., Valdwin, J., and Singh, H. (2018). An electronic trigger based on care escalation to identify preventable adverse events in hospitalised patients. (2018). *British Medical Journal* 27: 241–246.

Burton, L. Anderson, G., and Kues, I. (2004). Using electronic health records to help coordinate care. *The Millbank Quarterly* 82(3): 457–481.

Chan. K, Fowles. J, and Weiner, J. (2010). Electronic health records and the reliability and validity of quality measures: A review of the literature. *Medical Care Research and Review* 67(5): 503–527.

Clarke, A., Watt, I., Sheard, L. et al. (2017). Implementing electronic records in NHS secondary care organisations in England:

policy and progress since 1998. *British Medical Bulletin* 121(1): 95–106.

Coorevits, P., Sundgren, M., Klein, G. et al. (2013). Electronic health records: new opportunities for clinical research. *Journal of Internal Medicine* 274(6): 547–560.

Courtwright, K., Bayes, B., Singh, J. et al. (2018). Prognosticating Outcome and Nudging Decisoons with Electronic Records in The ICU (PONDER-ICU) Trial: Implemenattion in a Learning Health System (trial in progress).

DeMellow, J. and Kim, T. (2018). Technology-enabled performance monitoring in intensive care: An integrative literature review. *Intensive and Critical Care Nursing* 48: 42–51.

Department of Health & Social Care (2018). *Guidance to the Ionising Radiation (Medical Exposure Regulations 2017)*. London: DHSS.

Dexter, R., Perkins, S., Overhage M. et al. (2001). A computerized reminder system to increase the use of preventive care for hospitalized patients. *New England Journal of Medicine* 345(13): 965–970.

Donyal, P., O'Grady, K., Jacklin, A. et al. (2007). The effects of electronic prescribing on the quality of prescribing. *British Journal of Clinical Pharmacology* 65(2): 230–237.

Intensive Care Society (2019) (2nd Ed). Guidelines for the Provision of Intensive Care Services. www.ficm.ac.uk/sites/ficm/files/documents/2021-10/gpics-v2.pdf (acessed July 2022).

Islam, M., Poly, T., and Li, Y. (2018). Recent advancement of clinical information systems: Opportunities and challenges. *Yearbook of Medical Informatics.* 27(1): 83–90.

Flatow, N. Ibragimova, C. Divino, D.S. et al. (2015). Quality Outcomes in the Surgical Intensive Care Unit after Electronic Health Record Implementation. *Applied Clinical Informatics* 6(4): 611–618.

Kaewprag, P., Newton, C., Vermillion, B. et al. (2017). Predictive models for pressure ulcers from intensive care unit electronic health records using Bayesian networks. *Medical Informatics and Decision Making* 7(2): 82–91.

Kruse, C., Smith, B. Vanderlinden, H., and Nealand, A. (2017). Security techniques for the electronic health records. *Journal of Medical Systems* 41(127).

National Audit Office (2013). Digital Britain 2: Putting Users at the Heart of Government's Digital Services. https://www.nao.org.uk/report/digital-britain-2-putting-users-at-the-heart-of-governments-digital-services/ (accessed March 2022).

The National Health Service (2019). The Long Term Plan. https://www.longtermplan.nhs.uk/wp-content/uploads/2019/08/nhs-long-term-plan-version-1.2.pdf (accessed December 2020).

Nursing and Midwifery Council (2018) The Code: Professional Standards of Practice and Behaviour for Nurses, Midwives and Nursing Associates. https://www.nmc.org.uk/standards/code/ (accessed March 2022).

Palabindala, V. Pamarthy, A., and Jonnalagadda, N. (2016). Adoption of electronic health records and barriers. *Journal of Community Hospital Internal Medicine Perspectives.* 6(5).

Pederson, N., Rasmussen, L., Petersen, J. et al. (2017). A critical assessment of early warning score records in 168,000 patients. *Journal of Clinical Monitoring and Computing* 32(1): 109–116.

Royal College of Physicians. (2017). National Early Warning Score (NEWS) 2: Standardising the assessment of acute-illness severity in the NHS. https://www.rcplondon.ac.uk/projects/outputs/national-early-warning-score-news-2 (accessed 15 December 2020).

Shortliffe, E. (1999). The evolution of electronic medical records. *Academic Medicine* 74(4): 414–419.

The Royal College of Anaesthetists 2021. Guidelines for the Provision of Anaesthetic Services. Chapter 7: Guidelines for the Provision of Anaesthesia Services in the Non-theatre Environment.

The Royal College of Nursing (2019). *Record Keeping: The Facts*. London: RCN.

Supady A., Weber, E., Rieder, M. et al. (2021). Cytokine adsorption in patients with severe COVID-19 pneumonia requiring extracorporeal membrane oxygenation (CYOV): a single centre, open=label, randomised, controlled trial. *The Lancet.* 9(7): 755–762.

Wang, Y., Lu, X., Li, Y. et al. (2020). Clinical course and outcomes of 344 intensive care patients with COVID-19 *American Journal of Respiratory and Critical Care Medicine* 201(11).

Wright, D., Mackenzie, M., Buchan, I. et al. (1991). Critical incidents in the intensive therapy unit. *Lancet.* 14: 676–681. https://www.ficm.ac.uk/ICCQIP (accessed November 2020).

114

Chapter 11

Pharmacology

Sadie Diamond-Fox and Alexandra Gatehouse

Aim

The aim of this chapter is to provide the reader with an introduction to some of the pharmacological principles and therapies that may be encountered within the critical care environment.

Learning outcomes

After reading this chapter the reader will be able to:

- Have gained an understanding of the principles of pharmacology including pharmacokinetics and pharmacodynamics.
- Understand key classes of drugs utilised within the critical care environment pertaining to the respiratory, cardiovascular, haematological, renal, gastrointestinal, central nervous and immune systems and their related pharmacology.
- Understand the side effects of common pharmacotherapy utilised within critical care and how to acknowledge and respect that this should be taken in to account when counselling the patient and/or their carers to reach an informed decision regarding their evidence-based care.
- Have gained an understanding of the current evidence base behind key recommendations of pharmacotherapy management of common disorders that may require critical care intervention.

Test your prior knowledge

- Describe the four principal pharmacological processes.
- Describe the mechanisms in which drugs may exert their actions.
- Name four common drug classes used within critical care.
- Describe the formula commonly used to calculate the infusion rate for sympathomimetic drugs.
- Name a national resource that may be used if drug toxicity is suspected.

Fundamentals of Critical Care: A Textbook for Nursing and Healthcare Students, First Edition. Edited by Ian Peate and Barry Hill.
© 2023 John Wiley & Sons Ltd. Published 2023 by John Wiley & Sons Ltd.
Companion website: www.wiley.com/go/peate/criticalcare

Introduction

Pharmacotherapy can be the cornerstone of treatment for multiple disease processes, particularly for those requiring critical care admission. To practise safe medicines management, the healthcare professional is required to possess an understanding of the core pharmacological concepts including the interaction between chemical and physiological processes. This chapter provides a brief introduction to some of the core concepts concerning pharmacology, and the targets sites to which pharmacotherapy may be applied to treat various disease processes. Chapter 13 provides an in-depth discussion of medicines management within critical care.

Healthcare professionals have a professional obligation to ensure safe, evidence-based care is provided to their patients and to minimise potential harm. The prescribing, administration and subsequent titration and monitoring of medications, commonly referred to as medicines management/optimisation, is no exception. Those involved in this area of patient care should familiarise themselves with good practice guidance (NICE, 2015; RPS, 2020). There are also multiple up-to-date resources provided by The UK's Medicines and Healthcare Products Regulatory Agency (MHRA) Drug Safety Updates (https://www.gov.uk/drug-safety-update) and 'MedicinesComplete', a definitive online resource for drug and healthcare information which brings together the world's leading resources to provide healthcare professionals with expert and unbiased knowledge to make the best clinical decisions on the use and administration of drugs and medicines (https://about.medicinescomplete.com/).

Step 2 competencies: national standards

Elements of the following Critical Care Networks-National Nurse Leads (CC3N) (2015) competencies are covered within this chapter:

2.1.9 – Respiratory system associated pharmacology
2.3.3 – Renal system associated pharmacology
2:4.3 – Gastrointestinal associated pharmacology
2.5.3 – Neurological system associated pharmacology

Principles of pharmacology and pharmacotherapy

Pharmacology concerns the scientific principles of how drugs (xenobiotics) exert their effects upon the body through a complex combination of chemical processes, physiology and pathophysiology with the resulting aim being to translate these complex processes into a therapeutic effect. This area of biomedical science is an important discipline as it aids in the discovery of novel therapies to fight pathophysiological disease processes, improving medication safety and effectiveness and understanding the implications that an individual's genes (pharmacogenetics) have upon the effectiveness of medicines.

Pharmacotherapy concerns the use of a drug's therapeutic effect in the treatment of diseases. The safe selection of appropriate pharmacotherapy relies upon knowledge of pathological disease processes, as well as the pharmacokinetics and pharmacodynamics of the drugs selected. It is important that all healthcare professionals involved in the management and administration of medications possess a basic knowledge of pharmacotherapy, particularly those clinicians involved in the care of the critically ill patient as their tolerance for side effects is often greatly reduced. The Royal Pharmaceutical Society (2018 and 2019) has produced essential guides regarding the handling and administration of medicines in healthcare settings, this provides principles-based guidance to ensure the safe administration of medicines by healthcare professionals, an essential read for anyone practising in this area.

The processes of drug therapy

There are four main process of pharmacotherapy, each with important questions, that the clinician should consider when determining whether a drug will have a desired (therapeutic) effect. Due to complexity of each of these processes, it is beyond the scope of this chapter to examine each one in detail. However, Table 11.1 seeks to simplify and outline the interrelationships between them.

The following section of this chapter will examine the principles of drug action (pharmacodynamics) in more detail. Further supporting information can be found within additional texts by Neal (2020) and Peate and Hill (2021). An expert-driven guide to pharmacological targets and the substances that act on them can also be found here https://www.guidetopharmacology.org/.

The most common ways upon which drugs exert their effects can be found in Figure 11.1. The human body has multiple homeostatic control processes in order to maintain stability. Homeostasis partly relies on the maintenance of regulatory mechanisms via naturally occurring (endogenous) hormones (e.g. insulin), neurotransmitters (e.g. noradrenaline) or enzymes (e.g. angiotensin-converting enzyme) release or inactivation. These endogenous substances act mainly by binding to specific receptors (proteins) located on the surface of target cell membranes. The majority of drugs mimic this naturally occurring process by binding to cell receptor sites and either activate (agonist) or inactivate (antagonist) the resulting process. Alternative ways in which drugs exert their effects are via:

1. **Uptake blockers:** The blocking of the reuptake of certain neurotransmitter substances such as serotonin and noradrenaline by pre-synaptic neurones from the synaptic cleft via serotonin transporter (SERT) and the noradrenaline transporter (NAT).

Table 11.1   An overview of the four main processes of pharmacotherapy.

Process	Question for consideration	Factors that may affect the process

Pharmaceutical	Is the drug getting into the patient?	• Patient concordance with therapy
		• The physicochemical properties of the drug formulation:
		  – Amount of active drug
		  – Drug molecule size
		  – Bulking agents used
		  – Rate of disintegration of an orally given tablet
		  – Rate of dissolution drug particles in the intestinal fluid after oral administration
		• Bioavailability – fraction of an administered drug that reaches the systemic circulation and therefore able to reach the site of action

Pharmacokinetic	Is the drug getting to its site of action?	A – Drug absorption and systemic availability(bioavailability):
		• Drug-related factors
		• Patient-related factors
		• Environmental-related factors
		D – Drug distribution:
		• Drug–protein binding complexes
		• Tissue distribution, dependent on:
		  – Vascular permeability
		  – Regional blood flow
		  – Cardiac output
		  – Perfusion rate of the tissue in question
		M – Drug metabolism
		• Patient age, alcohol consumption and smoking
		• Cytochrome P450 enzymes
		• Phase 1 reactions
		• Phase 2 reactions
		• Liver, gut, kidney and/or lung function
		E – Drug excretion
		• Renal function (blood flow, glomerular filtration rate (GFR), urine flow rate and urinary pH
		• Gastrointestinal tract (GIT) and liver function

Pharmacodynamic	Is the drug producing the required pharmaceutical effect?	• Drug-receptor effects (most commonly via protein molecules located within the cell membrane) • Inhibition of transport processes and/or enzymes • Drug potency and receptor affinity • Drug efficacy • Drug interactions
Therapeutic	Is the pharmacological effect being translated in to a therapeutic effect?	• Positive or adverse effects • Pharmacological effects and rate of onset and duration • Drug-disease interactions • Tolerance, tachyphylaxis and desensitisation • Withdrawal

2. **Enzyme inhibitors:** Prevent the target enzyme from causing a specific chemical reaction within the cell. Examples of these types of drugs include acetylcholinesterase (AChE) inhibitors which prevent the breakdown of acetylcholine within the neuromuscular junction, resulting in acetylcholine accumulation which increases both the level and duration of the neurotransmitter action on muscle-activating function.

3. **Hormone inhibitors:** Inhibit or increase the release of endocrine hormones (e.g. insulin) or local hormones (e.g. histamine). Drugs in this class include the antihistamine chlorphenamine, which binds to the histamine H_1 receptor. This blocks the action of endogenous histamine, which subsequently leads to temporary relief of the negative symptoms brought on by histamine (itching, swelling, etc.)

Other important aspects of pharmacodynamics are the development of:

• **Tachyphylaxis:** concerns a rapid decrease in the effect of a drug with repeated administration over a short time period, resulting in diminished receptor sensitivity in response to repeated stimulation by a drug agonist.

• **Tolerance:** repeated administration requires increasing drug dose requirement, over a prolonged period of time causing target receptor down-regulation, deactivation and second-messenger changes. Intravenous infusion of

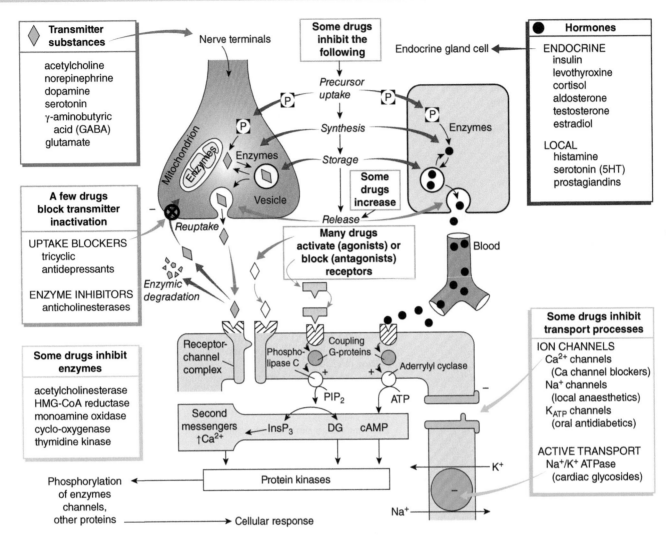

KEY

 Transmitter substances

 Agonists—activate a sequence of events (e.g. acetylcholine activates receptors in skeletal muscle = muscle contraction)

 Antagonists—bind to receptor, but don't activate it (e.g. angiotensin receptor blockers antagonise/block type 1 angiotensin II (AT₁) receptors on bloods vessels = blocks vascular smooth muscle contraction)

● **Hormones**

 Receptor—Two main types:

1. Intracellular receptors—found inside of the cytoplasm or nucleus of a cell (in the cytoplasm or nucleus, e.g. steroid hormone receptors)

2. Cell surface receptors—found in the plasma membrane. Several types exist:

   a. Ligand-gated ion channels
   b. G-protein coupled receptor—linked to second messengers which result in a physiological response such as vaso-constriction)
   c. Kinase-linked receptors (such as insulin receptors)
   d. Enzyme-linked receptors

Figure 11.1   Principles of drug actions. *Source:* Neil (2020) with permission from John Wiley & Sons.

glyceryl trinitrate (GTN) is known to result in both tachy-phylaxis and tolerance and is a complex phenomenon involving neurohormonal counter-regulation (known as pseudotolerance) as well as intrinsic vascular tolerance (Hegde et al., 2014).

- **Desensitisation:** a progressive reduction of a process called signal transduction which concerns the transmission of molecular signals from a cell's exterior surface receptors to its interior. Desensitisation can occur rapidly after receptor activation depending on the agonist and the signalling pathway involved. Opioid receptor desensitisation is a well documented phenomenon which results in reduction of their effectiveness.

Medication safety in critical care

It is incredibly important that any healthcare professional involved in the dispensing, administration or otherwise manipulation of pharmacotherapies be aware of the potential adverse effects that drug therapy can have upon the short and long-term function of organ systems. One of the main concerns of adverse effects of pharmacotherapy within the critical care population is upon the renal system. Certain drugs in patients with known reduced renal function can give rise to clinical deterioration due to (BNF, 2020):

- Drug toxicity – secondary to reduced renal excretion of a drug or its metabolites
- Increased drug sensitivity
- Poorly tolerated known side effects of drugs
- Certain drugs are ineffective when renal function is reduced

Therapeutic drug monitoring (TDM) via analysing plasma drug levels of certain drugs can aid in ensuring individualised drug therapy and avoid both sub-therapeutic and toxic plasma drug concentrations. NHS Trusts often have a medicines management policy that covers TDM which are often based upon *The Renal Drug Database* (https://renaldrugdatabase.com/), alternatively our specialist critical care pharmacist colleagues are an excellent source of this information. The National Institute for Health and Care Excellence (NICE) provides very useful guides within the British National Formulary regarding dosage adjustment for impaired renal function, and how to estimate renal function in those patients where a serum creatinine level has been obtained.

The selection of appropriate pharmacotherapy and safe prescribing practice is reliant upon knowledge of pathological disease processes, as well as the pharmacokinetics and pharmacodynamics of the drugs selected. One of the most common and potentially avoidable causes of acute and chronic renal damage is via pharmacotherapy itself. Drugs can cause renal damage in a number of ways, including altered renal blood flow, damage to the nephron or damage to the interstitial tissues. Figure 11.2 provides a

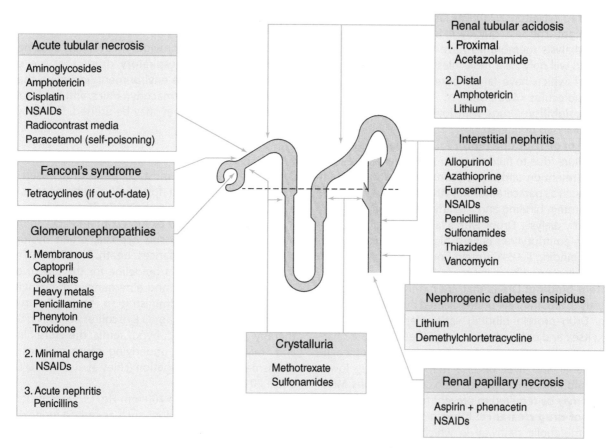

Figure 11.2 The adverse effects of certain drugs upon the kidney. *Source:* Peate and Hill (2021) with permissions from John Wiley & Sons.

non-exhaustive list of some of the adverse effects that pharmacotherapies can exert upon the kidneys.

6Cs: Communication

Good communication is critical to ensuring effective medicines management.

Drugs and dialysis

Patients with acute or chronic renal failure may require the initiation of renal replacement therapy (RRT) in the form of haemodialysis, filtration or hemodiafiltration. This is an important consideration when prescribing and monitoring pharmacotherapy in this patient population and the following aspects should be considered (Richards et al., 2012; Steddon et al., 2014):

- **Drug efficacy:** Removal of drugs and their metabolites via dialysis which can reduce their effectiveness.
- **Equipment and mode of RRT:** The type of filter and the size of the pores within the membrane will affect the rate of clearance of the drug by dialysis or filtration. The rate of flow of dialysis and/or filtration fluid will determine the rate of drug clearance and may affect serum electrolytes and fluid balance, in addition to drug effect and the volume of distribution.
- **Molecular weight:** Drugs have a molecular weight (measured in Daltons (Da)). The larger the drugs molecular weight, the less quickly it is cleared by dialysis. Haemodialysis membranes have relatively small pore sizes and will only clear molecules <500 Da, versus haemofilters which have larger pore sizes and can clear larger molecules <5000 Da.
- **Water solubility:** Drugs with low water solubility are poorly dialysed or filtered.
- **Volume of distribution (VoD):** VoD may be increased by renal failure (due to fluid retention) and liver failure (due to fluid retention and altered protein binding). Certain drugs (such as paracetamol and lithium) have a low affinity for protein binding and a relatively low VoD, so easily cleared by dialysis. Drugs with a large molecular weight (such as amitriptyline) have a high affinity for plasma protein binding (~96% protein-bound), a large VoD and are poorly cleared by dialysis.
- **Protein binding:** Drugs that are highly protein-bound (mostly to albumin) are poorly cleared by dialysis or filtration. Drug–protein binding varies depending on the drug itself and only unbound drugs (free drug) are pharmacologically active, exerting effects upon target receptors. Renal and liver disease may significantly lower serum albumin, elevating free drug concentrations. Monitoring may be required to prevent toxicity.
- **Route of drug clearance:** If hepatic metabolism is the major metabolic pathway in which a drug is broken down (metabolised) then the rate at which the drug is cleared by dialysis or filtration, in a patient with sufficient hepatic function, may be insufficient to have an effect upon total drug clearance.

Core drugs utilised within critical care

There are a plethora of pharmacological agents that the intensive care clinician has within their arsenal to treat the critically ill patient. It is beyond the scope of this chapter to describe and analyse them all, instead there is a focus on those that are deemed as essential by the World Health Organization (WHO, 2019; WHO and PAHO, 2020) and/or most commonly used within our current practice. There are a number of intravenous drugs mentioned within the following section of this chapter. ICU professionals should not only refer to local guidance but should consider adoption of national guidance in this area to ensure both patient safety and efficient use of resources (ICS, 2016).

6Cs: Care

High-quality care should always be at the centre of all work and practices when caring for patients.

Respiratory drugs

The following section provides an overview of some of the common classes of respiratory drugs that are utilised within the critical care environment, including the pharmacokinetics and pharmacodynamics, and the respiratory conditions in which they may be utilised. This is outlined in Table 11.2.

Oxygen

Oxygen is one of the most common drugs used within the healthcare setting for medical emergencies (Hiley et al., 2019; O'Driscoll et al., 2017). The aim is to correct hypoxaemia (low blood oxygen content PaO_2), in order to prevent subsequent tissue hypoxia, organ dysfunction, and in severe circumstances, death. The British Thoracic Society has produced a guideline for the use of oxygen in adults in healthcare and emergency settings with recommendations for administration, targeted saturation, monitoring and weaning (O'Driscoll et al., 2017). Oxygen therapy will only correct hypoxaemia, therefore diagnosis and treatment of the underlying cause requires timely assessment and investigation (Hiley et al., 2019; O'Driscoll et al., 2017).

Hyperoxaemia (PaO_2>100 mm Hg/13.3 kPa) is beneficial in specific clinical situations such as carbon monoxide and cyanide poisoning, spontaneous pneumothorax, cluster

Table 11.2   Common respiratory dugs utilised within critical care.

Drug class	Sub-class	Example drug names	Common *indications*/conditions
Oxygen			Any respiratory disorder resulting in low oxygen saturations requiring oxygen supplementation (see specific guidance for targets)
Bronchodilators	Short-acting beta-2 adrenergic receptor agonists (SABA)	*Salbutamol* *Terbutaline*	· Asthma · COPD · Bronchiectasis
	Long-acting beta-2 adrenergic receptor agonists (LABA)	*Salmeterol* *Formoterol*	· Asthma · COPD
	Muscarinic receptor antagonists	*Ipratropium* *Tiotropium*	
	Xanthines	*Theophylline* *Aminophylline*	
Mucolytics		*Carbocisteine* **Acetylcysteine**	· *Reduction of sputum viscosity in mechanically ventilated patients* · Bronchiectasis (non-Cystic Fibrosis related) · COPD
Stimulants		**Naloxone**	· *Overdose with opioids* · *Reversal of post-operative respiratory depression*

headaches and sickle cell crisis (O'Driscoll et al., 2017; Siemieniuk et al., 2018). However, there are both physiological and clinical risks of hyperoxaemia as outlined in Table 11.3. A clinical practice guideline for oxygen therapy in acutely ill adult medical patients recommends maintaining saturation levels ≤96%, and no oxygen therapy in the case of acute myocardial infarction or stroke patients with SpO_2 ≥92%. These groups should have target saturations of 90–92% (Siemieniuk et al., 2018).

Medicines management: oxygen

Oxygen is a drug and must be prescribed according to a targeted oxygen saturation range either on a paper or electronic drug chart (BNF, 2019; O'Driscoll et al., 2017). Ideally this should occur on hospital admission, but the absence of a prescription does not prohibit oxygen therapy in an emergency situation. Normal oxygen saturation levels are 94–98%; however, this can be affected by pre-existing comorbidities and age (Hiley et al., 2019; O'Driscoll et al., 2017). Administration and titration of oxygen should be performed by clinical staff that appropriately trained to detect and manage complications (WHO, 2016).

Bronchodilators

Bronchodilators are drugs primarily administered via inhalation to treat asthma, COPD and bronchiectasis. Oral and intravenous preparations are available but do not exert a direct, targeted affect and may have more adverse systemic effects such as tachycardia and arrhythmias. They exert their effects via parasympathetic (muscarinic (M_3)) or sympathetic (beta-adrenoceptor (β_2) receptors. Bronchodilators are classified into four groups: short-acting β_2 adrenergic receptor agonists (SABA), long-acting β_2 adrenergic receptor agonists (LABA), short and long-acting muscarinic receptor antagonists (SAMA, LAMA) and xanthines.

Examination scenario

The route of administration of bronchodilators will depend upon the severity of the bronchoconstriction and the resulting physical examination findings. Severe bronchoconstriction can result in minimal air movement throughout the respiratory tree and therefore administration of a bronchodilator such as salbutamol via the inhaled or nebulised route may prove to be inappropriate and a more systemic approach via intravenous administration may be required. In this case, the patient will need to be placed in a clinical area capable of continuous cardiac monitoring due to the potential deleterious cardiovascular effects (including myocardial ischaemia) that may be observed. Salbutamol can induce metabolic changes such as hypokalaemia and increased blood glucose levels. Diabetic patients must be regularly monitored for the development of hyperglycaemia and potential resulting ketoacidosis.

Table 11.3   Physiological and clinical risks of hyperoxaemia. *Source:* Based on O'Driscoll et al., 2017.

Physiological risks

- Decreased ventilation with worsening ventilation/perfusion matching
- Absorption atelectasis
- Vasoconstriction of coronary and cerebral arteries, reducing blood flow
- Decreased cardiac output
- Tissue damage from oxygen free radicals
- Increased systemic vascular resistance

Clinical risks

- Worsening or increased risk of type II respiratory failure
- Failure to recognise clinical deterioration
- Increased mortality – post cardiac arrest, stroke and myocardial infarction

Snapshot: Liu

Anthony is a 22-year-old admitted to hospital with an exacerbation of asthma due to a viral infection. He has a history of moderately severe asthma requiring numerous acute admissions to hospital this year. He is currently on a medical ward. At 1700 hours a Registered Nurse (RN) records the following information on his observation chart:

Airway (A): Airway is patent.
Breathing (B): Speaking in broken sentences. Oxygen saturations 88% (NEWS2 = 0), on 10 litres of oxygen via non-rebreathe mask (NEWS2 = 2), respiratory rate (RR) 28 breaths per minute (NEWS2 = 3). A polyphonic expiratory wheeze was heard in the lung fields.
Cardiovascular System (C): Blood Pressure (BP) is 130/81 mmHg (NEWS2 = 0), Heart Rate (HR) is 115 beats per minute (NEWS2 = 2), capillary refill time (CRT) is 3 seconds, he is warm to touch.
Disability (D) (neurological system), Patient is A (NEWS2 = 0) on the AVPU scale (see Chapter 14), body temperature (T) is 37.6°C (NEWS2 = 0).
Exposure (E) Adequate urine output. No abnormal examination findings.
Total NEW2 Score: 7.

Nursing actions:

- RN immediately informs the senior medic caring for the patient using the Situation Background Assessment Recommendation Response (SBARR) tool.
- Emergency assessment by the critical care outreach team is requested for consideration of transfer to the critical care unit.
- RN commences continuous monitoring of the patient's vital signs.

Diagnosis:

- Acute severe asthma exacerbation as characterised by increased respiratory rate, heart rate, and the inability to speak in full sentences.

- Patients with severe asthma who have had repeated attendances to the emergency department and/or multiple previous admissions (especially within the last year) are at high risk of developing near-fatal asthma and should be reviewed by a senior clinician.

6Cs: Courage

Critical care patients can often lack capacity due to the underlying disease process that has required them to be admitted to the critical care unit. It is important as healthcare professionals to have the courage to do the right thing for the people we care for and to advocate for them in instances when they are not able to do so themselves.

Mucolytics

Exacerbations of respiratory disorders may present to critical care areas with mucous hypersecretion due to goblet cell hyperplasia and hypertrophy. Mucolytics, such as Carbocisteine and Acetylcysteine, affect the proteins (mucins) secreted by the goblet cells, breaking them down and in turn reducing sputum viscosity, increasing mucous clearance. A recent Cochrane review identified that the use of Carbocisteine and Acetylcysteine are useful for reducing flare-ups, days of disability, and hospital admissions in people with COPD or chronic bronchitis (Poole et al., 2019).

Respiratory stimulants

The mainstay of respiratory stimulants within the adult critical care environment is Naloxone. It is indicated for the reversal of the central nervous system (CNS) and respiratory depressant effects of naturally derived or synthetic opioids post-acute overdose or intoxication.

Cardiovascular drugs

An understanding of cardiovascular system (CVS) physiology and neurohormonal control of blood pressure is essential in order to treat certain disorders affecting the cardiovascular system within critical care. The main indication for instituting CVS pharmacotherapy is to improve tissue perfusion. Pharmacotherapy targets used to treat conditions which lead to impaired tissue perfusion (e.g. cardiogenic or septic shock) is mainly upon the nervous system via adrenergic, muscarinic or phosphodiesterase receptors (see Table 11.4).

Learning event: reflection

Reflect upon the complications you have observed within your own practice for patients receiving sympathomimetic drugs.

Table 11.4 Receptors of the autonomic nervous system. *Source:* Chess-Williams, 2002; Hedge, 2006; Klabunde, 2012; Rattu, 2015.

| Site | Autonomic nervous system | | | |
| | Sympathetic | | Parasympathetic | |
	Receptor	Action (when activated)	Receptor	Action (when activated)
Heart	Beta$_1$	↑ Rate & contractility	Muscarinic (M$_2$)	↓ Rate & contractility
Blood vessels (vascular smooth muscle)	Beta$_2$	Dilatation/Relaxation	Muscarinic (M3)	Dilatation – Nitric oxide-induced
			Muscarinic (M3)	Contraction – Acetylcholine-induced
Bronchioles	Beta$_2$	Dilatation	Muscarinic (M3)	Contraction/Constriction
Kidney	Beta$_1$	Renin secretion		
Gastrointestinal tract smooth muscle – wall	Alpha$_2$ and Beta$_2$	Dilatation/Relaxation	Muscarinic	Contraction
Gastrointestinal tract smooth muscle – sphincter	Alpha$_1$	Contraction	Muscarinic	Relaxation

Inotropes/Inoconstrictors and vasoconstrictors

Catecholamines mediate their cardiovascular actions predominantly through alpha-1 (α1), Beta-1 (ß1), Beta-2 (ß2) or dopaminergic receptors. Figure 11.3 details some of the common drugs within this class that either cause vasoconstriction, increased heart rate (chronotropy) or increased force or energy of heart muscle contraction (inotrope). Further reading regarding this drug class includes several seminal guidelines and systematic reviews (Khanna and Peters, 2017; Rhodes et al., 2017; Russell, 2019; Van Valkinburgh et al., 2020).

Inodilators

Inodilators have inotropic effects, but also cause vasodilatation of the systemic vascular bed and/or the pulmonary vascular bed. They may act upon adrenergic receptors, inhibit phosphodiesterase enzymes, or both. Phosphodiesterase inhibitors (PDIs), like alpha-1 receptor blockers, have the potential to exert their effect upon multiple sites of the body, targeting disorders of the cardiovascular and respiratory system.

| Vasoactive Agent | Receptors (▓ =main effect) or action | Midrange dose effects | | |
		Inotropic contractility	Chronotrope (heart rate)	Vaso-constrictor
Inoconstrictors				
Epinephrine	α, β$_1$, β$_2$	++++	+++	++
Dopamine	α, β$_1$, β$_2$	+++	++	– to ++
Inodilators				
Dobutamine	α, β$_1$, β$_2$	+++	+	– to ±
Milrinone	PDI(↑cAMP)	+++	0	– –
Enoximone	PDI (↑cAMP)	+++	0	–
Vasoconstrictor				
Norepinephrine	α, β$_1$	+/++	0	++++
Phenylephrine	α, β$_1$	+	0	++++

PDI = phosphodiesterase inhibitor;
cAMP = cyclic adenosine monophosphate;
– = vasodilation

Figure 11.3 Properties of inotropic drugs.

Medicines management: sympathomimetic drugs

Sympathomimetic drugs such as adrenaline and noradrenaline are often prescribed in micrograms per kilogram, per minute (mcg/kg/min). The following formula should be used in order to calculate the desired infusion rate:

$$\text{IV infusion rate}\left(\frac{mL}{hr}\right) = \frac{\text{Dose}\left(mcg/kg/min\right) \times \text{weight}\left(kg\right) \times 60\,min/hr}{\text{Concentration}\left(\frac{mg}{ml}\right) \times 1000\,mcg/mg}$$

Anti-arrhythmics and anti-anginal

Antiarrhythmic drugs are used to either restore sinus rhythm in patients with arrhythmias, or control heart in patients whereby restoration of sinus rhythm cannot be achieved, for example atrial fibrillation. Anti-anginal drugs are often used in combination with anti-arrhythmics to optimising the balance of myocardial oxygen supply and demand and reduce incidences of myocardialischaemia.

Examination scenario: arterial blood pressure monitoring

Patients requiring continuous infusions of sympathomimetic drugs should have intra-arterial blood pressure and continuous electrocardiograph (ECG) monitoring in situ in order to assess the dynamic changes in haemodynamic stability that these potent agents can cause.

Figure 11.4 details some of the fundamental principles surrounding the use of arterial blood pressure monitoring.

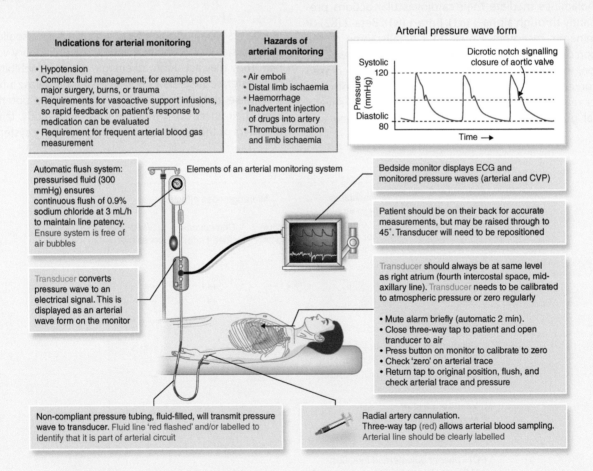

Figure 11.4   Arterial blood pressure monitoring.

Anti-hypertensives

There are several groups of antihypertensive drugs that reduce blood pressure by several different mechanisms. Figure 11.5 details some of the mechanisms anti-hypertensives exert their effects. Manipulation of the renin-angiotensin-aldosterone system is one of the most potent pharmacotherapy targets, producing systemic effects upon peripheral resistance, sympathetic outflow and electrolyte and water exchange within the kidney. This subject is explored in further detail within Chapter 24.

ß1-agonists	Tachycardia Arrhythmias Can precipitate angina or myocardial infarction in patients with coronary artery disvwease
ß2-agonists	Hypotension (due to peripheral vasodilatation) and reflex tachycardia Metabolic disturbances such as hyperglycaemia and hypokalaemia Agitation Tremor Diaphoresis (sweating)

125

Red Flags

Sympathomimetic drugs can have multiple adverse effects, dependent upon the pharmacological site of action, such as:

α1-agonists	Hypertension and reflex bradycardia Ischaemia and necrosis of digits
α2-agonists	Central nervous system depression Respiratory depression Bradycardia and hypotension Rebound hypertension if withdrawn rapidly after prolonged therapy

6Cs: Competence

Competence in healthcare means the individual must possess the necessary expertise, clinical knowledge, and technical knowledge to deliver treatments that are effective and based on research and evidence.

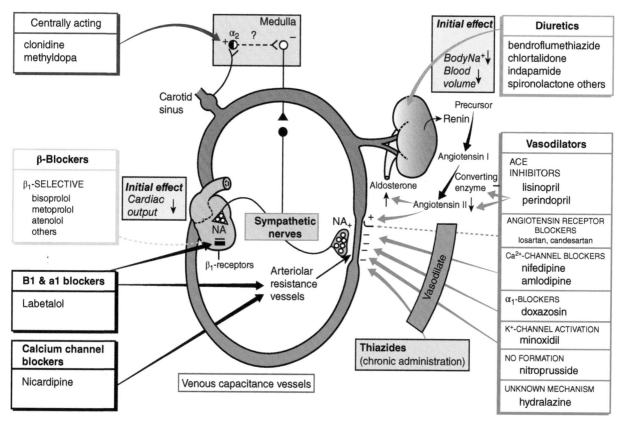

Figure 11.5   Antihypertensive agents and their location of action.

Haematological drugs

Anticoagulants

The most common anticoagulants that are used within critical care, unfractionated heparin (UFH) and low molecular weight heparins (LMWH). UFH has the benefit of being rapidly reversed, for instance in the case of haemorrhage, by protamine sulphate, however, LMWH are only partially reversed by protamine. The use of UFH and LMWH may lead to the development of heparin-induced thrombotic thrombocytopaenia syndrome (HIITS). This is more common with UFH and more likely to occur with higher doses and/or prolonged periods of time. It is characterised by a fall in platelet count, coupled with an extremely hypercoagulable state and carries a significant mortality rate (Nicholas et al., 2020).

6Cs: Clinical Investigations

The British Society for Haematology recommend that the therapeutic effect of UFH and LMWH is monitored using the plasma Anti-Xa assay (Kitchen et al., 2014). Monitoring of LMWH used for prophylaxis of thromboembolic events is not routinely required, unless there are concerns regarding drug clearance in renal failure, or drug distribution in extremes of weight range. To ensure the correct result,

the specimen must be collected within the correct time frame post heparin administration. This is particularly important for LMWH and a specimen should generally be obtained 3–4 hours post administration. Local guidance should always be followed in regard to assay timings and dosage adjustments.

Renal drugs

Knowledge of renal anatomy, physiology and common renal diseases within critical care is essential for assessment and management of patient's renal status. This will be explored in further depth in Chapter 24. The following section provides an overview of the classes of renal drugs, including the pharmacokinetics and pharmacodynamics, and the renal conditions in which they may be utilised. This is outlined in Table 11.5.

Diuretics are the main stay treatment of multiple conditions which lead to fluid retention and formation of interstitial oedema, with the overall aim to increase excretion of sodium and water via the kidneys. They exert their effect upon electrolyte and water balance within nephrons via either co-transporter pumps, antagonising the effects of aldosterone, or inhibiting transport of bicarbonate (see Figure 11.6). Diuretics are classed according to their site of action and include loop diuretics, thiazide diuretics, osmotic diuretics, potassium-sparing diuretics, aldosterone antagonists and carbonic-anhydrase inhibitors.

Table 11.5 Common renal drugs.

Drug class	Sub-class	Example drug names	Common conditions
Diuretics	Loop Diuretic	Furosemide Bumetanide	- Fluid retention/oedema - Hypertension
	Thiazides & related diuretics	Bendroflumethiazide	- Hypertension - Heart failure
		Indapamide	- Hypertension
	Osmotic	Mannitol	- Cerebral oedema and raised intra-ocular pressure
	Potassium-sparing & Aldosterone antagonists	Amiloride	- Oedema - Potassium conserving diuretic in hypertension, congestive heart failure or hepatic ascites
		Spirinolactone	- Oedema - Ascites - Nephrotic syndrome - Heart failure - Hypertension - Primary hyperaldosteronism - Potassium conserving diuretic
	Carbonic-anhydrase inhibitors	Acetazolamide	- Reduction of intra-ocular pressure - Glaucoma - Epilepsy

Table 11.5   (Continued)

Drug class	Sub-class	Example drug names	Common conditions
Electrolyte disorders	Phosphate binders	*Sevelamer* *Lanthanum*	• Hyperphosphataemia in chronic renal failure
	Vitamin D supplementation	*Alfacalcidol*	• Severe renal impairment • Rickets • Hypocalcaemia due to hypoparathyroidism or pseudohypoparathyroidism
		Calcitriol	• Renal osteodystrophy
	Potassium binders	*Calcium polystyrene sulfonate* *Sodium polystyrene sulfonate*	• Hyperkalaemia in renal failure
	Potassium supplements	*Sando-K°*	• Potassium depletion
	Bicarbonate supplements	*Sodium bicarbonate*	• Chronic acidotic states

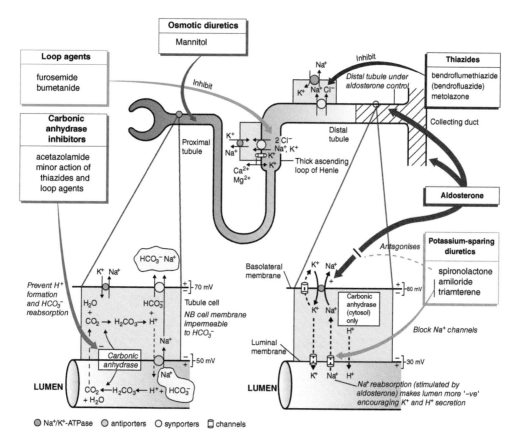

Figure 11.6   Site of diuretic effects upon the nephron.

Fluids and electrolytes

Fluids

Fluids are one of the most common treatments administered in critical care. Intravenous fluids may be utilised for resuscitation and electrolyte replacement and are viewed as drugs, and so should be prescribed accordingly so. The aim of fluid resuscitation is restoration of end-organ perfusion and physiological imbalance (Martin et al., 2018). This will be discussed further in Chapter 20.

The National Institute for Health and Care Excellence (2013) clinical guideline (CG174) has made key recommendations with regard to intravenous therapy, based upon the five Rs – resuscitation, routine maintenance, replacement, redistribution and reassessment. The guideline also contains a useful algorithm for intravenous fluid therapy for adults in hospital which may be used to guide administration. Specific disease processes may result in fluid and electrolyte losses or abnormal distribution requiring the use of crytalloids or colloids.

Electrolytes

Electrolyte disorders can occur as a result of altered homeostasis of the renal system, multiple disease processes (adrenal gland dysfunction, gastrointestinal dysfunction, etc.) or iatrogenic causes such as pharmacotherapy (i.e. potassium depletion due to loop diuretics). Derangement can manifest in severe organ dysfunction and principle treatments involve either replacement or the promotion of excretion. The primary or underlying cause should be addressed to unnecessary long-term treatment strategies.

Derangement of potassium is managed with potassium binders or supplements in hyperkalaemia or hypokalaemia. Oral sodium bicarbonate is recommended for patients with chronic kidney disease to manage metabolic acidosis. Phosphate binders, calcium supplements and vitamin D supplements are commonly used in combination in chronic renal disease due to the altered calcium and phosphate metabolism.

> ## 6Cs: Clinical Investigations
> Renal failure is common in critical care and may be present upon admission, develop during the patient's stay or be chronic in presentation, all of which will affect the clearance of drugs that are excreted renally. Drug dosages may need to be reduced or dosing intervals increased to prevent drug toxicity, drug sensitivity and side effects. Renal impairment may be mild, moderate or severe and may be monitored with serum creatinine, estimated glomerular filtration rate (eGFR) and urine output.

Gastrointestinal drugs

Knowledge of gastrointestinal (GI) tract anatomy, physiology and common GI disorders within critical care is essential for assessment and management. This will be explored in further depth in Chapter 22. The following section provides an overview of the classes of gastrointestinal drugs, including the pharmacokinetics and pharmacodynamics, and the GI conditions in which they may be utilised. This is outlined in Table 11.6.

Table 11.6   Common gastrointestinal drugs.

Drug class	Subclass	Example drug names	Common conditions
Antidiabetic drugs	Insulin	*Actrapid* *Humulin I* *Insulin glargine*	· Diabetes mellitus (DM)
	Biguanide	*Metformin*	· Type 2 DM · Polycystic ovary syndrome
	Sulphonlurea	*Glicazide*	· Type II DM
Stress ulcer prophylaxis	H$_2$-histamine antagonists	*Omeprazole* *Lansoprazole*	· *Helicobacter pylori* · Gastro-oesophageal reflux disease · Oesophagitis · Prophylaxis, benign or NSAID-associated gastric/duodenal ulcer
	Proton pump inhibitors	*Ranitidine*	· Prophylaxis, benign, stress or NSAID-associated gastric/duodenal ulcer · Gastric acid reduction in surgical procedures
Anti-emetics	5HT$_3$ antagonists	*Ondansetron*	· Emetogenic chemotherapy and radiotherapy · Prevention and treatment of post-operative nausea and vomiting
	Dopamine antagonists	*Metoclopramide* *Prochlorperazine*	· Radiotherapy-induced or post-operative nausea and vomiting · Hiccup
Laxatives	Osmotic laxatives	*Lactulose* *Polyethylene glycol*	· Constipation · Heptatic encehalopathy
	Stimulant laxatives	*Senna* *Bisacodyl* *Glycerol*	· Constipation
	Faecal softeners	*Docusate*	

Insulin

Glycaemic control within critical care is often challenging and associated with an increased risk of morbidity and mortality. Hyperglycaemia is a common complication due to pre-existing conditions, such as diabetes mellitus (DM), genetic disorders, infection, medications (steroids), parenteral nutrition or critical illness stress-induced hyperglycaemia. Conflicting evidence surrounds blood glucose targets and management strategies. In a landmark trial, tight glucose control increased mortality whilst moderate control improved survival rates (Finfer et al., 2009). In hospital, the recommended target blood glucose is 6–10 mmol/L, accepting a range of 4–12 mmol/L (Joint British Diabetes Societies for Inpatient Care, 2014).

Under normal physiological conditions, raised plasma glucose stimulates the release of insulin from islet β-cells in the pancreas. This binds to receptors in cell membranes, increasing glucose uptake by cells in the muscle, liver and adipose tissue, inhibiting of fat and glycogen breakdown, increasing protein synthesis and inhibiting of gluconeogenesis.

Diabetes is a metabolic condition resulting in hyperglycaemia due to insulin deficiency (Type 1) or insulin resistance (Type 2) (Leach, 2014). Secondary diabetes may occur due to other disease processes including endocrine conditions and pancreatitis.

Type 1 DM is associated with β-cell destruction due to viral, autommimune or genetic factors, presenting in younger individuals, resulting in insulin deficiency and ketoacidosis, if left untreated. Insulin therapy is essential and regimens incorporate combinations of short-acting, biphasic and long-acting preparations.

Insulin resistance occurs in Type 2 DM and management includes diet alone or diet and oral hypoglycaemic medications, biguanides and or sulphonylureas. Biguanides increase peripheral glucose utilisation and uptake as well as decrease hepatic production of glucose e.g. metformin. The sulphonylureas, such as glicazide, close the potassium ATP channels, stimulating insulin release. Other oral hypoglycaemic agents include incretin analogues, glucosidase inhibitors and glitazones, which increase insulin release, delay absorption of glucose and increase sensitivity to insulin respectively. The newest group of drugs are the sodium-glucose co-transporter 2 (SGLT2) inhibitors which inhibit renal glucose tubular reabsorption but tend to be stopped in critical illness due to their mechanism of action. Insulin may be required in the long term or during periods of acute illness.

Red Flag

Three diabetic emergencies may be managed within critical care – hypoglycaemia, diabetic ketoacidosis (DKA) and hyper-osmolar hyperglycaemic state (HHS). The most common cause of hypoglycaemia is diabetic medica-tions, other causes in critical care include renal and liver disease, sepsis and drug overdose. Clinical manifestations include neurological deterioration and management strategies incorporate oral glucose or carbohydrate, if the patient is conscious, or intravenous glucose.

DKA occurs in Type 1 DM wherein insulin deficiency results in hyperglycaemia, metabolic acidosis, ketosis, electrolyte disturbance, dehydration and haemodynamic instability. Emergency treatment includes fluid resuscitation and intravenous insulin. Life-threatening hypokalaemia may occur following insulin therapy and should be replaced in early management.

HHS is uncommon, occurring in elderly patients with Type 2 DM. It is characterised by hyperglycaemia, pseudo-hypernatraemia, and hyperosmolality usually without ketosis and metabolic acidosis. Rapid fluid replacement and reduction of blood glucose may cause cerebral oedema and osmotic demyelination and therefore management should be conservative with cautious fluid resuscitation and intravenous insulin.

H₂-histamine antagonists and proton pump inhibitors (PPIs)

Stress-related mucosal injury may occur in critically ill patients, leading to ulceration and upper gastrointestinal (GI) bleeding. Advances in critical care, in addition to stress ulcer prophylaxis (SUP), have significantly reduced the incidence of clinically significant bleeding but pharmacological management is not without risk, including ventilator-acquired pneumonia and clostridium difficile infection. The literature is controversial, however, the most recent large multicentre trial concluded that the incidence of clinically important GI bleeds was lower with the use of a PPI (Krag et al., 2018).

H_2 antagonists and PPIs reduce acid secretion from the gastric parietal cells thereby preventing mucosal damage and reducing the risk of clinically significant bleeding. H_2 antagonists block the histamine receptor, whilst PPIs inhibit the gastric hydrogen-potassium ATPase (H+/K+ ATPase) pumps enzyme system.

Anti-emetics

Vomiting and nausea have multifactoral causes and the underlying causes include drugs (cytotoxics, opioids, antibiotics), neurogenic (migraine, raised intracranial pressure), vestibulocochlear (infection, ischaemia, motion), GI (postoperative ileus, obstruction, analgesics, infection, hiatus hernia), inflammation (pancreatitis, hepatitis), sepsis and pregnancy (Grahame-Smith and Aronson, 2002; Leach, 2014). Once precipitating factors have been addressed, antiemetic drugs may provide symptom relief by exerting their effects at various target sites.

129

Medicines management

Within critical care, patients are susceptible to prolongation of the QT interval, potentially causing cardiac arrhythmias such as Torsades de Pointes and cardiac arrest. Risk factors include age, gender, electrolyte disturbances and medications. A 12-lead electrocardiogram should be performed on admission to critical care and the QT interval assessed prior to administration of medications known to cause prolongation. Ondansetron and metoclopramide both increase this risk and, although this may be relatively higher for ondansetron as it is widely utilised, the absolute risk remains low (Freedman et al., 2014).

Laxatives and anti-diarrhoeal drugs

Gastrointestinal function is complex and it is an important determinant of outcome within critical care (Blaser et al., 2012). Constipation is defined as impairment of peristalsis leading to the inability to pass stool for three or more consecutive days, with no mechanical obstruction, regardless of bowel sounds, and occurs in 5–90% of critically ill patients (Vincent and Preiser, 2015). Contributing factors include abdominal surgery, sepsis, neuromuscular disease including spinal cord injury, dysmotility, immobility, medications (opioids, diuretics), electrolyte disturbances and hypovolaemia. Early protocolised care may improve outcome and prevent complications. Laxatives are classified according to their action and include osmotic (lactulose, polyethylene glycol), stimulant (senna, bisacodyl, glycerol) or softeners (docusate, glycerol) laxatives. Enemas may be required if oral or rectal laxatives are ineffective.

Diarrhoea is common in critical care, being defined as three or more loose or liquid stools in a day, greater than 200–300 mLs (Blaser et al., 2012; Leach, 2014). The causes of diarrhoea include medications (laxatives, antibiotics), infection (gastroenteritis, clostridium difficile), intestinal dysfunction, ischaemic colitis, constipation (overflow diarrhoea), enteral feeds, sepsis and malabsorption (pancreatitis, inflammatory bowel disease) and complications include loss of skin integrity, dehydration and electrolyte imbalance. The primary cause should be addressed with fluid and electrolyte replacement as required. Anti-diarrhoeal drugs may provide symptom relief.

Neurological drugs

Knowledge of central nervous system anatomy (CNS), physiology and common CNS disorders within critical care, is essential for assessment and management. This will be explored in further depth in Chapters 12, 14 and 15. The following section provides an overview of the classes of CNS drugs, including the pharmacokinetics and pharmacodynamics, and the CNS conditions in which they may be utilised. This is outlined in Table 11.7.

Analgesics

Within critical care a vast majority of patients report moderate to severe pain during their admission, the causes of which may be multifactorial including pre-existing conditions or acute conditions such as post-operative, neurological, trauma, invasive procedures or routine care (Narayanan, Venkataraju and Jennings, 2016). Recognition, assessment and management is essential in order to minimise the deleterious effects of pain, and subsequently intensive care morbidity, mortality and length of stay in critical care and the hospital. It is beyond the scope of this chapter to discuss detailed physiological mechanisms of pain, assessment and management and this is explored in Chapter 12.

Opioids

Pain receptors transmit pain information to the dorsal horn of the spinal cord, this is in turn conveyed to the brainstem and brain, via relay neurons. Opioid peptides inhibit the activity of these relay neurons, mimicking the effects of endogenous opioid peptides, acting as complete or partial agonists at the opioid receptor, producing analgesia.

Non-opioid analgesics

Non-steroidal anti-inflammatory drugs (NSAIDs) may be utilised in the treatment of mild to moderate pain, in addition to having antipyretic and anti-inflammatory effects. Their mechanism of action is inhibition of cyclo-oxygenase (COX), an enzyme, which prevents the synthesis of prostaglandins which are implicated in the inflammatory response and pain mediation. NSAIDs are of limited use within critical care as the GI-adverse effects, such as gastritis and bleeding and increased risk of myocardial infarction, outweigh the benefit.

Paracetamol is widely used for its analgesic and antipyretic properties but does not exert any significant anti-inflammatory actions. Its mechanism of action is not fully understood but is thought to cause COX inhibition.

Neuropathic pain is caused by damage or disease that affects the nervous system in the absence of nociceptive stimuli, either centrally central (multiple sclerosis, spinal cord injury, stroke, Parkinson's disease) or peripherally (diabetic neuropathy, herpes zoster infection, Guillain–Barré, cancer, amputation).

Epidural and regional anaesthesia

Over the last decade there has been a significant shift towards the use of regional anaesthesia in critical care due to the significant side effects of systemic opioids.

Table 11.7   Common CNS drugs.

Drug class	Subclass	Example drug names	Common conditions
Analgesics	Opioid	*Morphine* *Fentanyl* *Codeine phosphate*	- Pain - Pulmonary oedema - Myocardial infarction - Dyspnoea at rest or cough in palliative care - Mechanical ventilation - Acute diarrhoea
	Non-opioid	*Ibuprofen* *Paracetamol*	- Pain and inflammation - Pyrexia
	Neuropathic analgesics	*Gabapentin* *Amitriptyline*	- Peripheral neuropathic pain - Seizures (gabapentin) - Depression (amitriptyline) - Sleep (amitriptyline)
	Local anaesthetics	*Lidocaine* *Levobupivicaine*	- Acute post-operative pain, labour pain - Surgical anaesthesia – peripheral nerve block, Caesarean section, lumbar epidural - Regional anaesthesia – nerve block - Cardiopulmonary resuscitation (lidocaine) - Ventricular arrhythmias (lidocaine)
Sedatives and anxiolytics	Sedative	*Propofol*	- Sedation - Status epilepticus
	Anxiolytic	*Midazolam*	- Premedication - Confusion and restlessness in palliative care
Muscle relaxants	Non-depolarising neuromuscular blocking	*Atracurium* *Rocuronium*	- Neuromuscular blockade for intubation, surgery, critical care
Anticonvulsants	Benzodiazepines	*Lorazepam* *Midazolam*	- Status epilepticus
	Antiepiletics	*Phenytoin* *Levetiracetam*	- Status epileticus - Prevention and treatment of seizures
Antideliriogenics	Atypical antipsychotics	*Haloperidol* *Olanzapine*	- Acute delirium - Psychoaffective disorder - Nausea and vomiting (haloperidol)

Indications for regional anaesthesia include surgery (thoracotomy, laparotomy, limb fractures/amputation), acute pancreatitis and procedures (chest drain) and options include thoracic epidural, paravertebal block, rectus sheath blocks and other various nerve blocks (Venkataraju and Narayanan, 2016). Local anaesthetic drugs are administered either by subcutaneous infusion or single dose, infiltration around a single nerve or nerve plexus or epidural anaesthesia. It is not without risk, and complications include failure of placement, local anaesthetic toxicity, risk of infection and epidural haematoma. Local anaesthetic drugs block sodium channels in nerves preventing the generation of action potentials.

Sedatives and anxiolytics

Sedative requirements in critical care are dependent upon invasive procedures, the need for or optimisation of mechanical ventilation, agitation, seizures, oxygen consumption as well as management of raised intracranial pressure and temperature (Leach, 2014). Adequate sedation is primarily achieved via combinations of anaesthetic drugs, benzodiazepines and opioids. This will be explored in depth in Chapter 12.

Muscle relaxants

Short-term neuromuscular blockade is utilised within critical care to facilitate intubation, transfers, prone positioning and procedures. Infusions of these drugs may be required to manage ventilator dysynchrony, severe respiratory failure, raised intracranial pressure and shivering during therapeutic hypothermia. Prolonged neuromuscular blockade is not without complication including critical care weakness and serious cardiovascular events. Non-depolarising drugs, such as rocuronium and atracurium, antagonise the effects of acetylcholine at the muscle endplate preventing depolarisation and contraction.

Learning event

Snapshot

John is a 65-year-old admitted to critical care with type I respiratory failure due to a community-acquired pneumonia. Three days ago he was intubated, mechanically ventilated and sedated due to increasing oxygen requirements. He was paralysed with an atracurium infusion due to ventilator dysynchrony. On the ward round this morning the infusions of sedation and opioid, propofol and morphine, were reduced. In the last 5 minutes John's heart rate and blood pressure have increased significantly. The RN at the bedside completes a full assessment, contacts a member of the medical team and increases the rate both of the propofol and morphine infusions as well as giving a bolus of each medication. John's heart rate and blood pressure normalise once more.

It is concluded that John's sedation was inadequate whilst he was still paralysed. Due to his improvement in his ventilator failure a plan is made to stop the atracurium infusion first with adequate time given before the sedatives are then reduced.

Anticonvulsants

Status epilepticus (SE) is defined as 5 or more minutes of either continuous seizure activity or repetitive seizure activity without recovery of consciousness (BMJ, 2020). Generalised pharmacological management includes a benzodiazepine as first-line treatment then an anticonvulsant, as second line treatment. If seizure activity persists infusions of propofol and or midazolam may be required.

Medication management

Therapeutic drug monitoring ensures that plasma concentrations are high enough to produce a clinical response but low enough to prevent toxicity or side effects. Phenytoin requires measurement of plasma concentrations to guide therapy. The target range for optimum response is 10–20 mg/litre (or 40–80 micromol/litre) (BNF, 2020). Plasma concentration should be interpreted with care in the elderly, during pregnancy, renal failure and other disease processes that may result in hypoalbuminaemia, as reduced protein binding will decrease phenytoin plasma concentration. Metabolism of phenytoin occurs primarily in the liver via oxidation. Drugs that induce or inhibit these enzymes will also affect plasma concentration.

Antideliriogenics

Delirium is associated with increased hospital mortality, prolonged critical care stay and hospital length of stay, in addition to development of post-critical care cognitive impairment in adult critical care patients (Barr et al., 2013). Early recognition of delirium is key to management and this will be explored in depth in Chapter 15.

Pharmacological management of delirium within critical care utilises neuroleptic drugs. A Cochrane Review recently concluded that dexmedetomidine, an alpha$_2$ agonist, was the most effective in reducing the duration of delirium, with atypical antipsychotics being second (Burry et al., 2019). Atypical antipsychotics, such as haloperidol and olanzapine, exert their effects by antagonising dopamine receptors in the brain. In the UK, the A2B trial is currently investigating continuous infusions of intravenous alpha$_2$ agonists, dexmedetomidine and clonidine, for use as an alternative to propofol for sedation, outcomes of which include time to successful extubation and duration of delirium, as well as quality of sedation and analgesia.

Immunomodulatory drugs

Within critical care, immunomodulatory drugs are utilised to treat a wide range of disease processes and conditions. These drugs exert their effects via treatment of diseases caused by infection (bacterial or fungal) or viruses, suppression of the immune system or prevention of infection. The following section provides an overview of the classes of immunomodulatory drugs, including the pharmacokinetics and pharmacodynamics, and the conditions in which they may be utilised. This is outlined in Table 11.8.

Antibacterial agents

One of the commonest causes of admission to critical care is infection and the initial choice of antibiotics is dependent upon several factors including the disease, the patient, the organisms and the drugs utilised. Critical care patients are susceptible to nosocomial infections, which confer significant morbidity and mortality due to several risk factors, including patient-related factors such as age, disease acuity, pre-morbid conditions, surgery, trauma and burns as well as healthcare such as invasive procedures, recent antimicrobial therapy, immunosuppressive treatment, stress ulcer prophylaxis, transfusion, parenteral nutrition and length of critical care stay (Edwardson and Cains, 2019).

Antimicrobial resistance is becoming a global problem and features within critical care due to selective pressures from regular antibiotic use. This is compounded by the transmission of nosocomial transmission of resistant organisms. This has been addressed by the introduction of care bundles and more appropriate use of antibiotics. Antimicrobial stewardship focuses on knowledge of local resistance patterns, early targeted therapy and source control, timely

Table 11.8   Common immunomodulatory drugs.

Drug class	Subclass	Example drug names	Common conditions
Antibacterial agents	Inhibition of bacterial cell wall synthesis · Penicillins · Cephalasporins · Carbopenems · Tetracyclines	*Flucloxacillin,* *piperacillin tazobactam* *Cefuroxime* *Meropenem* *Vancomycin*	· Sepsis · Complicated infections involving urinary tract, bone, lungs, heart, CNS, bowel, skin or soft tissue · Clostridium difficile · Surgical prophylaxis
	Inhibition of bacterial nucleic acid synthesis · Sulphonamides · Quinolones · Nitromidazoles · Rifampicin	*Ciprofloxacin* *Metronidazole* *Trimethoprim*	· Crohn's disease · Lower respiratory tract infection in cystic fibrosis · Infections involving urinary tract, lungs, bowel, liver, skin, ear or eyes · Surgical prophylaxis
	Inhibition of bacterial protein synthesis · Aminoglycosides · Tetracyclines · Macrolides · Oxalizidones	*Gentamicin* *Doxycyline* *Clarithromycin* *Linezolid* *Chloramphenicol*	· Infections involving urinary tract, lungs, bowel, heart, CNS, liver, skin, ear or eyes · Surgical prophylaxis
Antifungals	· Polyenes · Trazoles · Echinocandins	*Amphotericin* *Fluconazole* *Caspofungin*	· Fungal infections · Prevention of fungal infections in immunocompromised patients · Treatment of systemic fungal infections in patients with neutropenia
Antivirals	· Inhibit nucleic acid synthesis · Inhibitors of viral DNA polymerase · Inhibition of exit · Delayed chain terminator	*Aciclovir* *Oseltamivir* *Resdemivir* *Immunoglobulins*	· Viral infections · Prevention and treatment of influenza · COVID-19
Corticosteroids	Glucocorticoids	*Prednisolone* *Hydrocortisone* *Dexamethasone*	· COPD · Thyrotoxic crisis · Asthma · Adrenocortical insufficiency · Anaphylaxis · Ulcerative colitis · Myaesthenia gravis · Bacterial meningitis · Nausea and vomiting · Cerebral oedema · COVID-19
Immunoglobulins	Vaccines Human immunoglobulins		· Vaccines · Guillain–Barré · Myaesthenia gravis · Septic shock

de-escalation of broad-spectrum drugs, with shorter duration and appropriate dosing.

6Cs: Commitment

Being highly committed to our patients helps to improve their quality of care and experience as well as that of other patients.

Antibacterial agents exert their effects via several mechanisms – impairment of bacterial cell wall synthesis, bacterial protein synthesis or bacterial nucleic acid synthesis. They are considered either bactericidal, the organism is killed, or bacteriostatic, bacterial growth is inhibited.

Antifungals

There is an increasing incidence of fungal infections within critical care. Risk factors include those who are immunocompromised, people who are respiratory compromised (cystic fibrosis, bronchiectasis, chronic obstructive airways disease), invasive procedures (lines, parenteral nutrition, prosthetics), increased use of antimicrobials and contamination of body compartments with gut lumen contents (Beed et al., 2014). Antifungals exert their effect on the virus cell wall (echinocandins, imadazoles, triazoles, polyenes) or inhibit DNA or RNA synthesis (flucytosine).

Antiviral drugs

The incidence of viral infections within critical care is increasing due to the development of more effective diagnostic testing and emergence of novel pathogens. Immunocompromised patients are more at risk from viral infections, whether this is apparent prior to critical care or as a consequence. Viral infections commonly affect the respiratory system or the central nervous system. Recently novel viruses have emerged such as Severe Acute Respiratory Syndrome (SARS), Middle East Respiratory Syndrome (MERS) and Coronavirus (COVID-19), which resulted in a worldwide pandemic.

Antivirals exert their effects via inhibition of virus penetration into the cell, inhibition of uncoating of the virus once in the cell, inhibition of neuraminidase preventing new viron exit from the cells as well as interference with DNA or RNA synthesis and replication.

Corticosteroids

The use of corticosteroids (glucosorticosteroids, glucocorticoids or steroids) within critical care remains controversial. Anti-inflammatory effects are utilised in anaphylaxis, airway oedema, exacerbation of asthma or COPD, raised intracranial pressure due to cerebral tumour, *Pneumocystis* pneumonia or bacterial meningitis (*Streptococcus pneumonia*). The most recent Cochrane review concluded that there is moderate certainty of evidence for the use of corticosteroids in reducing 28-day and hospital mortality in sepsis (Annane et al., 2019). In acute critical illness or chronic disease states, cortisol may be depleted and replacement with exogenous forms of corticosteroids may be required in adrenal crisis, myxoedema coma and peri- and post-operatively. Glucocorticoids stimulate the synthesis of anti-inflammatory gene proteins and inhibit the synthesis of inflammatory gene proteins via the glucocorticoid receptor.

Immunoglobulins

Vaccines or human immunoglobulins are given to provide active immunisation against specific infectious diseases. Viruses have superficial antigens against which specific vaccine antibodies act, preventing their entry into the host cell. They provide immunisation against bacterial or viral infections. Consideration should be given to immunisation history in trauma patients, with penetrating injuries (tetanus), and head injuries with cerebrospinal fluid leak (pneumococcal), admitted to critical care, with administration prior to discharge, if appropriate.

Intravenous immunoglobulins may also be utilised within critical care under special circumstances in the treatment of Guillain–Barré, myasthenia gravis, inflammatory diseases and more rarely septic shock. They contain human antibodies and are prescribed by specialist doctors.

Toxicology

Since 2012 in England and Wales there has been a steep upward trend in deaths related to drug poisoning, with a similar picture in Northern Ireland, Scotland and Northern Europe (Office for National Statistics, 2020). Drug poisoning accounted for 4,393 deaths in 2019 according to the Office for National Statistics, two thirds of which were due to drug misuse, with 50% due to opiates. The emergence of new psychoactive substances, such as 'legal highs' or synthetic cannabinoids, as well as cocaine, have also been implicated.

Suicide death rates, within the England and Wales remain high, with self-poisoning accounting for 16–32% of deaths (Office for National Statistics, 2020). The UK National Poisons Information Service developed an online poisons information database, TOXBASE, in 1999 which is routinely employed in the management of patients presenting with poisoning.

Management of drug poisoning includes supportive care and certain strategies including identification of the drug and specific treatment, removal of the drug from the GI tract and prevention of absorption, enhanced drug elimination and psychiatric assessment. Admission to critical care may be necessary for ongoing resuscitation and management of the airway, cardiorespiratory system, temperature, fluid and electrolyte balance, seizures and renal function. However, specific therapies such as haemodialysis to remove drugs, highly specialised treatment of specific drugs and close monitoring may only be conducted within critical care.

Orange Flag

Self-poisoning may be accidental or intentional. Patients treated in critical care following overdose may require assessment and psychological support from the Liaison Psychiatry Team prior to discharge to the ward or home.

6Cs: Compassion

Compassion, also known as 'intelligent kindness', requires the delivering of care to be focused around several key aspects; empathy, respect, dignity, recognising people's emotions and forming therapeutic relationships with patients based on empathy.

Snapshot

Jobi is a 28-year-old lady who presented to the emergency department at 0800 hours having taken a paracetamol overdose at 1800 hours the previous evening. She recently lost her job, has been feeling 'low', took an overdose and is now remorseful. Jobi thinks that she has taken approximately 40 tablets (20 grams) of paracetamol. Blood tests demonstrated a paracetamol level of 280 mg/L and an infusion of N-acetylcycteine (NAC) was commenced at 0900 hours. Jobi was transferred to the monitoring unit but had worsening bloods at 1900 and so was admitted to the critical care unit for closer monitoring and ongoing management. On arrival the RN receives a handover from the ward staff and completes a full assessment as follows:

Airway (A): patent

Breathing (B): self-ventilating on room air, saturations 92%, respiratory rate 22, chest is clear on auscultation, speaking in short sentences

Circulation (C): Heart rate 112 beats per minute, Blood pressure 95/46 mmHg, capillary refill time 4 seconds, cool peripherally

Disability (D): drowsy but rousable to voice on the AVPU scale, blood glucose is 3.6, body temperature is 36.7°C

Exposure (E): she reports feeling nauseated and on abdominal examination she has bowel sounds present with abdominal pain in the right upper quadrant, the NAC infusion is being administered via a peripheral cannula.

Nursing actions

- Administer oxygen via nasal cannulae.
- Request urgent medical review highlighting concerns regarding new oxygen requirement, increased respiratory rate, hypotension, low blood glucose.
- Set up a flush bag in anticipation of the placement of an arterial line.
- Once line placed send admission bloods and arterial blood gas.
- Continue the paracetamol o verdose protocol with a plan to send repeat blood tests, specifically full blood count, urea and electrolytes, liver function tests and INR, 2 hours prior to the third NAC infusion finishing.
- Provide personal patient care.
- Discuss clinical situation with patients and update family on admission.
- Consider referral to Psychiatric Liaison team.
- Await medical review and further plans for management.

Conclusion

As a student healthcare practitioner working within the critical care environment, you will undoubtedly be involved in the care of a number of patients requiring different pharmacological interventions as part of their treatment pathway. Medicines management for the critical care population can be very complex and has the potential to have detrimental effects. As such, it is crucial that the healthcare professionals involved in supporting this patient group have a sound understanding of the pathophysiological, pharmacological and evidence base that underpins the promotion of safe and effective care.

Take home points

1. Healthcare professionals involved in medicines management should have an understanding of the four key pharmacological principles in order to promote safe and effective patient care.
2. One of the main concerns of adverse effects of pharmacotherapy within the critical care population is upon the renal system.
3. Therapeutic drug monitoring aims to individualise drug therapy and avoid both sub-therapeutic and toxic plasma drug concentrations.
4. The Renal Drug Database is an excellent, evidence-based resource for safe and effective medicines management in the critically ill population.

References

Akbari, P. and Khorasani-Zadeh, A. (2019). Thiazide diuretics. *Stat Pearls*. https://www.ncbi.nlm.nih.gov/books/NBK532918/ (accessed December 2020).

Anandaciva, S. (2020). Critical care services in the English NHS. https://www.kingsfund.org.uk/publications/critical-care-services-nhs#activity (accessed September 2020).

Annane, D., Bellissant, E., Bollaert, P.E. et al. (2019). Corticosteroids for treating sepsis in children and adults (Review). *Cochrane Database of Systematic Reviews* 12. doi: 10.1002/14651858.CD002243.pub4.

Barr, J., Fraser, G., Puntillo, K. et al. (2013). Clinical practice guidelines for the management of pain, agitation and delirium in adult patients in the intensive care unit. *Critical Care Medicine* 41: 263–306.

Beed, M., Sherman, R., and Holden, S. (2014). Fungal infections and critically ill adults: Continuing education in anaesthesia. *Critical Care & Pain* 14(6): 262–267.

Blaser, A.R., Malbrain, M.L.N.G., Starkopf, J. et al. (2012). Gastrointestinal function in intensive care patients:

135

terminology, definitions and management. Recommendations of the ESICM working group on abdominal problems. *Intensive Care Medicine* 38: 384–394.

British Medical Journal Best Practice Guidance (2020). Status epilepticus. https://bestpractice.bmj.com/topics/en-gb/3000127/pdf/3000127/Status%20epilepticus.pdf (accessed December 2020).

BNF: British National Formulary (2020). Prescribing in renal impairment. https://bnf.nice.org.uk/guidance/prescribing-in-renal-impairment.html (accessed December 2020).

Burry, L., Hutton, B., Mehta, S. et al. (2019). Pharmacological interventions for the treatment of delirium in critically ill adults (Review). *Cochrane Database of Systematic Reviews*. doi:10.1002/14651858.CD011749.pub2.

Cavallazzi, R., Saad, M., and Marik, P. (2012). Delirium in the ICU. https://pubmed.ncbi.nlm.nih.gov/23270646/ (accessed December 2020).

Chess-Williams, R. (2002). Muscarinic receptors of the urinary bladder: detrusor, urothelial and prejunctional. *Auton Autacoid Pharmacol* 22(3): 133–145. doi: 10.1046/j.1474-8673.2002.00258.x.

Critical Care Networks-National Nurse Leads (CC3N) (2015). National Competency Framework for Registered Nurses in Adult Critical Care. Step 2 competencies. https://www.cc3n.org.uk/uploads/9/8/4/2/98425184/02_new_step_2_final.pdf (accessed December 2020).

Cook, D.J., Fuller, H.D., Guyatt, G.H. et al. (1994). Risk factors for gastrointestinal bleeding in critically ill patients. *New England Journal of Medicine* 330: 377–381.

Diamond-Fox, S.L. and Gatehouse, A. (2021). Medications and the renal system. In: *Fundamentals of Pharmacology: For Nursing and Healthcare Students* (ed. I. Peate and B. Hill), 225–284. Wiley.

Dutton, H. and Finch, H. (2018). *Critical Care Nursing at a Glance*. Wiley-Blackwell.

Edwardson, S. and Cairns, C. (2019). Nosocomial infections in the ICU. *Anaesthesia & Intensive Care Medicine* 20(1): 14–18.

Finfer, S., Chittock, D.R., Su, S.Y. et al. (2009). Intensive versus conventional glucose control in critically ill patients. *New England Journal of Medicine* 360(13): 1283–1297.

Freedman, S.B., Ulkeryk, E., Rumantir, M. et al. (2014). Ondansetron and the risk of cardiac arryhtmias: a systematic review and postmarketing analysis. *Annals of Emergency Medicine* 64(1): 19–25.

Graeme-Smith, D.G. and Aronson, J.K. (2002). *Oxford Textbook of Clinical Pharmacology and Drug Therapy*, 3e. Oxford: Oxford University Press.

Hardinge, M., Annandale, J., Bourne, S. et al. (2015). British Thoracic Society guidelines for home oxygen use in adults. https://thorax.bmj.com/content/thoraxjnl/70/Suppl_1/i1.full.pdf accessed November 2020 (accessed March 2022).

Hedge S.S. (2006) Muscarininc receptors in the bladder: from basic reasearch to therapeutics. *Br J Pharmacol* 147(Suppl 2): S80–S87. doi: 10.1038/sj.bjp.0706560.

Hegde, H.V., Jagadish, N. & Raghavendra Rao, P. (2014). An ultra-rapid development of tachyphylaxis to nitroglycerin. *Indian Journal of Anaesthesia*. https://www.ncbi.nlm.nih.gov/pmc/articles/PMC4296377/ (accessed November 2020).

Hiley, E., Rickards, E., and Kelly, C.A. (2019). Ensuring the safe use of emergency oxygen in acutely ill patients. *Nursing Times* 115: 18–21.

Hill, A.T., Sullivan, A.L., Chalmers, J.D. et al. (2019). British Thoracic Society Guideline for Bronchiectasis in Adults. https://thorax.bmj.com/content/74/Suppl_1/1 (accessed September 2019).

Huang, H., Jiang, W., Wang, C. et al. (2018). Stress ulcer prophylaxis in intensive care unit patients receiving enteral nutrition: a systematic review and meta-analysis. *Critical Care*. https://ccforum.biomedcentral.com/articles/10.1186/s13054-017-1937-1 (accessed October 2020).

ICS: Intensive Care Society (2016). Medication Concentrations in Adult Critical Care Areas. V2.2. https://www.ics.ac.uk/ICS/ICS/Blogs/New_Standard_Medication_Concentrations_in_Adult_Critical_Care_Area.aspx (accessed November 2020).

Joint British Diabetes Societies for Inpatient Care (2014). The use of variable rate intravenous insulin infusion (VRIII) in medical inpatients. https://www.diabetes.org.uk/resources-s3/2017-09/Use%20of%20variable%20rate%20intravenous%20insulin%20infusion%20in%20medical%20inpatients_0.pdf (accessed December 2020).

Kelesidis, T., Mastoris, I., Metsini, A., and Tsiodras, S. (2014). How to approach and treat viral infections in ICU patients. *BMC Infectious Diseases* https://bmcinfectdis.biomedcentral.com/articles/10.1186/1471-2334-14-321 (accessed December 2020).

Khanna, A. and Peters, N.A (2017). The Vasopressor Toolbox for Defending Blood Pressure. https://www.sccm.org/Communications/Critical-Connections/Archives/2017/The-Vasopressor-Toolbox-for-Defending-Blood-Pressu (accessed November 2020).

Kitchen, S., Gray, E., Mackie, I. et al. (2014). Measurement of non-coumarin anticoagulants and their effects on tests of haemostasis: Guidance from the British Committee for Standards in Haematology. *British Journal of Haematology* 166(6): 830–841. doi: 10.1111/bjh.12975.

Klabunde, E. (2012). *Cardiovascular Physiology Concepts*. 2e. Philadelphia: Lippincott Williams and Wilkinson.

Krag, M., Perner, A., Wetterslev, J. et al. (2015). Prevalence and outcome of gastrointestinal bleeding and use of acid suppressants in acutely ill adult intensive care patients. *Intensive Care Medicine* 41: 833–845.

Leach, R. (2014). *Critical Care Medicine at a Glance*, 3e. Wiley-Blackwell.

Lei, M. & Huang, C.L.-H. (2018). Modernized Classification of Cardiac Antiarrhythmic Drugs. *Circulation* 138: 1879–1896. doi: 10.1161/CIRCULATIONAHA.118.035455.

Joint British Diabetes Societies for Inpatient Care (2014). The use of variable rate intravenous insulin infusion (VRIII) in medical patients. https://www.diabetes.org.uk/resources-s3/2017-09/Use%20of%20variable%20rate%20intravenous%20insulin%20infusion%20in%20medical%20inpatients_0.pdf (accessed October 2020).

Martin, C. Cortegiani, A. Gregoretti, C. et al. (2018). Choice of fluids in critically ill patients. *BMC Anesthesiology* https://link.springer.com/article/10.1186/s12871-018-0669-3 (accessed October 2020).

Narayanan, N., Venkataraju, A., and Jennings, J. (2016). Analgesia in intensive care: Part 1. *BJA Education* 16(2): 72–78.

National Institute for Health and Care Excellence (2013). Intravenous fluid therapy in adults in hospital. Clinical Guideline 174. https://www.nice.org.uk/guidance/cg174 (accessed October 2020).

National Institute for Health and Care Excellence (2014). Chronic Kidney disease in adults: assessment and management. Clinical guideline 182. https://www.nice.org.uk/guidance/cg182 (accessed December 2020).

National Institute for Health and Care Excellence (2015). Medicines optimisation: the safe and effective use of medicines to enable the best possible outcomes. NICE guideline [NG5]. https://www.nice.org.uk/guidance/ng5/chapter/Introduction (accessed November 2020).

National Institute for Health and Care Excellence (2017) Cystic fibrosis: diagnosis and management. NICE guideline [NG78] https://www.nice.org.uk/guidance/ng78 (accessed November 2020).

National Institute for Health and Care Excellence (2017). Asthma: diagnosis, monitoring and chronic asthma https://www.nice.org.uk/guidance/ng80/chapter/Recommendations#principles-of-pharmacological-treatment (accessed November 2020).

National Institute for Health and Care Excellence (2019a). Asthma, acute. Levels of severity. https://bnf.nice.org.uk/treatment-summary/asthma-acute.html (accessed November 2020).

National Institute for Health and Care Excellence (2019b). Chronic obstructive pulmonary disease in over 16s: diagnosis and management. https://www.nice.org.uk/guidance/ng115 (accessed November 2020).

Neal M.J (2016). *Medical Pharmacology at a Glance*, 8e. Section 14. Wiley & Sons.

Neal, M.J (2020). *Medical Pharmacology at a Glance*, 9e. Wiley-Blackwell.

Nicolas, D., Nicolas, S., Hodgens, A. et al. (2020). Heparin induced thrombocytopenia. https://www.ncbi.nlm.nih.gov/books/NBK482330/ (accessed December 2020).

O'Callaghan, O. (2017). *The Renal System at a Glance*, 4e. Wiley & Sons.

O'Driscoll, B.R., Howard, L.S., Earis, J. et al. (2017). British Thoracic Society guideline for oxygen use in adults in healthcare and emergency settings. *Thorax* 72(S1): 1–90.

Office for National Statistics (2020). Suicides in England and Wales: 2019 registrations. https://www.ons.gov.uk/peoplepopulationandcommunity/birthsdeathsandmarriages/deaths/bulletins/suicidesintheunitedkingdom/2019registrations#:~:text=In%202019%2C%20a%20total%20of,(10.5%20deaths%20per%20100%2C000) (accessed December 2020).

Peate, I. and Hill, B. (2021). *Fundamentals of Pharmacology: For Nursing & Healthcare Students*. Wiley-Blackwell.

Poole, P., Sathananthan, K., and Fortescue, R. (2019). Mucolytic agents versus placebo for chronic bronchitis or chronic obstructive pulmonary diease. *Cochrane Database of Systematic Reviews* 7 (Art. No.: CD001287). https//doi.org/10.1002/14651858.pub.6.

Public Health England (2015). Respiratory disease: applying All Our Health. https://www.gov.uk/government/publications/respiratory-disease-applying-all-our-health/respiratory-disease-applying-all-our-health (accessed September 2020).

Public Health England (2019). National Poisons Information Service. Report 2018/19. https://www.npis.org/Download/NPISAnnualReport2018-19.pdf (accessed December 2020).

Rattu, M. (2015). Pharmacists' role in managing male urinary incontinence. www.upharmacist.com/article/pharmacists-role-managing-male-urinary-incontinence (accessed December 2020).

Rhodes, A., Evans, L., Waleed, A., et al (2017). Surviving Sepsis Campaign: International guidelines for management of sepsis and septic shock: 2016. *Intensive Care Medicine* 43: 304–377.

Richards, D., Aronson, J., Reynolds, D.J., and Coleman, J. (2012). *Oxford Handbook of Practical Drug Therapy*. 2e. Oxford: Oxford University Press.

RPS: Royal Pharmaceutical Society (2020). Medicines optimisation hub https://www.rpharms.com/resources/pharmacy-guides/medicines-optimisation-hub (accessed November 2020).

Russell, J.A. Vasopressor therapy in the critically ill patient with shock. *Intensive Care Medicine* 45: 1503–1517.

Siemieniuk, R.A.C., Chu, D.K., Kim, L.H. et al. (2018). Oxygen therapy for acutely ill medical patients: a clinical practice guideline. https://www.bmj.com/content/363/bmj.k4169 (accessed December 2020).

Steddon, S., Ashman, N., Chesser, A., and Cunningham, J. (2014). *Oxford Handbook of Nephrology and Hypertension*, 2e. Oxford: Oxford University Press.

The National Health Service (2019). *The NHS Long Term Plan*. https://www.longtermplan.nhs.uk/wp-content/uploads/2019/08/nhs-long-term-plan-version-1.2.pdf (accessed September 2020).

The Royal Pharmaceutical Society of Great Britain (2019). Professional guidance on the administration of medicines https://www.google.com/url?sa=t&rct=j&q=&esrc=s&source=web&cd=&cad=rja&uact=8&ved=2ahUKEwjRw5Ld14TtAhUSZMAKHV4tBRoQFjAAegQIBhAC&url=https%3A%2F%2Fwww.rpharms.com%2FPortals%2F0%2FRPS%2520document%2520library%2FOpen%2520access%2FProfessional%2520standards%2FSSHM%2520and%2520Admin%2FAdmin%2520of%2520Meds%2520prof%2520guidance.pdf%3Fver%3D2019-01-23-145026-567&usg=AOvVaw3WJECAmdHj_zgNWOIiTAQa (accessed November 2020).

The Royal Pharmaceutical Society of Great Britain (2018). Professional guidance on the safe and secure handling of medicines. https://www.rpharms.com/recognition/setting-professional-standards/safe-and-secure-handling-of-medicines/professional-guidance-on-the-safe-and-secure-handling-of-medicines (accessed November 2020_.

VanValkinburgh, D. Kerndt, C.C. Hashmi, M.F. (2020). Inotropes and Vasopressors. StatPearls. https://www.ncbi.nlm.nih.gov/books/NBK482411/ (accessed November 2020).

Vaughan Williams, E.M. (1970). Classification of antiarrhythmic drugs. In: *Symposium on Cardiac Arrhythmias* (ed. E. Sandoe, E. Flensted-Jensen, and K.H. Olsen), 449–472. Elsinore: Astra.

Venkataraju, A. and Nararayan, M. (2016). Analgesia in intensive care: Part 2. *BJA Education* 16(12): 397–404.

Vincent, J.L. and Preiser, J-C. (2015). Getting critical about constipation. *Practical Gastroenterology* https://www.practicalgastro-digital.com/practicalgastro/august_2015?pg=7#pg7 (accessed December 2020).

World Health Organisation (2016) *Oxygen Therapy for Children*. https//apps.who.int/iris/bitstream/handle/10665/204584/9789241549554_eng.pdf;jesssionid=20408069BC3191A6FC42826A2CEAA000?sequence=1 (accessed December 2020).

WHO: World Health Organization (2019). The 2019 Expert Committee on the Selection and Use of Essential Medicines. https://www.who.int/groups/expert-committee-on-selection-and-use-of-essential-medicines/essential-medicines-lists (accessed November 2020).

WHO: World Health Organization & PAHO: Pan American Health Organization (2020). Essential Medicines List for Management of Patients Admitted to Intensive Care Units with Suspected or Confirmed COVID-19 Diagnosis. https://iris.paho.org/handle/10665.2/52191 (accessed November 2020).

Chapter 12

Anaesthesia and sedation

Lorraine Mutrie and Iain Carstairs

Aim

The aim of this chapter is to explore the use of anaesthesia and sedation in the critical care environment. It will provide the reader with an evidence-based understanding of the indications, assessment and nursing care and management of the patient requiring anaesthesia and sedation.

Learning outcomes

After reading this chapter the reader will be able to:

- Identify the indications for sedation and anaesthesia in the critical care environment.
- Name commonly used drugs for sedation and anaesthesia.
- Describe the pharmacology of commonly used drugs associated with anaesthesia and sedation critical care.
- Discuss the nurse's role in sedation assessment and management.
- Explain the risks and side effects of sedation and anaesthesia.

Test your prior knowledge

- Can you explain the difference between sedation and anaesthesia?
- Can you identify 5 reasons why patients require sedation?
- When caring for a patient requiring continuous sedation, what observations should you monitor and why?
- Can you name any sedation scoring tools used in clinical practice?
- Can you name one of each of the following drugs?
  - Induction agent
  - Muscle relaxant
  - Benzodiazepine
  - Opioid

Fundamentals of Critical Care: A Textbook for Nursing and Healthcare Students, First Edition. Edited by Ian Peate and Barry Hill.
© 2023 John Wiley & Sons Ltd. Published 2023 by John Wiley & Sons Ltd.
Companion website: www.wiley.com/go/peate/criticalcare

Introduction

Sedation and anaesthesia are commonly used therapies within the critical care unit (CCU) with many patients thought to require them during their critical care stay (Laws and Rudall, 2013). Anaesthesia is the process of inducing loss of sensation and/or awareness, and sedation can be described as the action of administering a sedative drug to produce a state of calm or sleep. The established view is that sedation allows better tolerance of invasive procedures, improves synchronisation with mechanical ventilation, facilitates tight control of physiological parameters, increases patient safety and reduces physiological stress for critically unwell patients (Whitehouse et al., 2014).

The medications used to sedate patients produce short-term side effects including haemodynamic instability and delirium and the long-term effects of sedative drugs have been linked as causative factors to a decline in cognitive function, the incidence of post-traumatic stress disorder, depression and delirium (Aitken et al., 2018; Jones, 2010). It is therefore essential that nurses are knowledgeable and skilled in this area of practice. Sedation and anaesthetic management requires:

- Knowledge of drug administration
- Understanding of the pharmacological agents used for sedation
- Assessment of the patient using recognised observation and sedation measurement tools
- Awareness of how sedation impacts direct care and post-critical care management.

Step 2 competencies: National Standards

2.1.4   Medications used in the process of patient intubation

2.1.5   Management of the patient requiring invasive ventilation

2.1.9   The assessment and administration of pharmacological agents used to facilitate mechanical ventilation

2.2.1   Haemodynamic effect of drugs used in anaesthesia and sedation

2.4.2   Impact of anaesthetic and sedative drugs on the gastrointestinal system

2.5.3   Pharmacological effects of anaesthetic and sedative agents on the neurological system

2.8.1   The long-term impact of sedation practices

Critical Care Networks-National Nurse Leads (CC3N), 2015

Indications for sedation and anaesthesia

Sedation and anaesthesia are mainstays of critical care practice, and the Intensive Care Society (ICS) (Whitehouse et al., 2014) highlight that the term 'sedation' is used to cover the continuum of medication prescribed to reduce anxiety (anxiolysis) to deep unresponsiveness that is similar to that of a general anaesthetic. This continuum covers the many levels of sedation that could be required by critically unwell patients and it is first essential to understand the difference between sedation and anaesthesia.

> ## 6Cs: Care
> A hallmark of quality care is recognising and treating the patient as an individual.

Anaesthetics are a group of drugs that cause a controlled loss of sensation and/or a loss of awareness to facilitate interventions. Anaesthesia is that loss of sensation and the two most common types of anaesthetic are local anaesthetic and general anaesthetic (National Health Service, 2018). Local anaesthetics are used to numb a specific area of the body, to prevent pain and facilitate minor procedures. In the critical care environment examples of the use of local anaesthetics are:

- To relieve post-operative pain
- To reduce pain and sensation during invasive procedures, for example insertion of a vascular access devices or insertion of a chest drain.

A general anaesthetic is a reversible state of unconsciousness in a controlled environment that is typically used for performing procedures including surgery (Shorthouse, 2017). The combination of anaesthetic agents administered for general anaesthesia invoke a state of amnesia, analgesia and muscle relaxation that can lead to loss of airway reflexes. Airway reflexes provide airway protection and therefore a general anaesthetic leaves the patient vulnerable to aspiration of gastric contents if the stomach is full. To reduce this risk, patients are required to fast pre surgery, and cease all fluid intake for a minimum of 2 hours prior to surgery (National Institute for Health and Care Excellence, 2020). This fasting helps to reduce stomach contents so that induction of anaesthesia can be controlled, using calculated drug dosages (often on patient body weight), and allowing for clear progression through each stage of anaesthesia based on patient observation (titrating to effect) (Yentis et al., 2018).

In the CCU, the most common need for a general anaesthetic is tracheal intubation (the insertion of an endotracheal tube into the patient's airway; see Chapter 16), but other indications can include insertion of tracheostomy, endoscopic procedures and complex changes of dressings. Inducing a state of general anaesthesia in a critically unwell patient requires a modified approach to that of a patient that is having planned surgery. Whilst preparing for planned surgery, a patient's condition is optimised to minimise any risks associated with the surgery and anaesthetic. In critically unwell patients, optimisation is often not an option as they present with life-threatening organ dysfunction that requires immediate intervention. These patients will require Rapid Sequence Induction (RSI) of anaesthesia, a process where the patient progresses through the stages of anaesthesia rapidly by administering the anaesthetic agents in quick succession, without titrating to effect. A more detailed explanation about the processes involved in RSI for tracheal intubations can be found in Chapter 16, but in relation to the drugs used to induce anaesthesia during this event, it is recommended that a fast-acting induction agent is administered to a predetermined dose, that a rapidly acting opioid should be considered alongside this to minimise the side effects of the induction agent, and that this should be followed by administration of a rapid onset neuromuscular blocking agent (NMBA) at a pre-determined dose. Further information about these drugs can be found later in this chapter.

Medicines management 1

Process of drug administration in RSI:

- Administration of a suitable fast-acting induction agent
- Sequentially followed by administration of a fast-acting neuromuscular blocker
- Once a patient is successfully intubated, plans for continuous sedation should be made.

N.B. Additional medication to ensure patient stability might be indicated; for example, medication to increase blood pressure.

Snapshot 1

Renuka is a 56-year-old admitted to hospital with community-acquired pneumonia. She was transferred from the Emergency Department to the CCU as a level 2 patient 2 hours ago. Despite being given antibiotics and receiving non-invasive ventilation, her arterial blood gases have deteriorated, and her breathing is becoming more laboured. Renuka has no significant past medical history. The registered nurse immediately escalates her concerns to the doctor on duty after recording the following observations for Renuka:

Airway (A): Airway is patent. The patient can speak in broken sentences.

Breathing (B): Oxygen saturations 92% (NEWS2 = 2), oxygen therapy increased from 50% to 65% (via non-

invasive ventilator) since last observations (NEWS2 = 2). Respiratory rate 28 breaths per minute (NEWS2 = 3). The patient is using accessory muscles of breathing and sitting in a tripod position.

Circulation (C): Blood pressure 115/65 mmHg (NEWS2 = 0), heart rate 116 beats per minute (NEWS2 = 2), capillary refill time 3 seconds, and she is warm to touch.

Disability (D): Patient is Alert on the ACVPU scale (NEWS2 = 0). Body temperature is 38.2°C (NEWS2 = 1).

Exposure (E): no abnormal findings.

Total NEWS2 score: 10.

Diagnosis:

- Deterioration in respiratory function despite appropriate intervention.
- Patient requires invasive mechanical ventilation.
- Patient will require RSI of anaesthesia to secure her airway to provide invasive ventilation.

Nursing actions:

- Inform nurse in charge of patient deterioration and need for intubation.
- Ensure that the patient and relatives understand plan of care.
- Gather equipment for intubation, including drugs for RSI.
- Ensure that all observations and diagnostic tests results are available to the intubating practitioner, and that the patient has adequate haemodynamic monitoring in place. Examples of diagnostic tests include Arterial Blood Gases (ABGs) and Urea and Electrolyte blood results (U & Es).
- Nurse in charge to establish appropriate team present and check role allocation for safe RSI (see Chapter 16).
- Set up ventilator and confirm safety checks have been carried out and passed.
- Request prescription for and set up ongoing sedation infusions.
- Update nursing notes.

An emerging approach to anaesthesia in the CCU is regional anaesthesia (RA). Regional anaesthesia allows for numbing of a larger or deeper part of the body (Royal College of Anaesthetists (RCoA), 2020). This approach to anaesthesia is largely an approach to targeted pain management in awake patients; however, it can provide an alternative approach to continuous sedation and administration of systemic opioids, thereby minimising the risks associated with these drugs. Although further evidence of its use in critical care is required, specific examples of RA in the critical care environment include (Venkataraju and Narayanan, 2016):

- Management of rib fractures
- Patients undergoing laparotomy
- Pancreatitis
- Vasospasm
- Hip fractures.

Sedation can be described as an induced state of reduced consciousness (Yentis at al, 2018) that can range from a very light level of sedation (for example, a premedication prescribed to relax a patient prior to surgery) to a deep level of sedation similar to a general anaesthetic (to facilitate the prone positioning of a patient for example). Sedative medications in the CCU can be prescribed and administered as either bolus doses or as continuous infusions, the latter being the most prevalent. It is a common misconception that all invasively ventilated patients require sedation, and that ventilation is the only reason to sedate. Indications for sedative use are many and varied, and sedation should always be considered in relation to individual patient factors. Common indications can be found in Box 12.1.

Box 12.1   Indications for sedation.

Facilitation of mechanical ventilation	Invasive mechanical ventilation requires insertion of a tracheal tube to secure the airway; a tube passed down the trachea to just above the tip of the carina. A tracheal tube, particularly an orally inserted tube, can induce a cough or gag reflex. Sedation can help the patient to tolerate the tube preventing patient self-extubation (Woodrow, 2019).
	During invasive mechanical ventilation, ventilator delivered breaths and patient demand for breaths should match otherwise patient-ventilator dysynchrony can occur. This dysynchrony, also known as 'fighting the ventilator' can have adverse effects on the patient. This can be minimised with the use of sedation (Pierce, 2007).
Prevent discomfort, stress, and anxiety	There are many reasons why patients in critical care suffer from discomfort, stress, and anxiety. They include: - Pain from procedures and interventions (surgery, invasive devices, non-invasive ventilation, dressing changes, tracheal suction, mobilisation with muscle myopathy) - Environmental factors (white noise from machinery, staff noise) - Communication challenges - Emotional response to critical illness (i.e., fear)
To facilitate treatment and procedures	Examples of procedures include, but are not limited to: - Tracheal suction - Insertion of invasive devices (chest drain, arterial line, central line) - Bronchial lavage - Dressings changes or minor surgical procedures - Prone positioning - Inverse ratio ventilation
Promote sleep	Sleep hygiene is commonly affected in critically unwell patients. Sedative drugs can be used to increase total sleep time, but they can also alter normal circadian sleep pattern (Whitehouse et al., 2014). The Clinical Practice Guidelines for the Prevention and Management of Pain, Agitation/Sedation, and Delirium, Immobility and Sleep Disruption in Adult Patients in the ICU (PADIS) (Devlin et al., 2018) identify that there are no sedative drugs that are recommended for sleep promotion, but dexmedetomidine can be used for overnight sedation for haemodynamically stable patients. Because many factors that affect sleep are modifiable (noise, light, interruptions for care), it is prudent to modulate the environment first.
To treat confusional states	Delirium is a common presentation associated with critical illness and although not a routine recommendation, dexmedetomidine can be used for patients where agitation is preventing weaning from mechanical ventilation (Devlin et al., 2018).

To prevent awareness during administration of neuromuscular blocking agents (NMBAs)	NMBAs relax skeletal muscle but do not offer any sedation. Administration of NMBAs without sedation has been associated with a feeling of going back and forth (between life and death), suffering unusual dreams, a loss of control including being tied down and being scared, almost dying and feeling cared for (Ballard et al., 2006), as the patient is unable to move, but is aware.
As a treatment	Sedation can prevent secondary brain injury following primary neurological insult by reducing metabolic demand. It can also offer myocardial protection for patients that have known myocardial dysfunction.
	Sedatives can also be used in the treatment of status epilepticus.
	Despite optimal sedation being associated with a reduction in metabolic demand and modification of the stress response, it is not an indication for use (Whitehouse et al., 2014).

Anaesthetic and sedative medications

There is currently no one drug that fits the ideal drug profile to provide sedation in the CCU and anaesthetic agents are frequently used in conjunction with analgesics to induce sleep and deliver pain relief. Time of onset, side effects and duration of action of the drug are all aspects that should be considered when choosing which agents to administer.

Medicines management 2

Context-sensitive half time refers to the time it takes for the drug concentration in blood plasma to reduce by 50% after an infusion of the drug has discontinued. This is different to the half-life of a drug as it also takes into account drug accumulation within tissue. The impact of context-sensitive half time in sedation is as follows:

- Low context-sensitive half time = short period of time between discontinuation and wake up
- Moderate context-sensitive half time = moderate period between drug discontinuation and wake up
- Long context-sensitive half time = long period of time between drug discontinuation and wake up
- Context insensitive half time = no residual effect after infusion discontinued

---

Sedative drugs

There are a range of drugs used to sedate ranging from drugs designed specifically as induction or anaesthetic agents, to those whose primary function is as pain relief. Below is a brief overview of some of the drugs used for sedation in critical care.

Propofol

The anaesthetic agent propofol is the most used drug for sedation purposes on the CCU. It manipulates neurotransmission by increasing the effect of neuro inhibitory neurotransmitters. Propofol has a rapid onset, is easy to titrate and has only a moderate increase in context-sensitive half time (see box Medicines management 2). It is an inexpensive drug that both medical and nursing staff are comfortable using but it does generate well known side effects including arterial and venous vasodilatation, myocardial depression, hypertriglyceridemia, and the rarer Propofol Infusion Syndrome (PRIS). When caring for a patient receiving a propofol infusion nurses must remain vigilant for signs of hypotension, cardiac dysfunction, and a metabolic acidosis. A propofol adjusted feeding regimen should also be considered to reduce lipid intake.

Midazolam

Benzodiazepines should be avoided for sedation in adults in CCU as their respiratory depressive effects are associated with longer wake up times and longer time to extubation (Devlin et al., 2018), and they can increase likelihood of delirium (Jones, 2010). Where a benzodiazepine is indicated, midazolam is most frequently used. It has a relatively good speed of wake-up in comparison with other benzodiazepines; however, it still poses a risk of accumulation due to its active metabolites. Its mode of action is to enhance neuro inhibition, acting on benzodiazepine-specific receptors.

Thiopentone

Thiopentone (thiopental sodium) is a thiobarbiturate that is classically combined with suxamethonium for use in RSI. Thiopentone has a rapid onset but a long context-sensitive half-life, therefore is not suitable for continuous infusion of sedation. Although it causes less vasodilation than propofol, side effects include histamine release, worsening of bronchospasm and caution should be used when using in unstable patients. Thiopentone is contraindicated in acute porphyria (a rare blood disorder).

Ketamine

Ketamine is a slower onset anaesthetic agent than propofol and thiopentone. It can be used for induction of anaesthesia, analgesia and sedation for short procedures. The slower onset of this drug could lead to awareness in the patient if used incorrectly during RSI. The benefits of ketamine include maintenance of cardiovascular stability, maintenance of airway reflexes, bronchodilation (beneficial in difficult to treat asthma) and its analgesic effect. Contraindications to its use are the head injured patient and acute porphyria.

Etomidate

Etomidate is a rapid onset induction agent that causes minimal cardiovascular depressant effects and minimal histamine release. Despite this, it is not recommended for use in critically unwell patients as it causes immunosuppression after the first bolus dose.

Opioids

Opioids are primarily used for their analgesic effects however most do have additional sedative benefits. Their main side effects are histamine release, hypotension and respiratory depression. Opioids target opioid receptors and mimic the inhibition of pre- and post-synaptic responses that occur in naturally occurring opioids. Morphine has a long context-sensitive half time and accumulates during liver and renal failure. Fentanyl is a shorter acting synthetic opioid but if administered as a continuous infusion does have a long context-sensitive half time unlike alfentanil, which has a reduced context-sensitive half time when compared with both morphine and fentanyl. Remifentanil, a synthetic opioid, is a fast-acting opioid analgesic that has a context insensitive half time.

Dexmedetomidine

Dexmedetomidine is a sedative agent that has more recently been introduced to CCU sedation practice and has several potential benefits over the previously discussed agents. Its mechanism of action is to inhibit noradrenaline release by acting as a specific alpha-2 agonist. This reduces the risk of respiratory depression in the short term and reduces the negative effect of the stress response. Dexmedetomidine produces an analgesic and anxiolysis effect that promotes a state of patient arousal that allows for an alert, communicative state. Despite the potential benefits demonstrated, the use of dexmedetomidine to replace the standard sedatives has not been widely accepted into practice. This could be as a result of its current limited generalisability to all patient groups, and the longer-term risk of tachyphylaxis (desensitisation to a drug) and agitation limiting its suitability for long-term sedation. Nonetheless, consideration should be given to its role as an adjunct to reduce sedation accumulation.

Medicines management 3

The medications administered for pain relief, sedation and anaesthesia all have a different mechanism of action, half-life and context-sensitive half time. When used in combination it is important to consider the effect of concurrent medications and the potential for drug interactions.

Examination scenario 1

The inclusion of allied health professionals in the Guidelines for Provision of Intensive Care Services (GPICs) (ICS, 2019) highlights the need for a multidisciplinary approach to care for all critically unwell patients. An example of this is the expert dietician input required when patients are sedated with propofol, especially at higher doses. Propofol has a high lipid content that should be considered when nutritional requirements are calculated for patients that are being enterally or parenterally fed. Dietician review should take place early in the patient's critical care stay, and a review requested when sedation needs change.

143

Neuromuscular blocking agents and reversal agents

Neuromuscular blocking agents (NMBAs) are drugs that are designed to work at the neuromuscular junction to stop nerve impulse transmission, causing skeletal muscle to relax. NMBAs do not have any sedative or analgesic effect therefore in critical care they are usually administered as a bolus dose as part of the RSI process for intubation, or when short-term muscle relaxation is required. They are commonly referred to as muscle relaxants or paralysing agents. There are two types of muscle relaxants: non-depolarising and depolarising. Non-depolarising NMBAs compete with acetylcholine (ACh) for receptor sites at the neuromuscular junction to block nerve impulse transmission and can be reversed. Depolarising NMBAs cause depolarisation by mimicking ACh at the ACh receptor sites and cannot be reversed (British National Formulary, 2021; Yentis et al., 2018). The neuromuscular junction is the synapse between the presynaptic motor neurone and the postsynaptic membrane.

Suxamethonium

Suxamethonium is a depolarising NMBA that is traditionally used in RSI and is typically used alongside thiopentone but can be used with other induction agents. It is often the muscle relaxant of choice for emergency intubation as it is fast-acting and quick to wear off (approximately 3 minutes) but its side effects include transient hyperkalaemia, bradycardia, increased intraocular pressure, malignant hyperpyrexia (a dangerous complication of general anaesthesia), suxamethonium apnoea (prolonged time of effect caused by an alteration to the enzyme that breaks down the drug) and myalgia.

Rocuronium

Rocuronium is a non-depolarising NMBA and its use has increased since the introduction of the reversal agent sugammadex. Its onset of action is determined by the dose administered, and a dose of 0.9–1.2 mg/kg will provide intubating conditions required for emergency RSI (within 60 seconds) compared to a standard dose of 0.6 mg/kg that will provide slower onset of muscle relaxation. Duration of action with the RSI dose ranges from 45–60 minutes. This prolonged time makes availability of a reversal agent essential to prevent complications associated with a 'can't intubate, can't oxygenate' scenario (see Chapter 16 for more details).

Atracurium

Atracurium is a non-depolarising NMBA. It is not routinely used as a bolus drug for RSI in the critical care environment due to its slower onset of action, it is used for continuous infusion when longer-term muscle relaxation is required. Indications for longer-term muscle relaxants include facilitation of prone positioning, difficult to ventilate patients and reduction in metabolic demand due to shivering in hypothermic patients (including targeted temperature management). Atracurium does not accumulate in renal and liver impairment, making it a suitable choice for patients with organ failure.

Sugammadex

Sugammadex is the reversal agent for rocuronium. It works by encapsulating the rocuronium on the ACh receptor at the neuromuscular junction to rapidly reverse any residual effect of the drug. To reverse the RSI dose of rocuronium, a dose of 16 mg/kg of sugammadex is needed. This would reverse the effects of the rocuronium should a 'can't intubate, can't oxygenate' scenario present. Calculating the required dose of sugammadex prior to administration of rocuronium would be prudent.

Neostigmine

Neostigmine works by reducing the breakdown of ACh so that more ACh is available to compete with residual NMBA at the receptor site. It is the first-line reversal agent used in anaesthetic practice, but it is not effective for reversing the RSI dose of rocuronium and cannot reverse the effects of the depolarising NMBA suxamethonium.

Medicines management 4

Critical illness can alter the pharmacokinetics and pharmacodynamics of drugs causing unpredictability. This can be attributed to alterations in fluid balance, gastrointestinal absorbency, liver impairment and renal impairment leading to changes in drug metabolism, excretion and accumulation.

Clinical investigation 1

Prior to the use of suxamethonium, a recent blood potassium level should be available due to the risk of significant transient hyperkalaemia.

Clinical investigation 2

Minimum standards for patient monitoring during anaesthesia and sedation are:

Airway (A): Ability to maintain own airway or presence of patent tracheal tube/ airway adjunct.

Breathing (B): Respiratory rate, oxygen saturation, waveform capnography (for RSI and intubated patients).

Circulation (C): Continuous ECG monitoring, regular non-invasive blood pressure monitoring if invasive blood pressure monitoring not in use.

Disability (D): Regular GCS scoring (including pupil reaction), sedation assessment tool, pain assessment tool, delirium assessment tool.

Exposure (E): Nothing specific to anaesthesia and sedation.

Snapshot 2

Steven, a 65-year-old, has been admitted to CCU as a level 3 patient following an out-of-hospital cardiac arrest. He had return of spontaneous circulation after receiving bystander cardiopulmonary resuscitation (CPR) and defibrillation by paramedics. He was intubated at the scene. His 12-lead ECG and troponin blood tests suggest that his cardiac arrest was the result of myocardial infarction. A chest X-ray on admission to the Emergency Department confirmed ETT placement, and multiple left-sided rib fractures thought to be sustained during CPR. He has been admitted to critical care for post cardiac arrest management including targeted temperature management. On admission to the CCU the registered nurse performs a full A–E assessment. For this patient, it is unlikely that a NEWS2 scoring system would be used as care has already been escalated to a level of higher dependency with increased observation, and the interventions that the patient is receiving are not addressed within this scoring system. Instead, the registered nurse would document observations and infusions on the critical care specific observations chart or e-record.

Airway (A): Airway protected with size 8.0 cm endotracheal tube (ETT), measuring 23 cm at the lips.

Breathing (B): Ventilated using a pressure support mode (see Chapter 16). Respiratory rate set at 18 breaths per minute with sporadic spontaneous effort from patient. No added breath sounds on auscultation. Has not required tracheal suction.

Circulation (C): Blood pressure 92/ 47 mmHg, heart rate 126 beats per minute, capillary refill time 4 seconds. Patient is cool to touch. Dobutamine infusion running at 5 mcg/kg/min and noradrenaline infusion at 4 mL/hr. Intravenous fluid therapy at 80 mL/hr.

Disability (D): Patient responds to Verbal command on the ACVPU scale. GCS recorded as 8 (Eye opening to sound = 3, No verbal response with ETT = 0, Motor response = 5). Pupil size 3, equal and reactive to light. Propofol infusion running at 10ml/hr. Richmond Agitation and Sedation Scale score = −2.

Exposure (E): Patient has BMI 42. Current temperature 38.7°C.

Diagnosis:

Patient requires active cooling to achieve normothermia.

Nursing actions:

- Registered nurse to set up equipment for targeted temperature management.
- Consider nutritional needs of patient.
- Alert medical team to patient responsiveness and request sedation review.
- Ensure next of kin understand plan of care.
- Update nursing notes.

Sedation management

Targeted sedation

Depth of sedation can be divided into light, moderate and heavy and historically patients requiring sedation on critical care have been heavily sedated via a continuous infusion of intravenous sedative agents (Jackson et al., 2009). This method of sedation results in difficult patient arousal, increased context-sensitive half times relative to the duration of the infusion and has been proven to be an independent predictor of increased duration of mechanical ventilation, increased intensive care stay and increased time to hospital discharge (Kollef et al., 1998). Deep, continuous and excessive sedation can lead to a delay in patient waking and increase difficulty performing and interpreting daily neurological examinations. If prolonged, delayed waking could prompt unnecessary neurological investigations thus exposing the patient to radiation and the risk of associated transfer complications.

Optimal sedation is difficult to determine but aims to provide patient comfort and compliance whilst reducing the incidence of both short- and long-term complications of sub-optimal sedation (see Box 12.2). The use of heavy sedation is considered the most common form of sub-optimal sedation (Jackson et al., 2009) and since the Kollef et al. (1998) study there has been a shift towards lighter levels of sedation.

6Cs: Compassion

Providing dignity and respect whilst a patient is sedated is essential to compassionate care.

6Cs: Courage

The knowledge and ability to discuss patient treatment strategies, and advocate on behalf of the patient for safe and high-quality care.

Examination scenario 2

When patients are sedated it can be difficult for them to communicate their needs and preferences to you. To gather this information, you could ask their next of kin to complete a 'This is me' document.

The 'This is me' tool was designed by the Alzheimer's Society to record details about a person who is not able to easily share this information themselves. It can be used in any care setting to find out about a person's cultural and family background, important information about their life, and any preferences and routines they might have. This can facilitate holistic, individualised and patient-centred care.

Although not researched, using the 'This is me' document can create a sense of involvement in care for relatives, and it can help staff to build therapeutic relationships by providing known talking points to engage patients.

The 'This is me' document can be found at https://www.alzheimers.org.uk/get-support/publications-factsheets/this-is-me.

The critical care nurse is responsible for titrating sedation based on their assessment of the patient. Depth of sedation can be measured subjectively using validated sedation scales such as the Richmond Agitation-Sedation Score (RASS), Ramsey Sedation Scale (RSS), Riker Sedation-Agitation Scale (SAS) or Motor Activity Assessment Scale (MAAS), or objectively with using physiological tools including Bispectral Index (BIS) monitoring, patient electroencephalogram (EEG) or Auditory Evoked Potentials (Whitehouse et al., 2014). The objective measurements available are useful as adjuncts to

145

sedation measurement but subjective measurements of sedation are deemed best despite the risk of bias and inter-individual variability (Devlin et al., 2018; Sessler et al., 2002; Whitehouse et al., 2014). The RASS tool has demonstrated to have high reliability and validity when carried out by nurses trained in its use and has been accepted in many CCUs (Sessler et al., 2002). RASS (see Box 12.3) is a 10-level scale which has four levels of anxiety (+1 to +4); one level to denote a calm and alert state (0) and five levels of sedation (−1 to −5). It is assumed that a score of anything but zero will result in further investigation and management of the underlying cause, including titration of sedative medications. The RASS is also used in collaboration with the Confusion Assessment Method for the ICU (CAM-ICU) in the assessment for delirium (Whitehouse et al., 2014).

6Cs: Competence

A competent practitioner can select the correct assessment tool for any given situation.

Box 12.2   Consequences of sub-optimal sedation.

Over sedation	Under Sedation
Increased duration of ventilation	Agitation
Increased length of CCU stay	Increased oxygen demand and utilisation
Increased risk of ventilation acquired pneumonia	Reduction in ability to tightly control physiological factors
Risk of barotrauma	Increased nursing input and staffing
Gastric function altered	Not appropriate for all patients
Increased risk of thromboembolism	Potential increase risk of adverse events
Decreased physical function	Increased ventilation dysynchrony
Increased risk of delirium	
Link to decreased cognitive function	
Increased risk of post-traumatic stress disorder	

Box 12.3   Richmond Agitation-Sedation Score (RASS).

Score	Definition	Description
+4	Combative	Violent, combatitive, dangerous
+3	Very agitated	Pulls/removes tubes, aggressive
+2	Agitated	Frequent non-purposeful movement/ patient-ventilator dysynchrony
+1	Restless	Anxious/ apprehensive, movement not aggressive or vigorous
0	Alert and calm	
−1	Drowsy	Eye opening to voice, sustained eye contact for >10 seconds
−2	Light sedation	Less than 10 seconds awakening
−3	Moderation sedation	Movement or eye opening to voice, no eye contact
−4	Deep sedation	No response to voice, movement or eye opening to physical stimulation
−5	Unarousable	No response to voice or physical stimulation

Sedation-reducing strategies

Lighter levels of sedation can allow the patient to retain the ability to communicate and be involved with care (Whitehouse et al., 2014). It can also lead to reductions in

- Number of days ventilated
- Hospital length of stay
- Total amount of sedation administered

(Kress et al., 2000; Girard et al., 2008; De Wit et al., 2008; Strom et al., 2010).
   Strategies to reduce sedation include the following.

Sedation interruption

The process of sedation interruption involves stopping all continuous sedative infusions daily to prevent the accumulation of sedative medications therefore resetting the context-sensitive half time of the drug. During the interruption, neurological evaluation can take place including delirium screening (see Chapters 6 and 15). It is recommended that sufficient staff should be available during any episode of sedation interruption as patient reaction can be unpredictable (physical and haemodynamic). Whilst daily sedation interruption makes pharmacological sense, it may not be suitable for patients that require muscle relaxants, are unstable haemodynamically, have high ventilator requirements, or those with raised intracranial pressure (Laws and Rudall, 2013).

Protocolised sedation

Protocolised sedation is when the nurse titrates the sedation rate to reach a specific sedation target (for example to keep a patient at RASS score −2), instead of administering the infusion at the same rate as it is started.

Analgesia first

The concept of analgesia first aims to minimise or entirely eradicate the use of sedative agents with a focus on improved pain management.

6Cs: Commitment

Continuous improvement in care requires you to keep up to date with current research and evidence for practice.

Snapshot 3

It is 3 days since Steven was admitted to the CCU following his cardiac arrest. His targeted temperature management treatment is completed, and early indicators suggest a good neurological recovery. His noradrenaline has been discontinued but dobutamine infusion continues. At the ward round the medical team have requested that you begin to 'wake and wean' Steven, beginning with a sedation interruption. For this, the nursing team will need to:

- Risk assess to plan optimum time to stop sedation. This should include assessing patient risk factors by performing A–E assessment, confirming all interventions that might require sedation are carried out prior to sedation hold, and assessing the ward environment to ensure adequate personnel available if any complications arise.
- Ensuring emergency airway trolley is available (and not in use at another bedspace) should the patient self-extubate.
- Use recognised scoring systems to assess the patient when sedation has been held (RASS, GCS, pain assessment tool, delirium assessment tool).
- Make a clear plan for restarting sedation, if required.
- Remembering the patient has fractured ribs, request a pain management review to facilitate pain free waking and weaning.
- Ensure that the patient and next of kin understand plan of care.
- Update nursing notes.

6Cs: Communication

Clear, simple instruction and explanation can help overcome the barriers of communicating with sedated patients.

Conclusion

Sedation and anaesthesia are mainstays of critical care practice and both can have an impact on the long- and short-term outcomes of the patient. It is important for nursing staff to understand the indications for sedation and anaesthesia, have knowledge of the drugs available for use and understand the need to effectively assess the sedated patient.

Red Flag

- Neurological assessment whilst a patient is sedated can be challenging. The normal mechanisms of assessing consciousness, cognition, brainstem function and motor function are impaired in the presence of anaesthesia and sedation. Changes to pupil size and reaction can help to identify changes to neurological function and indicate neurological decline therefore it is pragmatic to suggest regular pupillary assessment should take place (Sharshar et al., 2014).
- Unnecessary deep sedation has been shown to increase CCU mortality and morbidity (Kollef et al., 1998; Jackson et al., 2009).
- Sub-optimal sedation can be detrimental to a patient (see Box 12.2).

Orange Flag

- Many patients that are sedated will not be able to consent to care. Treatment should be in the best interests of the patient and in line with the Mental Capacity Act and Deprivation of Liberty safeguards. The main decision making is likely to be the lead clinician; however, decision making should be collaborative and therefore the registered nurse has an important advocacy role (Intensive Care Society and Faculty of Intensive Care Medicine, 2017).
- Patients that require sedation are at high risk of developing delirium. Strategies to prevent delirium should focus on early recognition, modification of environment, management of pain, and review of therapies before pharmacological intervention (PADIS, 2018).

Learning event: reflection

Reflect on your understanding of anaesthesia and sedation in the CCU.

Take home points

1. Sedation and anaesthesia are both used in CCU, and their use is different to the theatre environment.
2. There are many different classes of drugs that can be used for sedation and anaesthesia.
3. Sedation should be tailored to the patient.
4. Assessment of sedation is essential to provide safe and high-quality care.
5. Sedation reducing strategies should be considered.

References

Ballard, N. et al. (2006). Patients' recollections of therapeutic paralysis in the intensive care unit. *American Journal of Critical Care* 15(1): 86–94.

British National Formulary (2021). Neuromuscular blockade. https://bnf.nice.org.uk/treatment-summary/neuromuscular-blockade.html (accessed 3 January 2021).

Critical Care Networks-National Nurse Leads (CC3N) (2015). *National Competency Framework for Registered Nurses in Adult Critical Care. Step 2 Competencies*. https://www.cc3n.org.uk/uploads/9/8/4/2/98425184/02_new_step_2_final.pdf (accessed 3 January 2021).

Devlin, J. et al. (2018). The Clinical Practice Guidelines for the Prevention and Management of Pain, Agitation/ Sedation, and Delirium, Immobility and Sleep Disruption in Adult Patients in the ICU (PADIS). https://www.sccm.org/ICULiberation/Guidelines (accessed 3 January 2021).

De Wit, M., Gennings, C., Jenvey, W., and Epstein, S. (2008). Randomized trial comparing daily interruption of sedation and nursing-implemented sedation algorithm in medical intensive care unit patients. *Critical Care* 12(3): R70.

Girard, T., Kress, J., Fuchs, B. et al. (2008). Efficacy and safety of a paired sedation and ventilator weaning protocol for mechanically ventilated patients in intensive care (Awakening and Breathing Controlled trial): a randomised controlled trial. *The Lancet* 371(9607): 126–134.

Intensive Care Society and Faculty of Intensive Care Medicine (2017). Deprivation of Liberty Safeguards and Mental Capacity Act Guidance for Critical Care. https://www.ics.ac.uk/ICS/ICS/GuidelinesAndStandards/Guidelines_pg2.aspx (accessed 3 January 2021).

Intensive Care Society (ICS) (2019). Guidelines for the Provision of Intensive Care Services (GPICS). Version 2. https://ics.ac.uk/ICS/ICS/GuidelinesAndStandards/GPICS_2nd_Edition.aspx (accessed 3 January 2021).

Jackson, D. et al. (2009). The incidence of sub-optimal sedation in the ICU: a systematic review. *Critical Care* 13(6): R204.

Jones, C. (2010). Post-traumatic stress disorder in ICU survivors. *Journal of the Intensive Care Society* 11(2_suppl): 12–14.

Kollef, M. et al. (1998). The use of continuous IV sedation is associated with prolongation of mechanical ventilation. *Chest* 114(2): 541–548.

Kress, J., Pohlman, A., O'Connor, M., and Hall, J. (2010). Daily interruption of sedative infusions in critically ill patients undergoing mechanical ventilation. *The New England Journal of Medicine* 342(20): 1471–1477.

Laws, P. and Rudall, N. (2013). Assessment and monitoring of analgesia, sedation, delirium and neuromuscular blockade levels and care. In: *Critical Care Manual of Clinical Procedures and Competencies* (ed. J. Mallett, J. Albarran, and R. Richardson), 333–356. Chichester: Wiley Blackwell.

National Health Service (2021). Anaesthesia. https://www.nhs.uk/conditions/anaesthesia/ (accessed 3 January 2021).

National Institute for Health and Care Excellence (NICE) (2020). Perioperative care in adults. NICE guideline 180. https://www.nice.org.uk/guidance/NG180 (accessed 3 January 2021).

Pierce, L. (2007). *Management of the Mechanically Ventilated Patient*, 2e. Elsevier: Missouri.

Royal College of Anaesthetists (RCoA) (2020). *You and Your Anaesthetic*, 5e. https://www.rcoa.ac.uk/sites/default/files/documents/2020-05/02-YourAnaesthetic2020web.pdf (accessed 3 January 2021).

Sessler, C., Gosnell, M., Grap et al. (2002). The Richmond Agitation-Sedation Scale. Validity and Reliability in Adult Intensive Care Unit Patient. *American Journal of Respiratory and Critical Care Medicine* 166(10): 1338–1344.

Sharshar, T. et al. (2014). Neurological examination of critically ill patients: A pragmatic approach. Report of an ESICM expert panel. *Intensive Care Medicine* 40(4): 484–495.

Shorthouse, J. (2017). *A Dictionary of Anaesthesia*, 2e. Oxford: OUP.

Strom, T., Martinussen, T., and Toft, P. (2010). A protocol of no sedation for critically ill patients receiving mechanical ventilation: A randomised trial. *The Lancet* 375(9713): 475–480.

Venkataraju, A. and Narayanan, M. (2016). Analgesia in intensive care: part 2. British Journal of Anaesthesia Education 16 (12): 397–404.

Whitehouse, T., Snelson, C., and Ground, M. (eds) (2014). *Intensive Care Society Review of Best Practice for Analgesia and Sedation in the Critical Care*. https://www.ics.ac.uk/ICS/ICS/Guidelines AndStandards/Guidelines_pg2.aspx (accessed 3 January 2021).

Woodrow, P. (2019). *Intensive Care Nursing: A Framework for Practice*, 4e. London: Routledge.

Yentis, S., Hirsch, N., and Ip, J. (2018). *Anaesthesia, Intensive Care and Perioperative Medicine A–Z*, 6e. Edinburgh: Elsevier.

Chapter 13

Medicines management and drug calculations

Jan Guerin

Aim

The aim of this chapter is to provide the reader with an overview of fundamental knowledge of safe medicines management in the context of an adult CCU and to provide an explanation of formulae for mathematical calculations.

Learning outcomes

After reading this chapter the reader will be able to:
- Develop an understanding of accountability, legal and professional regulations applicable to the safe administration and management of pharmaceutical interventions.
- Understand the significance of avoidable medication errors.
- Apply and understand the role of human factors associated with medication errors, and the importance of risk assessments and safe nursing interventions throughout the administration process to reduce incidents.
- Understand the significance and value of ensuring the rights of medicine administration in clinical practice.
- Gain confidence in performing mathematical calculations required for prescriptions of methods of medication administration.

Test your prior knowledge

- Explain what is meant by the term 'medication'.
- 'Registered Nurse (RNs) need to possess an overall understanding of the medicine being administered.' What does this mean?
- What is the importance of Control Of Substances Hazardous to Health (COSHH) in safe medicines administration in critical care?
- How do you ensure the safe handling and disposal of sharps in clinical practice?
- When do you perform hand hygiene during the process of medication administration?

Fundamentals of Critical Care: A Textbook for Nursing and Healthcare Students, First Edition. Edited by Ian Peate and Barry Hill.
© 2023 John Wiley & Sons Ltd. Published 2023 by John Wiley & Sons Ltd.
Companion website: www.wiley.com/go/peate/criticalcare

Introduction

This chapter provides key information to afford embedding of essential knowledge and skills to support development of competency and confidence in carrying out the complex nursing responsibility of safe medication administration in the setting of an Adult CCU. Due to the subject content being extensive and taking into consideration the prior learning that is embedded during preregistration training, the primary focus will be on the administration of medications via the intravenous route (IV). The chapter content supports the learning outcomes of the National Competency Framework for Registered Nurses (RNs) in Adult Critical Care, Step 1 competencies, (CC3N, 2015).

National Competency Framework for Registered Nurses (RNs) in Adult Critical Care, Step 1 competencies (CC3N, 2015).

Summary of key areas of discussion are:

- National and local legislation, guidelines, protocols and policies for the administration of medication.
- Health and Safety regulations relevant to medicines administration in critical care.
- Legal requirements: acting in the patients' best interest.
- Process of administration in critical care and the importance of working within scope of practice.
- Preparation of medications/infusions.
- Importance of monitoring, titration and safe discontinuation of administration.
- Critical care medications and their effects on pre-existing comorbidities.
- Adherence to the safe practices used in critical care to minimise the risk of harm to the individual or reduce the risk of error in medication and fluid administration using the 5 Rs when administering any medication.
- Prepare and administer medications in critical care adhering to the following guidance: NMC Code (NMC, 2018), NMC Medicines Administration Standards (NMC, 2019) and CC3N Preparation in Advance Statement.
- Different routes and methods of administration and use of equipment.
- Competence in performing mathematical calculations.
- Identifying, managing and reporting signs of anaphylaxis.

Medicines management, as defined by the Medicines and Healthcare Regulatory Agency (MRHA) is the 'clinical-cost effective and safe use of medicines to ensure patients get the maximum benefit from the medicines they need, while at the same time minimising potential harm'. The patient is the key focus of targeted safe care, requiring monitoring, safe prescribing systems, on-going education and training for all staff.

It is a Nursing and Midwifery Council (NMC, 2018) requirement that all RNs and Nursing Associates (NAs) work within their scope of practice including ensuring ongoing continuous professional development (CDP). Training, education and competencies are necessary in order to gain fundamental knowledge, skill and build confidence in safely administering a multitude of medications in adult critical care. Furthermore, safe and effective medicines management requires strict adherence to policies/protocols with accountability, autonomy, delegation and the ability to deal with emergent situations. This competence required by the Royal College of Nursing and Royal Pharmaceutical Society (RPS and RCN, 2019) aligns with a definition cited by Roach (1992) as a state of possessing knowledge, clinical judgement skills, energy, experience and motivation that is the prerequisite to having the ability to respond safely and adequately to the demands of our professional responsibilities.

Safely managing medications in a critically ill patient population group is a complex, high risk and time-consuming task. This skill requires accuracy in managing complicated medication regimens along with complex drug calculations making the potential for a drug error more likely. Furthermore, the critically ill patient has alerted pathophysiology due to failing organs that greatly increases sensitivity to some medications. This combined problem of failing organs, unpredicted physiological responses also poses a risk for other drug-induced events that may result in a drug-induced anaphylaxis (DIA), acute kidney injury, liver toxicity, coagulopathies, gastrointestinal disturbance and neurological compromise.

Therefore, safe administration of medication requires a multifaceted set of skills:

- Cognition: knowing the pharmacology of the medication, applying evidence-based practice (EBP) protocols, performing mathematical drug calculations, understanding underlying patient pathophysiology as well as the positive and negative outcomes related to the medication intervention. Ensuring correct use of personal protective equipment (PPE) for medications that may be harmful to the healthcare worker (HCW).
- Clinical dexterity: Maintaining aseptic non-touch technique (ANTT) throughout the administration process whilst simultaneously dealing with competing demands requiring task – switching and multitasking.
- Psychomotor skills: Working in a bed space congested with equipment, safely accessing the route for administration that may have several ports and coordinating priming and connecting medical devices.

The physical demand and mental concentration for the HCW during the various processes are profuse. This involves critical thinking with clinical decision making for appropriateness to hold IV sedation (see Chapter 12), close observation of the patient during this time as well as the potential for speedy responses to safely administer a bolus and/or recommence the infusion should the patient become unstable.

Purpose of pharmacological interventions in the critically ill adult patient

The role of pharmacological interventions for the adult CCU patient is a strand of the patient-centred critical care bundle aimed at:

- Managing the physiological disorders of critical illness that occur secondary to an underlying pathological process, such as, antimicrobials to treat sepsis secondary to pancreatitis.
- Slowing the progression of the disease, for example, anti-hypertensives to control blood pressure and prevent further renal impairment.
- Relieving symptoms, for example, pain management with analgesia.
- Supporting normal physiological processes; supporting cardiovascular system stability with blood pressure optimisation using vasopressors.
- Destruction of toxic substances or ingested poisons, such as, antidote to reverse the effects of the toxic substance, preventing further organ damage.
- Life-saving – this includes oxygen therapy to manage hypoxaemia secondary to pulmonary compromise.
- Facilitate synchronous effective mechanical ventilation, including sedatives/ analgesics to optimise level of sedation and patient comfort.
- Facilitate advanced interventions for organ support modalities, for example, anticoagulation of the circuit used for continuous renal replacement therapy (CRRT).
- Prevent CCU-related complications, such as, proton pump inhibitors to prevent Curling's stress ulcer.
- Optimising nutritional support, this includes parental nutrition for patients with non-functioning gastro-intestinal system.
- Diagnosing underlying hormonal deficits that may be compounding the clinical state; tetracosactide testing to identify adrenal insufficiency.
- Optimising electrolyte balance by means of supplementation of potassium, sodium, calcium, magnesium and phosphate.

Fundamental knowledge of pharmacology is an absolute key requirement. Chapter 11 discusses pharmacology.

Legal and professional issues

The registered nurse (RN) is legally authorised to practise via their registration with the NMC in line with the NMC Code (NMC, 2018) and the various NMC standards. Accountability, to their employer is through their contract of employment where their job role and responsibilities are clearly stated. It is usual for health care providers (such as the National Health Service) to provide practitioners with vicarious liability provided the practitioner works within the scope of practice and within the job description as set out in the contract thus practising safely as per guidelines and policies.

In Chapter 3 legal and ethical issues are addressed and the importance of 'Duty of Care' is considered in detail. Should there be any breach either by act of omission or commission there may a case of negligence to answer. The outcome of negligence would be concluded, if the nurse had knowledge that their action, for example, administering the wrong dose of medication, would intentionally harm the patient/s.

Furthermore, RNs need to exercise professional accountability for their actions whether they are following instruction or using own initiative at all times. The RCN defines accountability as 'taking responsibility for your actions, always ensuring you are competent to do the activity you've been asked to perform and always putting patients'/ clients' interests first'. For the RN, this accountability requires recognising limitations, refraining from performing care that they are not confident or competent to deliver and being able to report an incident or raise a concern. It is essential that the nurse thinks before undertaking an action and not acting if instructions are not clear or understood and reaching out to seniors for support and guidance.

In CCU, the critically ill patient/s may lack capacity to make decisions and therefore is unable to provide informed consent for their medications for several reasons. These being severity of illness, acute confusion, acquired delirium, coma, tracheal intubation either endotracheal/tracheostomy or sedation. Therefore, the RN is required to exercise professional accountability in applying best interest decisions for their patient/s at all times.

As described by the (RPS, 2019) intravenous medicines administration involves a broad range of practitioners including the medical prescriber and pharmacist. Professional Guidance on the administration of medications in healthcare is co-produced by the RPS and RCN (2019).

Principles-based guidance is provided to ensure the safe administration of medications, the RPS is also jointly responsible for leadership and support of the pharmacy profession within England, Wales and Scotland. In the context of CCU, see the summary of the guidelines in (Table 13.1) (RPS and RCN, 2019).

Table 13.1 Overview of implementing RPS safe administration of medicines guidelines in CCU clinical practice.

Guideline	Application and rationale in CCU clinical practice
Patient-Specific Direction	· Electronic or paper prescription · Meets all legal requirements

Patient Group Direction (Prescription)	· Commonly used for Normal saline (NaCL) needed to flush and maintain patency of an intravenous (IV) device e.g.:
	  · Peripheral intravenous cannula (PIVC)
	  · Central venous catheter (CVC)
	  · Percutaneous Intravenous Central Catheter (PICC)
	  · Arterial Cannula (IABP)

Available literature resources with sufficient information about the medicine. Not sure what this means	· CCU drug handbook · CCU Unit bedside protocols · BNF · Medusa
Overall understanding of the medicine being administered including seeking appropriate advice.	· CCU drug handbook · CPD study days for CCU nurses · Clinical Pharmacist · CCU Nurse Educator.
Adherence to organisational policies for who can administer and/or delegate.	· Attainment of competency for safe non-supervised practice as per Step 1 competencies.
When administering exercise professionalism and professional judgement.	· This implies the accountability of the RN for their actions, non-actions and omissions during the process. · Maintaining accurate defensible documentation as this serves as a written record and provides continuity of care.
Achieve relevant professional and regulatory standards via training, assessment to achieve competency.	· Step 1 competencies signed off by your practice supervisor and assessor.

Follow organisational procedure to minimise risks associated with the handling or administration, for example, vasopressors	· Use of CCU standardised regimen protocols for
	  · Mixing of infusions
	  · Dosing
	  · Double pumping

Use only appropriate organisation approved equipment and devices.	· Medical device training and competency for IV infusions including: patient-controlled analgesia (PCAs) and epidurals.
Adverse drug reactions	· Follow organisational policy/procedure for reporting, such as, Datix reporting
Controlled Drugs (CDs)	· Adhere to legislation and organisational policies/procedures. · Double checking and signing by two RNs
Verbal orders	· Accepted under exceptional circumstances where a change or addition to administration details is required as a delay would compromise patient care and outcome. · Patient direction requires updating within 24 hours

Snapshot

During a nightshift RN Minti is responsible for administering the prescribed IV medications at 2200. Mrs Yo, the patient, is day 2 post-operatively following admission for hypovolemic shock secondary to a perforated duodenal ulcer. Mrs Yo's prescription order is for a dose of pantoprazole 40 mg IVI twice daily. The prescription chart is full as the day shift doctor did not get a chance to write up a new chart. How should RN Minti manage this situation?

Actions:
- Contact the Night CCU doctor on call to request an urgent prescription chart.
- Should the Medical Doctor (MD) be unable come to the unit immediately, take a two RN verbal prescription telephonically, adhering to local policy and procedure.
- Update the Nurse in Charge.
- Complete an incident report as prescription charts need to be valid for use and in date, as a delay in administering this medication would potentially cause further harm to Mrs Yo.
- Follow up to ensure the MD updated the prescription within 24 hours.

Collaborative multidisciplinary team working

Integral to all CCU settings is collaborative working between various specialities as this goes hand in hand with patient safety and outcome. Effective team working with good communication is associated with a strong safety culture. Furthermore, the Core Standards for Intensive Care Units (ICS, 2013) sets the standards for units providing care to Level 2 and Level 3 critically ill patients, with a standard requirement for a dedicated critical care pharmacist. Their role is to support the entire case mix of patients who are in conditions with extremes of physiology seen in critical illness resulting in severe and rapidly shifting pharmacokinetic and dynamic parameters (Borthwick, 2019). Further to this is the need to intercept and resolve medication errors, thus optimising the medication therapy, all of which improve quality, ensure safety, reduce costs and reduce mortality.

Medication errors

Medication interventions delivered are based on the premise to do good, thus optimising the patients' outcome and reducing mortality. However, CCU is a fast-paced healthcare environment and administration of medication is a highly complex, high-risk patient care intervention with potential for error. These errors may occur during any phase of the process of prescribing, transcribing, dispensing, administering, monitoring or recording with consequences ranging from no harm to harm to death. Fortunately, most patients remain safe; however, some sustain significant injury that results in either long-term damage with a resultant increase in length of stay. Consequences for the HCW may be loss of confidence by family, patient and public. For the HCW, emotional trauma may undermine self-esteem and negatively impact on clinical confidence within their roles. Therefore, robust, effective preventive strategies in CCU need to be implemented in order to reduce the risk of error, especially in this setting, where patients receive high-risk, complex and multiple medications. This echoes the goal driven by, the World Health Organization (WHO) (2017) third global Safety Challenge, medication without harm, focusing on reducing the substantial burden of iatrogenic harm associated with medications by 50% in the next 5 years. It is essential that national and local guidance is followed at all times.

Errors can occur in the stages of prescription, transcription, dispensing, administration and the need to continuously monitor. Errors identified:

- Wrong patient, route, dose and drug calculation
- Administration without a valid prescription
- Administration of medication to a patient with a known allergy

- Omitted doses
- Late/early administration
- Failure to record.

A systematic review conducted by Sutherland et al. (2017), of 2576 infusions administered in UK showed a total of 101 medication errors per 1000 administrations. The common cause for these errors were related to 'Errors of Wrong Rate'.

Based on the evidence, the administration of medication therefore always poses a risk, and even more in the context of CCU as it involves complex patient pathophysiology. It therefore requires a high level of knowledge of pharmacology, accuracy with mathematical calculations and overarching multidisciplinary team collaboration, all of which are subject to human factors in the context of this high-impact care environment.

Top tips for safer practice

- Safe keeping and storage of all medications in locked/coded cupboards.
- Separate look-alike packaging or ampoules.
- Use pre-filled syringes in emergency situations.
- Separate high dose ampoules with concentrated solutions from others eg. In Controlled Drug Cupboards (CDs) keep morphine sulphate 30 mg/2 mL and morphine sulphate 10 mg/2 mL in different spaces.
- Store intrathecal/epidural medications separately from IV fluids.
- Use dedicated pre-programmed syringe and volumetric pumps with alerts for minimum and maximum dosages for CCU medications.
- Use unit-specific standardised protocols and infusion regimens.
- Colour-coded standardised labelling for infusions, bags and giving sets.
- Unique ports to prevent lines intended for two different routes from being connected. These are interlocking mechanisms to distinguish enteral, intrathecal and IV routes.
- Specific labelling of ports.
- Double checking of all medications and mathematical calculations by two RNs (Camire et al., 2009).
- Barcode medication administration to provide a double check to verify medication dose, route, patient and dosing time

Communication:
- Avoid using abbreviations.
- Clear documentation.
- Good handover between staff using SBAR approach.
- Standardise procedures for drawing up of medications in dedicated areas that ensures adherence to Infection Control Policy, Epic3 Infection and Control policy (IPC) guidelines (Loveday et al., 2014).

154

- Prepare each medication in a different tray to avoid confusion.
- Minimise advance preparation of medication infusions or syringes.
- Discard unused/expired medications from the bed space.
- Standardise common processes or procedures, for example monographs for drugs.
- Decrease reliance on vigilance such as lengthy repetitive activities, because humans get bored.
- Review and simplify the processes – 'Simple is better'.

Overview of routes and methods of administering medications in CCU

There are various routes for the administration of medications. However, in critically ill patient/s, IV and enteral are the most frequent routes used. Clinical considerations for non-IV routes of administration in the critically ill patient is dependent on many factors.

Oral

The oral route, which is a convenient and cost-effective route (Dougherty and Lister, 2015), may be unsuitable, for the reasons of:

- Nil by mouth
- Presence of an endotracheal (ETT) or tracheostomy tube (TT)
- Reduced level of consciousness
- Non-functioning gastrointestinal tract
- Dysphagia with a high risk for aspiration
- Preparation only available in parental form

Topical

To treat localised disease;

- Steroid creams for chronic dermatitis
- Transdermal patches for:
  - Nicotine replacement,
  - Acute or chronic pain relief,
  - Chronic disease management eg. Parkinson's disease,
  - Glyceryl trinitrate (GTN) patch to offset excessive peripheral vasospasm and ischaemia secondary to high dose vasopressors

Sublingual

These have the advantage of being rapidly absorbed into the systemic circulation e.g. GTN. However, the intended therapeutic effect may not be achieved in the critically ill patient.

Rectal

Besides suppositories to relieve constipation and antiplatelet therapy with aspirin post cardiac surgery, this is the least preferred route despite a higher bioavailability than oral, this being due to a high leakage of medication as well as unpredictable absorption. Furthermore, this route is contraindicated in patients following bowel and rectal surgery, presence of leucopenia and thrombocytopenia.

Aerosolisation (nebulisation)

This route is used to achieve high concentrations of medication in the lung tissue. This route and method requires a suspension of liquid in a gaseous medium to be delivered via a device (Dhanani et al., 2016) The purpose is for treatment of a variety of respiratory diseases as well as being a portal for systemic therapy. The frequency may either be at set intervals or continuous via an aerosolisation device.

Clinical indications for aerosolisation

- Antibiotic therapy: Ribavarin and colistin for respiratory infections
- Mucolytic agents: Acetylcysteine to reduce mucus plugging of airways
- Bronchodilators: Salbutamol for bronchospasm
- Corticosteroids: Budesonide to reduce bronchial inflammation
- Prostacyclins: Epoprostenol for pulmonary hypertension
- Heliox: Upper airway oedema

Subcutaneous

Clinical considerations with medications administered via subcutaneous route:

- Accuracy for depth of injection is uncertain.
- Variable absorption due to vasoactive medications and haemodynamic instability eg heparin and insulin (Dörffler-Melly et al., 2002).

Intramuscular

Clinical considerations with medications administered via subcutaneous route:

- High risk for inadvertent administration into tissue due to muscle wasting rather than muscle affecting absorption.
- Increased risk for haematoma in anticoagulated and coagulopathic patients (Greenblatt and Allen, 1978).

Enteral

Enteral nutrition provides a route via an oro/naso gastric, Percutaneous Endoscopic Gastrostomy (PEG) or Percutaneous

155

Endoscopic Jejunostomy (PEJ) routes for nutrition. However, these tubes are also used for medications (BAPEN, 2017). Use of enteral tubes, using the method of gavage, poses some challenges as they are designed for food and liquids thus administering medication intended for oral use during continuous feeding requires the correct delivery method in order to prevent complications. A blocked enteral feeding tube being the most common problem.

Complications associated with blocked enteral tubes

- Blocked feeding tube secondary to incorrect medication administration which will have a direct impact on the patient's quality of life as they will be unable to receive their caloric needs via nutritional feed.
- Increased morbidity due to lack of access for time-sensitive medications such as anti-Parkinson meds.
- Reinsertion with potential harmful xray exposure to reconfirm position.

Furthermore, the RN/NA needs to follow protocols and clinical pharmacist advice and guidance as manipulated formulations may result in interactions with the feeding products, exposure of the active ingredients when capsule is removed or drug adherence to the inner lumen of the feeding tube.

Clinical considerations with medications administered via enteral route

1. Small fine-bore feeding tubes becoming easily clogged.
2. Variety of medications may not be crushed.
3. Splitting of tablets may lead to incorrect dosage.
4. Absorption in stomach and duodenum may be affected by bowel resection, gastroparesis, decreased splanchinic blood flow and ileus.
5. Holding of feed to optimise absorption via nasojejunal and jejunostomy tubes that bypass the duodenum, the principle site for the majority of medications leading to variable effects and first-pass metabolism eg. Warfarin, phenytoin and levothyroxine.

Kruer et al. (2014)

Intravenous

Intravenous (IV) medication administration may be defined as the therapeutic administration of a sterile preparation of medication directly into the patient's peripheral or central vein. This method requires the use of a vascular device that may be inserted either centrally or peripherally based on the identified need, clinical indication and length of intended time for use. These devices may be for therapeutic and/or for monitoring purposes. Safe and effective administration of IV medications relies on adherence to hospital policies along with procedural guidelines for Evidence-Based Practice as set out in the Royal Marsden Manual of Clinical Nursing Procedures (Lister and West-Oram, 2020) (Table 13.2).

Considerations: advantages of IV route for medications in CCU

- Non-functional gastro-intestinal tract.
- Life-saving medication preparations only available in IV form.
- Indicated for rapid onset of action for inducing sedation prior to intubation.
- Delivery of precise quantities of drug.
- Avoids first-pass effect so 100% bioavailability.
- Achieves optimal therapeutic effect as it affords immediate titrated dose adjustment.

The method of administration via IV route may be as a direct intermittent injection (Bolus administration). This method is for rapid onset of actions and uses a concentrated, small volume <20 mL either diluted or undiluted eg. pantoprazole or metoclopramide. Taking into account the labile condition of the critically ill patient, a dose administered too quickly or incorrectly may result in significant harm or death.

The second method is via intermittent infusion (short Infusion) of a volume of 25 to 250 mL of fluid/medication over a set period of time at prescribed intervals and then stopped until the next dose is required, e.g. erythromycin short infusion as a prokinetic. Mostly commonly used is the method of continuous infusion via an infusion device. The patient in CCU is most often prescribed multiple medications to be delivered via continuous (IV) infusion, which often exceeds the number of available lumens, i.e. CVC or IVC sites. This may require the co-administration which may be intermittent or continuous down the same lumen using a Y-site connector. This procedure has the risk to result in physiochemical incompatibilities which may result in adverse effects which ultimately harm the CCU patient (Mosopefoluwa et al., 2020).

Further to incompatibilities, several medications commonly used in CCU are considered to be high-risk medications and may compound medication errors due to complex multiple processes involved in the administration Titiesari et al. (2017) these medications are anticoagulants, sedatives, opiates and insulin. All these methods require knowledge of potential adverse effects and well as the safe preparation process. Hunter (2019) suggests the importance of standardised practices to reduce patient harm from errors as well as adverse events.

156

Table 13.2   Quick guide to vascular access devices used for IV medications.

Peripheral cannulae (IVC)	· Short-term (1–5 days) · Used for infusion of fluids, blood products, medications and parental nutrition · Relatively easy to insert and maintain
Midlines (PVAD)/'Long Cannula'	· Venous access in a large peripheral vein up to 20 cm i.e. basilic or cephalic vein · Used as an alternative in patients with unsuitable peripheral veins or those who have minimal suitable vessels and require therapy for a period of up to 6 months.
Central Venous Catheters (CVC) – Non Tunnelled	· Short term · Inserted into a large vein with the tip positioned into the superior vena cava · Short-term indication +/– 10 days. · Sites: Internal jugular, subclavian, basilic, cephalic or femoral veins. · Single or multi lumen (double/triple/quad or quin) · Indicated for monitoring of central venous pressure (CVP), administration of fluids, blood products, parental nutrition, short and long-term infusions. · Benefits: provides long-term access for vesicant drugs i.e. cytotoxic drugs · Multiple lumens afford numerous drugs to be administered simultaneously.
Peripherally Inserted CVC (PICCs)	· Short to long-term indication · Sites: Antecubital fossa veins/basilic or cephalic · Fine-bore catheters, either single or double-lumens · Tip position confirmed radiologically · Indicated when peripheral access is needed for infusion of vesicant or irritant medications/fluids, parental nutrition and hyperosmolar solutions.
Central inserted Catheters (CVC) – Tunnelled	· 'Hickmann lines' with large-bore silicone either single or double-lumen · Long-term infusion therapy (months to years) – chemotherapy and parental nutrition · Provide access for blood sampling · Sites: jugular or subclavian with tip in superior vena cava · Dacron cuff enables tissues to bond with the line creating a secure fixation and provides a mechanical barrier to limit bacterial migration.
Intraosseous (IO)	· IV access for effective route for Emergency situations for fluid resuscitation, drug delivery and laboratory evaluation · IO access obtained using a manual or drill-inserted (EZ-IO) device for insertion of specialised needles · Positioned into the medullary space. · Sites: Proximal tibia, distal tibia and distal femur · Used during cardiac arrest, decompensated shock when IV access not achievable
(Extra vascular) Epidural	· Neuroaxial opioids

157

Snapshot: IV Medication Clinical Skill competencies required by CCU HCWs

Types of prescriptions:
* Routine
* Variable rate
* Variable dose
* PRN
* STAT

Method of preparation:
* Reconstituting intravenous medication form a powder from a vial
* Drawing up of intravenous medication in liquid form from an ampoule
* Adding intravenous medication to a bag of fluid for infusion
* Using pre-prepared intravenous medications

Method of Administration:
* Administration of a timed bolus at the correct rate (IV bolus)
* Administration of an intermittent infusion via gravity – drops per minute, volumetric or syringe pump – mL/hour
* Administration of a continuous infusion via volumetric or syringe pump – mL/hour and dose per kg/hour or per minute/hour
* Double pumping where one infusion is substituted for another without interrupting the flow of the medication to the patient. For medications with a short half-life eg. Noradrenaline and adrenaline

The RN requires knowledge about the medication and preparation in order to reduce adverse events, complications. Prior to administering an IV medication, the nurse must have an understanding of a number of factors. There are specific patient populations/groups in the critical care environment that must be given particular consideration such as the older person and the obestric patient.

Clinical considerations

- Consider volume of medication in patients who are 'fluid restricted'
- Consider special precautions for patients with hypernatraemia eg. Ciprofloxacin and metronidazole
- Does the administration of this medication have a maximum dose per minute rate?
- Are there any special precautions during the administration eg. Phenytoin dose of >50 mg?
- Does the medication require an inline filter?

Rights of medication administration

The RN/NA is responsible for ensuring quality of patient care and safety at all times Elliot and Liu (2010). Edwards and Axe (2015) propose the 12 Rights of administration. However, for the purposes of applying these rights to CCU, these rights are further expanded based on the experience of the author of this chapter (Table 13.3)

Table 13.3   Rights of medication administration in the CCU patient

Right	Rationale
Right Patient	Correct identification via: Verbal confirmation from patient ID bracelet Prescription
Prescription	Check that the prescription is clearly written and unambiguous.
NOT Allergic	Check prescription chart. Check ID Band.
NOT Expired	Check expiry date on medication/IV fluid.
Right Medication	Drug name should be clear and correct. Use only generic names.
Right Time	Appropriate time(s) for effective outcomes: PRN, STAT, TDS, QDS, BD, Nocte, Mane or Continuous.
Right Dose	Correct drug calculation – double checked and signed. Do not divide unscored tablets. Check name of drug against the dosage of the medication to be administered.
Right Formulation	To be administered via the prescribed route e.g. capsule via enteral route.
Right Route	Enteral: oral, gavage Topical: skin, eyes, ears, vagina, rectum, inhaled Parental: subcutaneous, Intramuscular, intravenously.
Right Access	IVC PICC CVC Enteral feeding tube Endotracheal/tracheostomy tube
Right Maintenance	Ensure delivery continuity of critical short-half-life infusions.
Right Reconstitution of drug	Correct diluent used.
Right Formulae Calculation	Correct formulae with double checking of calculation.
Right Indication	Consider mode of action of medication. Part of the patient's clinical need.
Right Infection Control Principles	ANTT for IV drug preparation. Applying Epic3 Guidelines to reduce hospital-acquired infections (HAIs).
Right Education	Informed consent for patient.
Right to Refuse	Consider best interest decisions.
Right Assessment	Use SBAR for decision making.

(Continued)

158

Table 13.3 (Continued)

Right	Rationale
Right Evaluation	Assess for positive and negative effects of the treatment.
Right Documentation	Sign administration of all medications. Make a clear, accurate and immediate record of all medicine administered, intentionally withheld or refused by the patient, ensuring that any written entries and the signature are clear and legible; it is also a responsibility to ensure that a record is made when delegating the task of administering medicine.
Right Medical Device	Volumetric pump, syringe pump or syringe driver.
Right to correct titrating or weaning infusion dosages	Titrates and weans safely as per protocol.
Right to delivering of a bolus doses	Administers bolus as prescribed.
Right to Pro Ne rata (PRN)	Supplementing electrolytes to achieve optimal serum levels. Administer as per local policy.

Managing and reporting a medication error

The RN is required to report an error that is always in the best interests for the safety of the patient at hand. Reporting forms part of *quality assurance and risk management*, thus making it mandatory to report all drug errors and near misses irrespective of whether or not the patient came to harm. There are systems in place to analyse these incidents and learn from them. These findings are then converted into lessons learned that result in quality and safety improvements.

Near misses and never events

A 'near miss' as described by the WHO (2005) is when a patient is exposed to a hazardous situation when no harm or injury is sustained due to early detection. In contrast, 'preventable events' should not occur as they are preventable if national guidance and recommendations are adhered to by all HCWs. These preventable events are the 'never events'. NHS Improvement (2018a) has published a never-events policy and framework which supports HCWs to deliver safe, high-quality, compassionate care that is financially sustainable. If a breach occurs, this is interpreted as a failure of the care delivery process as guidance and recommendations have not been followed.

Never events for medications are:

- Mis-selection of a strong potassium solution
- Administration of medication by the wrong route
- Overdose of insulin due to abbreviations or use of incorrect device
- Overdose of methotrexate for non-cancer use
- Mis-selection of high-strength midazolam during conscious sedation

Snapshot: drug error scenario

RN Pokky has completed taking handover of Mr Jibby, admitted with sepsis. Mr Jibby is intubated, sedated with several infusions running. During RN Pokky's routine patient and bed space safety check, she is handed over a calculated dose of noradrenaline of 0.20 mcg/kg/min. When she calculates the dose she gets a result of 0.25 mcg/kg/min. RN Pokky observes that Mr Jibby's invasive blood pressure reading is 175/80 mmHg.

Action to be taken in best interests and safety of Mr Jibby:

- Seek support from senior RN to ensure Mr Jibby is safe.
- Recalculate the rate and dose ensuring that the weight entered into the syringe pump is correct.
- Review the chart and syringe pump history to look for range of doses administered.
- Cautiously correct the administration rate taking into account noradrenaline's pharmacokinetic and pharmacological properties. Reduce the dose in small increments in order to achieve the target blood pressure, e.g. MAP 60–70 mmHG.
- Following Mr Jibby's safety, i.e. blood pressure within target range, escalate medication error, patient concerns and actions to nurse in charge.
- Complete an incident report via Datix as this will provide a lesson learned for other staff in order to prevent the error occurring again.
- Document the incident and patient effects if any in the care records.
- Ensure Duty of Candour for Mr Jibby. This involves apologising to Mr Jibby and telling him that the medication was set at the incorrect rate, and that the rate was adjusted to the correct dose, along with the short- and long-term effects of this medication error.

Important! RNs are accountable for reporting errors as this results in improving practice as it affords an opportunity to change practice and formulation of an action plan to prevent it happening again (Johnstone and Kanitsaki, 2006). Providing a Duty of Candour is a statutory duty for all health care providers registered with the Care Quality Commission (CQC, 2015).

Anaphylaxis

Anaphylaxis is a severe, life-threatening, generalised or systemic hypersensitivity reaction secondary to several triggers (RCUK, 2016) which may be induced secondary to drugs, foods, bites and stings. In general, in the UK, it is estimated that anaphylactic reactions to occur in 1:1333 people, resulting in 20 deaths per year (RCUK, 2016)

In specific relation to medications administration in CCU, is the consequence of a drug-induced anaphylaxis (DIA). This may be a life-threatening condition occurring post intake of a common CCU medication via any route (Table 13.4) (Blanca-Lopez et al., 2015)

Pathophysiology and clinical manifestations of DIA

Making a diagnosis in of anaphylaxis CCU can be challenging due to the complexity of organ dysfunction, multitude of medications infusing simultaneously and existing labile status of the CCU patient. The RN needs to be observant for red flags during medication administration, this is an acute deterioration superimposed on the patients underlying pathology. This is a challenge and requires expert clinical judgement skills that are acquired overtime through experience and clinical practice. The RN should use of the ABCDE approach in order to make a rapid clinical judgement to timeously escalate for medical intervention with regards to anaphylaxis.

Table 13.4   Known common medications causing anaphylaxis

Antibiotics:
Beta-Lactams:
Amoxicillin
Non-Beta Lactams:
Fluoroquinolones: Ciprofloxacin and moxifloxacin
Amphotericin
Vancomycin

Anaesthetics:
Suxamethonium
Vercuronium
Atracurium

Others:
Non-steroidal anti-inflammatories (NSAIDs)
Angiotensin-converting enzyme inhibitors (ACEIs)
Colloids: Gelatins
Protamine sulphate
Vitamin K
Radiocontrast media
Proton pump inhibitors (PPIs)
Opioids – morphine

Table 13.5   ABCDE approach.

A
Airway swelling – pharyngeal/laryngeal oedema
Hoarse voice
Stridor

B
Sudden onset of shortness of breath (SOB)
Audible wheeze
Increasing peak airway pressure (PAP) with reduction in tidal volume (vT) in intubated and mechanically ventilated patient
Steep fall in oxygen saturations from baseline
Increasing etCO$_2$
Cyanosis
Respiratory arrest in non-ventilated patients

C
Signs of shock:
Pallor and clamminess
Sudden increase in heart rate: tachycardia/atrial fibrillation/premature ventricular ectopics
Hypotension
Decreased Glasgow Coma Scale (GCS) score or RASS
Arrhythmia with cardiac arrest

D
Alterations in level of consciousness

E
Skin and or mucosal changes: subtle or dramatic
Erythema
Urticaria
Angioedema

Management for DIA

Management for DIA focuses on:

1. Early identification and escalation of high index of suspicion for DIA (see Table 13.5)
2. Removing the trigger – stop the medication
3. Support hemodynamic stability with vasopressors and IV fluids
4. Stop histamine release with an IV antihistamine
5. Reduce inflammation with IV corticosteroids
6. Implement RCUK guidelines for managing shock secondary to anaphylaxis.

Medication calculation formulae

In this second part of this chapter, the focus is on the mathematical drug calculations commonly used in the Adult CCU setting.

These calculations are:

1. Rounding decimals up/down to required decimal place/s or whole number.
2. Converting from one unit to another.
3. Understanding the relevance of displacement values in clinical practice.

4. Calculating 'Drugs in volume and dose required'.
5. Calculating 'Rate, time and volume for infusions'.
6. Calculating 'Stated rate of dose (per minute)'.
7. Calculating 'Drip rate in drops per minute'.
8. Calculating 'Drugs doses expressed in ratio'.
9. Calculating 'Drugs doses expressed in percentage'.
10. Calculating a 'Flow rate for a given dose in micrograms/ kg/min'.
11. Calculating 'micrograms/kg/min for a given flow rate'.

Mastering this skill to achieve confidence and accuracy in mathematical drug calculations along with gaining fundamental knowledge of pharmacology is difficult for all new CCU RNs. Therefore, review the suggested learning guidelines (Table 13.6) to support your development and embed safe practice as part of your accountability and responsibility in order to decrease the potential for a 'preventable event' or 'near miss'.

Table 13.6 Suggested learning guidelines for a new RN in CCU to achieve accuracy and confidence in mathematical drug calculations.

Prior preregistration training, learning, theory and practice gained during formal training courses in order to achieve qualification as a RN.

Competence attained in mathematical drug calculations for oral/ enteral/aerosolised/subcutaneous and intramuscular administered drugs during preregistration training with your academic assessor and practice Supervisor/s and Assessor.

Completion Step 1 competencies: 1.8 Medicines Administration with support from your practice Supervisor/s, Assessor and CCU Nurse Educator to attain sign off competencies.

Attendance and active participation in hospital mandatory training IV study day/s and workshops for safe medication administration.

Practice drug calculations with support from Supervisor/s/Assessor using sample patient direction prescriptions.

Practise, Practise and Practise!

Work under the supervision of supervisor/s to gain confidence in managing medications for your allocated critically ill patient.

1. Decimals and rounding

A calculation for a specific medication may result in a number containing a decimal point (Figure 13.1) Lack of understanding of the decimal point is a risk for a serious medication error if it is misplaced and this misinterpretation could result in the 'wrong dose' being administered.

When a calculation for a medication or intravenous (IV) fluid results in a number with decimal places, the result is either rounded to a whole number or 1 to 2 decimal places depending on the type of medication or IV fluid prescribed. Rounding is necessary for programming a rate-controlled infusion pump to deliver millilitres per hour (mL/hr). Furthermore, rounding to a whole number is necessary for the delivery of IV fluid via an infusion set with a drop factor. The mathematical rules for rounding are:

- To be able to round up/down to the required decimal place/s, we need to look at the decimal place NEXT to what is being asked.
- If the one you are looking at is between 0–4, the answer (What is being asked), stays the same.
- If the one you are looking at is between 5–9, you add (1) one to the
- answer.

Worked example

7.7324 = 8 rounded to whole number
    = 7.7 rounded to one decimal place
    = 7.73 rounded to second decimal place
    = 7.732 rounded to third decimal place

2. Converting from one unit to another

When calculating a prescribed dose always convert *all weights into the same unit* before starting your drug calculation.

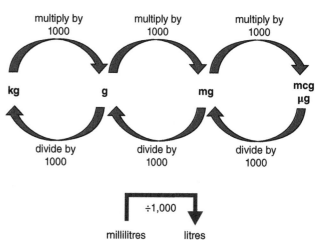

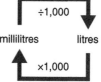

Hundred Thousands	Ten Thousands	Thousands	Hundreds	Tens	Ones	Decimal point ↓	Tenths	Hundredths	Thousandths	Ten-thousandths	Hundred-thousandths
						•					

Figure 13.1 Decimal place value chart. *Source:* Socoratic.org.

Example: grams (g), milligrams (mg), micrograms (mcg), nanograms (ng) or all volume into the same units e.g. Litre (L) or millilitre (mL)

Tip!

To convert big to small, think big, therefore go ahead and multiply.
e.g. 2 litre = 2000 mL
Versus
To convert small to big, think small, therefore go ahead and divide.
e.g. 700 micrograms = 0,7milligrams (700 divided by 1000 = 0.7)

4. **Drugs in volume and dose required**
This method is used for calculating a medication dose as a volume. During preregistration training it may have been referred to as 'What I want, divided by what I got, times the volume':

$$\frac{\text{Dose required}}{\text{Stock available}} \times \text{Volume}$$

Worked CCU clinical example:
Prescription: 750 mg vancomycin IV stat.
Stock available: 1000 mg vancomycin reconstituted with sterile water to a total volume of 20 mL. Calculate the volume to be administered.

$$\frac{750\,\text{mg}}{1000\,\text{mg}} \times 20\,\text{mL} = 15\,\text{mL}$$

5. **Calculating rate, time and volume**
In practice, this calculation is usual for intravenous fluids prescribed over *hours*, for example crystalloids, colloids, parental nutrition or medications in volume infused via a rate-controlled infusion pump. Alternatively, it may also be used for short infusions of medications to be infused over *minutes* for example, IV paracetamol.

a. **Calculating rate per hour**

$$\text{Rate}\left(\text{mL / hour}\right) = \frac{\text{Volume}\left(\text{mL}\right)}{\text{Time (hours}}$$

Prescription: 1000 mL 5% dextrose IV over 12 hours via a rate-controlled infusion pump. Calculating the rate to be set.

$$\frac{1000\,\text{mL}}{12\,\text{hours}} = 83.33\,\text{mL / hr}$$

rounded to whole number = 83 mL/hr

b. **Calculating total volume to be infused**
This is a useful calculation when planning maximum total fluid intake targets.
Clinical application:

- Fluid restricted
- Setting hourly fluid removal via Continuous Renal Replacement therapy (CRRT).
- Titrating an hourly dose for a continuous infusion of IV Furosemide.
- Rationalising total IV fluid requirements involved in medication preparation.

Total volume= Volume (mL) × Time (hours)

Worked CCU clinical example:
Mrs Jazz has an infusion of IV Plasmalyte running at a rate of 120 mL/hour via a rate-controlled infusion pump. Calculating the total volume that will be infused in 10 hours.
120 mL × 10 hours = 1200 mL in 10 hours

c. **Calculating total time for infusion to be complete**

$$\text{Total time}(\text{hours}) = \frac{\text{Volume}}{\text{Rate}}$$

Worked CCU clinical example:

Miss Violet, has an infusion of 1000 mL dextrose/saline running at a rate of 125 mL/hour via a rate-controlled infusion pump. Calculating the total time for the prescribed volume to be complete.

$$\frac{1000\,\text{mL}}{125\,\text{mL}/\text{hr}} = 8\,\text{hours}$$

d. **Calculating rate per hour for volume over minutes**

$$\text{Rate per Hour} = \frac{\text{Volume required}(\text{mL}) \times 60(\text{Time})}{\text{Time}(\text{minutes})}$$

6. **Calculating a stated rate (dose per minute)**

Several medications have a maximum safe dose/concentration for infusion per minute/hour, for example:

- Furosemide
- Potassium chloride
- Vancomycin

$$\text{Stated dose mL / hour} = \frac{\text{Total Volume to be infused} \times \text{Dose (max dose)} \times 60\,(\text{minutes})}{\text{Total Dose Required}}$$

Worked clinical CCU example:

Prescription: 250 mg IV furosemide added to NACL to a total volume of 50 mL.

Infused via a syringe pump at a dose no greater than 4 mg/minute.

$$\frac{50\,\text{mL} \times 4\,\text{mg}(\text{max dose}) \times 60\,\text{minutes} = 12000}{12000}$$

$$\frac{12000}{250}$$

$$= 48\,\text{mL / hour}$$

7. **Calculating a drip rate in drops per minute**

This method of delivering a volume of IV fluid/medication involves the use of a manual infusion controller.

Common sizes:

- Macrodrip tubing for 15 drops/mL
- Macrodrip tubing for 20 drops/mL

- Microdrip tubing for 60 drops/mL commonly used in CCU for arterial and central line NACL flush sets.

It is essential for the CCU RN to be competent using this method as an alternative when there may be a shortage of infusion devices during a surge of admitted CCU patients, such as during the COVID-19 pandemic. Therefore, the use of this manual method could be used for IV fluids and TPN.

Tips:

- The drop factor is the number of drops contained in 1 mL.
- When calculating, the answer is always rounded to a whole number.

Worked CCU clinical examples:

a. **Calculating drip rate in drops/minute**

$$\text{Drops per minute} = \frac{\text{Volume}(\text{mL}) \times \text{Drip factor}}{\text{Time}(\text{hour}) \times 60}$$

Worked clinical CCU example:

Prescription: 1000 mL IV Plasmalyte over 8 hours via a giving set with a drip factor of 20 drops/minute. Calculating the drip rate to be set.

1000 mL × 20 drops/mL = 20,000

8 hours × 60 minutes = 480

$$= \frac{20,000}{480} = 480 = 41.66 \text{ rounded to a whole number}$$

= 42 drops per minute

b. **Calculating drip rate over minutes**

This is a common method used for short duration infusions i.e. antibiotics:

$$\text{Drops / minute} = \frac{\text{Volume}(\text{mL}) \times \text{Drip factor}}{\text{Time}(\text{minutes})}$$

Worked clinical CCU example:

Prescription: IV paracetamol 1 g/50 mL over 30 minutes via a giving set with a drip factor of 15 drops per minute. Calculating the drip rate to be set.

$$\frac{50\,\text{mL} \times 15 = 750}{30} = 25 \text{ drops per minute}$$

163

c. **Calculating (time) duration of the infusion**

(Time) Duration for completion =

Step 1: $\dfrac{\text{Drop rate/min}}{\text{Drip factor} = \text{mL/min}}$

Step 2: $\dfrac{\text{Total volume to be infused}}{\text{mL/min}}$

Step 3: $= \dfrac{\text{Time in minutes}}{60 = \text{HOURS}}$

Mrs Jenkins, is receiving an infusion of 100 mL Ciprofloxacin at 42 drops per minute via an infusion set with a drip factor of 20 drops/mL. Calculating the time for this infusion to complete.

1. $\dfrac{42}{20} = 2.1$ mL/min

2. $\dfrac{100}{2.1} = 48$ minutes

d. **Calculating drip rate in drops per minute when prescribed as mL/hour**

$$\text{Drops/minute} = \dfrac{\text{Rate}(\text{mL/hour})(\text{prescribed}) \times \text{Drop factor}}{60\,(\text{minutes})}$$

Worked clinical CCU example:
Prescription: 1000 mL NACL IV at a rate of 130 mL/hour via a giving set with a drip factor of 20 drops per minute. Calculating the drops per minute.

$130 \times 20 = 2600$

$\dfrac{2600}{60} = 43$ drops per minute

8. **Drugs expressed in ratio**
This is the concentration of a dilute solution. These are usually emergency CCU medications such as adrenaline in prefilled syringes used in cardiac arrest or anaphylaxis.
Tips:

- May be expressed as a weight to volume ratio (w/v)
- The '1' in a ratio always means 1 g in 1000 mL or 100 mg in 100 mL

CCU Emergency drug examples:
Adrenaline 1:1000 prefilled syringe = 1 mg in 1 mL
Adrenaline 1: 10000 prefilled syringe = 1 mg in 10 mL

9. **Drugs expressed in percentage**
These medications/fluids are expressed as an amount of a substance out of a possible 100, for example, 10% glucose w/v means 10g of glucose in every 100 mL.
Common CCU medications expressed as % are:

Lignocaine 1% = 1g in 100 mL
Glucose 5% = 5g in 100 mL
NACL: 0.9% = 0.9g in 100 mL
Saline 0.45% = 0.45g in 100 mL
Calcium gluconate 10% (10g/100 mL = 1g/10 mL = 100 mg/mL)
Magnesium sulphate 20% (20g/100ml = 2g/10 mL = 200 mg/mL)
Magnesium sulphate 50% (50g/100 mL = 5g/10 mL = 500 mg/mL)

$$\dfrac{\text{Volume} \times \text{Percentage}\,(\%)}{100} = \text{Grams}$$

Learning event

In clinical practice, magnesium sulphate is most often prescribed in mmol.
However, magnesium sulphate stock is available expressed as a %.
The conversion is:

10% magnesium sulphate/10 mL = 100 mg/mL
100 mg = 0.4 mmol/mL
10 mL = 4.06 mmol/mL

Worked clinical CCU example:
Prescription: 5% glucose 500 mL IV over 6 hours. Calculating the total amount of glucose that will be administered in 6 hours.

$$\dfrac{500\,\text{mL} \times 5}{100} = 25\text{g}$$

10. **Calculating flow rate for a given dose in micro-grams/milligrams/nanograms/kg/min**
This is a frequently used mathematical calculation that needs to be mastered. The dose delivered per minute is titrated to achieve a desired therapeutic effect. e.g. haemodynamic parameter such as Mean Arterial Blood pressure (MAP) or level of sedation as per the Richmond Agitation-Sedation Score (RASS).
Types of medications are concentrated in strength, diluted in smaller volumes and act within narrow therapeutic margins.

Drug examples are:

- Haemodynamics: adrenaline, dopamine. dobutamine, noradrenaline and milrinone.
- Heart rate: isoprenaline
- Anticoagulation: flolan

$$\frac{\text{Rate}}{(\text{mL}/\text{hour})} = \frac{\text{Micrograms}/\text{kg}/\text{min} \times \text{weight}(\text{kg}) \times 60}{\text{concentration}(\text{micrograms}/\text{mL})}$$

Worked clinical CCU example:

Prescription: Adrenaline IV as a continuous infusion at a dose of 0.2mcg/kg/min.

Reconstitute 4 mg Adrenaline in 5% glucose to a total volume of 50 mL.

Patient weight: 80 kg

1. Determine the dose required per hour:

   0.2 mcg (dose required) × 80 kg × 60 (time) = 960 mcg of adrenaline per hour.

2. Convert 4 mg adrenaline = 4000 mcg divided by 50 mL (volume) = 80 mcg/mL.

$$\frac{960\,\text{mcg}}{80\,\text{mcg}} \times 1 = 12\,\text{mL}/\text{hr}$$

d. **Calculating micrograms/milligrams/nanograms/ kg/min for a given flow rate**

   It is part of daily routine for an CCU RN taking handover between shifts to complete a bedside safety check which includes checking the rate and dose for all infusions so ensure they correlate with the prescription chart and CCU observation chart.

$$\frac{\text{Micrograms}}{/\text{kg}/\text{min}} = \frac{\text{rate}(\text{mL}/\text{hour}) \times \text{concentration}(\text{mcg}/\text{mL})}{\text{weight}(\text{kg})\,\text{divided by}\,60\,(\text{minutes})}$$

Worked clinical CCU example:

Miss Jazz is receiving an infusion of 4 mg adrenaline in 5% glucose in a total volume of 50 mL running at 6.5 mL/hour via an infusion pump. Patient weight: 72 kg

Convert 4 mg = 4000 mcg divided by 50 mL (volume) = 80 mcg/mL (concentration)

6.5 mL × 80mcg/mL divided by 72 kg (weight) divided by 60 (time) = 0.12mcg/kg/min

Displacement

Displacement occurs when reconstituting a powder for injection e.g. Meropenem (antibiotic) with a solvent e.g. NACL, the net result is an increase in the volume caused by the displacement value of the powder. This has no effect on the amount of drug administered provided that the entire contents of the vial is administered to a single patient following reconstitution. Importantly, displacement is brand specific, please check the manufacturer's instructions for reconstitution.

This is not a main concern working in an adult CCU however, displacement values for powders for intravenous injection become important when only part of the reconstituted vial it to be administered, this may occur when a smaller dosage is required in the neonate baby. If displacement is not taken into account it may result in under-dosing (Dixon and Evans, 2006).

Conclusion

The content presented in this chapter evidences that the safe administration of medications in CCU requires confidence, knowledge and practice of skill in order to prevent errors as well as to optimise the therapeutic effects and hence the outcome for the adult patient with critical illness. Furthermore, providing a safe and therapeutic environment for the patient involves a collaborative multidisciplinary team approach between the prescribing intensivist/medical doctor, specialist medical teams and the clinical critical care pharmacist. Best practices for this specialised group of patients involve promoting a culture of patient safety by means of standardisation of intravenous medication concentrations for infusions, use of infusion medical devices with pre-programmed dosing and robust use of approved regimens to decrease the margin for error.

RNs are pivotal in their roles in the custodianship as well as administration of medications as part of their role responsibilities. However, this high-risk task necessitates further development with a good foundation of knowledge of pharmacology.

Take home points

1. Proficiency in performing mathematical drug calculations is *essential* for accurate and safe medication administration.
2. Keep up to date with changes and drug safety bulletins.
3. Implement interventions to decrease distractions.
4. Implement the 'Rights of medication administration'.

165

5. Do not to document the dose *before* administration.
6. Evaluate effectiveness of administered medications.
7. Use standardised IV dosing regimens, eg dopamine infusion prescribed using microgram/kilogram/min.
8. Use infusion pumps and syringe pumps for accuracy in dose and volume delivery.
9. Report medication errors via Datix.
10. Expand knowledge and skill of fundamentals of pharmacology for CCU medications.

References

Blanca-Lopez, N., Plaza-Seron, M., Cornejo-Garcia, J.A. et al. (2015). Drug-induced anaphylaxis. *Current Treatment Options in Allergy* 2: 169–182. https://link.springer.com/article/10.1007/s40521-015-0055-z.

British Association for Parenteral and Enteral Nutrition (BAPEN) (2017). Administering medicines via enteral feeding tubes. https://www.bapen.org.uk/nutrition-support/enteral-nutrition/medications (accessed March 2022).

Borthwick, M. (2019). The role of the pharmacist in the intensive care unit. *Journal of the Intensive Care Society* 20(2): 161–164. https://journals.sagepub.com/doi/pdf/10.1177/1751143718769043 (accessed March 2022).

Care Quality Commission (CQC) (2015). *Regulation 20: Duty of Candour.* https://www.cqc.org.uk/guidance-providers/regulations-enforcement/regulation-20-duty-candour (accessed March 2022).

Critical Care Networks – National Nurse Leads (CC3N) (2015). National Competency Framework for Registered Nurses in Adult Critical Care. Version 2: 2015. https://www.cc3n.org.uk/uploads/9/8/4/2/98425184/01_new_step_1_final__1_.pdf (accessed March 2022).

Dhanani, J., Fraser, J.F., Chan, H.K. et al. (2016). Fundamentals of aerosol therapy in critical care. *Critical Care* 20(269). https://ccforum.biomedcentral.com/articles/10.1186/s13054-016-1448-5 (accessed March 2022).

Dixon, A. and Evans, C. (2006). Intravenous therapy: Drug calculations and medication issues. *Journal Infant.* (3) 110–114.

Dougherty, L. and Lister, S. (2015). *The Royal Marsden Hospital Manual of Clinical Nursing Procedures.* Wiley-Blackwell.

Dörffler-Melly J., de Jonge E., Pont A.C. et al. (2002). Bioavailability of subcutaneous low-molecular-weight heparin to patients on vasopressors. *Lancet.* 359(9309): 849–850.

Edwards, S. and Axe, S. (2015). The ten 'R's of safe multidisciplinary drug administration. Nurse prescribing. 13 (8): 352–360.

Elliot, M. and Liu, Y. (2010). The nine rights of medication administration: an overview. *British Journal of Nursing* 19(5): 300–305. doi: 10.12968/bjon.2010.19.5.47064.

Greenblatt, D.J. and Allen, M.D (1978). Intramuscular injection-site complications. *JAMA* 240(6): 542–544.

Hunter, S., Considine, J., and Manias, E. (2019). Nurse management of vasoactive medications in intensive care: A systematic review. *Journal of Clinical Nursing* 29(3–4): 381–392.

Intensive Care Society (ICS) (2013). *The Intensive Care Society – Guidelines and Standards.* https://www.ficm.ac.uk/sites/default/files/Core%20Standards%20for%20ICUs%20Ed.1%20(2013).pdf (accessed 25 November 2020).

Johnstone, M.J. and Kanitsaki, O. (2006). The ethics and practical importance of defining, distinguishing and disclosing nursing errors: a discussion paper. *International Journal of Nursing Studies* 43(3): 367–376.

Kruer, R.M., Jarell, A.S., Latif, A. (2014). Reducing medication errors in critical care: a multimodal approach. *Journal of Clinical Pharmacology* 6: 117–126.

Lister, S. and West-Oram, S. (2020). *The Royal Marsden Manual of Clinical Nursing Procedures: Procedural Guidelines for Evidence Based Practice,* 10e. Wiley Blackwell.

Loveday, H.P., Wilson, R.J., and Pratt, M. (2014). epic 3: National Evidence-based Guidelines for preventing Healthcare-Associated Infections in NHS Hospitals in England. Journal of Hospital Infection. https://improvement.nhs.uk/documents/847/epic3_National_Evidence-Based_Guidelines_for_Preventing_HCAI_in_NHSE.pdf

Moniz, P., Coelho, L., and Povoa, P. (2020) Antimicrobial stewardship in the intensive care unit: The role of biomarkers, pharmacokinetics, and pharmacodynamics. *Advances in Therapy* 38: 164–179. https://link.springer.com/article/10.1007/s12325-020-01558-w.

Mosopefoluwa, S., Oduyale, M., Patel, N. et al. (2020). Co-administration of multiple intravenous medicines: Intensive care nurses' views and perspectives. *Nursing in Critical Care.* https://onlinelibrary.wiley.com/doi/full/10.1111/nicc.12497.

NHS Improvement (NHSi) (2018a). *Never Events Policy and Framework.* https://www.england.nhs.uk/wp-content/uploads/2020/11/Revised-Never-Events-policy-and-framework-FINAL.pdf (accessed March 2022)

NHS Improvement (NHSi) (2018b). *Never Events List 2018.* https://www.england.nhs.uk/wp-content/uploads/2020/11/2018-Never-Events-List-updated-February-2021.pdf (accessed March 2022)

Nursing and Midwifery Council (2018). The Code: Professional Standards of Practice and Behaviour for Nurses, Midwives and Nursing Associates. https://www.nmc.org.uk/standards/code/ (accessed March 2022).

Nursing and Midwifery Council (NMC) (2019). Standards for medicines management. https://www.nmc.org.uk/standards/standards-for-post-registration/standards-for-medicines-management/1999.999 (accessed March 2022).

Roach, T. (1992). A preoperative assessment and education programme: Implementation and outcomes. *Patient Education and Counselling* 25(1): 83–88.

Royal Pharmaceutical Society (RPS) and Royal College of Nursing (RCN) (2019). Professional Guidance on the Administration of Medicines in Healthcare Settings. https://www.rcn.org.uk/workingwithus/-/media/royal-college-of-nursing/documents/working-with-us/endorsements/professional-guidance-on-the-administration-of-medicines-in-healthcare-settings.pdf (accessed March 2022).

Titiesari, Y.D., Barton, G., Bothwick, M. et al. (2017). Infusion medication concentrations in UK's critical care areas: Are the Intensive Care Society's recommendations being used? *Journal of the Intensive Care Society* 8(1): 30–35.

Chapter 14

Neurological critical care

Samantha O'Driscoll

Aim

To help the reader to understand the neurological system in health and the management of altered neurology in critically ill patients.

Learning outcomes

After reading this chapter the reader will be able to:
- Demonstrate awareness of the underpinning anatomy and physiology of the brain and nervous system.
- Understand the importance of timely and accurate neurological monitoring in the critically unwell, and how to perform this.
- Understand the pathological changes that can lead to deterioration in patient condition, and indicators of these.
- Understand the fundamental principles governing maintenance of Intracranial Pressure (ICP) and Cerebral Perfusion Pressure (CPP) in health.
- Gain a basic understanding of the medications used to optimise neurological function in the critically unwell.

Test your prior knowledge

- What two systems combine to make the nervous system?
- What three components are assessed for a Glasgow Coma Score?
- What is the name given to the fluid flowing around the brain and spinal cord?
- Which part of the brainstem houses the respiratory centre?
- What medications can affect consciousness?

Fundamentals of Critical Care: A Textbook for Nursing and Healthcare Students, First Edition. Edited by Ian Peate and Barry Hill.
© 2023 John Wiley & Sons Ltd. Published 2023 by John Wiley & Sons Ltd.
Companion website: www.wiley.com/go/peate/criticalcare

Introduction

This chapter discusses the effects of critical illness on neurology, focusing on timely assessment and management of patients with neurological impairments. Whilst impairment can arise as a result of congenital abnormalities, this chapter focuses on acquired or acute brain injuries (ABI), such as traumatic brain injury (TBI), stroke (haemorrhagic and ischaemic) and brain lesions (e.g. tumours or cysts). The uniting factor in these conditions is the impact they have on neurological function. Long-term neurological impairment can severely impact quality of life; ability to live independently; maintain relationships and continue to work in the same way the patient was able to prior to the acute brain injury (O'Keeffe et al., 2020; Watkin et al., 2020). It is crucial that those with neurological impairments are assessed and treated in a timely manner to optimise remaining brain function, prevent further deterioration and achieve the best possible outcome.

Step 2 competencies: National standards

2:5.2 Assessment, Monitoring and Observation

Demonstrate your knowledge using a rationale through discussion, and the application to your practice:

- Comprehensive neurological assessment, recording findings, optimising treatment within prescribed limits and escalating problems to appropriate MDT members:
  — Glasgow Coma Scale (GCS) assessment and accurate documentation.
  — Pupil response (size, shape and reactivity).
  — Indications for CT scanning according to local, national and professional guidance.
  — Signs and symptoms of raised ICP

Neurological anatomy and physiology

Functions of the nervous system

The nervous system is a highly complex arrangement made up of billions of functional units. On a basic level, these functional units work together to integrate information gathered from both the internal and external environment, and elicit a response. On a more complex level, they are the platform on which thoughts and emotions are built, and on which our ability to plan, process and communicate is founded. These functional units are highly specialised cells known as neurones. Neuronal structure is varied and is dependent on their function. Figure 14.1 depicts a multipolar neurone.

The key parts of a neurone are: dendrites which receive the action potential; cell body; the axon, along which the action potential travels; and axon terminals, allowing delivery of the action potential to the next neurone or muscle. Neurones are supported by glial cells which differ in structure and can perform a variety of functions.

The transfer of information is possible due to changes in the cell environment, known as an *action potential*. The presence of ions (Na^+, K^+ and Ca^{2+}) inside a neurone provide a small amount of electrical charge at rest. When the neurone is stimulated, the ions move rapidly across the cell membrane causing an increase in the electrical charge and the generation of an action potential. This process is replicated along the cell membrane, allowing the electrical impulse to travel along the neurone like a wave, onto the next neurone and so on. The axons of motor and sensory neurones in the PNS are wrapped in a protein layer known as a myelin sheath (Figure 14.1). This provides electrical insulation allowing the action potential to travel faster along the axon. Depending on location and function of the neurone, an action potential can travel up to 130 m/s, resulting in rapid transfer of information through the nervous system.

Understanding of the concept of an action potential is crucial when nerves are damaged by disease, or their action is subdued by medication, such as with paralysing agents.

Medications management: atracurium

Atracurium is a neuromuscular blocking agent (NMBA). This class of drugs are also known as paralysing agents, they inhibit the efferent motor pathway for skeletal muscle contraction by blocking the action potential. They are used when it is necessary for the patient to be completely still, as in surgery; or when muscular contraction may be interfering with treatment, allowing full control of a patient's ventilation when mechanically ventilated. In patients with neurological injury, paralysing agents result in a reduction of neural activity and therefore reduced blood flow to the brain and a reduction in ICP. As paralysing agents block the action of all skeletal muscles, the patient must always be deeply sedated. A lack of adequate sedation can result in 'awake paralysis': an awareness of events around the person but being completely unable to move or communicate.

The central and peripheral nervous systems

The nervous system can be subdivided into the central nervous system (CNS; the brain and spinal cord) and peripheral nervous system (PNS; all other nervous tissue)

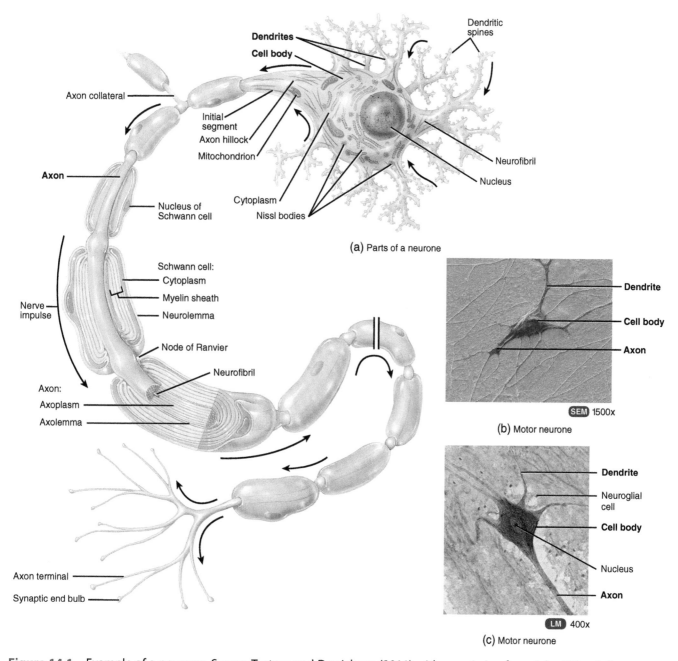

Figure 14.1 Example of a neurone. *Source:* Tortora and Derrickson (2011) with permission from John Wiley & Sons.

(Figure 14.2). Neurones that deliver information to the CNS about a stimulus are known as afferent or sensory neurones and make up the somatic nervous system (SNS). Those carrying information to the PNS to affect a change (such as contraction of a muscle) are efferent or motor neurones. The motor neurones that deliver impulses to skeletal muscles are under voluntary control whereas motor control of visceral organs is involuntary. Within the organs, neurones deliver impulses to smooth muscle, cardiac muscle and glands, controlling responses such as heart rate, respiratory rate, pupil dilation and blood flow. The sensory and motor neurones within those organs make up the autonomic

nervous system (ANS), and this can be further subdivided into the sympathetic and parasympathetic nervous systems – innervation of each cause opposing responses (Figure 14.3).

Central nervous system

Structure and function of the brain

The brain is an exceptionally complex and specialised organ, which can be observed in anatomically distinct regions (Figure 14.4). The largest part of the brain is the cerebrum, divided into frontal, parietal, occipital and temporal lobes

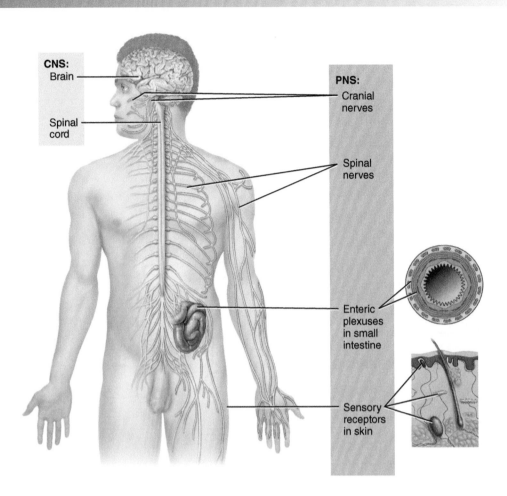

Figure 14.2 Subdivision of the nervous system into PNS and CNS. *Source:* Tortora and Derrickson (2011) with permission from John Wiley & Sons.

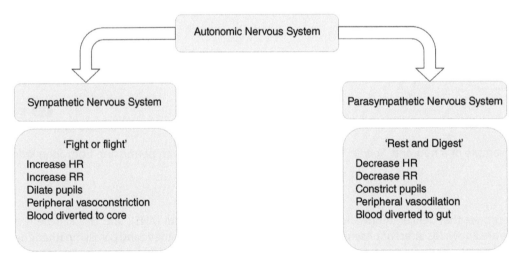

Figure 14.3 Division of the autonomic nervous system.

(Figure 14.5a). Within each lobe are zones controlling specific functions. The location of these areas was elucidated by K. Brodmann in 1909, the numbers respond to the mapping, still in use today (Amunts et al., 2020; Amunts and Zilles, 2015) (Figure 14.5b). The structure and function of the brain is discussed in Box 14.1.

Meninges

The brain and spinal cord are wrapped in three distinct layers of protective coverings called meninges. The inner most layer is the pia – this thin membrane wraps closely to the surface of the brain, folding in along the many gyri of the cerebrum and continuing along the spinal cord.

The middle layer is the arachnoid layer – consisting of collagen and elastic fibres and named for its web-like appearance. The outer layer is the dura – a tough, fibrinous layer which continues along the spinal cord as far as S2. The meninges offer physical protection to the brain and spinal cord, provide pathways for blood vessels and channel cerebrospinal fluid.

Cerebrospinal fluid (CSF)

Cerebrospinal fluid (CSF) is a water-based liquid produced in chambers of the brain known as the lateral ventricles. The brain contains four ventricles, with a lateral ventricle in each of the hemispheres. CSF flows through the ventricles, around the brain and spinal cord. It acts as a shock-absorber, protecting the brain from impacting the inside of the skull and as an infective defence (Tortora and Derrickson, 2017).

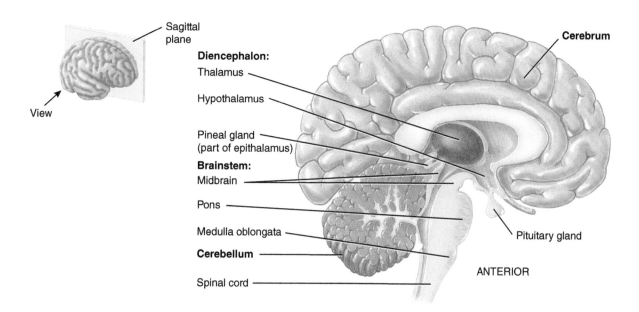

Sagittal section, medial view

Figure 14.4 Anatomical regions of the brain. *Source:* Tortora and Derrickson (2011) with permission from John Wiley & Sons.

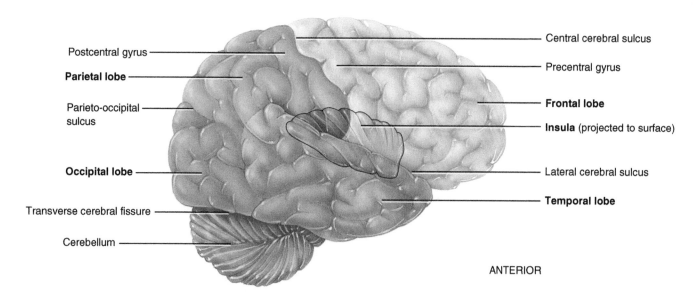

(a) Right lateral view with temporal lobe cut away

Figure 14.5 (a) Lobes of the cerebrum. (b) Functional areas of the brain. *Source:* Tortora and Derrickson (2011) with permission from John Wiley & Sons.

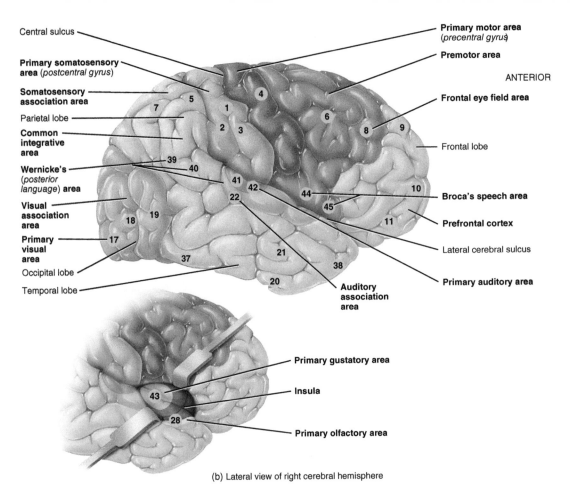

(b) Lateral view of right cerebral hemisphere

Figure 14.5 (Continued)

Box 14.1 Structure and function of the brain.

Structure	Sub-structure	Function
Cerebrum		The distinctive folded surface is formed of grooves, known as gyri, which provide an increased surface area. The cerebrum is bisected into right and left hemispheres along the longitudinal fissure, resulting in two halves.
	Frontal lobe	Higher function such as personality, cognition, intelligence and memory. The frontal lobe also contains the primary motor area, involved in muscle control. The ability to process speech is also based here in the left lobe, in a region known as Broca's area.
	Parietal lobe	Contains the sensory cortex. Involved with processing sensory information and integrating this with information from other areas. An area that complements Broca's area is Wernicke's area – located in the left parietal lobe. This area gives understanding to words as they are processed.
	Temporal lobe	Contains the primary auditory area and auditory association area, involved with sound processing. Also areas involved with visual processing and memory, specifically with facial recognition.
	Occipital lobe	Primary visual and visual association areas. Involved with visual processing and recognition.
Diencephalon	Thalamus, hypothalamus, epithalamus	The hypothalamus plays a strong regulatory role in the ANS, releasing hormones such as anti-diuretic homone (ADH).
Cerebellum		Controls fine motor movement and balance.
Brainstem	Midbrain, Pons, Medulla	Primitive regulatory centres for survival. Autoregulation of cardiovascular and respiratory systems. Involved in arousal and consciousness.

Cerebral blood flow

The brain receives approximately 15–20% of the cardiac output (Williams and Leggett, 1989), which is essential to provide oxygen and glucose to cells in order to produce adenosine triphosphate (ATP) for cellular activity. In the brain, this is primarily geared toward movement of ions across cell membranes, facilitating action potentials and transmission of nerve impulses (Clarke and Sokoloff, 1999). The amount of oxygen and glucose needed to maintain cellular function is known as the basal metabolic rate (BMR). As neuronal activity increases, so too does BMR and homeostatic mechanisms must respond ensuring an adequate supply of oxygen, glucose and nutrients to meet demand. One such mechanism is the baroreceptors (pressure sensors) located in the internal carotid arteries. The blood supply to the brain is predominantly via the vertebral and internal carotid arteries, subdividing into smaller branches to feed specific regions of the brain. Fluctuations in pressure in the internal carotid arteries, detected by the baroreceptors, triggers autoregulatory processes that aim to maintain a steady-state blood pressure, ensuring brain tissue remains perfused. For the transported nutrients and oxygen to pass from the arterial supply to the cells, they must pass the blood-brain barrier. This protective wall is a line of defence to reduce the risk of infection and harmful substances passing into the brain. The permeability of the blood-brain barrier allows for the movement of oxygen, glucose and smaller lipid- and water-soluble molecules only. Venous drainage occurs via dural venous sinuses: pockets formed between the dural layers allowing blood to collect into a channel and drain into the internal jugular veins.

Monro–Kellie hypothesis

The brain is surrounded by the skull, providing a physical defence to the soft, delicate structure of the brain. However, this rigidity results in a lack of flexibility to tolerate fluctuations in the pressure within. The Monro–Kellie Hypothesis explains the pressure within the skull (known as intracranial pressure; ICP) as a sum of the components housed within it:

$$ICP = Brain\ tissue + Blood + CSF$$

For ICP to remain constant, there must be reciprocal change between the 3 components making up the volume within the skull – brain tissue, CSF and blood. An increase in one of these without a decrease in another or both would cause an increase in ICP (Monro, 1783).

Regulation of CPP and ICP

In an average adult ICP is approximately 5–15 mmHg (Rangel-Castillo et al., 2008). Homeostatic regulation mechanisms control the volume of blood or CSF to maintain ICP within this range. For example, if an increase in blood flow to the brain was required, the volume of CSF within the skull can be reduced by diverting larger volumes around the lower portion of the spinal cord. The vascular system can accommodate changes in pressure by compressing smaller vessels and reducing the volume of venous blood in the brain (Woodward and Mestecky, 2011). This compensation is possible to a point, and is determined by the speed at which one component increases. Compensatory mechanisms are able to adapt to a slow-growing tumour, for example, better than a traumatic injury resulting in a large haemorrhage taking up the same volume.

The brain relies heavily on a constant supply of oxygenated blood for cellular function. An unmoderated increase in ICP will impede blood flow and perfusion of brain tissue and quickly result in loss of consciousness (Clarke and Sokoloff, 1999). Poor outcomes are noted with ICP >20–25 mmHg (Carney et al., 2016). The perfusion pressure to the brain is known as cerebral perfusion pressure (CPP) and can be demonstrated as a relationship between mean arterial pressure (MAP) and ICP.

$$CPP = MAP - ICP$$

Using this calculation, CPP will be reduced with an increase in ICP, a decrease in MAP, or both. Autoregulatory mechanisms are able to maintain parenchymal perfusion within a CPP of 50–150 mmHg (Rangel-Castillo et al., 2008). The management strategies for patients with raised ICP use this hypothesis, focusing on the reduction in ICP and maintenance of MAP in order to maintain CPP.

6Cs: Commitment

Providing the best care for patients requires a commitment to continually reflect on the evidence base.

Herniation of the brain

An uncompensated rise in ICP causes compression of collapsible structures within the brain such as the ventricles. Further increase in ICP will cause structures within the brain to begin to be pushed or 'herniate' into other spaces, along the path of least resistance (Woodward and Mesteky, 2010). Ultimately this will lead to brain tissue herniating through the foramen magnum, the opening in the skull through which the spinal cord passes (Figure 14.6). This causes compression of the brain stem and suppression of cardiovascular and respiratory function (see Red Flag: Cushing's Triad), eventually leading to death.

Red Flag: Cushing's Triad

When ICP is profoundly elevated the brainstem is compressed, reducing blood flow to the region and impeding function. The brainstem contains cardiac and respiratory centres – impairment will manifest as bradycardia, profound hypertension and apnoea. The combination of these three signs is known as Cushing's Triad, a sign of extensive neurological damage with a very poor prognosis.

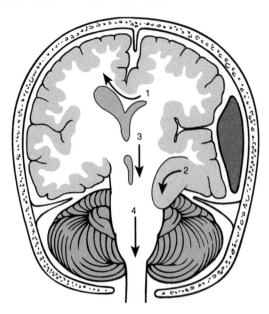

Figure 14.6 Brain herniation. *Source:* Woodward and Mestecky (2011) with permission from John Wiley & Sons.

Neurological assessment

For patients admitted with an ABI, the minimum acceptable documented neurological observations are: Glasgow Coma Score; pupil size and reactivity (Box 14.2); limb movements; respiratory rate; heart rate; blood pressure; temperature; and blood oxygen saturation (National Institute for Health and Care Excellence (NICE), 2014). Patients should be cared for in an area where staff are trained to perform these observations and escalate any deterioration. This may be a general hospital setting (such as an admissions unit; general medical ward) or neurological specialist area (such as neurology/stroke ward, Hyper-Acute Stoke Unit (HASU), High Dependency Unit (HDU) or Critical Care). The standardised track and trigger observation tool NEWS2 (Royal College of Physicians, 2017) has 'new confusion' included as a scoring classification, recognising that a change in baseline mental function of someone who is ill is a clear sign of clinical deterioration. As NEWS2 is not used for specific neurological function, most clinical settings will have a local Neurological Observation chart (such as the example in Figure 14.7)

6Cs: Competence

All practitioners have a duty of care to ensure they are competent to carry out the tasks required of their role.

The components incorporated in Neurological Observation will be discussed. These are observations that would be monitored as a minimum, and in some settings or clinical scenarios other observations may complement these.

Snapshot

Azami, 82 years year old, was admitted the previous day following a fall at home. Azami usually takes warfarin for atrial fibrillation. A CT scan on admission showed a small sub-dural haematoma. Azami was admitted to a neurological ward for observation. Over the course of the day Azami has become increasingly drowsy. At 1800h a Registered Nurse (RN) records the following information on the observation chart:

Airway (A): Snoring sounds, relieved by tilting Azami's head backwards using a head tilt chin lift manoeuvre.
Breathing (B): Oxygen saturations 92% (NEWS2 = 2), on room air (NEWS2 = 0), respiratory rate (RR) 12 breaths per minute (NEWS2 = 0).
Cardiovascular System (C): Blood Pressure (BP) is 110/65 mmHg (NEWS2 = 1), Heart Rate (HR) is 96 beats per minute (NEWS2 = 1), capillary refill time (CRT) is <2 seconds.
Disability (D) (neurological System), Patient responsive to pain (NEWS2 = 3), on the CAVPU scale, body temperature (T) is 37.0°C.
Exposure (E): Nil of note.
Total NEW2 Score: 7.

Nursing actions:
- The RN puts out a call for the Medical Emergency Team.
- With assistance, the RN uses an oropharyngeal airway to help open Azami's airway
- The RN applies oxygen mask with non-rebreathe bag to Azami's face, administering 15 L O_2/min

Diagnosis:
- Azami is taken for repeat CT scan of her head; shows expansion of the sub-dural haematoma, impairing Azami's level of consciousness.
- She is referred to Critical Care for HDU level care.

Glasgow Coma Scale

The Glasgow Coma Scale (GCS) is a tool used to assess level of consciousness (LOC). It is divided into three components: eye opening, verbal response and motor response. Since its inception in the 1970s, it has been adapted and modified, most recently in 2014. This adaptation removed the word 'pain' from the scale, replacing it with 'pressure' in response to the sentiment that inflicting pain on the patient is not something that should sit within healthcare. Clarification was also given to the verbal scale, updating the components to 'words' and 'sounds' (Table 14.1). The components of the GCS are assessed and scored on best observed response, out of a possible 15. The lowest possible score is 3/15, indicating deep coma, with 15/15 indicating normal consciousness.

The ROYAL MARSDEN
NHS Foundation Trust

Name: ....

Hospital No: .... NHS No: ....

Adult Neurological Observations

Date																								
Time																								

Glasgow Coma Scale					C = Eyes closed by swelling
	Eyes open	Eyes open spontaneously	4		
		Eye opening to speech	3		
		Eye opening to pain	2		
		No eye opening	1		
	Best verbal response	Orientated	5		T = Endotracheal tube or Tracheostomy
		Confused	4		D = Dysphasia
		Inappropriate words	3		LB = Language barrier
		Incomprehensible sounds	2		
		No verbal response	1		
	Best motor response (Record best arm)	Obeys commands	6		M = Muscle relaxant
		Localises pain	5		P = Paralysed
		Normal flexion to pain	4		
		Abnormal flexion to pain	3		
		Extension to pain	2		
		No motor response	1		
		Total GCS Score out of 15 *			

* See overleaf for guidance (Clinical Response)

Pupils				+ = Reacts
	Left	Size		− = No reaction
		Reaction		SL = Sluggish
	Right	Size		C = Eye closed
		Reaction		

Limb movement				Record right (R) and left (L) separately if there is a difference between the two sides
	Arms	Normal power		
		Mild weakness		
		Severe weakness		
		Flexion		P = Paralysed
		Extension		# = Fracture
		No response		
	Legs	Normal power		
		Mild weakness		
		Severe weakness		
		Flexion		
		Extension		
		No response		

Temperature°C

Pupil scale (mm)

● 1
● 2
● 3
● 4
● 5
● 6
● 7
● 8

230
220
210
200
190
180
170
160
150
140
130
120

Blood pressure ∧ ∨ 110
100
90

Pulse rate ● 80
70
60
50
40
35
30
25
20
15
10
5

Respiration (write number)

O₂ Sats																								
Inspired O₂%																								
Monitoring Frequency																								
Initials																								

Figure 14.7 Neurological observation chart.

175

Scoring the Activities of the Glasgow Coma Scale

Eye Opening Scored 1–4			Note
Spontaneously	4	Eyes open without need of stimulus	Normal pupils are spherical, usually at mid-position and have a diameter ranging from 1.5 to 6mm.
To speech	3	Eyes open to verbal stimulation (normal, raised or repeated)	**Look at both pupils together: size, equality and shape – monitor reaction to light.**
To pain	2	Eyes open to central pain only	
No eye opening	1	No eye opening to verbal or painful stimuli	

Verbal Response Scored 1–5			Note
Orientated	5	Able to accurately describe details of time, person and place	The absence of speech may not always indicate a falling level of consciousness. The patient may not speak English (though he/she can still speak), may have a tracheostomy or may be dysphasic. Some patients may need a lot of stimulation to maintain their concentration to answer questions, even though they can answer correctly.
Confused	4	Can speak in sentences but does not answer orientation questions correctly	
Inappropriate words	3	Speaking incomprehensible, inappropriate words only	
Incomprehensible sounds	2	Incomprehensible sounds following both verbal and painful stimuli	
No verbal response	1	No verbal response following verbal and painful stimuli	

Motor Response Scored 1–6			Motor response
Obeys commands	6	Follows and acts out commands, e.g. Lift up right arm	Normal Flexion Abnormal Flexion Extension Motor response is tested using the upper limbs since responses to the lower limbs may reflect spinal function.
Localises pain	5	Purposeful movement to remove noxious stimulus	
Normal flexion to pain	4	Flexes arm at elbow without wrist rotation in response to central painful stimulus	
Abnormal flexion to pain (Withdrawal from pain)	3	Flexes arm at elbow with accompanying rotation of the wrist into spastic posturing in response to central pain	
Extension to pain	2	Extends arm at elbow with some inward rotation in response to central pain	
No motor response	1	No response to central painful stimulus	

Evaluation of Painful Stimuli
Painful stimulus should be employed only if the patient does not respond to firm and clear commands. It is always important that the least amount of pressure to elicit a response is applied so as to avoid bruising the patient.

1. Trapezium squeeze – using the thumb and two fingers, hold 5 cms of the trapezius muscle where the neck meets the shoulder and twist the muscle. If the trapezius muscle is pinched the hand should move above the nipple line.
2. Supra-orbital pressure – to be performed only by health care professional competent in this method.
3. Sternal rub – not recommended for repeated assessment.

Clinical Response
If Glasgow Coma Score drops by 2 points or more or is <13 seek urgent assessment by medical team/critical care outreach and an anaesthetist, as this may indicate a neurological emergency. A drop of 1 point must also be considered as a significant change/deterioration and review sought from the nurse in charge/medical team. Any change, and action, should be documented in the patients notes.

Figure 14.7 (Continued)

6Cs: Compassion
Compassion lies at the heart of our profession – driving us to provide care, acknowledging the person, not just the patient.

Limb movement
The ability of a patient to move each limb, the power they are able to exert with it and the way the limb responds to stimulus provide valuable insight into neurological function or changes that may be occurring in the brain. As part of the GCS assessment the motor element identifies flexion or extension to stimulus (Table 14.2).

Table 14.1 Glasgow Coma Scale. *Source:* Based on Teasdale et al., 2014.

	Score	Response	Stimuli applied
Eyes	4	Spontaneous	
	3	To sound	Loud, firm use of preferred name to both ears (consider if hearing aids are normally used).
	2	To pressure	See section on stimuli for pressure response
	1	No response	
	NT	Not testable	Closed due to swelling, surgery, dressings etc.
Verbal	5	Orientated	Gives name, date, place
	4	Confused	Coherent speech but confused
	3	Words	Coherent single words
	2	Sounds	Moans/groans
	1	No response	
	NT	Not testable	Factor interfering with communication e.g. artificial airway
Motor	6	Obeys commands	Obeys two stage command (e.g. stick out tongue and put back in)
	5	Localising	Hand crosses midline towards stimulus
	4	Flexion	Moves arm rapidly toward body
	3	Abnormal flexion (decorticate)	See section on limb movement
	2	Extension (decerebrate)	See section on limb movement
	1	No response	
	NT	Not testable	Limiting factor e.g. paralysed, cast in situ etc.

Table 14.2 Limb movement. *Source:* Lister et al. (2020) with permission from John Wiley & Sons.

Limb response	Description
Normal flexion	Elbows bent, hands tucked towards the body.
Abnormal flexion (decorticate posturing)	Elbows bent, flexion of the wrists.
Extension (decerebrate posturing)	Elbows straight, arms rotated and wrists flexed away from the body.

Examination Scenario: assessing Glasgow Coma Scale

Assessment of the GCS has four steps:

1. Check for factors which may impede the patient's ability to interact with the assessor (such as a language barrier; hearing deficit).
2. Observe whether the patient demonstrates any component of the assessment spontaneously, such as watching the assessor approach with open eyes and greeting them verbally.
3. Stimulate those who do not respond spontaneously. Voice should be used first with clear, loud instructions given close to each ear. If there is no response to voice, the assessor should move to pressure. Starting with pressure on the fingertip (not the nail bed – this can cause bruising) with increasing intensity up to 10 seconds. The lower limbs should not be tested as there is a higher chance of misidentifying a spinal reflex as a response to pressure (Woodward and Mestecky, 2011). If no response is elicited, the assessor should apply pressure to the trapezius muscle, with increasing intensity again for up to 10 seconds (Teasdale and Jennett, 1974). Pressure to the sternum should not be applied, this can cause bruising.
4. Rate the response demonstrated to the Eyes, Verbal and Motor components. If the patient demonstrates varying responses, the best observed response should be used.

Pupillary assessment

Box 14.2 Pupil size, shape and reactivity.

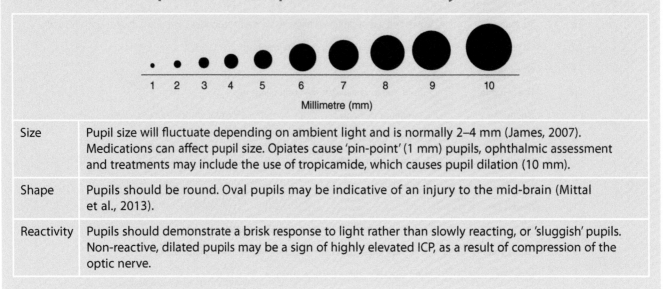

Size	Pupil size will fluctuate depending on ambient light and is normally 2–4 mm (James, 2007). Medications can affect pupil size. Opiates cause 'pin-point' (1 mm) pupils, ophthalmic assessment and treatments may include the use of tropicamide, which causes pupil dilation (10 mm).
Shape	Pupils should be round. Oval pupils may be indicative of an injury to the mid-brain (Mittal et al., 2013).
Reactivity	Pupils should demonstrate a brisk response to light rather than slowly reacting, or 'sluggish' pupils. Non-reactive, dilated pupils may be a sign of highly elevated ICP, as a result of compression of the optic nerve.

Examination Scenario: assessing pupil size and reactivity

The size, shape and reactivity of pupils should be assessed as part of a neurological examination. The procedure should be explained to the patient, and the patient encouraged to keep their eyes open. Wash hands. Gently hold the eyelid open if needed. Using a pen torch, shine the light across the pupil, observing for it to constrict briskly as the light passes. The opposite eye should show constriction at the same time. Wash hands. It may be difficult to detect pupil constriction in patients with dark irises. Ensuring the overhead lights are dimmed may aid this. Report and document findings.

Orange Flag: Delerium

Delirium is an acute change in cognitive function seen in >80% of ICU patients. Delirium in critically ill patients can be triggered by a range of factors including medications; physiological response to critical illness; disturbance of circadian cycle and unfamiliar environment. Patients experiencing delirium whilst in ICU are more likely to have a longer hospital stay and higher mortality 6 months post-discharge (Ely et al., 2004).

6Cs: Courage

It takes courage to care for patients with challenging behaviour.

Snapshot

Derek, 68 years old, was admitted to ICU following a car accident, sustaining a TBI. He was sedated and ventilated for 8 days and was extubated this morning. Prior to admission Derek worked full-time as a builder. He took medication for hypertension.

The nurse looking after Derek completed a CAM-ICU assessment to assess for indications of delirium.

Feature 1 – Acute onset of changes of fluctuations in mental status – is Derek's current mental status different from his baseline? Has mental status fluctuated in the last 24 hours?

Feature 2 – Inattention – Ask Derek to squeeze the nurse's hand when he hears the letter 'A'. Read the following letters:

SAVEAHAART

Inattention present with >2 errors.

Feature 3 – Altered level of consciousness – Present if Derek scores anything other than a RASS 0.

Feature 4 – Disorganised thinking – Ask Derek the following questions:

1. Does a stone float on water?
2. Are there fish in the sea?
3. Does one pound weigh more than two pounds?
4. Can you use a hammer to pound a nail?

Disorganised thinking present with >1 error.

Answering 'yes' to Feature 1 *and* 2, as well as *either* of Feature 3 or 4 indicates the presence of delirium, and should trigger local intervention strategy (Ely et al., 2001).

Signs and symptoms of increasing ICP

Appropriate documentation of neurological function can detect early warning signs of increasing ICP. The value itself is not necessarily a complication, but rather the impact on CPP, vascular occlusion, ischaemia and the progression towards herniation (Rosner and Daughton, 1990). Pathologies causing ICP to rise slowly, such as tumours and hydrocephalus, will demonstrate an onset of symptoms slower than rapidly changing pathologies such as a ruptured aneurysm (weakness in the wall of the artery) (Table 14.3).

Whilst the threshold for increased ICP is not absolute, negative outcomes are correlated with ICP >20–25 mmHg. Strategies to reduce ICP should be employed within this range (Carney et al., 2016). Appropriate monitoring and documentation of observations can demonstrate a change in patient condition – when used alongside clinical judgement, can guide the need for further investigations or treatment such as CT scanning. The indications for CT imaging of the brain are discussed in detail by NICE (2014).

Table 14.3   Signs and symptoms of increasing ICP.

Early	Late	Critical
Headache	Reduction in level of consciousness	Reduction in level of consciousness leading to loss of consciousness
Vomiting	Seizures	Loss of pupillary reactivity to light progressing to dilation without response
Seizures	Changes to pupil size and reactivity	Changes to respiratory pattern: Cheyne-Stokes/ Neurogenic hyperventilation
Focal neurological signs		Abnormal motor response – decorticate posturing progressing to decerebrate posturing
		Cushing's triad

Red Flag: fixed and dilated pupil

In patients who are sedated, frequent monitoring of pupil size, shape and reactivity is essential as normal neurological function cannot be assessed. Therefore, deterioration is more difficult to detect. The presence of a fixed and dilated or 'blown' pupil can indicate an acute intracerebral event. Pupillary constriction is controlled by the optic and oculomotor nerves. Compression of these nerves by, for example, an intraparenchymal bleed, inhibits function, resulting in a fixed and dilated pupil (Belliveau et al., 2020). This necessitates urgent medical review.

6Cs: Communication

Clear communication is a cornerstone of good care. It is particularly important when delays in escalation or treatment may result in irreparable neurological damage. Clear communication aids rapid investigation and intervention. A communication tool, such as SBAR or RSVP, can be used to convey information in a structured manner.

Clinical Investigations: computed tomography (CT) scan

A CT scan is a diagnostic tool using multiple layers of X-rays, which are reconstructed by a computer to give detailed 2D images of slices through the body. It provides essential information, guiding treatment and management strategies. The scan requires the patient to lie flat and still on a bed which passes through the scanner. Patients with a raised ICP may be confused and agitated, making it difficult to perform the scan. It may be necessary to give medication to keep the patient calm, allowing the scan to be completed safely.

Clinical Investigations: intracranial pressure monitoring

ICP can be directly monitored by inserting a sensor into the skull, allowing fluctuations in pressure of the tissue surrounding the sensor to be relayed to a monitor, providing a real-time ICP value. Some monitors also provide a wave form, providing further clinical information.

Primary and secondary brain injury

Primary brain injury occurs through a specific insult, for example, trauma to the brain tissue impacting its function, or a haemorrhage starving the tissue of oxygenated blood causing hypoxic damage. Secondary injury is caused by the body's response to the primary injury. When tissue is damaged, inflammatory processes cause swelling (oedema) to the area to protect it. When oedema occurs within the rigid box of the skull, this can exacerbate rising ICP, leading to further hypoxic damage. Whilst it is not possible to reverse the primary injury, secondary injury occurs over a period of hours to weeks from the original insult. Management strategies of ABI focus on optimisation of remaining neuronal tissue, mitigating the negative potential of secondary brain injury (Werner and Engelhard, 2007). The term 'neuroprotection' is often used to describe goal-directed therapy, focusing on protecting the remaining healthy brain tissue.

Management of raised ICP

Goal-directed therapy

When achieving neuroprotective targets, it may be necessary to sedate the patient to control their respiratory function with invasive ventilation such as an Endotracheal Tube (ETT) and insert an arterial line. An arterial line allows continuous blood pressure monitoring, safe use of vasoactive medication and close observation of arterial blood gas values. The values given in Table 14.4 outline target ranges between which the negative impact of secondary brain injury can be reduced.

If target ranges are not achieved if may be necessary to implement the management strategies now discussed.

Table 14.4 Neuroprotective target ranges.
Source: Carney et al., 2016; NICE, 2014.

Parameter target	Rationale
Oxygen $PaO_2 \geq 13$ kPa	To optimise blood flow to parenchyma, ensuring that an adequate amount of oxygen is available to tissue that may be compromised by reduced blood flow.
Carbon dioxide $PaCO_2$ 4.5–5 kPa	Carbon dioxide acts on endothelial smooth muscle to promote vasodilation. An elevated $PaCO_2$ will result in cerebral vasodilation, increased blood flow and raised ICP. A reduced $PaCO_2$ will cause vasoconstriction, reducing blood flow to the tissue and exacerbating ischaemia of the parenchyma.
ICP ≤ 22 mmHg	ICP >22 mmHg is associated with worsening neurological outcomes and mortality.
Temperature Normothermic	The autoregulatory response to pyrexia is vasodilation, which would increase cerebral blood flow, increasing ICP and reducing CPP. Research, however, no longer supports induced hypothermia as a management strategy in TBI — the evidence is not strong enough to outweigh the negative effects such as coagulopathies, infection and cardiac dysrhythmias, Instead, treatment should focus on the avoidance of pyrexia.

Red Flag: Raised ICP

Patients with ABI who are nursed in specialist areas may have ICP measured directly. The plan of care includes a threshold pressure, below which ICP should be maintained. Stimuli such as personal care, repositioning, suctioning and pain will cause an increase in ICP. ICP may 'spike' above this threshold and management strategies focus on reducing ICP below threshold. First-line treatments include correcting head alignment ensuring venous drainage, removing extraneous stimuli, ensuring $PaCO_2$ and temperature are within target ranges. Deepening level of sedation, addition of further sedatives, paralysing agents or osmotic medications may be necessary. If it is not possible to maintain ICP within the target range, CT imaging may be necessary to determine if neurosurgical intervention is necessary.

Fluid balance

Maintaining an accurate fluid balance is an integral part of ABI management. Fluid in the body is housed in either the intracellular or extracellular space. Extracellular fluid can be further categorised according to location within the body – within the vascular system as plasma, and in the space around cells as interstitial fluid, for example (Tortora and Derrickson, 2017). The movement of fluid between these spaces is controlled by opposing forces, generated by the presence of large molecules and a concentration gradient of electrolytes (see Box 14.3). When tissue is damaged an inflammatory response is triggered, leading to an increase in permeability of the cell membranes. There is a subsequent increase in interstitial fluid in the affected area, in the form of oedema. This is a physiological protection mechanism, designed to cushion the damaged tissue, preventing further injury. Within the skull, however, parenchymal oedema will exacerbate an increase in ICP, decrease in CPP and subsequent ischaemia.

Box 14.3 The forces contributing to movement of water between intra and extracellular spaces.

Osmosis	Osmolarity	Tonicity	Oncotic pressure
The movement of water from an area of high concentration to low concentration across a semi-permeable membrane.	A measurement of dissolved solute in a litre of fluid.	The force exerted by the dissolved solute that drives the osmosis of water.	The force exerted by large molecules in the plasma that contribute to tonicity.

Hypovolaemia causes a reduction in MAP and CPP, exacerbating ischaemia of neuronal tissue. In patients who have a cerebral aneurysm, a reduction in pressure in the cerebral arteries can result in vasospasm – a significant constriction of cerebral arteries causing a reduction in perfusion and ischaemic damage (Kolias et al., 2009). Medication can be given to relax the cerebral arteries, reducing the risk of vasospasm (nimodipine, see Medications management: nimodipine). Reducing the complications of hyper- or hypovolaemia, fluid therapy aims to achieve normovolaemia in patients with ABI.

Haemodynamic therapy

Treatment options can also include the manipulation of blood pressure to increase CPP, achieved either by increasing the intravascular volume by fluid therapy or by using vasoconstricting drugs. Drugs such as noradrenaline, adrenaline and metaraminol act on alpha-2 receptors in the peripheral vasculature, resulting in vasoconstriction and an increase in blood pressure. Maintaining adequate cerebral blood flow and CPP is a fundamental aspect of ABI care, and one of the best ways to reduce secondary brain injury (Carney et al., 2016). The threshold at which systolic blood pressure (SBP) should be maintained in patients with TBI is age adjusted, to highlight the expected pre-morbid baseline. Patients 15–49 years or those over 70 years SBP ≥ 110 mmHg, patients 50–69 years SBP ≥ 100 mmHg. In practice, this is often translated into a targeted CPP as invasive monitoring allows for accurate measurement. In patients with spontaneous intracerebral haemorrhage the target SBP should be maintained between 130–140 mmHg (NICE, 2019).

Vasoconstricting drugs can cause peripheral ischaemia and good nursing practice includes monitoring for signs of reduced peripheral perfusion. This should include the character of peripheral pulses, temperature of the limbs as well as observation of patients' hands and feet for changes in colour. It is important to remember, close attention should be paid to patients with darker skin tones, as subtle changes may be easy to miss.

Oncotic therapy

The movement of water as driven by the principles in Box 14.3 can be used as a management strategy to manage raised ICP as a result of cerebral oedema. The administration of solutions that are highly oncotic results in the movement of water from the intracellular and interstitial spaces into the intravascular space. Commonly used oncotic solutions include mannitol and hypertonic saline (2–5%). The benefit of these solutions in ABI management is widely accepted, however, current evidence does not support a specific regimen of either (Carney et al., 2016; Cook et al., 2020). Mannitol and hypertonic saline reduce ICP as a result of oncotic movement of water into the intravascular space, a reduction of blood viscosity and an increase in cerebral circulation. Mannitol has a diuretic effect; however, this can be problematic in patients with hypovolaemia, potentially negating the initial benefit of reduced ICP by reducing MAP and compromising CPP (Carney et al., 2016).

Orange Flag: altered body image

Patients who have experienced an ABI may have to come to terms with a long recovery for functionality, or the prospect of never regaining the function they had prior to injury. This can have huge psychological impact on the patient and their image of themselves. Psychological recovery should be supported as well as physical recovery.

Nursing care

Approaches to nursing care can aid in the reduction of ICP, or focus on avoidance of stimulation. In critically unwell patients it is necessary to provide episodes of care, such as insertion of invasive lines, personal care, medication administration, repositioning and suctioning. All interventions will result in stimulation of the patient as neuronal pathways relaying information to the CNS are engaged. When these pathways are activated, sympathetic innervation causes blood pressure to rise as the BMR of the cells is increased, in turn causing an increase in ICP. Several strategies can be employed to reduce this effect.

- Clustering care: Critically ill patients who are sedated and ventilated are completely dependent on healthcare staff. However, grouping together episodes of care and allowing the patient time to rest, unstimulated, in between assists in reducing transiently elevated ICP. This may include planning episodes of care so mouthcare is performed immediately prior to repositioning, for example.
- Patient positioning: Cerebral venous drainage occurs through the jugular veins. Keeping the patient's head in a neutral alignment (i.e. not tilted to either side and compressing right or left jugular vein) can optimise cerebral venous drainage, reduce cerebral blood volume and ICP (Ng et al., 2004). Ensuring the bed is kept at a 20–30° angle allows gravity to assist in venous drainage and reduce ICP. This may be achieved either by sitting the head portion of the bed up, or tilting the entire bed in a reverse Trendelenburg position. Clinical indication, such as the presence or absence of spinal injury dictates which is appropriate.
- Endotracheal ties: In order to safely maintain an endotracheal tube (ETT), it should be anchored externally. This may be via ties, extended around the patient's head. In patients with an ABI, these may compress the jugular veins and impede venous drainage and fixation devices such as this should be avoided. In the absence of specially designed ETT securing devices, self-adhesive fabric tape may be used to secure the ETT to the patient's cheeks, this will avoid impedance of venous drainage.
- Bowel care: Patients who are critically unwell are at high risk of constipation for a variety of reasons, including immobility and the effects of medications such as opiates. Constipation causes an increase in pressure in the abdominal cavity, impinging on the ability of the diaphragm to contract and therefore adequate ventilation. Using higher ventilatory pressures increases intrathoracic pressure, reduces the gradient for venous drainage, reduces blood pressure and ultimately negatively impacts on CPP.
- Sedation: Invasive lines and tubes, episodes of care and procedures all cause sympathetic stimulation and may result in an increase in ICP and reduction in CPP. In order to reduce the sympathetic response to stimuli patients are sedated (Table 14.5). Sedatives are titrated to achieve a target sedation level, such as the Richmond Agitation-Sedation Scale (Table 14.6). Daily sedation targets should be set for the patient. Chapter 12 discusses anaesthesia and sedation.

> ## 6Cs: Care
> Care of ourselves and our colleagues is just as important as the care we provide to the patient.

Snapshot

Faiza is a 59-year-old woman admitted to hospital following a spontaneous subarachnoid haemorrhage. Faiza is sedated, intubated and ventilated. Aside from treating Faiza's neurological status, all other aspects of Faiza's care should be supported by healthcare staff:

- Frequent eye and mouthcare to reduce risk of infection.
- Regular repositioning. Whilst sedated Faiza is at risk of developing pressure ulcer damage. All lines, tubes and medical devices should be checked, ensuring that they are not causing pressure damage (see also Chapter 6).
- Passive range of movement exercises to maintain joint mobility. Fazia is at risk of long-term nerve damage if joints are not adequately supported in position.
- Dietician review ensuring Faiza's nutritional requirements are met, most likely supported via a nasogastric feeding regimen.
- DVT prophylaxis, reducing risk of blood clots whilst immobile.
- Emotional and psychological support for Faiza.
- Support of Faiza's family during this critical time. They may have questions surrounding her progression or the possible outcomes for her.
- Close monitoring of observations and fluid balance. Observations outside of set targets should be managed and escalated. They may be an indication of deterioration.
- Documentation of all care provided to Faiza.

Transfer

If it is not possible for management strategies discussed to be achieved at the initial hospital, the patient should be transferred to a specialist centre, such as those with trauma, stroke or neurosurgical services (NICE, 2014). Patients should be transferred to a specialist centre if they display:

- GCS <8 following resuscitation
- Unexplained confusion for > 4 hours
- Rapid deterioration in LOC following admission
- Worsening focal neurological signs
- Seizure without full recovery
- Confirmed or suspected penetrating injury
- CSF leak

Medications to control intracranial pressure

Table 14.5 Commonly used medications in the management of ABI.

	Example	Action on ICP
Analgesia	Fentanyl, remifentanil, oxycodone	Reduces ICP by controlling sympathetic stimulation caused by pain. Reduces overall cerebral activity.
Sedation	Propofol, midazolam	Reduces cerebral activity and therefore basal metabolic rate, reducing and nutrient demand. Results in a reduced cerebral blood flow and ICP.
Neuromuscular blocking agents	Atracurium, rocuronium, suxamethonium	Reduces cerebral activity and basal metabolic rate. Also allows ventilatory compliance which can reduce intrathoracic pressure, ease cerebral venous drainage and reduce ICP.
Osmotic agents	Hypertonic saline, mannitol	Reduces ICP by managing cerebral oedema; promoting movement of fluid into intravascular compartment.
Anticonvulsants	Phenytoin, levetiracetam	Prevents seizures which would cause significant rise in cerebral activity, metabolic rate and blood flow leading to a rise in ICP

Table 14.6 Richmond Agitation-Sedation Scale. *Source:* Modified from Sessler et al., 2002.

+4	Overtly combative, violent, immediate threat to self or staff
+3	Pulls or removed tubes or catheters; aggressive
+2	Frequent, non-purposeful movement, fights ventilator
+1	Anxious but movements not aggressive or vigorous
0	Alert and orientated
−1	Drowsy, >10 seconds eye contact
−2	Rousable, <10 seconds eye contact
−3	Movement or eye opening but no eye contact
−4	Some movement to physical stimulus
−5	No response to physical stimulus

Learning event

Reflect on your understanding of the rationale behind nursing interventions aimed at reducing ICP.

The patient should have initial management and monitoring established prior to transfer and interventions should consider any potential deterioration during the transfer:

- Intubate and ventilate the patient prior to transfer if:
  - GCS ≤ 8 or loss of protective laryngeal reflexes or rapidly deteriorating LOC
  - Ineffective ventilation – PaO_2 < 13 kPa; $PaCO_2$ < 4 kPa or
  - > 6 kPa; irregular respiratory pattern
  - Unstable facial fractures
  - Copious bleeding into the oral cavity
  - Seizures
- Instigate drug or fluid therapy to maintain MAP >80 mmHg

Chapter 30 discusses transfer in more detail.

Medications management: propofol

Propofol, an anaesthetic drug used to reduce level of consciousness, has profound cardiovascular side effects, reducing blood pressure and heart rate, given by continuous infusion or bolus dose in either 1% or 2% preparations. Due to the effect on level of consciousness the patient should have an artificial airway in place or be administered by a health care practitioner who has been deemed competent in airway management.

Medications management: nimodipine

Nimodipine is a calcium channel blocker, causing relaxation of smooth muscle in the cerebral arterial walls, minimising the risk of vasospasm, used in the management of subarachnoid haemorrhage and cerebral aneurysms. Nimodipine is given via the enteral route, doses should not be omitted or delayed.

Medications management: phenytoin

Phenytoin, an anti-epileptic drug used for the prevention and management of seizure activity, has a therapeutic range requiring drug levels to be monitored. Optimum response is 10–20 mg/litre (BNF, 2020), given IV or enteral route; if administered via the IV route an in-line filter (0.22–0.50 micron) should be used at a rate not exceeding 50 mg/minute (BNF, 2020).

Conclusion

The care of patients who have experienced an ABI focuses on preventing further damage to the injured brain, optimising non-injured brain tissue. The brain is a highly complex organ, and failure to prevent further damage can have lifelong impact on the patient and their family. Careful neurological observation can highlight deterioration, triggering the need for further imagining or transfer to a specialist centre. Patients may require direct monitoring of ICP and advanced interventions to reduce it, such as sedation, paralysing agents or osmotic medications. If the patient is sedated, a sedation tool such as RASS should be used to identify target sedation level. These patients will be fully dependent on healthcare providers to meet fundamental care needs. These must be attended to whilst aiming to reduce unnecessary stimulus and elevation of ICP. The psychological impact of an ABI should also be considered, and validated tools which monitor for signs of delirium (such as CAM-ICU) should be used to reduce length of hospital stay and improve patient outcome.

Take home points

1. Brain tissue + CSF + blood = ICP is a key concept in the management of patients with ABIs.
2. Management strategies focus on reducing ICP and optimising uninjured brain tissue. Strategies should aim to keep ICP < 22 mmHg (Carney et al., 2016).
3. Close monitoring of neurological status and timely escalation of deterioration can drastically improve patient outcome.
4. Transfer to a specialist centre should be considered in hospitals without the services to manage neurological deterioration.
5. Sedatives and mechanical ventilation can be used to achieve targets aimed at protecting non-injured brain tissue.
6. Practitioners should be familiar with the medications used to manage ABI and their effect on ICP and level of consciousness.

References

Amunts, K., Mohlberg, H., Bludau, S., and Zilles, K. (2020). Julich-Brain: A 3D probabilistic atlas of the human brain's cytoarchitecture. *Science* 369(6506): 988–992. doi: 10.1126/science.abb4588.

Amunts, K. and Zilles, K. (2015). Architectonic mapping of the human brain beyond Brodmann. *Neuron* 88(6): 1086–1107. doi: 10.1016/j.neuron.2015.12.001.

Belliveau, A.P., Somani, A.N., and Dossani, R.H. (2020). *Pupillary Light Reflex*. https://www.ncbi.nlm.nih.gov/books/NBK537180/ (accessed March 2022).

Carney, N., Totten, A.M., Ullman, J.S. et al. (2016). *Guidelines for the Management of Severe Traumatic Brain Injury*, 4e. https://braintrauma.org/uploads/03/12/Guidelines_for_Management_of_Severe_TBI_4th_Edition.pdf (accessed March 2022).

Clarke, D.D. and Sokoloff, L. (1999). *Regulation of Cerebral Metabolic Rate*. https://www.ncbi.nlm.nih.gov/books/NBK28194/ (accessed March 2022).

Cook, A.M., Morgan Jones, G., Hawryluk, G.W.J. et al. (2020). Guidelines for the Acute Treatment of Cerebral Edema in Neurocritical Care Patients. *Neurocritical Care* 32(3): 647–666. doi: 10.1007/s12028-020-00959-7.

Ely, E.W., Bernard, G.R., Speroff, T. et al. (2001). Delirium in mechanically ventilated patients: Validity and reliability of the Confusion Assessment Method for the intensive care unit (CAM-ICU). *Journal of the American Medical Association* 286(21): 2703–2710. doi: 10.1001/jama.286.21.2703.

Ely, E.W., Shintani, A., Truman, B. et al. (2004). Delirium as a predictor of mortality in mechanically ventilated patients in the intensive care unit. *Journal of the American Medical Association* 291(14): 1753–1762. doi: 10.1001/jama.291.14.1753.

James, B. (2007). The pupils. In: *Ophthalmology: Investigation and Examination Techniques* (ed. B. James and L. Benjamin), 123–127. Elsevier. doi: 10.1016/B978-0-7506-7586-4.50015-5.

Kolias, A.G., Sen, J., and Belli, A. (2009). Pathogenesis of cerebral vasospasm following aneurysmal subarachnoid hemorrhage: Putative mechanisms and novel approaches. *Journal of Neuroscience Research* 87(1): 1–11. doi: 10.1002/jnr.21823.

Mittal, M.K., Rabinstein, A.A., and Wijdicks, E.F.M. (2013). Pearls and oysters: Oval pupil: Two observations. *Neurology* 81: e124–e125. doi: 10.1212/WNL.0b013e3182a9583b.

Monro, A. (1783). *Observations on the Structure and Functions of the Nervous System*. https://helda.helsinki.fi/handle/10250/2433 (accessed March 2022).

National Institute for Health and Care Excellence. (2014). *Head Injury: Assessment and Early Management: Clinical Guideline*. www.nice.org.uk/guidance/cg176 (accessed March 2022).

National Institute for Health and Care Excellence. (2019). *Stroke and Transient Ischaemic Attack in Over 16s: Diagnosis and Initial Management*. NICE.

Ng, I., Lim, J., Wong, H.B., Czosnyka, M. et al. (2004). Effects of head posture on cerebral hemodynamics: Its influences on intracranial pressure, cerebral perfusion pressure, and cerebral oxygenation. *Neurosurgery* 54(3): 593–598. doi: 10.1227/01.NEU.0000108639.16783.39.

O'Keeffe, F., Dunne, J., Nolan, M. et al. (2020). 'The things that people can't see': The impact of TBI on relationships: an interpretative phenomenological analysis. *Brain Injury* 34(4): 496–507. doi: 10.1080/02699052.2020.1725641.

Rangel-Castillo, L., Gopinath, S., and Robertson, C.S. (2008). Management of intracranial hypertension. *Neurologic Clinics* 26(2): 521–541. doi: 10.1016/j.ncl.2008.02.003.

Rosner, M.J. and Daughton, S. (1990). Cerebral perfusion pressure management in head injury. *Journal of Trauma – Injury, Infection and Critical Care* 30(8): 933–940. doi: 10.1097/00005373-199008000-00001.

Royal College of Physicians. (2017). National Early Warning Score (NEWS) 2: Standardising the assessment of acute-illness severity in the NHS. https://www.rcplondon.ac.uk/projects/

outputs/national-early-warning-score-news-2 (accessed 15 December 2020).

Lister, S., Hofland, J., and Grafton, H. (eds) (2020). *The Royal Marsden Manual of Clinical Nursing Procedures*, 10e. Wiley-Blackwell.

Sessler, C.N., Gosnell, M.S., Grap, M.J. et al. (2002). The Richmond Agitation-Sedation Scale: Validity and reliability in adult intensive care unit patients. *American Journal of Respiratory and Critical Care Medicine* 166: 1338–1344. doi: 10.1164/rccm.2107138.

Teasdale, G. and Jennett, B. (1974). Assessment of coma and impaired consciousness: A practical scale. *The Lancet* 304(7872): 81–84. doi: 10.1016/S0140-6736(74)91639-0.

Teasdale, G., Maas, A., Lecky, F. et al. (2014). The Glasgow Coma Scale at 40 years: Standing the test of time. *The Lancet Neurology* 13(8): 844–854. doi: 10.1016/S1474-4422(14)70120-6.

Tortora, G.J. and Derrickson, B.H. (2017). *Principles of Anatomy and Physiology*, 15e. John Wiley & Sons.

Watkin, C., Phillips, J., and Radford, K. (2020). What is a 'return to work' following traumatic brain injury? Analysis of work outcomes 12 months post TBI. *Brain Injury* 34(1): 68–77. doi: 10.1080/02699052.2019.1681512.

Werner, C. and Engelhard, K. (2007). Pathophysiology of traumatic brain injury. *British Journal of Anaesthesia* 99(1): 4–9. doi: 10.1093/bja/aem131.

Williams, L.R. and Leggett, R.W. (1989). Reference values for resting blood flow to organs of man. *Clinical Physics and Physiological Measurement* 10(3): 187–217. doi: 10.1088/0143-0815/10/3/001.

Woodward, S. and Mestecky, A.-M. (2011). *Neuroscience Nursing: Evidence-Based Practice* (Sue Woodward & Ann-Marie Mestecky, Eds.). Wiley-Blackwell.

Chapter 15

Cognition

Barry Hill and Sadie Diamond-Fox

Aim

This aim of this chapter is to provide the reader with an evidence-based understanding of cognition in the context of typical neurocognitive impairments experienced by patients in critical care concerning delirium and the importance of sleep.

Learning outcomes

After reading this chapter the reader will be able to:

- Have an awareness of cognition.
- Appreciate the complexities of cognition in the critical care environment.
- Understand delirium and its management strategies.
- Consider sleep and its importance on cognition.
- Discuss the current evidence-based management strategies for neurocognitive disorders within the critical care environment.

Test your prior knowledge

- Describe the components of consciousness.
- How many points does the Richmond Agitation-Sedation Scale have?
- Name the four components of the Confusion Assessment Method in ICU (CAM-ICU).
- Based upon current evidence, critically discuss two drugs that may be used in the treatment of ICU delirium.
- Differentiate between the two components of mental status; consciousness and cognition.

Fundamentals of Critical Care: A Textbook for Nursing and Healthcare Students, First Edition. Edited by Ian Peate and Barry Hill.
© 2023 John Wiley & Sons Ltd. Published 2023 by John Wiley & Sons Ltd.
Companion website: www.wiley.com/go/peate/criticalcare

Introduction

Advances in critical care have increased survival rates, but they have highlighted the need to reduce the morbidity of critical care patients and improve their short- and long-term functional outcomes. Frequently, especially for those with acute respiratory distress syndrome, present neurocognitive impairments that extend beyond the acute phase and hospital stay and lead to significant deficits in quality of life. These neurocognitive sequelae generate health and economic problems related to the dependency of survivors. Neurocognitive impairments may be understood as a manifestation of occult brain damage secondary to underlying pathophysiological mechanisms related to critical illness (Turon et al., 2013).

Cognitive impairment

The term 'cognitive impairment' refers to persistent deficits in the brain's ability to function effectively. People with cognitive impairment often have difficulties with memory, attention span, processing speed, and executive functioning, which involves organising, planning, and problem solving. Depending on the severity of the cognitive impairment, long-lasting consequences can negatively impact an individual's functioning in areas including work and school, social functioning, driving and the management of money and medication. In severe cases, it can limit independence and result in people being significantly more reliant on family, friends and institutional support of various kinds to function.

Orange Flag: Supporting family and friends

A recent review identified that relatives who witness a loved one experiencing an episode of ICU delirium (particularly hyperactive delirium), can experience significant distress and psychological morbidity, including post-traumatic stress disorder. The levels of psychological stress experienced by relatives have been suggested to be greater than that experienced by patients themselves. Patient and family support groups (such as ICUsteps in the UK – https://icusteps.org/) may aid in the long-term management of the psychological sequalae of this disease.

6Cs: Commitment

Being highly committed to patients helps to improve their quality of care and experience as well as that of other patients.

Cognitive impairment after critical illness may improve over time and some people improve completely while others slightly improve but never return to baseline. In certain instances, individuals continue a pattern of decline that is suggestive of dementia.

6Cs: Communication

Good communication is critical to ensuring effective management of neurocognitive disorders within the critical care environment and beyond.

Causes of cognitive impairment

According to the Network for Investigation of Delirium: Unifying Scientists (NIDUS) (2018) up to 80% of critical care patients develop cognitive deficits, making it a serious but under-recognised problem. Those most likely to development cognitive impairment are listed in Box 15.1. Risk factors for ICU-acquired long-term cognitive impairment (LTCI) in older adults include neurological dysfunction, infection or severe sepsis, and acute dialysis. Duration of delirium is a risk factor for LTCI for adults of any age.

Relatively little research has been undertaken on the causes of cognitive impairment after critical illness, but experts think the following factors, either by themselves, or in combination, may play a role:

- Inadequate brain oxygenation – common in mechanically ventilated patients
- Delirium
- Infections, which lead to inflammatory responses
- Glucose dysregulation
- Certain medical illnesses, which may themselves have direct effects on the brain
- Medications

Box 15.1 People most likely to get cognitive impairment.

Some individuals are likely to be more susceptible than others to developing cognitive impairment after critical illness. Individuals at greatest risk may include those who:

- Have pre-existing cognitive problems that make them especially vulnerable
- Are older people >65 years
- Have delirium for a long duration
- Require mechanical ventilation
- Have a diagnosis of sepsis or Acute Respiratory Distress Syndrome, (ARDS)
- Have lengthy and complex hospital and ICU stays

Signs of cognitive impairment

Depending on how severe the cognitive impairment symptoms are, signs of cognitive impairment (CI) are sometimes obvious and sometimes very subtle. In the ICU setting, CI may be evidenced by similar presentations as those observed post-discharge, such as; memory difficulties, disorders of attention, problem solving and an inability to perform more complex tasks.

6Cs: Courage

Critical care patients can often lack capacity due to the underlying disease process that has required them be to admitted to the critical care unit, therefore it is important that healthcare professionals have the courage to enable us to do the right thing for the people we care for and to advocate for them in instances when they are not able to do this themselves.

When thinking about such presentations in the context of the patient being discharged home, survivors of critical illness with cognitive impairment may:

- Display problems with memory including difficulties such as remembering names, finding words and remembering items from a shopping list.
- Forget events such as doctor's appointments or social engagements
- Ramble and lose focus in conversations
- Use poor judgement
- Feel easily overwhelmed by tasks or responsibilities that used to be easy to manage
- Have problems managing money or medications and make careless errors
- Act impulsively

6Cs: Compassion

Compassionate care requires empathy, respect and dignity.

The above presentations are now well documented to be part of a plethora of other health problems including muscle weakness, cognitive or brain dysfunction and/or mental health problems, that remain after a period of critical illness, a syndrome classified as post-intensive care syndrome (PICS).

Snapshot (case study)

Bindu is a 46-year-old female. She has is currently residing on a vascular surgical ward after having undergone a left-sided carotid endarterectomy over 24 hours ago.

Airway (A): Own.
Breathing (B): unsupported. Oxygen saturations 95% on room air, respiratory rate 20 breaths, chest is clear on auscultation, speaking in full sentences.
Circulation (C): Heart rate 128 (regular), Blood pressure 160/82 mmHg, capillary refill time 3 seconds, warm peripherally.
Disability (D): V on AVPU scale. New-onset unilateral limb weakness. Body temperature is 37.4°C.
Exposure (E): Abdomen soft, does not appear tender.
NEWS2: 6.

Nursing actions:
- Registered nurse to immediately inform the medical team caring for the patient
- Registered nurse to request urgent assessment by a clinician or team with core competencies in the care of acutely ill patients
- Minimum 1 hourly observations commenced

Delirium

Delirium is an acute, reversible organic mental syndrome with disorders of attention and cognitive function, increased or decreased psychomotor activity and a disordered sleep-wake cycle. It is commonly found in the critically ill (i.e. not always in ICU) with a reported incidence of 15–80%. The term 'ICU psychosis' is old-fashioned, inaccurate and not appropriate.

Three delirium subtypes have been characterised:

1. Hyperactive – Agitated, paranoid.
2. Hypoactive – Withdrawn, quiet, paranoid.
3. Mixed – Combination of hyperactive and hypoactive

The hyperactive form is usually well recognised, and the patient may be labelled as being 'agitated'. Such patients exhibit some or all the following features:

- Continual movement (fidgeting, pulling at clothes, catheters, or tubes, moving from side to side)
- Disoriented (in at least one aspect such as who they are or where they are)
- Commands may not be followed (complex commands followed less than simple ones)
- Patients who can communicate verbally may be unintelligible or make inappropriate responses. The patient may shout or call out
- Pain is exaggerated
- Abnormal vital signs

It is worth noting that people who have schizophrenia do not have cognitive defects and tend to have auditory,

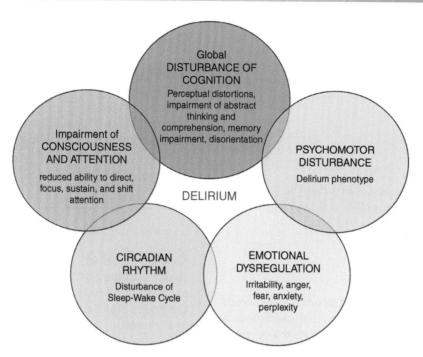

Figure 15.1 Delirium. *Source:* Maldonado (2017) with permission from John Wiley & Sons.

rather than visual hallucinations. The delirious patient may perceive the environment as hostile and try to escape, sometimes employing violence against staff or visitors.

Orange Flag: psychological sequalae of ICU delirium

ICU delirium can have profound and lasting psychological sequelae. There are multiple studies which have described the experience of ICU patients whom have suffered from delirium during their critical care stay, some of which tell a rather harrowing tale (Jones et al., 2001; Kiekkas et al., 2010; Samuelson et al., 2006; Van Rompaey, 2016).

The hypoactive form is often not well recognised and inappropriate therapy may be started if the patient is misdiagnosed as being depressed. Disorientation is common in delirium, but this is not a feature of depression. The behaviour of the delirious patient can change dramatically over hours or even minutes, giving rise to confusion amongst caregivers about the patient's actual mental state. See Figure 15.1.

Mixed delirium includes both hypoactive and hyperactive components. The patient with mixed delirium will often switch between the two presentations, which can make treatment strategies difficult.

Red Flag: new-onset delirium

Due to the plethora of potential causes, new-onset delirium requires urgent work-up. Baseline investigations should usually include full blood count (FBC), metabolic profile, fasting blood glucose, urinalysis and urine culture (Blanchard, 2020). A detailed clinical history and examination is used to rationalise further investigations and management.

Delirium is common in critical care patients and is associated with short- and long-term adverse outcomes (Bulic et al., 2020). It is important to acknowledge that delirium occurs in different healthcare settings, affecting between 15 and 20% of general hospital patients, and up to 80% of patients in a critical care unit such as ICU. Delirium has been associated with long-term disability following non-ICU hospitalisations and with poor outcomes following ICU admission including prolonged length of stay, cognitive impairment after hospital discharge, and increased odds of long-term disability in activities of living.

Clinical Investigation

Delirium can result in a prolonged period of cognitive dysfunction. For patients in whom delirium does not resolve, it is recommended that follow-up and continued assessment for possible dementia occurs (National Institute for Health and Care Excellence (NICE), 2018/2019). Clinical investigation for dementia primarily includes appropriate blood and urine tests to exclude reversible causes of cognitive decline and cognitive testing (such as 10-point cognitive screener (10-CS).

6Cs: Commitment

Being highly committed to patients helps to improve their quality of care and experience as well as that of other patients.

Risk factors

Known risk factors for developing delirium are numerous and commonly separated into factors that predispose a patient to delirium and others that precipitate the development of delirium (Table 15.1). According to Hayhurst et al. (2016), advanced age and baseline cognitive impairment have been consistently found to increase delirium risk across a variety of hospital settings. Similarly, patients with increased comorbid disease burden (especially respiratory disease) and frailty appear to be at higher risk. Thus, patients with lower cognitive and physical reserve likely possess decreased capacity to maintain normal brain functioning in response to stress (e.g., surgery, critical illness) and are, therefore, at higher risk for delirium. Similarly, a more significant systemic insult such as sepsis, prolonged mechanical ventilation, or major surgery (complex abdominal, hip fracture, and cardiac surgery), will increase risk of delirium compared to a lesser physiological insult. Increased pain levels have repeatedly been shown to increase delirium, especially in the post-operative setting, potentially due to heightened stress response and altered neurotransmission.

Risk factors for delirium are numerous and can be separated into predisposing patient factors and precipitating clinical factors.

Table 15.1 Delirium risk factors.

Predisposing factors	Precipitating factors	
Advanced age	Metabolic disturbances	Benzodiazepines
Baseline cognitive impairment	Hypotension	Opioids (meperidine, morphine)
Increased comorbid disease	Sepsis	Deep versus light sedation
Frailty	Poor pain control	Anticholinergics
Alcohol and drug abuse	Mechanical ventilation	Steroids
High severity of illness	Sleep disturbances	Surgery (abdominal, cardiac, hip)

Red Flag: Altered mental status (AMS)

AMS is a generalised term which encompasses alterations in conscious level and/or cognition. Alterations in either of these factors can be because of multiple factors, some of which can be life-threatening, therefore rapid assessment, stabilisation and subsequent investigation (may include computer tomography can of the cranium (CT head)) of the patient is required.

6Cs: Care

To demonstrate care in practice healthcare professionals, need to be considerate to a patient's beliefs, treat them with dignity, and work in accordance with their best interests.

Detection of delirium is under-recognised in the critically ill. The agitated patient is easily identified, but there are other differential diagnoses that may confuse the picture along with the fluctuating nature of the condition. An important step in the prevention of delirium in critically ill patients is the avoidance of either excessive or inadequate use of sedative and analgesic therapy. The use of validated sedation scoring systems is recommended when titrating sedative agents to the appropriate sedation level for each patient. There are three validated scoring systems that can be used in critically ill patients to monitor sedation and agitation. They are the Sedation-Agitation Scale (SAS), the Richmond Agitation-Sedation Scale (RASS) (Table 15.2) and the Motor Activity Assessment Scale (MAAS). These scales are 7-point (10 in case of RASS) scoring systems ranging from dangerously agitated to unrousable, with an aware and calm score in between. These scales go some way to identifying a patient with delirium as they can indicate several levels of agitation. A locally adopted scoring system should be used in all critically ill patients irrespective of their current sedative status. This continuous monitoring records the fluctuations in the patient's level of consciousness throughout their critical care stay. However, these scores are unable to identify all delirious patients and must be used in conjunction with specific delirium tests. Three delirium-screening tools have been validated in critically ill patients. The Intensive Care Delirium Screening Checklist (ICDSC) and the Delirium Detection Score (DDS) use an eight-feature checklist, while the Confusion Assessment Method for the Intensive Care Unit (CAM-ICU) uses a four-feature score. These tools aim to identify inattention, the single most important feature of delirium. When the CAM-ICU tool is used in conjunction with a sedation-agitation scoring system, two of the four features are already scored enabling rapid completion. This in turn increases the likelihood that the tool will be routinely accepted into clinical practice.

Examination scenario: the Richmond Agitation-Sedation Scale (RASS)

The RASS is a 10-point validated scale which is widely used within the ICU to assess patient's level of sedation. The scale is shown in Table 15.2.

Table 15.2 RASS.

Score	Description	
+4	*Combative*	Violent, immediate danger to self
+3	Very agitated	Aggressive. Pulls or removes tube(s) or catheter(s).
+2	Agitated	Frequent non-purposeful movements. May fight ventilator/ventilation.
+1	Restless	Anxious, apprehensive but movements are not aggressive or vigorous
0	Alert & calm	
−1	Drowsy	Not fully alert, but has sustained awakening tovoice (eye opening and eye contact (>10 seconds))
−2	Light sedation	Briefly awakens to voice(eye opening and eye contact (<10 seconds))
−3	Moderate sedation	Movement or eye opening to voice(no eye contact)
−4	Deep sedation	No response to voice, but movement or eyeopening to physical stimulation
−5	Unrousable	No response to voice or physical stimulation

Examination scenario: CAM-ICU

Multiple resources exist which detail the content and how to implement CAM-ICU in to clinical practice. It is beyond the scope of this chapter to cover them in detail, however, further resources can be found here: https://www.icudelirium.org/medical-professionals/delirium/monitoring-delirium-in-the-icu.

Assessment of CAM-ICU is split in to two steps:

STEP 1 – Sedation Assessment using Richmond Agitation-Sedation Scale

STEP 2 – Delirium Assessment

Step 2 is further divided in to four sub-steps/assessments:

1. Acute change of fluctuating course of mental status
2. Inattention
3. Altered level of consciousness
4. Disorganised thinking

6Cs: Competence

To provide competent care healthcare professionals must:

- Be mindful of the health and social needs of individual patients
- Possess the expertise, clinical knowledge, and technical knowledge to deliver care treatments
- Practice evidence-based care

Management of delirium

The management of delirium is an important and challenging facet of therapy when caring for critically ill patients. Delirium has recently been shown to be an independent predictor of increased mortality at 6 months and longer length of stay in ventilated intensive care patients. It is also associated with increased length of hospital stay and may predispose patients to prolonged neuropsychological disturbances after they leave intensive care.

Management of delirium within the ICU is complex and unfortunately there is no one single treatment that suits everyone. It is intensive for both ICU staff and patient's relatives and requires a multidisciplinary approach which primarily employs non-pharmacological strategies. The Pain, Agitation, Delirium, Immobility, and Sleep Disruption (PADIS) Guidelines (Devlin et al., 2018) adopts an evidence-based approach to the prevention, recognition and subsequent treatment of ICU delirium. The guidelines have been produced by world-renowned experts within the field and have since been adopted and adapted internationally.

Snapshot (case study)

Maria is a 39-year-old female of Brazilian descent. She has resided within the intensive care unit for the last 3 months following an emergency admission with COVID-19 pneumonitis. Maria was initially intubated and ventilated, but after a prolonged respiratory wean she is now self-ventilating, making good progress with her rehabilitation and was deemed ready for ward discharge on the morning ward round.

Airway (A): Own.

Breathing (B): Unsupported. Oxygen saturations 92% on room air, respiratory rate 35 breaths, chest is clear on auscultation, speaking in short sentences.

Circulation (C): Heart rate 132 (regular), Blood pressure 150/92 mmHg, capillary refill time 2 seconds, warm peripherally. Peripheral cannular in situ left hand.

Disability (D): +2 on RASS, making frequent non-purposeful movements. Blood glucose is 12.5 mmol/L, body temperature is 38.9°C.

Exposure (E): Maria had been reporting some suprapubic discomfort and irritation around her urinary catheter site earlier that day. The urine draining from her catheter now appears cloudy.

NEWS2: 8.

Nursing actions:

- Registered nurse to immediately inform the medical team caring for the patient
- Supplementary oxygen applied to maintain SpO₂ 94–98%
- Continuous monitoring of vital signs commenced
- Vascular accesses checked for patency
- Pain and delirium assessment performed
- Drug chart assessed for any recent administration of agents that may have precipitated this acute event
- Patient remains in critical care environment
- Initiation of an A-F bundle (Devlin et al., 2018) to address pain, agitation/sedation, delirium, immobility and sleep disruption whilst residing within the critical care environment

Pharmacological strategies for the treatment of ICU delirium may be required where appropriate, but there is currently little evidence to suggest a superior agent. Chapter 11 explores the pharmacological agents which may be utilised in more depth. The PADIS guidelines (Devlin et al., 2018) do not recommend the routine use of pharmacological agents to treat and/or prevent ICU delirium as there is little evidence to support their use. However, antipsychotics remain viable for short-term control of agitation (e.g., alcohol or drug withdrawal) or severe anxiety with need to avoid respiratory suppression (e.g., heart failure, COPD or asthma) (Vanderbilt University Medical Center, 2021).

Red Flag: toxidromes

Accidental or intentional poisoning from prescription drugs, illicit drugs, and/or alcohol, can cause acute changes in AMS. Rapid diagnosis is essential, and treatment will depend upon the suspected agent. A brief guide to

emergency treatment can be accessed here: https://bnf.nice.org.uk/treatment-summary/poisoning-emergency-treatment.html. More comprehensive guides can be accessed via www.toxbase.org.

Clinical investigation

The diagnosis of delirium is primarily based upon obtaining a patient history and performing a thorough clinical examination versus the use laboratory tests, or radiological investigations. However, there may be several co-existing factors causing new-onset delirium. A simple T.H.I.N.K alphabet checklist for delirium (Vanderbilt University Medical Center, 2021), a well recognised strategy internationally that focuses the healthcare professional to think about the possible underlying causes for delirium and some of the associated strategies for treatment:

T
Toxic situations:
  Congestive cardiac failure
  Shock
  Dehydration
  Deliriogenic medications
  New organ failure

H
Hypoxaemia

I
Infection
Immobilisation

N
Non-pharmacological interventions:
  Hearing aids
  Glasses
  Reorientation
  Sleep protocols
  Music (patient's choice!)
  Noise control
  Ambulation

K
K+ (potassium) or electrolyte disorders

These is a non-exhaustive list and each presenting condition requires appropriate investigation which may be supported by laboratory tests such as the measurement of inflammatory markers (white cell count, C-reactive protein and/or procalcitonin) and/or radiological studies such as computed tomography (CT) scan.

Medications management: haloperidol

A Cochrane Review suggested that the routine use of haloperidol for preventing ICU delirium is not an effective strategy. However, a large randomised, multi-centre, double-blind, placebo-controlled clinical trial is currently being conducted in Europe by Smit et al. (2020) which will analyse *Efficacy of haloperidol to decrease the burden of Delirium In adult Critically ill patients* (EuRIDICE trial). Although there is little current, quality evidence to support the use of haloperidol for prevention and/or treatment of ICU delirium, its use may still be observed in practice, therefore it is important to understand the common side effects of this agent. Haloperidol can cause QT interval prolongation which can give rise to the potentially fatal cardiac arrhythmia, Torsade de Pointes. It is important that a baseline electrocardiogram (ECG) is obtained prior to administering haloperidol, and at regular intervals during sustained use, to calculate the QT interval.

Medications management: dexmedetomidine

A Cochrane Review (Burry et al., 2019) concluded that the alpha2 agonist, dexmedetomidine, was the most effective in reducing the duration of delirium. Due to the receptor upon which this agent exerts its effect (alpha2), there are several potential side effects that need to be considered. Some of the most common side effects include (but are not limited to): hypotension, hypertension, bradycardia, atrial fibrillation and heart block, therefore the patient must be monitored closely and local practice area guidelines adhered to.

Medications management: antipsychotic and atypical/second-generation antipsychotic drugs

Antipsychotics (such as haloperidol) and atypical/second-generation antipsychotics (such as Olanzepine and Quetiapine) carry a potential risk for the prolonged QT interval, development of arrhythmias, extrapyramidal symptoms (Parkinsonism) and Neuroleptic Malignant Syndrome, particularly in the elderly population. NICE (2021) recommend the use of Screening Tool of Older Persons' potentially inappropriate Prescription (STOPP) criteria

(Gallagher et al., 2008) to aim to reduce the incidence of medicines-related adverse events from potentially inappropriate prescribing and polypharmacy. These are evidence-based criteria which can be found under the 'cautions' section of each drug within the British National Formulary: https://bnf.nice.org.uk/.

Source: Based on NICE.

Sleep

Dabrowska et al. (2018) identifies that sleep is indispensable for the regeneration of both body and mind. Nocturnal rest leads to the turning down of the nervous system and the regeneration of muscles, and results in physiological rest. Such regeneration is not observed in patients suffering from sleep disorders, which results in patients experiencing cognitive deficits and physical fatigue. Sleep disturbances in intensive care unit (ICU) patients have been studied worldwide for over 30 years. Factors contributing to sleep disturbances are still being identified, and therapeutic procedures aimed at the mitigation of such ailments are consequently being developed. What has been identified to date is that nocturnal rest of ICU patients is influenced by noise, pain experienced, discomfort, medication administered in the intensive care setting and the mode of mechanical ventilation. Sleep assessment is subjective in its nature; therefore, it is hard to perform in the ICU setting. As communication with a patient may be impeded, they are not able to provide clear information on their perceived rest and the most disturbing factors. Therefore, nocturnal rest is an issue commonly forgotten and frequently overlooked by healthcare professionals.

Assessment of sleep in ICU

The assessment of sleep in ICU patients has been performed using subjective and objective tools. Subjective tools include the Richard Campbell Sleep Questionnaire, self-reported sleep quality by patients and nurse, or clinician observations. These subjective tools, while they are simpler to use, are not reliable and can over- or underestimate the sleep quality and duration. Actigrapy, Bispectral Index (BIS) and polysomnography are the current available objective tools to measure sleep in critically ill patients. Polysomnography is gold standard. However, using polysomnography in ICU is fraught with challenges, including the skill, time and resources to apply the instrumentation, capture and analyse the data. The traditional polysomnography scoring systems used in sleep study reporting has been noted to be not as reliable in assessing sleep stages in patients who are in intensive care as compared to the non-ICU population due to the difficulties in voltage gain on signals and the influence of drugs such as benzodiazepines on electroencephalogram (EEG) signals. There is also compelling data to show that brain-derived neurotrophic factor (BDNF) is a blood biomarker of slow-wave sleep. Such novel biomarkers

193

may help in conjunction with polysomnography in assessing sleep quality in critically ill patients.

Reddy et al. (2020) identifies that regulation of sleep is processed by the homeostatic physiology of the circadian rhythm, also known as the sleep/wake cycle. Circadian rhythm is the 24-hour internal clock in the human brain that regulates cycles of alertness and sleepiness by responding to light changes in our environment. Human physiology and behaviour are shaped by the Earth's rotation around its axis. This biological circadian system has evolved to help humans adapt to changes in their environment and anticipate changes in radiation, temperature and food availability. Without this endogenous circadian clock, Homo sapiens would not be able to optimise energy expenditure and the internal physiology of the body.

Sleep quality in critical care settings is influenced by patient-related factors such as pain, stress, psychosis, circadian rhythm disturbances and organ dysfunction as well as critical care environmental-related factors such as ambient noise, alarms from monitoring devices, lighting, patient care activities, monitoring, diagnostic and therapeutic procedures. While the exact causal relation between sleep deprivation and adverse outcomes were not shown in critically ill patients, inadequate sleep was shown to be associated with mood changes including anxiety, depression, psychosis and delirium; a reduced pain threshold; impaired immunity; hormonal imbalances; and an impairment of inspiratory muscle endurance. Furthermore, a strong association between sleep disruption and mortality was proposed. While the clinical studies thus far have not shown a direct causal relation between sleep and mortality in critically ill patients, sleep deprivation was shown to increase mortality in the mice model of sepsis.

Factors related to patient and environment were implicated in poor sleep quality in ICU studies. Of these factors, environmental factors account to only 30% of arousals and awakenings. Indeed, when healthy volunteers were studied with polysomnography in an ICU, the quality of sleep appears to have been well preserved irrespective of the sound and light disturbance that are routinely noted in ICUs.

Management of sleep within the ICU can be challenging due to mitigation of noise and light disturbances. The use of music, scheduling of patients care activities, tapering of sedative drugs and daytime mobilisation have all been proposed as methods to aid the restoration of circadian rhythm (Reade and Liu, 2018).

Traditional pharmacological agents often used to promote sleep within the ICU include 'z drugs' such as Zopiclone, however these may be associated with increased incidences of delirium, particularly in the elderly population, and should be avoided. A review by Reade and Liu (2018) details a useful synopsis of the current evidence in this area and promotes the long-standing view of ICU professionals that 'sedation is a poor substitute for sleep'.

Medications management: melatonin

Melatonin, a naturally occurring 'sleep' hormone, that may also be administered as a medicinal agent (exogenous administration), has been the subject of a Cochrane Review and ongoing trials, the results of which are awaited (ClinicalTrials.gov, 2021). The review concluded that there is 'insufficient evidence to determine whether administration of melatonin would improve the quality and quantity of sleep in ICU patients'. However, there is no robust data for serious side effects (Tiruviopati et al., 2019) and so its use may be observed within the ICU. It is important to note that the timing and environmental factors prior to administration are important to promote the efficacy of the drug, such as:

1. Patient's dose to be taken 1–2 hours before bedtime.
2. Exposure to room light before bedtime room, light exerts a profound suppressive effect on melatonin levels and shortens the body's internal representation of night duration (Gooley et al., 2010), which can also have a negative effect upon exogenous administration (Emens and Burgess, 2015).

Snapshot (case study)

Princess is a 52-year-old female of Nigerian descent. She has recently been admitted to the high dependency unit (HDU) after undergoing an elective repair of an abdominal aortic aneurysm under general anaesthetic (GA) 1 day ago. She had reported having very little sleep during her first night on HDU.

Airway (A): Own

Breathing (B): unsupported. Oxygen saturations 88% on room air, respiratory rate 27 breaths, chest is clear on auscultation, speaking in short sentences

Circulation (C): Heart rate 110 (regular), Blood pressure 160/87 mmHg, capillary refill time 3 seconds, warm peripherally.

Disability (D): +1 on RASS, appears anxious and apprehensive but movements are not aggressive or vigorous. Blood glucose is 8 mmol/L, body temperature is 36.8°C

Exposure (E): Maria had been reporting some discomfort across her incision site. Her current pain score is reported as 10/10.

NEWS2: 10

- Registered nurse to immediately inform the medical team caring for the patient
- Supplementary oxygen applied to maintain SpO$_2$ 94–98%
- Continuous monitoring of vital signs commenced

- Pain and delirium assessment performed, and pain relief administered as indicated
- Drug chart assessed for any recent administration of agents that may have precipitated this acute event
- Initiation of an A-F bundle (Devlin et al., 2018) to address pain, agitation/sedation, delirium, immobility, and sleep disruption whilst residing within the critical care environment

Conclusion

As a student health care practitioner working with critically ill patients, you will undoubtedly be involved in the care of several patients with neurocognitive disorders, including ICU delirium. These disorders can be very complex and have the potential to have detrimental effects on a patient's chance of survival to hospital discharge. The causes of neurocognitive disorders can be multifactorial and often are interlinked with other comorbidities such as neurological and cardiovascular disease. The incidence of ICU delirium continues to be high despite multiple research and health improvement initiatives. As such, it is crucial that the healthcare professionals involved in supporting this patient group manage ICU delirium and potential PICS have a sound understanding of the causative factors, pharmacological and evidence base that underpins the promotion of safe and effective care.

Take home points

1. The incidence of neurocognitive impairment within the critical care population is high.
2. The neurocognitive sequelae of an intensive care admission can be extensive and can often impact upon a patient's quality of life long after ICU discharge.
3. Management of ICU delirium is not reliant on a 'magic bullet' and requires a multi-faceted and multidisciplinary approach.
4. The initiation of evidence-based pain, agitation/sedation, delirium, immobility, and sleep (PADIS) guidelines can aid in improving patient outcomes.

References

Blanchard, G. (2020). Assessment of altered mental status. BMJ Best Practice topics. https://bestpractice.bmj.com/topics/en-gb/843 (accessed 1 March 2021).

Burry, L., Hutton, B., Mehta, S. et al. (2019). Pharmacological interventions for the treatment of delirium in critically ill adults (Review). Cochrane Database of Systematic Reviews. doi: 10.1002/14651858.CD011749.pub2.

Bulic, D., Bennett, M., Georgousopoulou, E.N. et al. Cognitive and psychosocial outcomes of mechanically ventilated intensive care patients with and without delirium. Ann. Intensive Care 10, 104 (2020). doi: 10.1186/s13613-020-00723-2

Devlin, J.W., Skrobik, Y., Gélinas, C. et al. (2018). Clinical practice guidelines for the prevention and management of pain, agitation/sedation, delirium, immobility, and sleep disruption in adult patients in the ICU. Crit Care Med 46(9): e825–e873. doi: 10.1097/CCM.0000000000003299.

Emens, J.S. and Burgess, H.J. (2015) Effect of light and melatonin and other melatonin receptor agonists on human circadian physiology. Sleep Med Clin 10(4): 435–453. doi:10.1016/j.jsmc.2015.08.001.

Gallagher, P. and O'Mahony, D. (2008) STOPP (Screening Tool of Older Persons' potentially inappropriate Prescriptions): application to acutely ill elderly patients and comparison with Beers' criteria, Age and Ageing 37(6): 673–679. doi: 10.1093/ageing/afn197.

Gooley, J.J., Chamberlain, K., Smith, K.A. et al. (2011). Exposure to room light before bedtime suppresses melatonin onset and shortens melatonin duration in humans. J Clin Endocrinol Metab 96(3): E463–E472. doi:10.1210/jc.2010-2098.

Hayhurst, C.J., Pandharipande, P.P., and Hughes, C.G. (2016). Intensive care unit delirium: a review of diagnosis, prevention, and treatment. Anaesthesiology 125(6): 1229–1241. doi: 10.1097/ALN.0000000000001378

Jones, C., Griffiths, R.D., Humphris, G. et al. (2001). Memory, delusions, and the development of acute posttraumatic stress disorder-related symptoms after intensive care. Crit Care 29: 573–580.

Kiekkas, P., Theodorakopoulou, G., Spyratos, F., and Baltopoulos, G. (2010). Psychological distress and delusional memories after critical care: a literature review. Int Nurs Rev 57: 288–296.

Medrzycka-Dabrowska, W., Lewandowska, K., Kwiecień-Jaguś, K., and Czyż-Szypenbajl, K. (2018). Sleep Deprivation in Intensive Care Unit – Systematic Review. Open Medicine (Warsaw, Poland) 13: 384–393. doi: 10.1515/med-2018-0057

National Institute for Health and Care Excellence (2018). Dementia: assessment, management and support for people living with dementia and their carers. NICE guideline [NG97]. https://www.nice.org.uk/guidance/ng97/chapter/Recommendations#diagnosis (accessed 1 March 2021).

National Institute for Health and Care Excellence (2019). Delirium: prevention, diagnosis and management. Clinical guideline [CG103]. https://www.nice.org.uk/guidance/cg103/chapter/1-Guidance#ftn.footnote_6 (accessed 1 March 2021).

National Institute for Health and Care Excellence (2012). Prescribing in the elderly. https://bnf.nice.org.uk/guidance/prescribing-in-the-elderly.html (accessed 1 March 2021).

NIDUS (2018). Long-term cognitive impairment after ICU delirium: Common but under-recognized. https://deliriumnetwork.org/ltci-icu-delirium-blog/#:~:text=About%2030%2D80%25%20of%20ICU,severe%20sepsis%2C%20and%20acute%20dialysis (accessed 30 March 2021).

Reade, M. and Liu, D. (2018). Optimising sleep in the ICU. ICU Management & Practice 18(3). https://healthmanagement.org/c/icu/issuearticle/optimising-sleep-in-the-icu (accessed 1 March 2021).

Reddy, S., Reddy, V., and Sharma S. (2021). Physiology, circadian rhythm. In: StatPearls. Treasure Island (FL), StatPearls Publishing. https://www.ncbi.nlm.nih.gov/books/NBK519507/.

Samuelson, K., Lundberg, D., and Fridlund, B. (2006). Memory in relation to depth of sedation in adult mechanically ventilated intensive care patients. Intensive Care Med 32:660–667.

Smit, L., Trogrlić, Z., Devlin, J.W. on behalf of the EuRIDICE study group et al. (2020). Efficacy of halopeRIdol to decrease the burden of Delirium In adult Critically ill patiEnts (EuRIDICE): study protocol for a prospective randomised multi-centre double-blind placebo-controlled clinical trial in the Netherlands. BMJ Open 10: e036735. doi: 10.1136/bmjopen-2019-036735.

Tiruvoipati, R., Mulder, J., and Haji K. (2020). Improving sleep in intensive care unit: An overview of diagnostic and therapeutic options. *Journal of Patient Experience*. 697–702. doi:10.1177/2374373519882234

Turon, M., Fernandez-Gonzalo, S., Gomez-Simon, V. et al. (2013). Cognitive stimulation in ICU patients: should we pay more attention? *Crit Care* 17: 158. doi: 10.1186/cc12719

Vanderbilt University Medical Center (2021). Terminology and mnemonics. https://www.icudelirium.org/medical-professionals/terminology-mnemonics (accessed 1 March 2021).

Van Rompaey, B., Van Hoof, A., van Bogaert, P. et al. (2016). The patient's perception of a delirium: a qualitative research in a Belgian intensive care unit. *Intensive Crit Care Nurs* 32: 66–74. https://www.sciencedirect.com/science/article/pii/S096433971500021X?via%3Dihub (accessed 2 March 2022).

Chapter 16

Respiratory care: intubation and mechanical ventilation

Barry Hill and Lorraine Mutrie

Aim

The aim of this chapter is to provide the reader with an evidence-based understanding of contemporary respiratory care requirements for patients who are cared for in critical care settings.

Learning outcomes

After reading this chapter the reader will be able to:

- Demonstrate knowledge of respiratory care in the context of mechanical ventilation.
- Understand the different types of respiratory failure and the differences between them.
- Be introduced to the principles of intubation.
- Understand fundamental mechanical ventilation principles, ventilator modes, ventilator settings, risks of artificial ventilation, and weaning principles.
- Explore and develop knowledge for underpinning evidence base principles of mechanical ventilation using national guidelines and care bundles.

Test your prior knowledge

- Explain the two types of respiratory failure.
- What is meant by the term 'hypoventilation'?
- What is the difference between volume control and pressure control ventilation?
- What interventions can be used to prevent ventilator-associated pneumonia (VAP)?
- What is the difference between an endotracheal tube (ETT) and a tracheostomy?

Fundamentals of Critical Care: A Textbook for Nursing and Healthcare Students, First Edition. Edited by Ian Peate and Barry Hill.
© 2023 John Wiley & Sons Ltd. Published 2023 by John Wiley & Sons Ltd.
Companion website: www.wiley.com/go/peate/criticalcare

Introduction

Ventilation is the process by which gases move in and out of the lungs (Woodrow, 2019), during normal breathing we inhale room air that is oxygen (O_2)-rich and exhale the waste product carbon dioxide (CO_2). In critically unwell patients, self-ventilation may become inadequate and artificial ventilation may be required to either increase O_2 levels, decrease CO_2 levels or both. There are many conditions that lead to a patient requiring artificial ventilation and they include respiratory distress, neurological dysfunction and haemodynamic dysfunction, along with elective ventilation to provide therapy (for example repeated returns to theatre for surgery). The most common reasons for artificial ventilation in critical care include respiratory failure (covered in more detail in this chapter), and neurological distress causing loss of consciousness, the use of recreational drugs, sedatives, opioid medications, head injury and neurological disorders. Artificial ventilation can take the form of non- invasive ventilation (NIV) or invasive mechanical ventilation (IMV).

Invasive mechanical ventilation requires intubation and may be prescribed for patients who cannot maintain adequate oxygenation or ventilation or who need airway protection. The goal of IMV is to improve oxygenation and ventilation and to rest fatigued respiratory muscles. Mechanical ventilation is supportive therapy because it does not treat the causes of the illness and associated complications. However, ventilator support can buy time for other therapeutic interventions to work and allow the body to re-establish homeostasis. When using this life-saving intervention, clinicians should take steps to avoid or minimise risks and complications (for example ventilator induced lung injury (VILI)), which will be discussed in detail later.

Step 2 competencies: national standards

2:1.1 Function of the respiratory system
2:1.2 Assessment of the respiratory system and arterial blood gas analysis
2:1.3 Understanding of Non-invasive and invasive ventilation
2:1.4 Intubation for ventilation
2:1.5 Principles of invasive ventilation
2:1.7 Tracheostomy insertion
2:5.3 Medications for intubation

Medicines management: oxygen

Oxygen is a drug that can be administered in different concentrations and at different flow rates depending on patient need. It should be administered by trained staff, with reference to a target saturation (O'Driscoll, 2017). It is essential to interpret the observations of a critically ill patient in the context of their oxygen therapy; it is often easy to overlook the significance of this therapy when observations appear normal. When documenting oxygen therapy, care should be taken to ensure consistency between recording concentration as a percentage (i.e. 65%) or as a fraction (FiO_2 0.65).

Medicines management: ranitidine

Ranitidine is a specific histamine H_2 antagonist. It reduces the secretion of gastric acid with the aim of reducing the risk of stress ulcers and therefore gastro-intestinal bleeding in mechanically ventilated patients.

Respiratory failure

Respiratory function relies on gas exchange in the lungs, and this is determined by three factors (Woodrow, 2019):

1. Ventilation (V): breath size
2. Perfusion (Q): pulmonary blood flow
3. Diffusion: movement of gases across the tissue between pulmonary blood and alveolar air.

Inadequate gas exchange can lead to respiratory failure. There are two types of respiratory failure (O'Driscoll et al., 2017, for the British Thoracic Society):

- Type 1: oxygenation failure – hypoxia (PaO_2 <8 kPa) with normocapnia (normal $PCaO_2$ 4–6 kPa) or hypocapnia (low CO_2 because of increased respiratory rate)
- Type 2: ventilatory failure – hypoxia (PaO_2 <8 kPa) with hypercapnia ($PaCO_2$ >6 kPa).

See Figure 16.1.

The main pathophysiological mechanisms of respiratory failure are hypoventilation and ventilation/perfusion (V/Q) mismatch (Shebl and Burns, 2019):

Hypoventilation

Hypoventilation is a condition that arises when air entering the alveoli is reduced. This causes levels of oxygen (O_2) to decrease and the levels of carbon dioxide (CO_2) to increase. Hypoventilation may occur when breathing is too slow or shallow and is usually a consequence of other medical conditions such as neuromuscular disorders, head injury, chest wall abnormalities, obesity hypoventilation, and chronic obstructive pulmonary disease (Fayyaz and Lessnau,

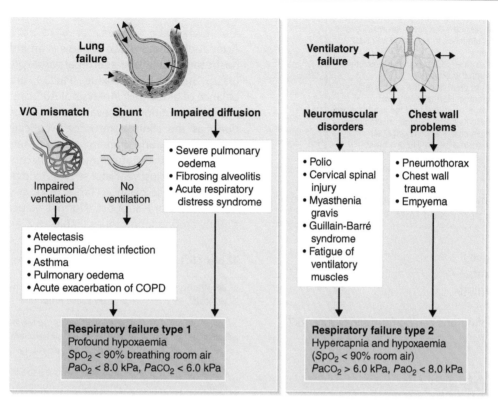

Figure 16.1 Respiratory failure and gas exchange. *Source:* Dutton and Finch (2018) with permission from John Wiley & Sons.

2018). It can also be caused by medications, such as sedatives, opioid-based analgesia and substances that depress brain function, for example alcohol and recreational drugs.

Hypoventilation leads to an abnormal retention of CO_2 in the blood due to poor gas exchange within the lungs. There can be a variety of underlying reasons for the poor exchange of CO_2, which results in higher CO_2 volumes in the bloodstream (hypercapnia), which then displaces and lowers the volume of O_2 carried in the blood (hypoxaemia) (Woodrow, 2019). The abnormal retention of CO_2 in the bloodstream is significant because it can lead to respiratory acidosis, whereby the pH level of the blood is raised making it too acidic. Consequently, cellular respiration is disrupted, and, in extreme cases, this will lead to type 2 respiratory failure (O'Driscoll et al., 2017).

Ventilation/perfusion (V/Q) mismatch

V/Q mismatch is the most common cause of hypoxaemia.

Shunt

Shunt or pulmonary shunt is one of the two contributors to V/Q mismatch (Woodrow, 2019). Generally, pulmonary shunt can occur in two ways: anatomical shunt and capillary shunt. Anatomical shunt happens when arterial blood returns to the pulmonary veins without passing through the pulmonary capillaries. A capillary shunt occurs when the blood passes through the capillaries of alveoli that are not ventilated

(Whitten, 2017). This poorly oxygenated blood subsequently returns to the heart, where it mixes with blood that has been oxygenated in well-ventilated areas of the lungs. Simply put, shunt is perfusion without ventilation.

Dead space

Dead space, total dead space or physiological dead space is the second contributor to V/Q mismatch (Woodrow, 2019). Generally, it has two components: anatomical dead space and alveolar dead space. Typically, anatomical dead space is the portion of the air that remains in the conducting airways where no gas exchange is possible. In comparison, alveolar dead space is the condition that results when the alveoli of the lungs have adequate ventilation and inadequate perfusion (Whitten, 2017). Simply put, dead space is ventilation without perfusion.

Work of breathing

Work of Breathing (WOB) is the amount of effort used to expand the lungs and the energy expended during breathing. It is determined by lung and thoracic compliance, airway resistance, and the use of accessory muscles for inspiration or forced expiration. In respiratory physiology, work of breathing = pressure × volume (WOB = P × V). There are five main factors that increase WOB, including.

- Lung and chest elasticity
- Lung compliance

- Compliance – the ease with which the lung stretches to accommodate tidal volume
- Resistance – the resistance to air flow through the airways
- Work of breathing – the energy required to breathe. Normally very low!
- Elasticity – the ability of the lung to recoil back to its normal shape on exhalation
- Tidal volume – the amount of air moving into the lung in one breath
- Minute ventilation = tidal volume × respiratory rate

Figure 16.2 Some useful definitions. *Source:* Dutton and Finch (2018) with permission from John Wiley & Sons.

- Airway resistance
- Rate of breathing
- Depth of breathing.

Some useful definitions can be found in Figure 16.2.

Snapshot 1

Zoe, a 23-year-old has been admitted to critical care with a reduced conscious level. Her friend has told you that they were at a party and that Zoe accepted a 'pill' from another person at the party. You record the following observations for Zoe:

Airway (A): Airway is patent. The patient can speak, but it is mumbled words.

Breathing (B): Oxygen saturations 89% (NEWS2 = 3), oxygen therapy 5 L/min O2 via simple face mask (NEWS2 = 2). Respiratory rate 10 breaths per minute (NEWS2 = 1).

Circulation (C): Blood pressure 115/65 mmHg (NEWS2 = 0), heart rate 96 beats per minute (NEWS2 = 1), capillary refill time 4 seconds, and she is cool to touch.

Disability (D): Patient is drowsy but respond to Verbal command on the ACVPU scale when you talk loudly to her (NEWS2 = 3). Body temperature is 36.2°C (NEWS2 = 0).

Exposure (E): no abnormal findings.

Total NEWS2 score: 10

Diagnosis:

Respiratory depression and reduced consciousness likely due to recreational drug use.

Nursing actions:

- Perform more detailed assessment of consciousness (GCS).
- Monitor airway.
- Consider arterial blood gas analysis and review oxygen therapy.
- Send urine sample for toxicology screen.

Arterial blood gases (ABGs)

Arterial blood gas (ABG) analysis is an indispensable diagnostic tool that measures arterial partial pressures of oxygen (PaO_2) and carbon dioxide ($PaCO_2$), and the acid/base balance of blood (pH). Analysis of ABG can help monitor the patient's condition and evaluate the response to interventions, as the clinical status of a critically ill patient can change rapidly and dramatically. By reviewing the patient's ABGs and clinical status, practitioners can use their clinical reasoning to adjust ventilator settings to improve oxygenation, blood acid-base balance (Table 16.1), or wean the patient from ventilatory support. Normal values for ABGs vary slightly among laboratories (Table 16.2, and Figure 16.3):

Table 16.1 The meaning of the ABG result.

Respiratory acidosis	Blood acid levels are too high, and the primary cause is from the respiratory system.
Metabolic acidosis	Blood acid levels are too high, and the primary cause is elsewhere in the body, not related to the respiratory system.
Respiratory alkalosis	Blood acid levels are too low, and the primary cause is from the respiratory system.
Metabolic alkalosis	Blood acid levels are too low, and the primary cause is elsewhere in the body, not related to the respiratory system.
Partial compensation	Blood acid levels are still abnormal, but the body has used compensatory buffer system to try to return them back to normal. See pathophysiology of the body's buffer system in Box 16.1.
Full compensation	The body has used its compensatory buffer systems to return the acid levels to normal.

Table 16.2 Normal arterial blood gas values.

pH: 7.35–7.45
PCO_2: 4.6–6.1 kPa,
PCO_2: 11.0–14.6 kPa.
HCO_3 22–28 mmol/l
Base −2–+2

Box 16.1   Physiology of the body's buffer system.

Carbon dioxide plays a remarkable role in the human body mainly through pH regulation of the blood. The pH is the primary stimulus to initiate ventilation. In its normal state, the body maintains CO_2 in a well controlled range of 4.6–6.1 kPa by balancing its production and elimination. In a state of hypoventilation, the body produces more CO_2 than it can eliminate, causing a net retention of CO_2. The increased CO_2 is what leads to an increase in hydrogen ions and a slight increase in bicarbonate, as seen by a

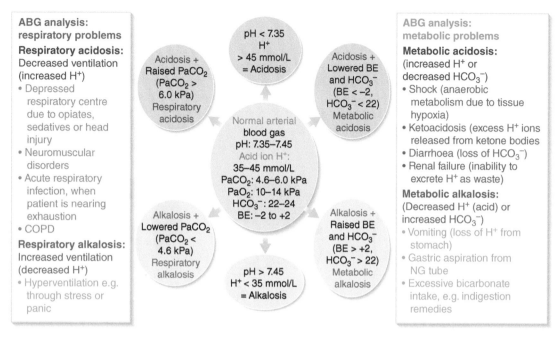

Figure 16.3 Problem identification using article blood gas analysis. *Source:* Dutton and Finch (2018) with permission from John Wiley & Sons.

right shift in the following equilibrium reaction of carbon dioxide:

$$CO_2 + H_2O \rightarrow H_2CO_3 \rightarrow HCO_3^- + H^+$$

The buffer system created by carbon dioxide consists of the following three molecules in equilibrium: CO_2, $H_2CO_3^-$, and HCO_3^-. When H^+ is high, HCO_3^- buffers the low pH. When OH^- is high, H_2CO_3 buffers the high pH. In respiratory acidosis, the slight increase in bicarbonate serves as a buffer for the increase in H^+ ions, which helps minimise the drop in pH. The increase in hydrogen ions inevitably causes a decrease in pH, which is the mechanism behind respiratory acidosis.

6Cs: Commitment

Learning new skills demonstrates your commitment, an example is blood gas analysis.

Clinical investigation 1

Arterial blood gases (ABG) can aid diagnosis (Figure 16.4) and help guide management of the patient, but they should only be carried out when there is an indication for them and not as a routine. It is recommended that you wait at least 20 minutes before taking an ABG if there have been changes to therapy (suction, changes to oxygen settings or ventilation, or significant positional changes) unless urgently required (Hennessey and Japp, 2016).

PaO_2: 10–13.5 kPa	Normal range
PaO_2: 8.0–10 kPa	Hypoxaemia probably due to VQ mismatch. Supplemental oxygen may be required. Check target oxygen saturations
$PaO_2 < 8.0$ kPa	Respiratory failure (profound hypoxaemia)
$PaCO_2 =$ 4.6–6.0 kPa	Normal range
$PaCO_2 < 4.6$ kPa	Hyperventilation (maybe due to hypoxemia). Increased minute ventilation has reduced partial pressure of CO_2 in arterial blood
$PaCO_2 > 6.0$ kPa	Hypoventilation: failure to maintain adequate minute ventilation
pH 7.35–7.45	Normal range
pH < 7.35	May be caused by increased CO_2 levels. Hypoventilation (respiratory acidosis)
pH > 7.45	May be caused by reduced level of CO_2. Hyperventilation (respiratory alkalosis)
HCO_3^- (bicarbonate) 22–26 mmol/L	Normal range
$HCO_3^- > 24$	Retention of bicarbonate by the kidneys probably due to chronically raised carbon dioxide in disorders such as COPD. The increased bicarbonate increases buffering, keeping the pH near normal range, despite a raised $PaCO_2$.

Figure 16.4 ABG analysis. *Source:* Dutton and Finch (2018) with permission from John Wiley & Sons.

Non-invasive ventilation (NIV)

Non-invasive ventilation provides respiratory support without the need to intubate a patient. It is a therapy that is used to treat acute hypercapnic respiratory failure and indications for use include reversible causes of hypercapnia (for example, pneumonia). NIV can be given as a treatment option to patients who have long-term conditions, patients who are receiving palliative care and patients at end of their life, when NIV can provide quality of life outcomes (Davidson et al., 2016). Oxygen and air are delivered with positive pressure at different points in the respiratory cycle via a mask that is fitted tightly to the patient's face, mimicking the inspiration and expiration phases of normal breathing (Figure 16.5).

The pressure that is provided during the inspiratory phase of breathing increases the volume of gas that the patient inhales and can increase the number of alveoli that have gas in them (recruitment), and the pressure that is provided during the expiratory phase of breathing prevents the alveoli from collapsing at the end of the patient's exhalation. This can therefore improve tidal volumes (the volume of air that moves in and out of the lungs during inspiration and expiration), increase functional residual capacity (FRC) (the volume of gas remaining in

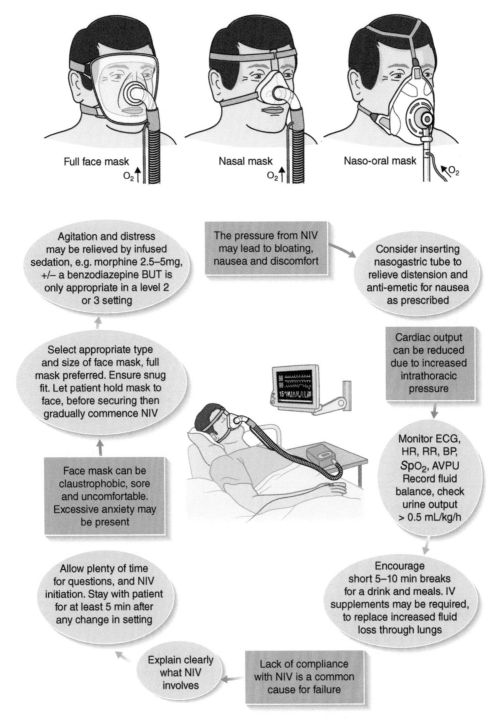

Figure 16.5 Mask options for CPAP and BIPAP; meeting the needs of the patient requiring NIV. *Source:* Dutton and Finch (2018) with permission from John Wiley & Sons.

the lung at the end of expiration) and reduce work of breathing. Practically, improving tidal volume can help to increase O_2 and reduce CO_2, increasing functional residual capacity supports diffusion of gases and work of breathing is reduced because less effort is required for the next breath in when the alveoli have residual air in them. Manufacturer trademarks mean that this two-level approach to pressure support has many names in practice, including BIPAP and IPAP/EPAP.

Non-invasive ventilation can completely control all the patients' breathing by delivering the number of breaths per minute that is set on the machine. This can be used when a patient is making minimal respiratory effort, but the patient must be able to protect their own airway. NIV can be used to support the patients' spontaneous effort of breathing by providing pressure in response to the patient starting to inhale themselves. This is referred to as pressure support and is often used with a safety back-up rate programmed into the ventilator so that if spontaneous effort reduces or ceases, the ventilator will provide those breaths. NIV can also provide a combination of both, which means that the patient will receive a mandatory number of breaths that are controlled by the ventilator, but those additional spontaneous breaths will also be supported.

The tight-fitting face masks that are used for NIV can be very uncomfortable for patients. This, along with the pressures that are blowing against their face with the aim of reaching the lung can make it difficult for a patient to tolerate this treatment. Providing clear explanations about this treatment is essential so that patients understand the importance of not removing the mask. By removing the mask, the work of recruiting the alveoli can be reversed. NIV can be delivered using a ventilator that is specifically designed for that purpose, or via a mechanical ventilator that can be used for invasive ventilation. Machines that are specifically designed for NIV have features built in that can help a patient to tolerate this therapy. They include:

1. Leak compensation: They can overcome the effects of air leaking from the face mask. This means that masks do not need to be overtightened. Overtightening of face masks is a common user error that can lead to pressure damage on the face, particularly the bridge of the nose when using a naso-oral mask (Davidson et al., 2016).
2. Rise time: Manipulating the time it takes the ventilator to reach the inspiratory (highest set) pressure can increase comfort for the patient.
3. Ramp time: The time it takes from applying the NIV to reaching the target inspiratory pressure. A gradual increase over 10–30 minutes can help the patient get used to the pressure and therefore improve tolerance (Dutton and Finch, 2018).

Treating patients with NIV can reduce the need for invasive mechanical ventilation, reduce length of hospital stay and reduce mortality. However, when NIV is commenced there should be a clear plan of ongoing care in place that has been developed with the patient. If NIV fails to improve the patient's condition, rapid escalation to emergency intubation might be needed and the decision to proceed to this intervention should be made in advance.

Snapshot 2

Andrew, a 55-year-old patient, was admitted to hospital with a community-acquired pneumonia. He has been cared for on critical care as a level 2 patient for two days, receiving non-invasive ventilation (NIV). Andrew is now reporting that he is tired, and that he is finding it harder to breathe. He complains of feeling pain in his chest that worsens when he is coughing, for which he is needing to remove his NIV mask regularly. The nurse performs an A–E assessment of the patient. For this patient, it is unlikely that a NEWS2 scoring system would be used as care has already been escalated to a level of higher dependency with increased observation, and the interventions that the patient is receiving are not addressed within this scoring system. Instead, the registered nurse would document observations and infusions on the critical care specific observations chart or e-record.

Airway (A): Patient is maintaining his own airway.

Breathing (B): Oxygen saturations 93%, respiratory rate 28 (ventilator set to deliver 12 breaths and patient adding 16 of his own). Non-invasive ventilator delivering pressure during inspiration and expiration to maintain an adequate tidal volume and positive end-expiratory pressure. The settings used are noted to be high and have increased throughout the day. Oxygen therapy via the ventilator is 65%. There is reduced air entry at his right base on chest auscultation.

Circulation (C): Blood pressure 138/ 65 mmHg, heart rate 98 beats per minute, capillary refill time 3 seconds. Patient is cool to touch. Intravenous fluid therapy at 80 mL/hr.

Disability (D): Patient is Alert on the ACVPU scale. Body temperature 37.4°C. Catheterised with urine output >0.5 mL/kg/hr. Copious amounts of green sputum noted to be in sputum pot.

Exposure (E): No abnormal findings.

Differential diagnosis:
- Worsening pneumonia
- Muscular pain affecting ability to breathe
- Sepsis
- Treatment ineffective because of regular removal of mask

Nursing actions:
- Communicate with the patient about what is happening
- Draw an ABG for blood gas analysis
- Consider change to ventilator settings to reduce work of breathing in line with critical care protocols and scope of practice
- Refer to medical team to review patient to consider intubation and ventilation

Continuous positive airway pressure (CPAP)

Continuous positive airway pressure (CPAP) is often referred to when discussing NIV, although it is different because it is indicated for the treatment of hypoxaemia. CPAP provides one continuous pressure to the airway throughout the whole of the respiratory cycle. Because it only uses one pressure, it is not able to mimic the inspiration and expiration of normal breathing. The pressure that is delivered is normally like the lower expiratory pressure of NIV. Although the pressure is being applied continuously its main action is when the patient is exhaling, by preventing the alveoli from collapsing at the end of exhalation. This increases FRC, thus improving PaO_2, and reduces the work of breathing.

The same machines and mask interfaces are usually used to deliver CPAP, and many of the complications of positive pressure ventilation (covered later in this chapter) are applicable to CPAP. However, a key difference is that the patient must be breathing spontaneously to receive CPAP because there is no inspiratory pressure set.

Learning event

Providing respiratory support using one pressure (CPAP, HFNC) will affect one gas. That one gas will be PO_2. This means that it will be useful in the treatment of Type 1 respiratory failure.

Providing respiratory support using two pressures (NIV) will affect two gases: PO_2 and CO_2. Therefore, this will be useful for Type 2 respiratory failure.

Intubation

Patients that require invasive ventilation will need to have an artificial airway, usually an endotracheal tube (ETT). An ETT is a flexible plastic tube that is inserted from the upper to the lower airway through the mouth or nose (Figure 16.6). The tube is placed to sit above the carina in the trachea so that both lungs can be ventilated. In special circumstances a specially designed tube can be placed further into the lungs, down one of the main bronchi and this would allow for only one lung ventilation. The process of placing the ETT tube is known as intubation. Critically unwell patients are normally so unwell that this procedure is carried out under urgent or emergency circumstances, making it a high-risk procedure. This procedure is usually undertaken at the patient's bedside in the critical care unit, but some patients may arrive to the department already intubated (from the emergency department, ward, or theatre).

Intubation in an emergency situation requires a distinctly different approach to when patients are intubated electively or as a routine approach to surgery, and this approach is called Rapid Sequence Induction (RSI). Approaches to RSI can vary depending on the person leading the procedure, but it includes the

Examination

When initiating any respiratory support, a Look, Listen, Feel approach should be used to assess its effectiveness:

- Look – at the patient's respiratory pattern and effort; ventilator observations and graphs; saturation levels
- Listen – to the patient's chest (auscultation)
- Feel – for equal chest expansion

High flow nasal oxygen

The use of high flow nasal cannula (HFNC) is more prevalent in practice, and offers an alternative to CPAP, as CPAP is associated with the same discomfort as NIV. HFNC can provide flows of oxygen up to 60 L/min and the high flow creates a resistance to exhalation. This creates a similar effect to CPAP by keeping the alveoli open to improve oxygenation (Dutton and Finch, 2018). Unlike CPAP, emerging evidence for HFNC indicates that if used early, it can reduce progression to hypercapnia and therefore reduce the need for NIV and if used after extubation from IMV, it can reduce the need for reintubation.

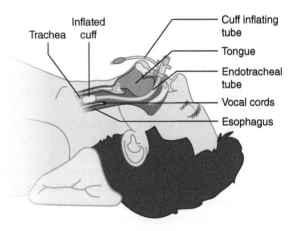

Figure 16.6   Cuffed endotracheal tube.

process of securing an airway whilst minimising time without ventilation and reducing the risk of aspiration of gastric contents by moving quickly between the phases of administering sedative medications, administering muscle relaxants, and inserting the ETT (see Chapter 12 for further information about gastric aspiration and the drugs used for RSI). A technique that nurses in critical care are sometimes trained to perform is cricoid pressure (CP). The application of CP can reduce the risk of regurgitation as it involves pressing firmly on the only full ring of cartilage in the respiratory tract to compress the oesophagus.

The RSI procedure requires a team of trained staff (nurses, doctors, advanced critical care practitioners (ACCPs), operating department practitioners (ODPs)) to work together to minimise the risk of complications during a stressful situation. The critically ill patient is usually unstable when they need to be intubated, and the procedure itself stops the patient from breathing by paralysing their muscles. If there are any complications during the procedure, and the airway cannot be inserted it can lead to an emergency called 'Can't Intubate, Can't Oxygenate (CICO)'. This can lead to oxygen deprivation for the patient resulting in risk of brain damage and death. Human factors including the environment, team behaviours and individual performance are also considered to put the patient at risk during this procedure (Higgs et al., 2017). Despite happening in a theatre environment, watching the case of Elaine Bromiley 'Just a routine operation' provides an example of what can go wrong during intubation. To minimise this risk, the Difficult Airway Society (DAS) provide guidelines for the intubation of critically unwell patients (Higgs et al., 2017), giving a standardised approach to planning for and carrying out intubation for critically unwell patients.

Red Flag

- Failure to intubate a patient can lead to a can't intubate, can't oxygenate (CICO) situation. A clear plan of care should be established before intubation attempts start. Failure to secure an airway and an inability to provide oxygen will result in the patient requiring emergency front of neck access (FONA). A cricothyroidotomy is the procedure of inserting a tube directly into the trachea in an emergency situation (Higgs et al., 2017).
- Secretions can block the internal diameter of a tracheal tube causing blockage. This can lead to partial or full airway obstruction. Assessment for humidification and suction is essential component of care to minimise this risk.
- Tracheostomies require additional care consideration and emergency algorithms that are beyond the scope of this chapter. The National Tracheostomy Safety Project (http://www.tracheostomy.org.uk) provides educational resources.
- Initiating any respiratory support should be done with a clear plan for escalation. This prevents the need for decision making during emergency situations.

After intubation, the patient requires an assessment to confirm that the ETT is in the trachea, as there is a risk that the tube is passed into the oesophagus because of the proximity. This leaves the patient unable to oxygenate their lungs. It is important to confirm the correct placement quickly and this is done using waveform capnography (see Clinical investigation 2 box). Chest auscultation and observing for chest movement are often used to indicate correct ETT placement but are not reliable enough to confirm this (Higgs et al., 2017). Chest x-ray is commonly used as an additional investigation to confirm ETT placement, but there can be a short delay whilst organising this procedure. Patients that are intubated usually need to have continuous sedation (see Chapter 12) so that they can tolerate the ETT.

A tracheostomy, an artificial opening directly into the wall of the trachea, is another method that can be used to intubate a patient. A small tube like an ETT is inserted and can be attached to a mechanical ventilator. Tracheostomies should be placed after day 10 if the patient is likely to require more than a few additional days of ventilation (Bice et al., 2015), if a patient requires regular tracheal suction, or a patient is not able to maintain their own airway (Waters and Mutrie, 2017). A patient is normally intubated with an ETT first, and a tracheostomy considered after monitoring patient progress for several days and making sure that they are stable enough to undergo the procedure. However, a tracheostomy can be the first choice for intubation if a patient has an upper airway obstruction. A tracheostomy can help to wean a patient from a ventilator because it is more comfortable than an ETT, this means that a patient can normally tolerate this tube better, reducing the need for sedation.

Clinical investigation 2

Waveform capnography is used to confirm placement of a tracheal tube by measuring carbon dioxide at the end of expiration (known as end-tidal CO_2; $ETCO_2$) and displaying it numerically and graphically. It represents the minimum and maximum concentration of CO_2 during each respiratory cycle.

Capnography monitoring is essential during intubation to confirm correct placement of a tracheal tube. Carbon dioxide is not normally present in the oesophagus but can be immediately after intubation therefore at least three full capnography traces must be witnessed before confirming that the tube is in the trachea.

Waveform capnography is part of the minimum monitoring requirements for a ventilated patient as it provides a real-time indicator of breathing. Absence of a trace can alert staff to a problem, prompting patient assessment (Kerslake and Kelly, 2017).

Examination

A tracheal tube must be secured around the head or neck to help prevent it becoming dislodged, but caution should be used when securing an ETT for a head injured patient (see also Chapter 14). The device used should offer enough support to provide security, but not too much that it contributes to risk of pressure damage to the mouth and face from the securing device or the tube itself.

6Cs: Confidence
The confidence to speak up can improve patient care.

Mechanical ventilation

A mechanical ventilator is a machine that assists a patient to breathe (ventilate) when they are unable to breathe on their own. The ventilator blows gas (air plus oxygen) into a patient's lungs. It can help by doing all the patient's breathing for them or by assisting their breathing.

The patient is connected to a ventilator via an artificial airway using either an endotracheal tube or a tracheostomy tube. This allows oxygen to be delivered directly to the lungs. An artificial airway is necessary when a patient is unable to breathe independently; when it is necessary to sedate and 'rest' someone who is critically unwell; or to protect the airway due to reduced consciousness (Eldridge and Paul, 2020). It maintains the airway so that O_2 can be inhaled into lungs, and CO_2 can be expelled from the lungs. It also offers access to the lower airways for suctioning and removal of secretions.

The ventilator can deliver higher concentrations of O_2 than that delivered by a mask or other devices. The machine can also provide what is called positive end-expiratory pressure (PEEP). This helps to hold the alveolar open preventing them from collapse at the end of expiration. Positive pressure ventilation is the most used in critical care units.

Historically, positive pressure ventilators were classified by their cycles as follows (Woodrow, 2019):

1. Time (controlled by rate or inspiration: expiration (I: E) ratio)
2. Volume (delivers gas until pre-set tidal volume is reached)
3. Pressure (delivers gas until pre-set airway pressure is reached)
4. Flow (speed in litres per minute at which the ventilator delivers breaths).

However, technological developments have led to more sophisticated modes of ventilation that can combine the most desirable features to provide safer ventilation for patients and minimise the risks associated with artificial and mechanical ventilation.

Mechanical ventilation is one of the most common interventions in intensive care (Scottish Intensive Care

Society (SICS), 2020) – it is often life-saving, but can have life-threatening physiological and psychological side effects (see 'Risks of mechanical ventilation' below). The main purpose of ventilation is to provide life support without causing harm to the patient. For this, it is essential that nurses have a sound knowledge of the fundamental underlying principles of mechanical ventilation because the variety of ventilator modes available, terminology, and manufacturer trademarks for these modes can cause confusion.

6Cs: Competence
Recognising your own limitations can help you to identify development needs.

Snapshot 3

Mohammed, 72 years old, was admitted intubated and ventilated following a low anterior resection. On admission, the nurse performs an A–E assessment of the patient. For this patient, it is unlikely that a NEWS2 scoring system would be used as care has already been escalated to a level of higher dependency with increased observation, and the interventions that the patient is receiving are not addressed within this scoring system. Instead, the registered nurse would document observations and infusions on the critical care specific observations chart or e-record.

Airway (A): Airway protected with size 8.0 mm endotracheal tube (ETT), secured and measuring 21 cm at the lips.

Breathing (B): Oxygen saturations 96%, ventilated with a volume control mode of ventilation and positive end-expiratory pressure. Oxygen is set at 55% and respiratory rate set at 18 breaths per minute with no spontaneous effort. On auscultation air entry is noted to be normal throughout.

Circulation (C): Blood pressure 116/ 58 mmHg, heart rate 101 beats per minute, capillary refill time 2 seconds. Patient is warm to touch. Intravenous fluid therapy at 125 mL/hr.

Disability (D): Patient is on continuous sedation of propofol 1% at 15 mL/hr and fentanyl 2 mL/hr. GCS 3. Body temperature 36.8°C.

Exposure (E): Abdominal wound dressing has a small amount of blood on it, a normal finding when a patient returns from theatre.

Patient plan documented in medical notes:
Overnight ventilation following prolonged surgery. Plan to wake patient, wean and extubate patient the next day.

Immediate nursing actions:
- Ensure bedside emergency equipment is available and working (prior to patient admission is best practice).

- Check gas supply and safety alarms on ventilator (before attaching to patient but prior to patient admission is best practice).
- Ensure minimum standard of monitoring in place and set alarm safety limits.
- Admission blood screen including arterial blood gas.
- Review ventilator settings.
- Initiate ventilator care bundle.
- Check volume of drug infusions to identify when they will need replaced.
- Confirm plan of care with relatives.

6Cs: Courage

The courage to ask for help can promote patient safety.

Artificial ventilation

Oxygenation relies on functional alveolar surface area and therefore is determined by:

1. Mean airway pressure
2. Inspiration time
3. Positive end-expiratory pressure (PEEP)
4. Fraction of inspired oxygen (FiO$_2$) and pulmonary blood flow

CO_2 removal requires active tidal ventilation and therefore is affected by:

1. Tidal volume
2. Expiratory time
3. Frequency and flow of breath
4. Resistance to expiration (gas trapping).

Minute ventilation (Vm)

Most ventilators will use respiratory rate (RR) and tidal volume (Vt) to work out a set minute volume (amount of air breathed in one minute). It is recommended to aim for a tidal volume of 6–8 mL/kg of ideal body weight, and a normal respiratory rate in adults is 12–20 breaths per minute (bpm) (Royal College of Physicians, 2017).

$$\begin{aligned} \text{Minute ventilation} &= \text{tidal volume} \,(450\,\text{mL}) \\ &\quad \times \text{respiratory rate} \,(16\,\text{bpm}) \\ &= \text{a minute volume setting of } 7200\,\text{mL} \end{aligned}$$

Fraction of inspired oxygen

Fraction of inspired oxygen (FiO$_2$) is the concentration of O$_2$ delivered to the patient. The FiO$_2$ ranges from 0.21 (room air) to 1 (100% O2). FiO$_2$ will be titrated to the patient's PaO$_2$ from their ABG.

Positive end-expiratory pressure (PEEP)

According to Elliot and Elliot (2018), normal physiological breathing prevents the alveoli from completely collapsing at the end of expiration because the epiglottis closes the airway, leaving a residual volume of air in the lungs. This is not possible if the larynx is permanently open because of the presence of an artificial airway. Positive end-expiratory pressure (PEEP) is applied to counteract this alveolar collapse and is the amount of pressure in the breathing circuit at the end of exhalation. The initial PEEP for patients admitted to CCU is usually between 5 cmH$_2$O and 10 cmH$_2$O (SICS, 2020). The amount of PEEP required can depend on multiple factors including how compliant lung tissue is. In prolonged ventilation, alveoli may continue to collapse because of several physiological and mechanical processes, such as lack of surfactant, sputum retention and endotracheal suctioning. Recruitment manoeuvres of intermittent higher levels of PEEP can help. Table 16.3 outlines the positive and negative issues associated with PEEP.

Volume control

The volume of a tidal breath is set in this mode for example, setting the ventilator to deliver a breath of 500 mL. Setting the rate is normally mandatory for this method of controlling ventilation, e.g. setting the Vt at 500 mL to be delivered at a rate of 14 bpm. The ventilator in this example is set to deliver a minute volume of 500 × 14=7 L/minute. The pressure needed to deliver this volume will depend on lung and chest wall compliance and will change breath to breath.

Pressure control

The pressure used to deliver the tidal breath is set in this mode for example, the ventilator is set to deliver a breath pressure of 25 cmH$_2$O. Setting the rate is normally mandatory for this method of controlling ventilation. For example, the set breath pressure may be at 25 cmH$_2$O to be delivered at a rate of 14 bpm. The tidal volume achieved in this mode of ventilation will depend on lung and chest wall compliance and will vary from breath to breath.

Table 16.3 Positive end-expiratory pressure (PEEP).

Positives	Negatives
Prevents atelectasis	Can cause barotrauma
Recruits collapsed alveoli	Gas trapping and hypercapnia
Facilitates oxygen exchange during expiratory pause, so improving oxygenation	Reduces venous return (increasing cardiac workload)
	Increased work of breathing on self-ventilating modes by increasing resistance to expiration

207

Inspiratory:Expiratory (I:E) ratio

The inspiratory:expiratory (I:E) ratio refers to the ratio of inspiratory and expiratory time. In normal spontaneous breathing the expiratory time is about twice the duration of the inspiratory time, this gives an I:E ratio of 1:2 (read as 'one to two'). This ratio is typically changed in patients with asthma due to the prolonged time of expiration (I:E of 1:3 or 1:4). Longer expiratory times can be used for patients who are in type 2 respiratory failure to expel excessive build-up of PCO_2.

Medicines management: salbutamol

Salbutamol is a selective beta$_2$ adrenoreceptor agonist. It works on bronchial smooth muscle, causing it to relax. Giving nebulised salbutamol to patients with reversible airway obstruction (for example asthma) can help to open their airways making it easier for them to breathe.

Inverse ratio

An inverse ratio is when the I:E ratio is 2:1 or higher and is typically used to ventilate non-compliant lungs. Pressure control modes of ventilation should be used when employing inverse ratios as the use of volume control modes might lead to 'breath dysynchrony stacking' (BDS) and increase airway pressure. BDS refers to the unintended high tidal volumes that occur due to incomplete exhalation between consecutive inspiratory cycles delivered by the ventilator (European Society of Intensive Care Medicine, 2020).

Synchronisation

Synchronisation is a feature of some modes of ventilation that allow the tidal volume to be delivered in synchrony with the patient's breathing. How ventilator synchrony works can vary between ventilator manufacturers, consulting the specific ventilator manual for a detailed description of the synchronisation method used is recommended.

Humidification

The upper airway provides 75% of the heat and moisture supplied to the alveoli and when bypassed, a humidifier is required to supply this missing heat and moisture. Restrepo and Walsh (2012) identified that when the upper airway is bypassed during invasive mechanical ventilation, humidification can prevent hypothermia, disruption of the airway epithelium, bronchospasm, atelectasis, and airway obstruction. While there is no clear consensus on whether additional heat and humidity are necessary when the upper airway is not bypassed, such as in NIV, humidification is highly suggested to improve comfort for IMV (Woodrow, 2019).

There are two main systems for warming and humidifying gases delivered to mechanically ventilated patients. Heated humidifiers operate actively to increase the heat and water vapour content of inspired gas and heat and moisture exchangers (HMEs) operate passively by storing heat and moisture from the patient's exhaled gas and releasing it to the inhaled gas.

Benefits of mechanical ventilation

The main benefits of mechanical ventilation are (American Thoracic Society (ATS), 2017):

- The patient does not have to work as hard to breathe – their respiratory muscles rest
- The patient is allowed time to recover in the hope that breathing becomes normal again
- It helps the patient receive adequate oxygen and clears carbon dioxide
- It preserves a stable airway and prevents injury from aspiration.

It is important to note that mechanical ventilation does not heal the patient. Rather, it allows the patient a chance to be stable while the medications and treatments help them recover.

Risks of mechanical ventilation

The main risks include (ATS, 2017):

- Haemodynamic instability: Positive pressure can reduce venous blood return, increasing right ventricular (RV) afterload, decreasing left ventricular (LV) filling and depressing cardiac output (CO), and overall organ perfusion (Wiesen et al., 2013)
- Infections: An artificial airway provides a route for bacteria to enter the patient's lungs. Wu et al. (2019) state that ventilator-associated pneumonia (VAP) is a hospital-acquired infection that occurs >48 hours after initiation of mechanical ventilation. It is a common complication of mechanical ventilation and has a high mortality rate. VAP results in increased time on a ventilator and increased hospital stay. This preventable complication has a detrimental impact on the patients chances of survival and the psychological wellbeing of them and their family members. Secondary to this, there are financial implications for hospitals and an increased demand on critical care beds and critical care services.
- Collapsed lung (pneumothorax): This can be difficult to recognise in a critically ill patient. Signs and symptoms include decreased breath sounds on one side, pulsus paradoxus, haemodynamic instability with tachycardia, hypotension, contralateral tracheal deviation, and sudden changes to airway pressures on the ventilator.

Although these clinical signs are unreliable, it can prompt radiographical investigation. A pneumothorax can be treated with a chest drain to draw out the extra air, re-expanding the lung.

- Lung damage: A major form of harm is from ventilator-induced lung injury (VILI) (Woodrow, 2019). The pressure used to push air into the lungs during ventilation can damage lung tissue, so it is important to use low pressure when possible. Very high levels of oxygen can also be harmful to the lungs. Jackson et al. (2019) identified that oxygen toxicity is due to the production of oxygen free radicals and this can cause inflammation and atelectasis. The clinician is encouraged to use the lowest FiO_2 that accomplishes satisfactory oxygenation (Jackson et al., 2019).
- Side effects of medications: Sedatives and pain medications can lead to delirium (see Chapter 12), and these side effects may continue after the medications have been discontinued. The healthcare team should use sedation scores and neurological screening tools to assess the patient's neurological function. Whilst sedated, patients remain in bed and this can lead to significant muscle wastage, the resultant weakness can be challenging to overcome.
- Inability to discontinue ventilator support: Sometimes the condition that led a patient to require mechanical ventilation does not improve, despite active treatment. When this happens, clinicians will discuss alternative treatments regarding continued ventilator support. Often clinicians will have these discussions with the patient's family because the patient may not be able to participate due to the severe nature of their illness and/or their lack of mental capacity. In situations where a patient is not recovering or is getting worse, a decision may be made to discontinue ventilator support and move to end-of-life care.

Ventilator care bundles

Ventilator-associated pneumonia is an important healthcare-associated infection (HCAI) that occurs in 10–20% of patients who are mechanically ventilated in the CCU (Hellyer et al., 2016). Although the exact attributable mortality has proved difficult to define, it has significant consequences, with increased mortality, length of CCU stay and hospital stay, and an increase in healthcare costs (Hellyer et al., 2016). Furthermore, within a global setting of worsening antimicrobial resistance, the treatment of respiratory tract infections represents a significant burden on antimicrobials in the ICU. The interventions below, recommended by Hellyer et al., (2016) provide a bundle of care thought to reduce the risk of VAP:

- Elevation of head of bed (30°–45°) to prevent aspiration
- Daily sedation holds (daily sedation interruption and assessment of readiness to extubate)
- Use of subglottic secretion drainage
- Avoidance of scheduled ventilator circuit changes

- Use of chlorhexidine mouthwash (in cardiac patients) because it has been shown to help decrease the incidence of VAP in combination with mechanical cleansing of the oral cavity (Lorente et al., 2007).

Prone positioning

Prone position (lying face down) is a position that a patient can be placed in to try to improve their gas exchange as lying face down can improve V/Q matching and reduce the gravitational effects of the heart on the lungs. A common reason for using the prone position is acute respiratory distress syndrome (ARDS), an inflammatory condition of the lungs that causes severe hypoxia. Turning a patient from supine to prone can be challenging because of the many tubes and wires that a critically unwell patient requires for their therapy, and because a patient requiring prone position is usually very ill. The Faculty of Intensive Care Medicine (FICM) (2019) note that there is currently a lack of evidence for an optimal method of proning a patient and the following recommendations are based on common themes that appear in the literature and intend to provide an example of safe and effective practice:

- Implement proning early in the course of the disease (<48 hours)
- Remain prone for 12–24 hours
- Ventilate using tidal volumes of 6–8 mL/kg
- Consider neuromuscular blocking agents
- Ensure the patient is in the centre of the bed and remove the slide sheet, ensuring counter traction on the patient to prevent them slipping off the bed
- Absorbent pad placed under patient's head to catch secretions
- Carefully position the patient's arms in the 'swimmer's position'. This involves raising one arm on the same side to which the head is facing, while placing the other arm by the patient's side. The shoulder should be abducted to 80° and the elbow flexed 90° on the raised arm. The position of both the head and arms should be alternated every 2 to 4 hours. The patient should be nursed at 30° in the reverse Trendelenburg prone position.

Prone positioning in COVID-19

Prone positioning is an established evidence-based practice in patients with typical ARDS undergoing IMV, but limited evidence exists in non-ventilated awake patients. In a multicentre, randomised controlled trial of patients with severe ARDS receiving IMV, prone positioning halved 28-day mortality rates (16% vs 32.8%, p<0.001) with no additional complications. Meta-analyses suggest that early prone positioning for 12–16 hours/day combined with low tidal volume IMV reduces mortality in severe hypoxic respiratory failure (Koeckerling et al., 2020).

Medicines management: neuromuscular blocking agents

Neuromuscular blocking agents (NMBAs) are administered during intubation. They provide short-term paralysis of patients by stopping nerve impulse transmission, causing skeletal muscle relaxation. Because of their action, they are commonly referred to as muscle relaxants or paralysing agents. See Chapter 12 for more information.

Weaning from mechanical ventilation

In patients with severe respiratory failure artificial ventilation may be life-saving but shortening ventilator time has been shown to reduce ventilation-related complications such as pneumonia, so actively pursuing liberation from mechanical ventilation (so-called 'ventilation weaning') is imperative in every ventilated patient. Prolonging ventilation unnecessarily is costly, in terms of both patient morbidity and healthcare costs.

There are no recognised criteria to wean ventilation, but the following should be considered (European Federation of Critical Care Nursing Associations, 2012; Mora Carpio and Mora, 2019; Woodrow, 2012):

- Improvement or resolution of the patient's underlying condition
- Adequate respiratory rate and gas exchange with minimal or no respiratory support. Specific respiratory parameters may include
  - PEEP 5 cmH$_2$O, FiO$_2$<0.5; pressure support 8–10 cmH$_2$O
  - Arterial blood pH: 7.35–7.45, PO$_2$: 11.0-14.4 kPa, PCO$_2$: 4.6–6.4 kPa
- Stable cardiovascular function
- An acceptable state of consciousness with GCS >8 so patient can protect own airway
- Adequately nourished
- Plan for secretion management (if needed)

After these criteria have been satisfied a spontaneous breathing trial (SBT) can be used. To perform this, two processes must be completed:

1. A sedation-hold trial should be done daily to assess readiness for extubation. This should be performed in every patient who is stable and in whom the indication for mechanical ventilation has resolved. During these daily trials, sedation is reduced to a minimum or eliminated until the patient is awake and co-operative but comfortable.

2. The second parameter is the SBT itself. To perform this, ventilator support should be reduced to a minimum. This can be done either via T-piece or pressure support ventilation (PSV). CPAP has been used in the past, although it has been suggested to be inferior to the other two methods. PSV has been identified as a superior weaning mode for performing SBTs among patients with simple weaning, when compared with T-piece and CPAP (Mora Carpio and Mora, 2019).

SBT should be performed for 30–120 minutes at a time, and the patient should be monitored closely for any signs of respiratory distress. This may include an elevated RR (>20 bpm), nasal flaring, obvious changes in body position, use of accessory muscles, shallow breaths, peripheral and central cyanosis, and compensated tachycardia (Bickley, 2016). If any of these signs are observed, the patient should be placed back on their prior ventilator settings. If the patient is deemed ready, the artificial airway should be removed, and the patient should be monitored closely. In patients with high risk for re-intubation, the use of non-invasive positive or high-flow nasal cannula should be considered. This needs to be communicated and explained to the patient and their family so that they are included in their decisions and have a clear understanding about what is happening, and the risks associated with such interventions.

Conclusion

Many patients admitted to critical care require respiratory support, and this can be provided non-invasively or invasively. Ventilation is a complex intervention that requires a multidisciplinary approach to care. Nurses caring for patients on mechanical ventilation require specialist knowledge and skills to monitor, identify and prevent the potential deleterious effects associated with it, so it is important to ensure that nurses caring for such patients have gained appropriate qualifications and experience. Student nurses and healthcare professionals are not required to have the underpinning knowledge and experience to look after complex critical care patients and are placed in this environment to gain exposure to the roles and responsibilities of the critical care team, as well as development fundamental knowledge about critical illness. Nurses that pick a career in critical care can undertake a post-registration academic programme specific to critical care nursing as part of their CPD, and there is an expectation that 50% of registered nurses working on each critical care unit have undertaken this study due to the complexity of providing such care.

Red Flag

- Failure to intubate a patient can lead to a can't intubate, can't oxygenate (CICO) situation. A clear plan of care should be established before intubation attempts start. Failure to secure an airway and an inability to provide oxygen will result in the patient requiring emergency front of neck access (FONA). A cricothyroidotomy is the procedure of inserting a tube directly into the trachea in an emergency situation (Higgs et al., 2017).
- Secretions can block the internal diameter of a tracheal tube causing blockage. This can lead to partial or full airway obstruction. Assessment for humidification and suction is essential component of care to minimise this risk.
- Tracheostomies require additional care consideration and emergency algorithms that are beyond the scope

of this chapter. The National Tracheostomy Safety Project (http://www.tracheostomy.org.uk) provides educational resources.
- Initiating any respiratory support should be done with a clear plan for escalation. This prevents the need for decision making during emergency situations.

Orange Flag

- Non-invasive and invasive ventilation are both uncomfortable therapies and patients that have received these treatments often report feelings of fear when faced with future hospital admissions.
- Invasive ventilation is a risk factor for delirium.

211

Take home points

1. Ventilation is a common therapy on critical care that can be provided non-invasively or invasively.
2. Invasive ventilation requires intubation; a high-risk procedure that must be carried out by appropriately trained staff.
3. Understanding normal respiratory function is essential to understanding how artificial ventilation works.
4. Nursing care for patients that require artificial ventilation requires a whole-body system approach that includes holistic care.
5. As a student you would be expected to demonstrate fundamental respiratory care skills on critical care patients under direct supervision by a qualified supervisor. Your placement will offer you a learning opportunity to generate knowledge and clinical skills in relation to respiratory failure and the need for artificial ventilation within the context of critical care.

References

American Thoracic Society (2017). Mechanical ventilation. *Am J Respir Crit Care Med* 196(2): 3–4. doi: 10.1164/rccm.1962P3.

Bice, T., Nelson, J.E., and Carson, S.S. (2015). To trach or not to trach: Uncertainty in the care of the chronically critically ill. *Seminars in Respiratory and Critical Care Medicine* 36(6): 851–858. doi: 10.1055/s-0035-1564872

Bickley, L. (2016). *Bates' Guide to Physical Examination and History Taking*. Wolters Kluwer Health.

Davidson, C., Banham, S., Elliott, M. et al. (2016). BTS/ICS Guidelines for the Ventilatory Management of Acute Hypercapnic Respiratory Failure in Adults. https://www.brit-thoracic.org.uk/quality-improvement/guidelines/niv/ (accessed March 2022).

Dutton, H. and Finch, J. (2018). *Acute and Critical Care Nursing at a Glance*. Oxford: Wiley Blackwell.

Eldridge, L. and Paul D. (2020). How an endotracheal tube is used: understanding the purpose, procedure, and possible risks. https://www.verywellhealth.com/endotrachealtube-information-2249093 (accessed 9 April 2020).

Elliot, Z.J. and Elliot, S.C. (2018). An overview of mechanical ventilation in the intensive care unit. *Nurs Stand*. 32(28): 41–49. doi: 10.7748/ns.2018.e10710.

European Federation of Critical Care (2012). Nursing associations (EfCCNa). Position statement on nurses' role in weaning from ventilation. https://tinyurl.com/u2zevkb (accessed 9 April 2020).

European Society of Intensive Care Medicine (2020). Exposure to high tidal volumes from breath stacking dyssynchrony

in ARDS. https://tinyurl.com/r55eudw (accessed 9 April 2020).

Faculty of Intensive Care Medicine and Intensive Care Society (2019). Guidance for prone positioning in adult critical care. https://tinyurl.com/t4suctq (accessed 9 April 2020).

Fayyaz, J. and Lessnau KD. What causes hypoventilation? 2018. https://www.medscape.com/answers/304381-169243/what-causes-hypoventilation (accessed 9 April 2020).

Hellyer, T.P., Ewan, V., Wilson, P., and Simpson AJ. (2016). The Intensive Care Society recommended bundle of interventions for the prevention of ventilator-associated pneumonia. *J Intensive Care Soc* 17(3): 238–243. doi: 10.1177/1751143716644461.

Hennessey, I. and Japp, A. (2016). *Arterial Blood Gases Made Easy*, 2e. Edinburgh: Elsevier.

Higgs, A., McGrath, B., and Goddard, C. (2017). Guidelines for the management of tracheal intubation in critically ill adults. *British Journal of Anaesthesia* 120(2): 323–352. https://bjanaesthesia.org/article/S0007-0912(17)54060-X/fulltext#%20.

Jackson, C.D., Muthiah MP. (2019). What is oxygen toxicity in mechanical ventilation? *Medscape* https://tinyurl.com/wrfu5qn (accessed 9 April 2020).

Kerslake, I. and Kelly, F. (2017). Uses of capnography in the critical care unit. *British Journal of Anaesthesia Education* 14(5): 178–183.

Koeckerling, D., Barker, J., Mudalige, N.L. et al. (2020). Awake prone positioning in COVID-19. *Thorax* 75: 833–834.

Lorente, L., Blot, S., and Rello J. (2007) Evidence on measures for the prevention of ventilator-associated pneumonia. *Eur Respir J* 30(6): 1193–1207. doi: 10.1183/09031936.00048507.

Mora Carpio, A.L., and Mora, J.I. (2019). Ventilator management. NCBI. https://tinyurl.com/uzrq2my (accessed 9 April 2020).

O'Driscoll, B.R., Howard, L.S., Earis, J. et al. (2017). British Thoracic Society guideline for oxygen use in adults in healthcare and emergency settings. *Thorax* 72(S1): 1–90.

Restrepo, R.D. and Walsh, B.K. (2012). American Association for Respiratory Care. Humidification during invasive and non-invasive mechanical ventilation. *Respir Care* 57(5): 782–788. doi: 10.4187/respcare.01766.

Royal College of Physicians. (2017). National Early Warning Score (NEWS) 2: Standardising the assessment of acute-illness severity in the NHS. https://www.rcplondon.ac.uk/projects/outputs/national-early-warning-score-news-2 (accessed 15 December 2020).

Scottish Intensive Care Society (SICS) (2020). Mechanical ventilation. https://tinyurl.com/vdfphts (accessed 9 April 2020).

Shebl, E. and Burns, B. (2019). Respiratory failure. NCBI. https://tinyurl.com/uyr5fgw (accessed 9 April 2020).

Waters, D. and Mutrie, L. (2017). Tracheostomy care. In: *Respiratory Care* (ed. V. Gibson and D. Waters), 185–198. CRC Press.

Wiesen, J., Ornstein, M., Tonelli, A.R. et al. State of the evidence: mechanical ventilation with PEEP in patients with cardiogenic shock. *Heart (British Cardiac Society)* 99(24): 1812–1817. doi: 10.1136/heartjnl-2013-303642.

Whitten C. (2017). Ventilation perfusion mismatch. https://airwayjedi.com/2017/01/06/ventilation-perfusionmismatch/ (accessed 11 April 2020).

Woodrow P. (2019). *Intensive Care Nursing: A Framework for Practice*, 4e. London: Routledge.

Wu, D., Wu, C., Zhang, S., and Zhong, Y. (2019). Risk factors of ventilator-associated pneumonia in critically ill patients. *Front Pharmacol* 10: 482. doi: 10.3389/fphar.2019.00482.

Chapter 17

Lung function in critical care

Rana Din and Joyce Smith

Aim

The aim of this chapter is to provide the reader with an evidence-based understanding of the function of the lungs for patients who are cared for in the critical care setting.

Learning outcomes

After reading this chapter the reader will be able to:

- Gain an appreciation of the importance of lung function.
- Understand the anatomical structures of the respiratory system.
- Understand the principles of gas exchange.
- Understand regularly encountered pathophysiological conditions of the lungs.

Test your prior knowledge

- Can you name the structures of the upper and lower conducting airways that convey inspired air to the lungs?
- What is meant by the terms 'anatomical dead space' and 'alveolar dead space'?
- The percentage of oxygen within room air is. . .
- The percentage of carbon dioxide within room air is. . .
- The percentage of nitrogen within room air is. . .
- What are the normal oxygen saturations of a healthy adult?
- Name the physiological process that allows the movement of oxygen and carbon dioxide within the respiratory membrane

Fundamentals of Critical Care: A Textbook for Nursing and Healthcare Students, First Edition. Edited by Ian Peate and Barry Hill.
© 2023 John Wiley & Sons Ltd. Published 2023 by John Wiley & Sons Ltd.
Companion website: www.wiley.com/go/peate/criticalcare

Introduction

Chapter 17 explores the importance of understanding the structure and function of the lungs when caring for patients who are critically ill. It is essential to understand the function of the lungs in caring for patients who are in respiratory distress. The primary function of the lungs is to allow oxygen to move from the air into the capillaries and carbon dioxide to move out. The lungs act as a reservoir for blood and also filter unwanted material from the circulation (West and Luks, 2020). Deterioration of the patient's lung function has been recognised as one of the first indicators of acute illness (Royal College of Physicians 2017) and one of the main reasons patients are admitted to critical care.

Step 2 competencies: National standards

2:1.1 Respiratory Systems (Critical Care Networks-National Nurse Leads (CC3N) 2015)
   Demonstrate your knowledge using a rationale through discussion, and the application to your practice.

- The anatomy and physiology of the upper and lower respiratory systems
- Internal and external respiration
- Cellular respiration
- Acid-base balance
- Ventilation/perfusion (VQ) mismatch

Anatomy and physiology

On inspiration air enters the lungs via the conducting airways and continues into the lungs. The carina is at the base of the trachea and separates into the left and right main bronchi. The right bronchus is shorter, wider and more vertical than the left bronchus. This is because it shares the left side of the thoracic space with the heart (see Figure 17.1).

The lungs are situated within the thoracic (chest) cavity on either side of the heart and major vessels. The lungs are protected by the thoracic cage that consists of the ribs, sternum, and vertebrae (Peate, 2018). The tip of each lung, the apex, lies about 25 mm above the level of the middle third of the clavicle and the base of the lungs is just above the diaphragm (Waugh and Grant, 2018). The lungs are separated by the mediastinum between the parietal and visceral pleurae, two thin protective membranes that surrounds each lung. The parietal pleura lines the wall of the thorax and the visceral pleura lines the outer surface of each lung. In between the two pleura is the pleural cavity that contains a small amount of serous fluid that lubricates the surface of the pleura allowing them to slide over each other and causes the two pleural layers to adhere together as the lungs change size and shape. Therefore, the lungs are held in place tightly to the wall of the thorax. This ensures that when the thorax expands, the lungs also expand, allowing air to enter (Marieb and Keller, 2018).

Each lung is a separate cavity therefore if one lung is punctured, for example a pneumothorax, the other lung will

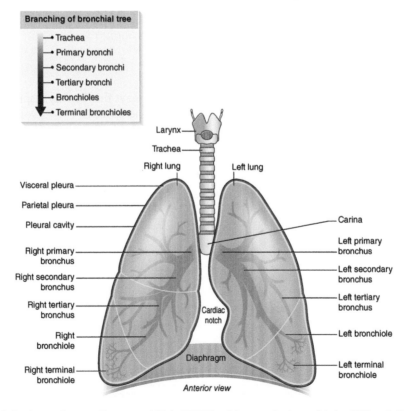

Figure 17.1   Picture of the lung. *Source:* Peate and Nair (2015) with permission of John Wiley & Sons.

remain inflated. A pneumothorax occurs if air enters the pleural space causing a partial or complete lung collapse. A traumatic pneumothorax occurs when the ruptured pleura remains open creating a one-way valve. As each breath draws in more air into the pleural space, the one-way valve prevents air leaving on expiration. Therefore, increased intrathoracic pressure on the side of the pneumothorax may shift the mediastinum (located between the lungs) towards the opposite side (Morton and Fontaine, 2013; Woodrow, 2019). Each lung is a separate cavity therefore it is important to assess each lung separately.

Red Flag

It is important on visual inspection of the chest to check the central position of the trachea. As deviation to one side could suggest a mediastinal shift, indicating a tension pneumothorax that requires urgent medical intervention.

Learning event: reflection

Reflect on how much you understand about a pneumothorax and insertion of a chest drain.

The most important muscle for breathing is the diaphragm that separates the chest cavity from the abdomen. On inspiration the diaphragm contracts downwards. It increases the length and diameter of the chest cavity, therefore reducing the pressure within the lungs. At the same time the external intercostal muscles contract, raising the

rib cage upwards and outwards, therefore increasing the thoracic space. When the intrapulmonary pressure falls below atmospheric pressure this allows air to passively enter the lungs. When the diaphragm relaxes due to the natural elastic recoil of the lungs, air is pushed out during expiration. Therefore, air moves from an area of high pressure to an area of low pressure.

After entering both lungs the main bronchi subdivide into smaller branches as they penetrate deeper into the lungs, finally ending at the terminal bronchiole which divide into respiratory bronchioles leading to the alveolar ducts which are lined with alveoli (Peate and Nair, 2015; West and Luks, 2020). Covering the alveoli are a network of tiny blood vessels called capillaries (see Figure 17.2). Due to the incredibly thin barrier between the air and capillaries oxygen can move from the alveoli into the blood and carbon dioxide can easily move from the capillaries into the alveoli to be exhaled.

This is the only section within the lungs that gas exchange occurs and is known as the respiratory zone (West and Luks, 2020).

Composition of air

Air is a mixture of gases, 0.04% carbon dioxide, 21% oxygen and 78% nitrogen. Each gas exerts part of the total pressure proportional to its concentration and recorded as P, for example PO_2, PCO_2. Atmospheric pressure at sea level is 760 mmHg or 101.3 kilopascals (Table 17.1).

Alveolar gas

Gas exchange takes place through the respiratory membrane located in the alveoli. The composition of the gas in the alveoli is significantly different from the atmosphere, as there is an increase of water content.

215

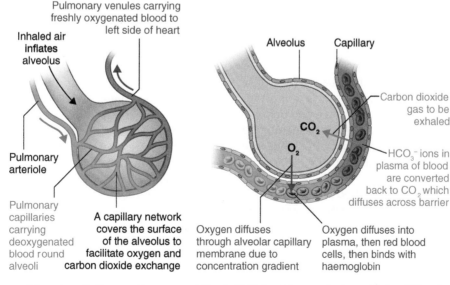

Figure 17.2 Picture of the alveoli. *Source:* Dutton and Finch (2018) with permission of John Wiley & Sons.

Table 17.1   Partial pressures of gases.

Gas	Oxygenated Blood	Deoxygenated Blood	Alveolar
Oxygen	13.3 kPa 100 mmHg	5.3 kPa 40 mmHg	13.3 kPa 100 mmHg
Carbon dioxide	5.3 kPa 40 mmHg	5.8 kPa 44 mmHg	5.3 kPa 40 mmHg
Nitrogen	76.4kPa 573 mmHg	76.4kPa 573 mmHg	76.4kPa 573 mmHg

Table 17.2   Inspired and expired air.

	Inspired air in %	Expired air in %
Oxygen	21	16
Carbon dioxide	0.04	4
Nitrogen	78	78

Table 17.3   Lung volumes.

Total lung capacity (TLC)	6,000 mL
Tidal volume (TV)	500 mL
Iinspiratory reserve volume (IRV)	3,100 mL
Expiratory reserve volume (ERV)	1,200 mL
Vital capacity (VC) calculation TV+IRV+ERV	4,800 mL
Residual volume (RV)	1,200 mL

Expired air

This is a mixture of atmospheric and alveolar air (see Table 17.2). There is a reduction of the oxygen content and increased carbon dioxide content. It is important to be aware of the reduced oxygen content especially in the context of having to deliver mouth to mouth resuscitation.

Lung volumes

An understanding of lung volumes and capacities is important when assessing the lung function of acutely ill patients. In a healthy adult the normal respiratory rate is between 12–20 breaths per minute (Royal College of Physicians, 2017). The total amount of air that the lungs can hold is approximately 6000 mL and this is called the total lung capacity (TLC). TLC is subdivided into actual and potential volumes of air and will depend on the age, sex and height of the patient. With each respiration around 500 mL of air is moved in and out of the lungs with each breath and is called the tidal volume (TV). However, the lungs have a capacity of extra inhalation and exhalation if needed for example in exercise or singing. The inspiratory reserve volume (IRV) is the potential for a person to inhale much more air than is taken in during a normal breath. The amount of air taken in forcibly over the tidal volume is around 3,100 mL. The expiratory reserve volume (ERV), approximately 1,200 mL, is the amount of air that can be forcibly exhaled after expiration. A small amount of air after expiration remains in the lungs and this is called the residual volume (RV). The residual volume around 1,200 mL is important because it allows gas exchange to continue and helps to keep the alveoli open. Vital capacity (VC) is the combined amount of air that can move in and out of the lungs (see Table 17.3). VC is calculated by adding the TV + IRV + ERV = 4,800 mL.

In health care settings one method of evaluating a patient's lung function is by spirometry, which assesses how much air the patient can breathe out. The minute volume (MV) is a volume that is also included in the settings for mechanical ventilation. To calculate the minute volume, it is the total amount of air entering or leaving the lungs in one minute. For example, the tidal volume 500 mL × the respiratory rate 12 breaths per minute = 6000 mL (Credland, 2017; Marieb and Keller, 2018; Woodrow 2019).

For lung function to be effective it is dependent on four distinct phases Pulmonary ventilation, external respiration, transport of gases and internal ventilation.

Pulmonary ventilation

This is the process by which air must move in and out of the lungs so that gases are exchanged in the alveoli. For example, the pressure within the lungs and the atmospheric pressure are the same before inspiration. On inspiration the thorax expands, and the intrapulmonary pressure falls below atmospheric pressure, Boyle's Law relates to the pressure exerted by gas and is inversely proportional to its volume. In other words, the higher the pressure, the lower the volume; the higher the volume, the lower the pressure. Therefore, as the thorax expands, intrathoracic pressure falls below atmospheric pressure (Credland, 2017; West and Luks, 2020).

On inspiration the diaphragm and external intercostal muscles contract, causing the diaphragm to be pulled down and the external intercostal muscles pull the rib cage outwards and upwards. This increase in the size of the thoracic cavity and reduced intrathoracic pressure creates a pressure gradient between the atmosphere and the lungs. The pressure within the lungs falls below 760 mmHg atmospheric pressure and air enters the lungs. The pressure inside and outside of the lungs then equalise. However, when the pressure within the lungs is greater than the atmospheric pressure, the lungs contract following a natural elastic recoil of the lungs and air is expelled (expiration).

Expiration is a passive process; however, inspiration and expiration become an active process for acutely ill patients with impaired lung function. Acutely ill patients with impaired lung function will use their abdominal, scalene, sternocleidomastoid, trapezius and pectoral muscles, known as the accessory muscles of respiration, to increase the volume of air in and out of the lungs. It is important when assessing patients to observe if they are using their accessory muscles as this may indicate that they are struggling with their breathing as in normal breathing the accessory muscles are not used.

External respiration

External respiration is the process of gas exchange, between the pulmonary blood and alveoli, including oxygen loading and carbon dioxide unloading. Gas exchange takes place at the thin alveolar-capillary membrane by a process of diffusion. The alveoli are grapelike clusters of air-filled sacs at the end of the respiratory passages and there are about 500 million pulmonary alveoli, which are about 1/3 mm in diameter. Alveoli consist of type 1 and type 2 epithelial cells. Type 1 cells form the alveolar walls through which gas exchange occurs and type 2 cells produce surfactant, a surface-active lipoprotein that coats the alveoli. During inspiration the alveolar surfactant allows the alveoli to expand and prevents alveolar collapse (Marieb and Keller, 2018).

Ventilation/Perfusion

Oxygen moves from the alveoli into the pulmonary capillaries; thus, blood leaving the lungs to travel to the pulmonary veins and the left side of the heart should be saturated with oxygen. By the process of diffusion carbon dioxide moves from the capillaries to the alveoli to be exhaled and eliminated from the body. Fick's Law is the principle that describes the movement of oxygen and carbon dioxide across the respiratory membrane of the alveoli (Peate and Nair, 2015). Diffusion of oxygen takes place from the alveolus into the pulmonary capillaries and carbon dioxide from the capillaries into the alveolus. According to Fick's Law diffusion is when the movement of a gas from an area of high concentration to an area of low concentration. This is determined by gas solubility, molecular weight, surface area, concentration differences and membrane thickness (Wheeldon, 2018).

Gas exchange in any healthy lung is dependent on adequate ventilation and adequate circulation (perfusion). Ventilation in a healthy adult at rest would equate to 4 L/min and pulmonary blood flow would be 5 L/min. During strenuous exercise there can be 15-fold increase in ventilation and a 6-fold increase in cardiac output. The rate at which respiratory gases can diffuse is proportional to the following:

- The total surface area
- The thinness of the respiratory membrane
- The magnitude of the partial pressure
- The solubility of the gas.

The structure of the alveolar-capillary membrane is incredibly thin less than 0.4 µm plus the millions of alveoli also provide a huge surface area of approximately 70 m². This large surface area allows for rapid gas exchange. Venous blood entering the capillary network of the lungs can equilibrate with alveolar air in approximately 0.2 seconds. Carbon dioxide is far more soluble than oxygen and therefore diffuses much faster. Nitrogen is not soluble and therefore does not cross the respiratory membrane.

However, there are occasions when deoxygenated blood arrives at the capillary membrane but does not uptake oxygen, this is referred to as a shunt. In the normal healthy lung this accounts for a very small percentage of blood flow to the lungs. There are pathophysiological conditions that result in a significant and often life-threatening shunt. Diffusion of gases may be impeded by thickening of the alveoli or loss of functional alveoli in conditions such as emphysema and pulmonary oedema and these would result in a shunt. This explains why that some patients in critical care despite being given a very high concentration of oxygen remain hypoxic, as venous deoxygenated blood arrives at the alveoli but is unable to pick up oxygen and then returns to the circulation deoxygenated (West and Luks, 2020).

For example, the alveoli surface area of the lungs is expansive and contains a network of pulmonary capillaries for gas exchange to take place. The partial pressure of oxygen (PO_2) within the alveolus is greater than the partial pressure of oxygen (PO_2) of incoming blood, therefore oxygen moves from the alveoli into the capillaries.

Equally the partial pressure of carbon dioxide (PCO_2) of venous blood is higher in the pulmonary capillaries than the PCO_2 within the alveoli therefore carbon dioxide diffuses into the alveolus and is exhaled by the lungs. Oxygen and carbon dioxide are both soluble in water and therefore easily diffused as the alveoli membrane is very thin which allows oxygen to enter the blood stream and carbon dioxide to leave. External respiration therefore converts oxygenated blood in the lungs before the blood returns to the left side of the heart.

Transport of gases

For gas exchange to take place the alveoli need a constant supply of both oxygen and pulmonary blood flow (Marieb and Keller, 2018). Oxygen is attached to the haemoglobin within the red blood cell each haemoglobin molecule binds to a maximum of four oxygen molecules. The percentage of haemoglobin carrying oxygen is measured as an oxygen saturation (SaO_2). The actual amount of oxygen carried by the haemoglobin in arterial blood is called the arterial oxygen content and is determined by the oxygen saturation levels SaO_2 In clinical practice you will be familiar with checking the patient's oxygen saturation levels using a pulse oximeter that measures the pulse and the saturation of haemoglobin in arterial blood.

Carbon dioxide is the end product of cellular metabolism and diffuses into the blood and involves three distinct phases. Around 10% is carried within plasma and when it reaches the lungs it is diffused into alveolar air and exhaled. There is 20% attached to haemoglobin which has a greater affinity for carbon dioxide than oxygen. This enables the release of oxygen as carbon dioxide is being created in the tissues. As carbon dioxide levels increase, the amount of oxygen binding to the haemoglobin will be reduced causing hypercapnia. The remainder of carbon dioxide will be transported in blood plasma as bicarbonate ions (HCO_3).

Internal respiration

Internal respiration is the process of gas exchange of oxygen and carbon dioxide between the blood and tissue cells. Cellular respiration is the process involved in converting oxygen and glucose to produce energy in the form of adenosine triphosphate (ATP). ATP is an important source of energy for metabolic processes including aerobic respiration. The cells also produce water and carbon dioxide as a waste product. As the cells use oxygen continuously, the concentration of oxygen is always lower within the tissues than the blood. Adequate oxygenation of blood is dependent on effective ventilation which allows the flow of air to and from the lungs. Pulmonary perfusion is the blood flow through the lungs via the pulmonary artery and capillaries to the heart. Diffusion is the exchange of gases under the influence of a pressure gradient (Marieb and Keller, 2018). The alveolar-capillary membrane is where gaseous exchange takes place. Blood entering the pulmonary capillaries comes from the right side of the heart, is low in oxygen and high in levels of CO_2 that it has collected from body tissues (Colbert et al., 2019).

Nursing and Midwifery Council (NMC, 2018a, 2018b)

22.3 Keep your knowledge and skills up to date.
  Nursing Associates: 3.11 demonstrate the ability to recognise when a person's condition has improved or deteriorated by undertaking health monitoring

6Cs: Competence

Knowledge and understanding of lung function are a key requisite when caring for critically ill patients. To provide care effectively and with competence, the nurse is required to ensure they are up to date with current practice.

Snapshot: control of breathing

Breathing is a combination of voluntary and involuntary responses. However, it is predominantly an involuntary act controlled by the rhythmic respiratory centre which is located in the brain stem (see Figure 17.3). If the nerve pathway was transacted above the first three cervical nerves (C3), it would result in total respiratory paralysis (Montague et al., 2005).

Voluntary control of breathing is necessary to aide with other processes such as vocalisation. It is also required during times of danger such as water immersion or hiding from threats. There are also marked changes in the respiratory pattern in various emotional states such as crying and laughing.

Respiratory rhythm is generated within the brain and carried to the spinal cord via three separate pathways.

- **Voluntary pathway:** Impulses are conveyed from the cerebral cortex to the medullary respiratory centre. However, the ability to not breathe is limited by the build-up of carbon dioxide (CO_2) and hydrogen ions (H^+) in body fluids.
- **Involuntary pathway:** This tracks in the dorsolateral region of the spinal cord. Voluntary and involuntary breathing occurs at the spinal cord level. Disease within the brain stem or spinal cord can destroy voluntary control but leave the involuntary pathway unaffected. Therefore, a patient that is unconscious may still breathe.
- **Tonic influences:** Within the medulla there are areas that help with the extent to which the various respiratory muscles contract and relax.

Red Flag

Paradoxical breathing often referred to as 'see saw' breathing and is a sign of respiratory distress. As the patient attempts to breathe the chest and the abdomen will move in opposite directions with each breath, this may be caused by a blockage within the airway.

- **Pnuemotaxic area:** Regulates the amount of air taken in one breath
- **Apneustic area:** Prolongs inhalation. However, when the pneumotaxic area is active it overrides the signal from the apneustic area.
- **Medullary rhythmicity area:** Controls rhythm. During normal breathing inhalation is approximately 2 seconds and exhalation is 3 seconds.
- **Chemoreceptors:** Changes in the partial pressure of oxygen and carbon dioxide effects simulation and inhibition of breathing. In normal physiology carbon dioxide is the predominant driver in respiration. An increase in carbon

dioxide concentration results in an increase of hydrogen ions that stimulate the chemoreceptors which in turn stimulate breathing. However, in some chronic respiratory conditions and at extreme altitude oxygen can have a significant influence on respiration. These changes are stimulated by alterations in the chemical composition of the blood and specific receptors located within the body.

- **Central chemoreceptors:** These are located within the brainstem and can detect levels of carbon dioxide within the blood. In normal physiology a rise in carbon dioxide levels will result in an increase in the respiratory rate and

depth, thus allowing the carbon dioxide to be exhaled. Within the critical care setting the levels of carbon dioxide in the blood help clinicians regulate the rate and depth of breathing with artificial ventilation.

- **Peripheral chemoreceptors:** These are located in the internal and external carotid arteries (see Figure 17.4). A drop in blood flow in the carotid artery can lead to hypoxia, hypercapnia and decrease in blood pH, resulting in receptor simulation. In turn this will stimulate ventilation in an attempt to remove the excess CO_2, maintain blood pH and homeostasis and prevent organ damage.

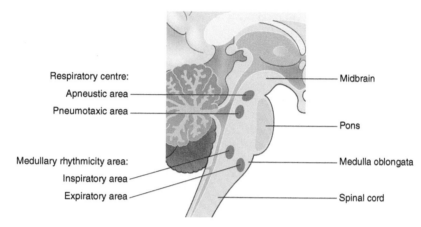

Figure 17.3   Picture of the respiratory centre. *Source:* Peate and Nair (2015) with permission of John Wiley & Sons.

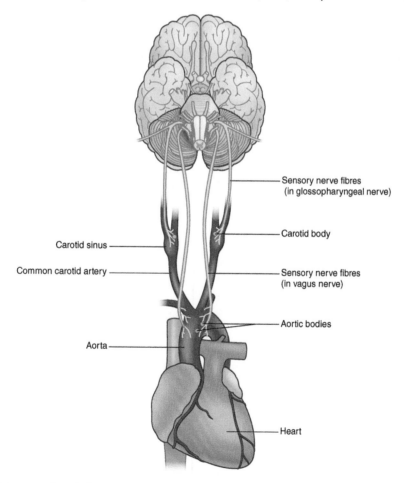

Figure 17.4   Picture of the peripheral chemoreceptors. *Source:* Peate and Nair (2015) with permission of John Wiley & Sons.

Red Flag

It is important to note that very high levels of PCO_2 will depress the central nervous system and respiratory centre and could be fatal unless artificial ventilation is initiated.

6Cs: Commitment

The role of any nurse caring for patients with lung failure requires constant vigilance to ensure their safety and best outcome. Therefore, there is a need for commitment to maintain the National Standards.

Assessment of lung function

It is critical that a thorough and complete assessment is made of the patient's respiratory status. It is important where possible that the patient is rested and unaware that the examination is taking place. The look-listen-feel assessment is recommended by the Resuscitation Council UK (RCUK, 2015).

- **Look:** The respiratory rate should be measured for a full minute. One breath comprises of one inspiration and expiration. The depth, rate and symmetry of the chest wall should be observed. Skin colour could also be an indication of adequate ventilation. Simultaneously observing the level of consciousness is crucial as high or low levels of oxygen and carbon dioxide can affect the level of awareness.
- **Listen:** Normal breathing should be quiet, and any added noises and the location should be noted. Additional noises such as wheezes may be an indication there is some disturbances in the flow of air into or out of the lower respiratory airways. Snoring and gurgling may be an indication that there is an obstruction in the upper airways.
- **Feel:** It may be necessary check the symmetry and depth of breathing through placing both hands on either side of the anterior aspect of the patient's chest. By placing the thumbs close together either side of the sternum it is possible to visualise the extent to which the patient's chest expands. Asymmetry may be indicative of pneumonia or a pneumothorax.

Learning event: reflection

Reflect on the importance of look, listen and feel when assessing a critically ill patient.

Examination: Respiratory assessment: Inspection:

In normal breathing the predominant muscle is the diaphragm which contracts during inspiration. Chest movement should be equal, bilateral and symmetrical. The contraction of muscles other than the diaphragm is referred to as use of the accessory muscles. Contraction of the scalene and sternocleidomastoid muscles lifts the clavicles and ribs; this is frequently encountered in patients with chronic obstructive pulmonary disease (COPD). Some patients with COPD and dyspnoea may develop the habit of pursing their lips during expiration. This is characterised by tightening of the lips and contracting cheeks upon expiration. Patients may find this technique helps relieve the effects of breathlessness. Changes in the pattern and the respiratory rate could be an indication of deterioration that requires further investigation or reporting to a senior colleague. During advanced stages of COPD, some patients may develop a barrel-chested appearance. This is a result of increases in the anteroposterior diameter of the chest.

Clinical investigation: pulse oximetry

Pulse oximetry should be undertaken in all breathless and acutely ill patients and oxygen saturation levels should be maintained between 94% and 98% for most acutely ill patients or 88–92% for patients who are at risk of hypercapnia. Further clinical assessment is required if the saturation falls by $\geq 3\%$ of the target range (O'Driscoll, Howard and Earis, 2017).

Red Flag

Cyanosis is a result of deoxygenated haemoglobin, which results in a bluish tinge to the skin or mucous membrane. It can be categorised as central or peripheral. Central cyanosis can be observed on the tongue and lips as these tissues are covered with mucosa. As the distance from the heart to the tongue is relatively short, the cyanosis could be a result of a heart condition or lung disease. Peripheral cyanosis is frequently seen in the fingers or toes and in the absence of central cyanosis is potentially due to inadequate circulation.

Medications management

Oxygen therapy should be regarded as medication and is prescribed for hypoxaemic patients to increase alveolar oxygen tension and decrease the work of breathing. In most acutely ill patients, the aim is to achieve oxygen saturations of 94–98%. On occasions there may be a requirement with patients who have chronically higher than normal carbon dioxide levels to have target saturations of 88–92%.

Clinical investigation: assessment of respiratory sounds (auscultation)

An understanding of the anatomy and physiology of the respiratory system is essential for performing chest auscultation. The Nursing and Midwifery Council (2018a) has included chest auscultation in the Standards of Proficiency for Registered Nurses in preparation for registration. It is important that practitioners have a good level of competence when using the stethoscope. The essential parts of the stethoscope are identified (see Figure 17.5)

The bell of the stethoscope is recommended for use above the clavicles when listening for sounds that are generated from the apex of the lung. The bell helps identify high pitch sounds. The diaphragm is used for the rest of the chest and will help identify low pitched sounds.

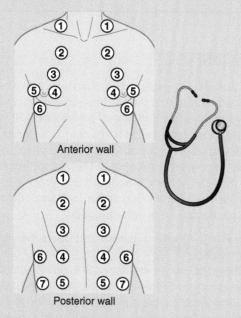

Figure 17.5 Auscultation. *Source:* Dutton and Finch (2018) with permission of John Wiley & Sons.

Normal breath sounds (vesicular)

These sounds are described as rustling and are heard directly over the lung fields, unlike the noise generated over the trachea, whose sound is referred to as bronchial.

Red Flag

Bronchial sounds should not be heard over the lung fields, and could be a sign of lung injury

---

Absent Sounds

This may be a result of consolidation in the lung, which can form a blockage in the lower or upper airways. A pneumothorax could also result in absent breath sounds. The movement of air in and out of the lungs can be restricted due to bronchospasm as sometimes experienced in asthma. The intensity of the noise of breath sound should be noted as this may be a useful sign of improvement or deterioration. It is important to adequately assess breath sounds in critically ill patients following endotracheal intubation as a method of assessing the correct positioning of the endotracheal tube (ET) and therefore adequate ventilation.

Red Flag

It should be noted that absent breath sounds could be a medical emergency and require further investigations, such as blood gas analysis and/or chest x-ray.

Wheeze

It is important that the nurse can identify the region of the wheeze and determine if it is present during inspiration or expiration. It may be a result of pathological deterioration, for example in worsening asthma. It could also be a consequence of an obstruction in the airway. It is imperative that the nurse assesses the efficiency of any medication that is administered such as bronchodilators by assessing if there has been a change to the sounds within the chest.

221

Medications management

Salbutamol (beta2-agonists short-acting) is a broncho-dilator therapy.

Indications: To reverse airway constriction caused by obstructive airway disease such as asthma. Salbutamol relax bronchial smooth muscle by stimulation of β-adrenoreceptors. Salbutamol can be given as an inhaler, tablet or intravenous infusion.
Inhalation of nebulised solution:

Adults 5 mg repeat every 20–30 minutes or when required, give via oxygen-driven nebuliser if available. In patients with acute asthma, the nebulised route (oxygen-driven) is recommended.

Oxygen-driven nebulisers are preferred for nebulising β2 agonist bronchodilators because of the risk of oxygen desaturation while using air-driven compressors (BTS and SIGN, 2019)

Side effects: Arrhythmias; headache; hypokalaemia (with high doses); muscle spasms; nasopharyngitis; nausea; palpitations; rash; tremor. (British National Formula (BNF), 2021).

Crackles

The location and volume of the crackles should be noted as these are abnormal breath sounds. They may be a product of excessive secretion production frequently experience with pneumonia and chronic lung conditions (Proctor and Rickards, 2020).

The work of breathing

This is the degree of effort that is required to move air in and out of the lungs. In a resting state less than 1% of the metabolic rate is used. This can increase to 3% during exercise; however, this may be up to 50% in severe respiratory disease (Montague et al., 2005). This demonstrates why patients become exhausted and frequently need supplementary support with their breathing.

The two concepts that must be considered when assessing a patient's lung function and ability to move air in and out of the lungs are compliance and resistance.

Compliance

This describes the extent to which the lungs can distend. Compliance is influenced by the stiffness or flexibility and three anatomic boundaries which are the anterior, posterior, and abdominal wall. In normal physiology the lungs can expand easily. However, in certain respiratory diseases such as emphysema there is an increase in compliance. The increase in compliance is detrimental as this impedes the natural recoil of the lungs.

Resistance

This can be described as the pressure of effort required to allow the flow of gas into the airways. This may be influenced by obstructions or narrowing of the airways, for example in the episode of acute asthma the patient will find it difficult in breathing due to the inadequate airflow and the resistance that has been caused by the narrowing of the airway.

Emphysema

This is characterised by a destruction of lung parenchyma that leads to an irreversible increase in the air spaces beyond the terminal bronchioles. This leads to abnormal enlargement of the alveoli. The result is a reduction of the surface areas for the exchange of oxygen and carbon dioxide. Smoking is known to be a major antagonist in developing emphysema.

Red Flag

In chronic respiratory disease the hypercapnic (raised carbon dioxide) drive may have become depressed and therefore less responsive to a decrease in ventilation. Therefore, it is the hypoxic (low levels of oxygen) reflex that stimulates breathing. Caution should be taken when administering oxygen to patients who may have chronic higher than normal levels of carbon dioxide within their blood as this may impact on their ability to breathe adequately.

Snapshot

John Walters is 68 years old, married with 2 children. He has been admitted to the Medical Assessment Unit, following a referral by his General Practitioner (GP). In the last couple of days, he has had a cold and a productive cough with copious amounts of yellow/green sputum. Despite a course of antibiotics, he was not improving. Past medical history diagnosed six years ago with emphysema. On admission to the unit John is distressed and says he cannot breathe properly.

Airway (A): Airway is patent but speaking in short sentences.

Breathing (B): oxygen saturations 87% on air (NEWS2 = 1), respiratory rate (RR) 24 breaths per minute (NEWS2 = 2). Shallow breathing but equal chest expansion at the apex but consolidation at the bases, using his accessory muscles.

Cardiovascular System (C): Blood Pressure (BP) is 102/60 mmHg (NEWS2 =1), Heart Rate (HR) is 102 beats per minute (NEWS2 = 1), capillary refill time (CRT) is 3 seconds, he is cool to touch. Urinalysis not recorded.

Disability (D) (neurological system), A (NEWS2 = 0), on the ACVPU scale. Blood glucose 6 mmol/l, pupils equal and reacting to light, Pain score 2 out of 3.

Exposure (E) Top-to-toe assessment, skin cool to touch. Body Temperature (T) is 38.3°C tympanic (NEWS2 = 1).

Total NEW2 Score: 6.

Nursing actions:
- RN escalates to the Senior medical team: (SBAR)
- Tripod position
- Prescribed oxygen and nebulisers
- Physiological observations every 15 minutes
- Pain assessment
- Sputum sample for culture and sensitivity
- Commenced a fluid balance chart
- Diagnostic tests including full blood tests and blood cultures were taken
- Arterial blood gas (ABG)
- Referral to physiotherapist
- Consent to inform relatives

Diagnosis:
- Exacerbation of COPD due to a chest infection.
- John is becoming fatigued due to increased respiratory effort.

Medications management

Prednisolone is a corticosteroid which has an anti-inflammatory effect which can help to ease inflammation in the airways, although the effect can take several hours to work.

Indications: Moderate to severe asthma and acute exacerbation of chronic pulmonary disease especially if breathlessness interferes with daily activities.

Dose: Mild to moderate acute asthma, adult 40–50 mg daily for at least 5 days, IV route with hydrocortisone is preferable in near-fatal asthma. For acute exacerbation of chronic obstructive pulmonary disease (if increased breathlessness interferes with daily activities) by mouth 30 mg daily for 7–14 days (British National Formula (BNF), 2021).

Side effects: Common; weight gain, indigestion, sleep problems, restlessness, anxiety, fluid retention, alterations in mood and excessive sweating.

6Cs: Compassion

Compassion when caring for patients with long-term lung conditions requires nurses to deliver care with empathy, respect, and dignity. So, compassion is about treating patients with intelligent kindness, empathy and is central to how patients perceive their care.

Asthma

This is characterised by short-term episodes of bronchoconstriction which result in a contraction of the smooth muscle. This can present as wheeze, shortness of breath, chest tightness and cough (Papi et al., 2018). Studies of fatal and near-fatal asthma show pronounced thickening of the airway walls, oedema and mucus plugs (King et al., 2018). The inflammation of the mucosa can lead to plugging of the small airways. Early pharmacological interventions include the administration of salbutamol which works by relaxing smooth muscle. Ipratropium bromide will block activity of the parasympathetic nerve and reduce reflex component of an asthmatic attack

Clinical examination

A sputum sample is a useful indicator of lung pathology as any disruption in the flow of air within the lungs can cause respiratory failure. Sputum samples are obtained using a non-invasive or invasive method (Shepherd, 2017). A non-invasive method involves the nurse explaining to the patient the purpose of obtaining a sputum sample and gaining informed consent. An invasive method is the endotracheal closed suctioning technique when patients are ventilated. When obtaining a sputum sample, it is important to note the colour, viscosity and amount. The sample is then sent to microbiology for culture and sensitivities within four hours or in line with clinical guidelines.

Snapshot

Jenny Travis is 20 years old and has just commenced a degree at university. Diagnosed with asthma when she was at junior school, her condition had been well controlled with salmeterol inhalers. Following the first exam Jenny and her friends went out to celebrate later that evening her friends brought Jenny to Accident and Emergency (A&E).

Admitted to the Medical Assessment Unit. On admission Jenny is speaking in short sentences and is visibly anxious.

Airway (A): Airway is patent, but Jenny is speaking in short sentences with an audible wheeze on inspiration and expiration.

Breathing (B): Oxygen saturations 93% on air (NEWS2 = 2), respiratory rate (RR) 26 breaths per minute (NEWS2 = 3). Depth shallow but equal chest expansion using her accessory muscles.

Cardiovascular System (C): Blood Pressure (BP) is 140/80 mmHg (NEWS2 = 0), Heart Rate (HR) is 110

beats per minute (NEWS2 = 1), capillary refill time (CRT) is 2 second, she is cool to touch.

Disability (D) (neurological system), A (NEWS2 = 0), on the ACVPU scale. Blood glucose 6 mmol/l, pupils equal and reacting to light, Pain score 2 out of 3.

Exposure (E): Top-to-toe assessment, skin cool to touch but no abnormal findings. Body Temperature (T) is 37.3°C tympanic (NEWS2 = 0).

Total NEW2 Score: 7.

Nursing actions:
- RN escalates to the senior medical team: (SBAR)
- Provide reassurance to relieve anxiety
- Position Jenny in high Fowler's position
- Oxygen and nebulisers as prescribed
- Physiological observations every 15 minutes
- Pain assessment
- Sputum sample for culture and sensitivity
- Diagnostic tests including full blood tests and blood cultures also venous blood gas
- Commenced on fluid balance chart
- Consent to inform parents
- Education on self-management skills

Diagnosis:
- Asthma is poorly controlled on the present medication
- Review medication
- History of previous attacks
- Pulmonary function test

Medications management

Aminophylline is a bronchodilator that relax the muscles in the bronchial tubes (air passages) of the lungs.

Indications: Early intervention in severe and acute asthma.

Pharmacokinetics: The mode of action involves enzyme activity inhibition in bronchial smooth and easing constriction. Aminophylline is metabolised by the liver; therefore, it is important that the nurse is aware of the patient's medical condition specifically for any signs of liver and/or cardiac failure. Measurement of plasma-theophylline concentration is advised to prevent symptoms of toxicity. Administration is by slow intravenous injection.

For adults, recommended dose is 250–500 mg (max. per dose 5 mg/kg), to be followed by intravenous infusion. Please note for elderly patients the dose should be 300 micrograms/kg/hour, adjusted according to plasma-theophylline concentration (British National Formula (BNF), 2021).

Side effects: Potentially serious hypokalaemia (low serum potassium). Plasma-potassium concentration should therefore be monitored in severe asthma.

6Cs: Care

Caring for patients with reduced lung function requires nurses to listen and respect the patient's individual needs so as to deliver person-centred high-quality care in line with evidence-based clinical practice.

Obstructive sleep apnoea

During sleep skeletal muscle tone is reduced. This also occurs in the upper airways, however patients diagnosed with obstructive sleep apnoea it is more pronounced and leads to periods of airway obstruction. One of the major contributing factors is obesity. Patients experience poor sleep patterns and prolonged tiredness that can result in suddenly falling asleep during the day, which is particularly dangerous in some occupations such as driving. Treatment for sleep apnoea may necessitate the application of pressure through a Continuous Positive Airway Pressure (CPAP) mask to maintain the opening of the upper airways.

6Cs: Communication

The role of the nurse in communication with patients with lung failure may be compounded by mechanical obstructions such as CPAP masks or ET tubes. The patient may also be receiving medication that inhibits hearing and comprehension. The critical care nurse must find tools that can overcome these obstacles.

Orange Flag: psychological implications of compromised lung function

The nature of the treatment which may include the insertion of an endotracheal tube or tight-fitting face mask will remove the patient's ability to verbally communicate. The loss of speech as a means of communication frequently leads to a sense of vulnerability (Engström et al., 2013).

Prone positioning

The traditional method of caring for patients in critical care is in the semi-recumbent position or lying on their back with the head raised. However, gravitational forces can increase pulmonary oedema and atelectasis in the dependent posterior lung zones.

Recent studies by Guérin et al. (2020) and Venus et al. (2020) have indicated the benefits of prone positioning of patients who are hypoxic. Pneumonia is one of the commonest causes of admission to critical care and frequently leads to hypoxic respiratory failure. The lung can become 'wet' during pneumonia – this increases the pressure, squeezing gas out of the dependent (posterior) part of the lung. An analogy is a wet sponge, when all the water is at the bottom of the sponge, depressing the small holes of the sponge and there is a loss of aeration due to the weight of the fluid (oedema). Placing a patient in the prone position has been demonstrated as an effective intervention. The prone position is turning the patient face down which can result in physiological changes that improve oxygenation. These changes include a greater recruitment of the posterior zones of the lung allowing for increase exchange across the respiratory membrane. Prone positioning also allows a more equal distribution of stress forces caused by the diaphragm (Woodrow, 2019).

Orange Flag: psychological implications of compromised lung function

Breathlessness is a common symptom for patients requiring critical care and the psychological impact is underestimated by nurses and physicians (Haugdahl et al., 2017). The experience of dyspnoea is unique to each individual and therefore it is important that the clinician wherever possible should develop a therapeutic relationship with the patient to minimise the stress of breathlessness. It has been reported that there is increased anxiety within patients that have been mechanically ventilated (Rose et al., 2014). It has also been stated that patients that have experienced episodes of dyspnoea have higher anxiety and delusional memories of their admission to critical care.

6Cs: Courage

Caring for patients with lung disease at times can be very difficult and a certain amount of courage is required when informing patients and relatives that there may be a need for clinical interventions such as ventilation. Courage is also required when informing patients and/or relatives that the clinical interventions to assist lung function are failing. It is important that the nurse has the courage to escalate concerns when a patient has difficulty in breathing.

Conclusion

An understanding of how the lungs function is essential for nurses to develop further their knowledge and skills. A thorough assessment including the psychological impact for patients with impaired lung function is important when caring for acutely ill patients who may require non-invasive and invasive ventilatory support.

Take home points

1. The key function of the lungs is to permit oxygen to move from the air into the capillaries and carbon dioxide to move out.
2. Deterioration of the patient's lung function is seen as one of the first indicators of acute illness.
3. The nurse is required to undertake a thorough assessment of the patient who has issues with their breathing.
4. The psychological impact of breathlessness can be underestimated by nurses.
5. The role of the nurse in communication with patients with lung failure can be hindered by mechanical obstruction, for example, CPAP masks or ET tubes.
6. A sputum specimen is a useful indicator of lung pathology.
7. Treating patients with intelligent kindness and empathy is key to how they perceive their care.

References

British National Formulary (BNF) (2021). https://bnf.nice.org.uk/ (accessed 16 December 2020).

British Thoracic Society: SIGN (2019). British guideline on the management of asthma: A national clinical guideline. https://www.brit-thoracic.org.uk/quality-improvement/guidelines/asthma/ (accessed March 2022).

Colbert, B., Ankney, J., and Lee, K. (2019). *Anatomy & Physiology for Health Professions: An Interactive Journey*, 4e Essex: Pearson.

Credland, N. (2017). Respiratory anatomy and physiology. In: *Respiratory Care* (ed. V. Gibson and D. Waters), 1–14. London: Taylor & Francis.

National Competency Framework for Registered Nurses in Adult Critical Care (2015). Step 2 Competencies. Version 2: Critical Care Networks-National Nurse Leads (CC3N) https://www.cc3n.org.uk (accessed March 2022).

Dutton, H. and Finch, J. (2018). *Acute and Critical Care Nursing at a Glance*. Oxford: Wiley Blackwell.

Engström, Å., Nyström, N., Sundelin, G., and Rattray, J. (2013). People's experiences of being mechanically ventilated in an ICU: *Intensive & Critical Care Nursing* 29: 88–95. https://doi.org/10.101.

Guérin, C., Albert. R.K., Beitler, J. et al. (2020). Prone position in ARDS patients: Why, when, how and for whom. *Intensive Care Medicine* 46(12): 2385–2396.

King, G., James, A., Harkness, L., and Wark, P.A.B. (2018). Pathophysiology of severe asthma: We've only just started. *Respirology* 23(3): 262–271.

Haugdahl, H.S., Dahlberg, H., Klepstad, P., and Storli, S.L. (2017). The breath of life. patients' experiences of breathing during and after mechanical ventilation. *Intensive & Critical Care Nursing* 40: 85–93.

Marieb E.N. and Keller S.M. (2018). *Essentials of Human Anatomy & Physiology*, Global Edition, 12e. Essex: Pearson.

Montague, S., Watson, R., and Herbert, R. (2005). *Physiology for Nursing Practice*, 3e. Edinburgh: Elsevier.

Morton, P.G. and Fontaine D.K. (2013). *Essentials of Critical Care Nursing: A Holistic Approach*. London, Lippincott Williams & Wilkins.

Nursing and Midwifery Council (2018a). Future nurse: standards of proficiency for registered nurses, London: NMC. https://www.nmc.org.uk/standards/standards-for-nurses/standards-of-proficiency-for-registered-nurses/ (accessed March 2021).

Nursing and Midwifery Council. (2018b). The Code: Professional standards of practice and behaviour for nurses, midwives, and nursing associates. https://www.nmc.org.uk/standards/code/ (accessed 16 December 2020).

O'Driscoll, B.R., Howard, L.S., Earis, J., and Mak, V. (2017). BTS Guideline for Oxygen Use in Adults in Healthcare and Emergency Settings. *Thorax* 72. http://dx.doi.org/10.1136/thoraxjnl-2016-209729.

Papi, A. Brightling, C. Pedersen, S.E., and Reddel, H.K. (2018). Asthma. *The Lancet* (British Edition) 391.10122: 783.

Peate, I. (2018). Anatomy and physiology, 10. The respiratory system. *British Journal of Healthcare Assistants* 12(4): 178–181. doi:10.12968/bjha.2018.12.4.178.

Peate, I. and Evans, S. (2020). *Fundamentals of Anatomy and Physiology for Nursing and Healthcare Students*, 3e. Oxford: Wiley.

Peate, I. and Nair, M. (2015). *Anatomy and Physiology for Nurses at a Glance*. Oxford: Wiley-Blackwell.

Proctor, J., Rickards, E. (2020). How to perform chest auscultation and interpret the findings. *Nursing Times* 116(1): 23–26.

Resuscitation Guidelines UK (2015). www.resus.org.uk/resuscitation-guidelines (accessed 16 November 2020).

Rose, L., Nonoyama, M., Rezaie, S., and Fraser, I. (2014). Psychological wellbeing, health related quality of life and memories of intensive care and a specialised weaning centre reported by survivors of prolonged mechanical ventilation. *Intensive & Critical Care Nursing* 30(3): 145–151.

Royal College of Physicians. (2017). National Early Warning Score (NEWS) 2: Standardising the assessment of acute-illness severity in the NHS. https://www.rcplondon.ac.uk/projects/outputs/national-early-warning-score-news-2 (accessed 15 December 2020).

Shepherd, E. (2017). Specimen collection 4: procedure for obtaining a sputum specimen. *Nursing Times*.113(10): 49–51.

Venus, K., Munshi, L., and Fralick, M. (2020) Prone positioning for patients with hypoxic respiratory failure related to COVID-19. *Canadian Medical Association Journal* (CMAJ) 192.47. E1532–E1537.

Waugh, A. and Grant, A. (2018). *Ross and Wilson Anatomy & Physiology: in Health and Illness*, 13e. London: Elsevier.

West, J.B. and Luks, A.M. (2020). *West's Respiratory Physiology: The Essentials*, 11e. Philadelphia: Wolters Kluwer.

Wheeldon, A. (2018). The person with a respiratory disorder. In *Nursing Practice: Knowledge and Care*, 2e (ed. I. Peate and K. Wild.), 635–634. Oxford: John Wiley & Sons.

Woodrow, P. (2019). *Intensive Care Nursing*, 4e. London: Taylor & Francis.

Chapter 18

Cardiac physiology

Paul Sinnott

Aim

In this chapter we will review normal cardiac physiology and in doing so explore the impact of critical illness on cardiovascular function. Importantly, we will also focus on the role of the critical care practitioner in supporting patients with cardiovascular dysfunction.

Learning outcomes

After reading this chapter the reader will be able to:

- Review the functions of the cardiovascular system.
- Describe relevant anatomy of the heart and great vessels.
- Explore cardiovascular physiology in the context of the critically ill adult.
- Discuss therapies which support the cardiovascular system.
- Explore the implications of critical care therapies e.g. positive pressure ventilation on cardiovascular physiology.

Test your prior knowledge

- Can you name the four valves of the heart? Why are they important for normal cardiac function?
- What are the differences in structure between the left and right ventricle? Can you account for these variations?
- Can you identify the main contributors to cardiac output and how we might manipulate these in clinical practice?
- Are you able to identify three important diseases that affect the cardiovascular system?
- List as many drugs as you can that influence the cardiovascular system.

Fundamentals of Critical Care: A Textbook for Nursing and Healthcare Students, First Edition. Edited by Ian Peate and Barry Hill.
© 2023 John Wiley & Sons Ltd. Published 2023 by John Wiley & Sons Ltd.
Companion website: www.wiley.com/go/peate/criticalcare

6Cs: Competence

It is important you have both the knowledge and skills to effectively care for your patient.

Introduction

The human cardiovascular system can perform extraordinary feats. The heart will beat 2.5 billion times during an average lifespan, circulating the entire blood volume through 60,000 miles of arteries, capillaries and veins every six seconds. The statistics for cardiovascular disease are equally staggering. Despite significant improvements in both prevention and treatment, cardiovascular disease remains the leading cause of death globally (WHO, 2017). Within the United Kingdom it is estimated that 7.4 million people are living with cardiovascular disease and is responsible for more than a quarter (27%) of all death and a leading cause of admission to critical care units (BHF, 2020).

In addition, critical care units are also seeing an increase in patients admitted having experienced cardiac arrest, with the British Heart Foundation estimating there are 30,000 out-of-hospital cardiac arrests every year (BHF, 2020). Whilst survival remains low, with the advent of bystander cardiopulmonary resuscitation and automated defibrillation, many of these patients now survive to hospital and require admission to critical care units.

It is also important to note that whilst patients may not be admitted due to primary cardiovascular disease, the vast majority of critically ill patients will require some degree of cardiovascular support, with the Intensive Care National Audit and Research Centre (ICNARC, 2019) identifying 89% of all patients as requiring some degree of cardiovascular support.

It is then clear that cardiovascular disease is an important cause of both morbidity and mortality in critically ill adults. As such the critical care practitioner must have an awareness of important pathologies and demonstrate competence in cardiovascular monitoring and therapies.

Critical Care Competencies: National standards

1:3.1 Anatomy & Physiology (Critical Care Networks-National Nurse Leads (CC3N), 2015a)

You must be able to demonstrate essential knowledge of:

- Structure and function of the heart (include chambers and valves)
- Identify major/minor blood vessels
- Oxygenated/deoxygenated blood flow

2:2.1 Assessment, Monitoring & Observation (Critical Care Networks-National Nurse Leads (CC3N), 2015b)

You must be able to demonstrate your knowledge through discussion, and the application to your practice:

- Determinants of the normal cardiac cycle
- Determinants of cardiac output
- Determinants of blood pressure
- Determinants of central venous pressure
- Normal Cardiac conduction pathway
- Effects of ventilation on the cardiovascular system

Functions of the cardiovascular system

The cardiovascular system has several key functions including:

- **Transport:** The movement of nutrients, gases and waste products around the body is crucial for cellular respiration and organ function.
- **Communication:** Utilising various hormone systems to communicate throughout the body e.g. antidiuretic hormone is released in the brain (hypothalamus) stimulating water reabsorption in the kidney.
- **Thermoregulation:** The manipulation of blood flow to the skin allows the regulation of temperature.
- **Protection:** Within the blood, components of the immune and coagulation system protect against infection and blood loss in the advent of injury.

Red Flag: chest pain

Chest pain is a common presentation in critically ill patients. It is crucial that patients are thoroughly investigated, whilst many causes of chest pain are relatively benign it is also associated with life-threatening conditions such as myocardial infarction and aortic dissection (Robertson et al., 2013)

6Cs: Commitment

You must have the commitment to gain the knowledge and skills required to care for critically ill patients.

Anatomy of the heart and great vessels

The heart lies within the mediastinum in the centre of the thorax with the apex projecting into the left hemithorax. It is protected by the sternum anteriorly and the vertebral column posteriorly. In essence the heart is a pump for two

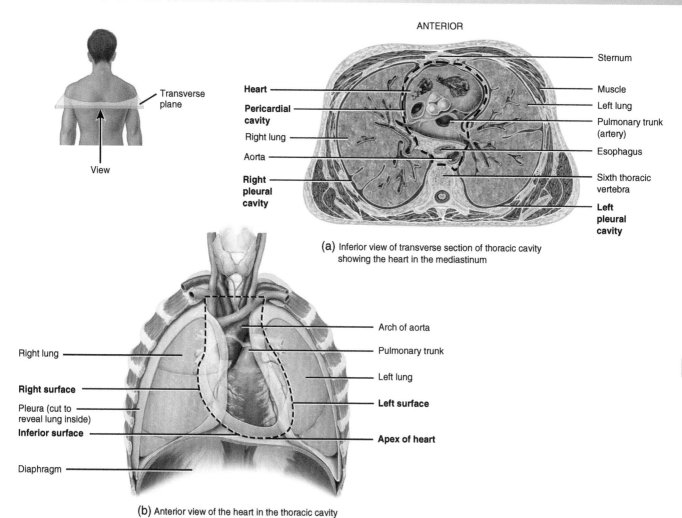

Figure 18.1 Position of the heart and associated structures. *Source:* Tortora and Derrickson (2017) with permission of John Wiley & Sons.

interconnected circulations (pulmonary and systemic). The right side of the heart receives deoxygenated blood from the systemic circulation via the inferior and superior vena cava and pumps this blood to the lungs via the pulmonary arteries. The left side of the heart receives oxygenated blood from the lungs through the pulmonary veins and pumps this blood to the systemic circulation via the aorta (see Figure 18.1).

Pericardium

The heart is surrounded by the pericardium. The outer fibrous pericardium is a tough connective tissue layer providing protection and points of attachment to anchor the heart within the mediastinum. The serous pericardium consists of two layers (parietal and visceral), the parietal layer lines the inner surface of the fibrous pericardium and the visceral layer the outer surface of the heart. These two layers are separated by a small amount of pericardial fluid with allows the heart to contract in a low-friction environment. Disease can occur if these layers become inflamed (pericarditis) or excessive

pericardial fluid accumulates (pericardial effusion) potentially leading to cardiac tamponade, a life-threatening condition where compression of the right ventricle prevents filling during diastole and can lead to cardiac arrest (see Figure 18.2).

Layers of the heart

The wall of the heart can be divided into three distinct layers, the outermost epicardium, which is formed by the visceral pericardium and covers a layer of adipose (fatty) tissue which supports the coronary blood vessels. The myocardium forms the bulk of the heart wall and consists primarily of myocytes, cardiac muscles cells which are packed with myofibrils, contractile proteins which allow the myocytes to contract. Myocytes are arranged in bundles which wrap around the heart to allow effective cardiac contraction. Finally, the innermost layer is the endocardium, a layer of endothelial cells which forms the inner surface of the heat and joins with the endothelial lining of the large vessels and the cardiac valves. Inflammation or infection of this layer can result in endocarditis.

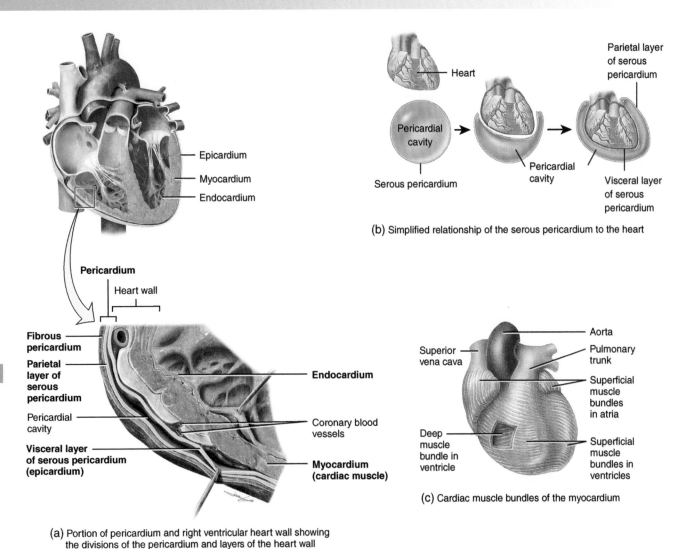

Figure 18.2   Pericardium and heart wall. *Source:* Tortora and Derrickson (2017) with permission of John Wiley & Sons.

Chambers of the heart

The heart is separated into four chambers, two atria and two ventricles. The atria receive venous blood from the systemic circulation to the right atria via the vena cava and the from the lungs to the left atria from the four pulmonary veins. The atria are separated by the intra-atrial septum, which contains the remnants of the foramen ovale, an important structure which allows blood to cross the heart during fetal development. The foramen ovale should close during the first 12 months of life but in some individuals the opening persists into adulthood (patent foramen ovale). This can increase the risk of strokes in these individuals as clots which form in the venous circulation can cross the heart and be embolised into the systemic circulation.

The two ventricles receive blood from the atria during diastole and are 'topped up' by the atria contracting. The left ventricle pumps blood to the systemic circulation through the aorta and the right ventricle to the lung via the pulmonary artery. The morphology (shape) of the left and right ventricle are quite different, which is to be expected if you consider the 'work' they both do. The left ventricle must generate higher systemic pressures to be able to pump blood around the body whereas the right ventricle must generate significantly less pressure to perfuse the pulmonary vasculature (lungs). As a result, the left ventricular wall is significant more muscular than the right (see Figure 18.3).

Valves of the heart

The heart valves ensure unidirectional flow through the heart and are essential for normal cardiac function. They are comprised of a connective tissue core and covered with the same endothelial lining that constitutes the endocardium of the heart. There are two types of valve: the atrioventricular valves which separate the atrial from the ventricles and the semilunar valves which separate the ventricles from the aorta and pulmonary artery.

The two atrioventricular valves separate the atria from the ventricles with the mitral valve on the left and tricuspid on the right. These valves are open when the heart is at rest (diastole) allowing blood to fill the ventricles and close when

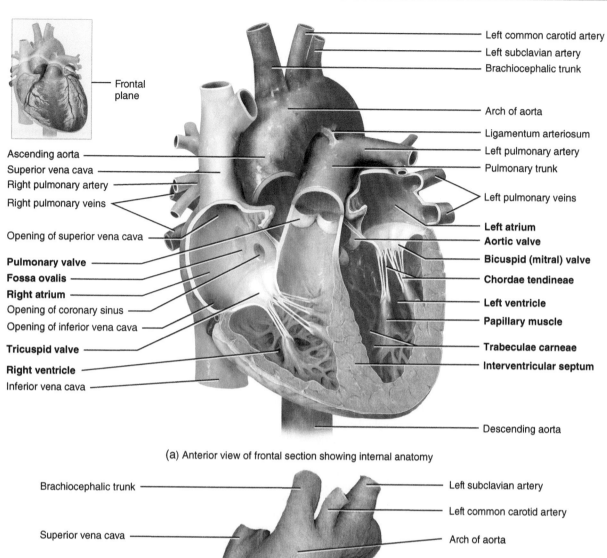

Frontal plane

Left common carotid artery
Left subclavian artery
Brachiocephalic trunk

Arch of aorta
Ligamentum arteriosum
Left pulmonary artery
Pulmonary trunk

Left pulmonary veins

Ascending aorta
Superior vena cava
Right pulmonary artery
Right pulmonary veins

Opening of superior vena cava

Pulmonary valve
Fossa ovalis
Right atrium
Opening of coronary sinus
Opening of inferior vena cava

Tricuspid valve

Right ventricle
Inferior vena cava

Left atrium
Aortic valve
Bicuspid (mitral) valve
Chordae tendineae

Left ventricle

Papillary muscle

Trabeculae carneae
Interventricular septum

Descending aorta

(a) Anterior view of frontal section showing internal anatomy

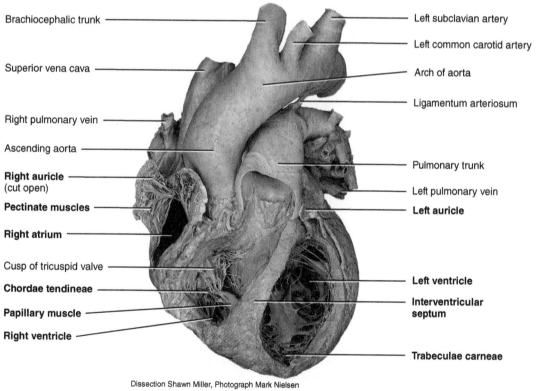

Brachiocephalic trunk

Superior vena cava

Right pulmonary vein

Ascending aorta

Right auricle
(cut open)

Pectinate muscles

Right atrium

Cusp of tricuspid valve

Chordae tendineae

Papillary muscle

Right ventricle

Left subclavian artery

Left common carotid artery

Arch of aorta

Ligamentum arteriosum

Pulmonary trunk

Left pulmonary vein

Left auricle

Left ventricle

Interventricular septum

Trabeculae carneae

Dissection Shawn Miller, Photograph Mark Nielsen
(b) Anterior view of partially sectioned heart

Figure 18.3 Internal structures of the heart. *Source:* Tortora and Derrickson (2017) with permission from John Wiley & Sons.

231

ANTERIOR

Transverse plane

View

Right ventricle

Interventricular septum

Lumen

Lumen

Left ventricle

Dissection Shawn Miller, Photograph Mark Nielsen

(c) Inferior view of transverse section showing differences in thickness of ventricular walls

Figure 18.3 (Continued)

the heart begins to contract (systole). Because the atrioventricular valves stop the backflow of blood into the atria during systolic contraction, they have elaborated sub-valvular structures, the chordae and papillary muscles, which act as guy ropes supporting the valves. Damage to the mitral sub-valvular structures, for example papillary muscle rupture because of myocardial infarction, can result in severe regurgitation (backflow), leading to life-threatening heart failure (see Figure 18.4).

The two semilunar valves stop the backflow of blood into the ventricles after contraction (systole). The aortic valve prevents backflow into the left ventricle and the pulmonary valve the right. Aortic stenosis (narrowing of the valve) is the most common valvular abnormality and significantly increases the workload of the left ventricle during systole, eventually leading to heart failure, angina and syncope (loss of consciousness because of reduced blood flow to the brain).

Coronary circulation

The coronary arteries and veins supply and drain blood to and from the heart muscle (myocardium). The coronary arteries are the first branches arising from the ascending aorta and divide many times creating an intricate network of collateral vessels ensuring a good blood supply. The coronary veins drain blood from the heart muscle and return it to the right atria via the coronary sinus. When considering the blood supply to the heart it is important to note a key difference when compared to the rest of the circulation. The perfusion of organs around the body takes place during systole. However, as the heart is contracting during systole there is limited blood flow through the coronary arteries. It is not until the heart begins to relax at the start of diastole that the diastolic pressure in the aorta drives blood through the coronaries arteries thus perfusing the heart. As such, regarding coronary perfusion, diastolic pressure is the key determinant of blood flow (see Figure 18.5).

6Cs: Care

Despite the advanced monitoring and therapies within a critical care environment the nursing care we deliver is just as important.

6Cs: Examination scenario: heart sounds

Auscultation of heart sounds can help diagnose diseases of the heart valves.

Heart sounds consist of two distinct sounds: S_1, the closure of the tricuspid and mitral valves, and S_2, the closure of the aortic and pulmonary valves. The closure of these valves gives rise to the characteristic "lub dub" heard on auscultation.

Additional noises (murmurs) in between these two sounds can often indicate turbulent blood flow through damaged heart valves.

Snapshot: chest pain

Peter is a 56-year-old patient who was admitted to the Surgical High Dependency Unit following a Whipple's procedure (pancreaticoduodenectomy) for cholangiocarcinoma. He has a past medical history of diabetes (type II), hypertension and hypercholesterolemia. The day after his operation he is complaining of central crushing chest pain which is radiating down his left arm.

Airway (A): Patent.

Breathing (B): Nasal high flow oxygen (FiO$_2$ 0.6), Respiratory rate 26 bpm (2), SpO$_2$ 100%.

Circulation (C): Sinus Tachycardia (120 bpm), BP 150/92 mmHg (0), capillary refill time 4 sec, cool peripheries, sweating (diaphoretic), Tympanic temperature 36°C (0).

Disability (D): Patient is alert (0), complaining of central chest pain (8/10).

Exposure (E): Nil of note.

NEWS2 score: 6.

Impression

In this case study Peter's pain is characteristic for cardiac ischaemia which is often described as

- Central/Retrosternal
- Heavy/Crushing in nature
- Radiates into the left arm or jaw
- Is associated with nausea, dyspnoea (shortness of breath) and diaphoresis (sweating)

Care plan

- Inform medical team
- Regular clinical observations
- 12-lead ECG (to look for signs of ischaemia)
- Routine bloods including troponin (troponin in the blood would suggest myocytes have been damaged)
- Consider glyceryl trinitrate spray (GTN) followed by intravenous morphine if the pain does not resolve
- Patient with cardiac ischaemia should be prescribed aspirin if there are no contraindications
- Titrate oxygen to maintain a SpO$_2$ > 94%

Can you think of any patient groups who may not present with pain even if suffering from cardiac ischaemia?

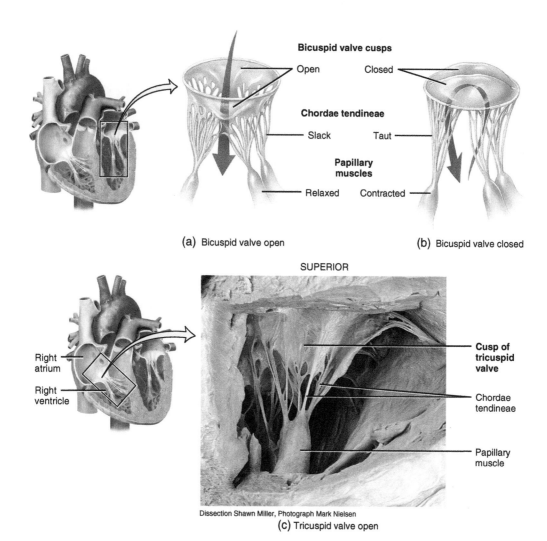

(a) Bicuspid valve open

(b) Bicuspid valve closed

(c) Tricuspid valve open

Dissection Shawn Miller, Photograph Mark Nielsen

Figure 18.4 The heart valves. *Source:* Tortora and Derrickson (2017) with permission from John Wiley & Sons.

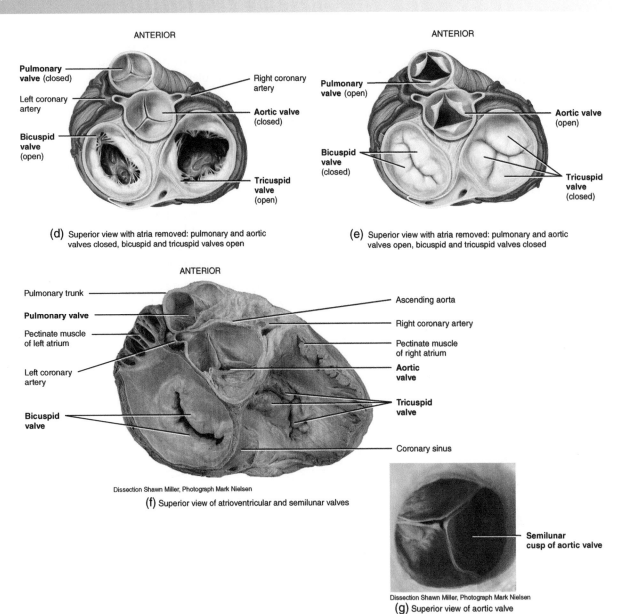

234

ANTERIOR

Pulmonary valve (closed)
Left coronary artery
Bicuspid valve (open)

Right coronary artery
Aortic valve (closed)
Tricuspid valve (open)

(d) Superior view with atria removed: pulmonary and aortic valves closed, bicuspid and tricuspid valves open

ANTERIOR

Pulmonary valve (open)
Bicuspid valve (closed)

Aortic valve (open)
Tricuspid valve (closed)

(e) Superior view with atria removed: pulmonary and aortic valves open, bicuspid and tricuspid valves closed

ANTERIOR

Pulmonary trunk
Pulmonary valve
Pectinate muscle of left atrium
Left coronary artery
Bicuspid valve

Ascending aorta
Right coronary artery
Pectinate muscle of right atrium
Aortic valve
Tricuspid valve
Coronary sinus

Dissection Shawn Miller, Photograph Mark Nielsen

(f) Superior view of atrioventricular and semilunar valves

Semilunar cusp of aortic valve

Dissection Shawn Miller, Photograph Mark Nielsen

(g) Superior view of aortic valve

Figure 18.4 (Continued)

Condition: angina pectoris

Angina pectoris is characterised as chest pain caused by myocardial ischaemia. It is most often caused when the coronary arteries narrow and stiffen because of atherosclerosis, an inflammatory process which results in fatty plaque formation in muscular arteries. The reduction in blood flow because of these plaques leads to a decrease in oxygen delivered to the myocardium, with the resultant ischaemia triggering the sensation of pain. Treatment includes medication to reduced myocardial oxygen demand (beta-blockers) and promote coronary artery vasodilation (glyceryl trinitrate).

Medications management: glyceryl trinitrate (GTN)

Nitrates in both short- and long-acting preparations are used to treat patients with angina pectoris. Nitrates work by inducing vasodilation in both arteries and veins. Venodilation reduces the amount of blood returning to the heart (preload) which in turn reduces myocardial workload and therefore myocardial oxygen demand. Arterial dilation is thought to improve blood flow through the coronary arteries, improving myocardial oxygen delivery. Side effect can include dizziness, hypotension, and headaches. (BNF, 2020; Neal, 2016)

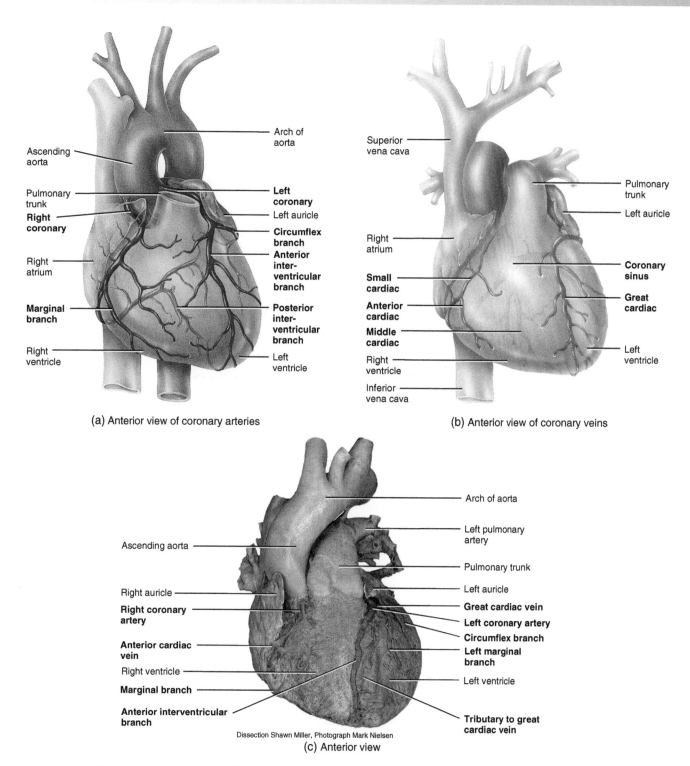

Figure 18.5   The coronary circulation. *Source:* Tortora and Derrickson (2017) with permission from John Wiley & Sons.

Cardiac conduction system

Throughout the heart there are specialised conduction tissues. These play a crucial role as the cardiac pacemaker but also provide rapid conduction pathways which allow the heart to contract in a co-ordinated manner e.g. right and left ventricle contracting together.

The main cardiac pacemaker, the sinoatrial node is found in the right atrium. Cells within the node are 'autorhythmic',

that is, they are capable of stimulating myocytes (depolarisation) with no external input. Indeed, this why a transplanted heart continues to beat despite the nervous supply to the heart being cut (denervation). The intrinsic rate of sinoatrial firing can, however, be influenced by both neural and hormonal input allowing the regulation of heart rate. Following triggering of the sinoatrial role and the subsequent depolarisation and contraction of the atria the atrio-ventricular

235

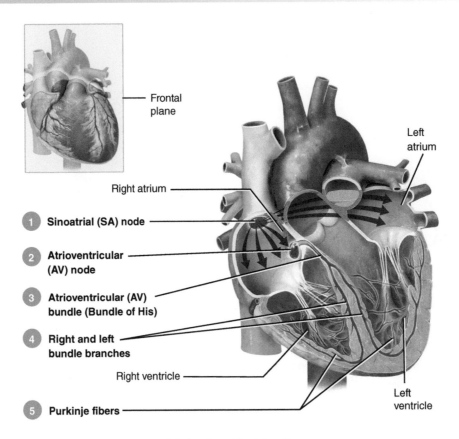

Figure 18.6   The cardiac conduction system. *Source:* Tortora and Derrickson (2017) with permission of John Wiley & Sons.

node conducts the cardiac depolarisation to the ventricles. From the atrioventricular node the signal spreads down specialised conduction pathways, the common, left and right bundle branches to the bottom of the heart (apex). From here the wave of depolarisation spreads up ventricles, again assisted by specialised conduction pathways, the Purkinje fibres. These pathways are key in ensuring ventricular contraction is both efficient and coordinated (See Figure 18.6).

Clinical investigations: 12-lead electrocardiogram (ECG)

The electrocardiogram records the electrical activity produced by the contraction of the heart muscle. There are normal waveforms associated with each element of the cardiac cycle (P,QRS,T waves). Changes to the shape and timings of these waveforms can give an indication of a cardiac abnormality.

The 12-lead ECG differs from continuous cardiac monitoring in that it uses 10 physical leads to generate 12 views of the heart and could be more usefully called a '12-view electrocardiogram'.

Each of these views can be thought of as a camera looking at a specific anatomical segment of the heart, thus allowing clinicians to pinpoint where in the heart the abnormality lies. We will explore using the ECG to identify arrhythmias in the next chapter.

Red Flag: medication errors

The incidence of medication errors is highest amongst patients within critical care units when compared to general wards (Wilmer et al., 2010). The reasons for this are multifactorial but include the frequency and complexity of drug administration in these areas. In this chapter we have discussed several high-risk medications including noradrenaline, which if incorrectly administered, could result in life-threatening complications. The critical care nurse is key in the prevention of such errors through the maintenance of high standards and the adoption of safe practices.

The cardiac cycle

The cardiac cycle describes a series of electrical and mechanical events which occur throughout each heartbeat, resulting in the ejection of blood from both the right and left ventricles. It can be separated into distinct phases: diastole during which the heart is in a relaxed state allowing it to fill with blood, and a second phase systole where the myocardium is contracting. The contraction of the atria shortly followed by the contraction of the ventricles in conjunction with the heart valves ensures a unidirectional flow of blood through the heat, resulting in systolic ejection of blood into the systemic and pulmonary circulations.

1. In Figure 18.7 we join the cardiac cycle during diastole where blood is returning to both atria. As the pressure in the atria increases the atrioventricular valves open, allowing blood from the atria to flow into the ventricles. This passive filling of the ventricles during diastole is responsible for 80% of the total ventricular volume. At the end of diastole, following stimulation from the sinoatrial node (depolarisation), the atria begin to contract. This contraction essentially 'tops up' the ventricles and is responsible for 20% of ventricular volume (atrial systole).

2. Following atrial contraction, depolarisation is transmitted through the atrioventricular node and down the specialised ventricular conduction pathways, resulting in a wave of contraction spreading from the apex of the heart (ventricular systole). This leads to a sharp rise in ventricular pressure which forces the atrioventricular valves shut. Pressure continues to increase within the ventricles and eventually exceeds the pressure on the other side of the semi-lunar valves (aortic & pulmonary) forcing them open, allowing blood to be ejected into the systemic and pulmonary circulation. It is important to remember that the pressures generated during systole are significantly different when comparing the left (~120 mmHg) and the right (~15 mmHg) ventricles.

3. At the end of systole, the ventricles relax, leading to an immediate drop in ventricular pressure. As the pressure in the aorta and pulmonary artery (diastolic pressure) is now greater than ventricular pressure, the semi-lunar valves are forced shut. This heralds the start of diastole as the atria and ventricles begin to fill again.

Condition: acute coronary syndrome

Acute coronary syndromes encompass a group of clinical symptoms caused by the partial or complete occlusion of a coronary artery. This occlusion most often occurs because of the rupture of an atherosclerotic (fatty) plaque triggering the formation of a blood clot (thrombus). We differentiate between the three acute coronary syndromes by characteristic changes to the 12-lead ECG and the measurement of troponin, a cardiac biomarker that is only present in the blood after the myocardium is damaged.

The acute coronary syndromes are:

- Unstable angina
- Non-ST elevation myocardial infarction (NSTEMI)
- ST elevation myocardial infarction (STEMI)

Treatment includes unblocking the culprit coronary artery using coronary angioplasty and drugs to prevent the formation of more clots, dual anti-platelet therapies (DAPT) e.g. aspirin and ticagrelor (Gurbel et al., 2014, Kumar and Cannon, 2009)

Medications management: ticagrelor

Ticagrelor is an orally administered drug which reduces platelet aggregation and therefore inhibits the formation of clots. Unsurprisingly the main adverse effect is bleeding (BNF, 2020, Neal, 2016).

In combination with aspirin, ticagrelor has been found effective in reducing further ischaemic events in patients who have suffered a myocardial infarction or had a stent inserted to unblock a coronary artery (Wallentin et al., 2009, Yusuf et al., 2001, Chen et al., 2005).

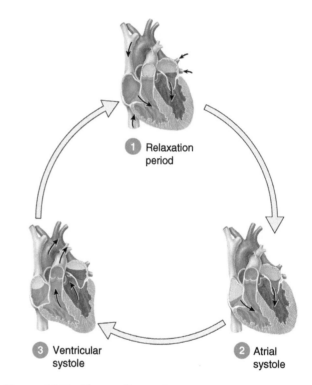

1 Relaxation period

3 Ventricular systole

2 Atrial systole

Figure 18.7   The cardiac cycle.

Cardiac output and blood pressure

Cardiac output is defined as the amount of blood ejected by the heart per minute with a normal cardiac output at rest between 4–6 l/min. It is determined by two factors, heart rate and stroke volume, the amount of blood ejected per beat (Figure 18.8).

Heart Rate (HR) × Stroke Volume (SV) = Cardiac Output (CO)
70 bpm × 70 mls = 4.9 L/min

Figure 18.8   Cardiac output.

Cardiac output can increase significantly to meet metabolic demands by altering both heart rate and stroke volume with some athletes able to increase their cardiac output to over 30 l/min. Cardiac output is intrinsically linked with blood pressure which can be defined as the pressure blood exerts on the walls of the arteries and is influenced by cardiac output, blood viscosity and systemic vascular resistance (SVR), the degree of vasoconstriction in the circulation.

Red Flag: Venous thromboembolism (VTE)

Veno-thromboembolic phenomena such as deep vein thrombosis and pulmonary embolism are both a common, potentially serious complication of critical illness with Minet et al. (2015) reporting an incidence of up to 27% in autopsy studies. It is therefore important when caring for critically ill patients that the nurse is observing for the signs of VTE and ensuring treatments such as low molecular weight heparin and mechanical thromboprophylaxis are administered.

Regulation of heart rate

The regulation of heart rate allows cardiac output to match metabolic demand and respond to physiological stressors such as hypovolemia. Remember, the sinoatrial node is autorhythmic and left to its own devices would depolarise 80–100 times per minute. This intrinsic heart rate, however, can be influenced by both neurological and biochemical mechanisms.

Neural regulation is controlled by the cardiovascular centre, part of autonomic nervous system found within the brain stem. This centre receives information from various tissues including baroreceptors in the major vessels (aorta and carotid) which detect blood pressure, proprioceptors in skeletal muscle and even the limbic system which accounts for the effect of emotional states, such as fear, on heart rate. Sympathetic neurones which project from the cardiovascular centre via the spinal cord to the cardiac conduction system and the myocardium increase heart rate (and cardiac contractility) by releasing the neurotransmitter, norepinephrine which stimulates Beta one adrenoreceptors (β_1) (see Table 18.1). Parasympathetic neurones carried via the vagus nerve synapse with the sinoatrial and atrioventricular nodes and decrease heart rate through the release of the neurotransmitter acetylcholine which acts on muscarinic receptors. These inputs are not on or off, there is a constant balance between sympathetic and parasympathetic activity regulating heart rate. Understanding these mechanisms allows us to manipulate heart rate in clinal practice. For example, in patients with an inappropriately slow heart rate (bradycardia) the drug atropine, which blocks the action of acetylcholine can lead to an increase in heart rate by reducing parasympathetic tone.

There are a number of biochemical factors that can also influence heart rate. Hormones such as epinephrine and norepinephrine have the same action as the sympathetic nervous system when released from the adrenal gland in response to exercise, stress and illness. Other hormones such thyroid and growth hormones can also lead to an increase in heart rate, as well as changes in temperature, with pyrexia resulting in an increased heart rate and hypothermia a decreased heart rate.

Table 18.1   An overview of the action of adrenoreceptors.

Receptor type	Location	Actions	Agonist drugs	Antagonist drug
Alpha – 1 (α_1)	Arterial smooth muscle Visceral smooth muscles Pupillary muscles	Smooth muscle contraction Vasoconstriction Pupil dilation	Norepinephrine	Doxazosin
Alpha – 2 (α_1)	Central nervous system	Inhibits the release of noradrenaline in the central nervous system Antihypertensive and sedative effects	Clonidine	
Beta – 1 (β_1)	Heart Kidney	Increase heart rate (chronotropy) Increase force of contractions (inotropy) Increase renin release	Dobutamine	Bisoprolol
Beta – 2 (β_2)	Bronchiole smooth muscle Liver Skeletal muscle	Bronchial dilation Vasodilation Inhibits insulin secretion	Salbutamol	

Stroke volume

There are three key contributing factors to stroke volume: preload, contractility and afterload.

Preload

Ventricular preload is essentially the pressure exerted on the ventricular wall by the volume of blood in the ventricle at the end of diastole, i.e. when the heart is at its fullest, end-diastolic volume (EDV). End-diastolic volume is a combination of two factors: the amount of blood that is left in the ventricle after the previous systolic contraction and the amount of venous blood returned to the heart. An import relationship exists between preload and stroke volume. Within a physiological range, increasing preload leads to an increase in ventricular contractility and therefore stroke volume (see Figure 18.9). This relationship was described by two physiologists, Otto Frank and Ernest Starting (the Frank–Starling Law). It is essential for normal cardiac function as it allows the heart to cope with an increase in preload without resulting in over-distention of the ventricle. This explains why hypovolemia (reduced pre-load) has such a deleterious effect on cardiac output and therefore blood pressure. The physiological mechanisms are complex, but a not unreasonable analogy would be that of an elastic band, the more you stretch the band the stronger the recoil. This analogue also helps to illustrate the limitations of the Frank–Starling relationship. If the ventricle is over-distended due to excessive preload the contractile fibres in the myocytes are disrupted and contractility reduces, the elastic band has snapped. We see this in patients who are fluid-overloaded and subsequently develop ventricular dysfunction (heart failure).

Contractility

Cardiac contractility is defined as the tension and velocity of myofibril shortening and can effectively be thought of as the strength of contraction. Several factors can affect contractility, preload as discussed above, the level of sympathetic activity from the autonomic nervous system and the adequacy of myocardial oxygen supply. Drugs that alter contractility are termed inotropes. They may have a positive inotropic effect, that is they increase contractility, examples would include epinephrine, dobutamine and digoxin (see Figure 18.9). Drugs with a negative inotropic effect such as beta-blockers reduced contractility. While this may sound counterintuitive, this is often a desired effect as it reduces myocardial oxygen demand for example in the treatment of angina or blood pressure when treating hypertension.

Afterload

Afterload is the resistance against the ejection of blood from the ventricle. Remember that during the cardiac cycle for the aortic and pulmonary valves, to open the ventricles must overcome the opposing pressure keeping the valves closed – this is effectively the afterload the ventricle is working against. Two important factors affect afterload: semilunar valve function and systemic vascular resistance. An increase in systemic vascular resistance or a narrowed valve (stenosis) can therefore increase afterload and lead to a reduction in stroke volume but also importantly increase ventricular work and therefore oxygen demand. Clinically, it is often beneficial to reduced afterload to support a struggling ventricle, for example in left ventricular failure, patients will often be prescribed glyceryl trinitrate (GTN), which results in both arterial and venous dilation. This often has the paradoxical effect of reducing blood pressure because of both a reduction in preload (venous dilation) and afterload (arterial dilation) but leads to an improvement in ventricular function as the struggling ventricle has to work less and therefore cardiac output can increase.

239

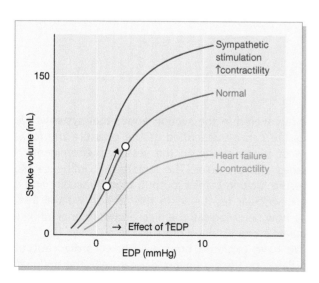

Figure 18.9 Frank–Starling relationship. *Source:* Jeremy and Roger (2017) with permission of John Wiley & Sons.

Medications management: dobutamine

Dobutamine is an intravenous inotropic drug. It exerts its effects predominantly by the activation adrenoreceptors in the heart leading to an increase in contractility and therefore stroke volumes. It can be used to improve cardiac output in patients with heart failure. Adverse effects include tachycardia and arrhythmia (BNF, 2020, Neal, 2016).

Snapshot: left ventricular failure

Mary is a 74-year-old female who had been admitted to the high dependency unit with severe shortness of breath. She has a history of heart failure, diabetes, hypercholesterolemia.

Airway (A): Patent.
Breathing (B): SpO$_2$ 84% (2), Oxygen via a non-rebreathe mask at 12 L/min (2), RR – 32 bpm (3), auscultation reveals bibasal crackles.
Circulation (C): Sinus Tachycardia (110 bpm) (1), BP 90/50 mmHg (2), capillary refill time 5 sec, cool peripheries, tympanic temperature 36.0 °C (0).
Disability (D): Patient is responding to voice (3), PEARL.
Exposure (E): Pitting oedema to lower limbs.
NEWS2 score: 13.

Investigations

Chest X-ray: Widespread pulmonary infiltrates consistent with pulmonary oedema.
Echocardiogram: Severe left ventricular systolic dysfunction, Ejection fraction < 30%.
NT-pro BNP: 2505 pg/ml.
Impression: Acute respiratory failure due to decompensated heart failure and pulmonary oedema.

Care plan

- Commence continuous positive airway pressure (CPAP).
- Titrate oxygen to maintain SO2 > 94%.
- Commence furosemide infusion and aim for negative fluid balance.
- Commence dobutamine infusion.

After reviewing the chapter try to explain the rational for Mary's care plan

Clinical investigations: B-type natriuretic peptide (NT-pro BNP)

B-type natriuretic peptide (NT-pro BNP) is a hormone released by cells in the wall of the heart when stretched because of fluid overload. Its action is to increase urine production and thus reduce fluid overload.

In patients who present with breathlessness it can be difficult to determine if the cause is due to heart failure causing pulmonary oedema or a primary respiratory problem. Measuring NT-pro BNP can help with this diagnostic conundrum, low levels of NT-pro BNP would exclude heart failure as the cause of breathlessness (NICE 2014, 2018; Oremus et al., 2014)

6Cs: Communication

Good communication is essential when working within large multidisciplinary teams in an often-stressful environment.

Condition: heart failure

Heart failure can be simply defined at the hearts inability to generate an adequate cardiac output. This results in two key problems which are responsible for the symptoms patient with heart failure experience.

There is inadequate perfusion of the tissue leading to lethargy, reduced exercise tolerance and organ dysfunction, e.g. renal failure. Secondly, because the heart is not able to eject blood from the ventricles the pressure during diastole (relaxation) increases, this increase in pressure results in 'back pressure' in the lungs resulting in breathlessness (pulmonary oedema) and also increased venous pressure in the system circulation leading to peripheral oedema.

We now have an understating that heart failure can be the result of either systolic dysfunction, the pumping ability of the heart or diastolic dysfunction where an abnormal stiff ventricle results in problems during filling, or often a combination of both. Because of this new understanding we now classify heart failure as either

- Heart Failure with Reduced Ejection Fraction (HFrEF) (Systolic)
- Heart failure with Preserved Ejection fraction (HFpEF) (Diastolic)

The regulation of blood pressure

We discovered in the section above that systemic blood pressure can be described as the pressure the forward flow of blood exerts on the vessels, predominantly the arteries and arterioles. The factors that influence blood pressure include cardiac output, blood viscosity and systemic vascular resistance. In this section we will investigate how neurological, chemical and hormonal influences regulate systemic blood pressure

We have explored previously how cardiac output is regulated by the cardiovascular centre in the brain stem. This centre plays an equally important role in the regulation of blood pressure. The cardiovascular centre receives input from blood pressure sensing baroreceptors, motion sensing proprioceptors and chemoreceptors that are able detect changes in the plasma concentration of oxygen, carbon dioxide and hydrogen ions (how acidic the blood is).

Baroreceptors in the aortic arch and the carotid arteries detect changes in blood pressure. A fall in blood pressure leads to a reduction in the frequency of nerve impulses to the cardiovascular centre which triggers several responses. A reduction in parasympathetic tone leads to an increase in heart rate. Simultaneously, there is an increase in sympathetic innervation, further increasing heart rate, ventricular contractility and stimulating vasoconstriction in arteries and arterioles. The combined effects lead to an increase in cardiac output and systemic vascular resistance and therefore blood pressure. This baroreflex is important in maintaining an adequate blood pressure in response to sudden changes in posture and blood volume. For example, the simple act of standing results in a sudden drop in cardiac preload as blood drains into the lower limbs. If left unopposed this would result in a significant drop in blood pressure and possibly loss of conscious due to poor cerebral perfusion (syncope). We see this response in individuals who exhibit postural hypotension. The baroreflex, however, results in an increase in both cardiac output and systemic vascular resistance thus restoring blood pressure.

Chemoreceptors provide a further mechanism by which blood pressure is regulated. These receptors within the aorta and carotid arteries can detect changes in oxygen, carbon dioxide and hydrogens ion levels. These receptors essentially detect the signs of physiological stress, hypoxia (low oxygen), elevated carbon dioxide levels and metabolic acidosis (increased hydrogen ion concentration). In response the cardiovascular centre increases blood pressure by boosting sympathetic output to compensate.

Finally, there are numerous hormone systems which help regulate blood pressure through changes in cardiac output, systemic vascular resistance or blood volume. It is beyond the scope of this chapter to discuss these in detail, but they are summarised in Table 18.2.

Examination scenarios: pulsus paradoxus

It is tempting to think that with the available monitoring technology within a modern critical care unit a physical patient assessment is unnecessary. This could not be further from the truth.

A good example is the palpation of a pulse. In the next chapter you will examine this further, but changes to pulse character can give vital information. A good example is pulsus paradoxus, a pronounced variation in pulse volume coinciding with respiration. The pulse volume increases during expiration and decreases during inspiration, whilst some variation is normal a significant difference can indicate several significant diseases which results in an increased pressure surrounding the heart e.g. accumulation of pericardial fluid (cardiac tamponade) or constrictive pericarditis (Robertson et al., 2013).

Table 18.2   Hormones involves in the regulation of blood pressure. Source: adapted from Tortora and Derrickson, 2017.

Hormone	Mechanism of action	Blood pressure
Epinephrine Norepinephrine	Released from the adrenal gland in response to sympathetic innervation. Results in an increase in heartrate (β_1), cardiac contractility (β_1) and systemic vascular resistance (α_1)	Increased
Angiotensin II	Reduced blood flow to the kidney triggers the renin-angiotensin system (RAS) which ultimately leads to the production of angiotensin II. Angiotensin II is a potent arterial vasoconstrictor and increases systemic vascular resistance.	Increased
Aldosterone	Released from the adrenal glands in response to angiotensin II and increased plasma potassium levels. Increases sodium reabsorption in the kidney which promotes water reabsorption and results in an increase in blood volume.	Increased
Antidiuretic Hormone	Release from the pituitary gland in response to dehydration (increased blood osmolarity) and angiotensin II. Increases water reabsorption in the kidney and results in an increased blood volume.	Increased
Natriuretic peptides	Released from cells within the atria and ventricles in response to over-distension (fluid overload). Inhibits the effects of renin and promotes water loss in the kidney.	Decreased

Snapshot: aortic dissection

Bill is a 66-year-old patient who has just been admitted to the intensive care unit. He presented to the emergency department with sudden onset severe chest pain which he describes as sharp and radiating to his back. His past medical history included hypertension and hypercholesteremia.

A CT aortogram demonstrates that Bill has suffered an aortic dissection and he is transferred to the intensive care unit for further management.

Airway (A): Patent.
Breathing (B): Respiratory rate 22 bpm (2), SpO$_2$ 96% on room air (0).
Circulation (C): Sinus tachycardia (125 bpm) (2), BP 225/105 mmHg (3), capillary refill time 3 sec, cool peripheries, left radial pulse noted to be weaker than right, calves – soft, non-tender, Tympanic temperature 36.8 °C (0).
Disability (D): Patient is alert (0), Complaining of chest pain (10 /10).
Exposure (E): Nil of note.
NEWS2 score: 7.

Aortic dissection is a life-threatening condition where a tear occurs in the intimal lining, separating out the layers of the aorta. Depending on the location of the dissection this can result in rupture or disruption of blood flow to vital organs.

What would your care priorities be?
Care plan:

- Monitoring of physiology observations including invasive arterial pressure monitoring.
- Management of Bill's hypertension, his elevated blood pressure increases the risk of further dissection and rupture.
- Management of Bill's pain, this will be contributing to his hypertension.
- Routine bloods including cross matching blood in case a blood transfusion is required.
- Monitoring for signs of poor organ perfusion e.g. cognitive function, urine output, peripheral pulses.

Expore the different types of classification for aortic dissection (Stanford vs DeBakey).

Condition: cardiomyopathies

Cardiomyopathies are a diverse group of diseases which affect the myocardium (heart muscle). Irrespective of the cause they can all result in severe heart failure. Cardiomyopathies are often classified by the changes in the shape of the ventricles seen because of the disease (Braunwald, 2017)

Types of cardiomyopathy:

- Dilated cardiomyopathy
- Hypertrophic cardiomyopathy
- Restrictive cardiomyopathy

The causes of cardiomyopathy are diverse and complex, examples include:

- Genetics (hypertrophic obstructive cardiomyopathy)
- Infection (viral cardiomyopathy)
- Toxins (alcoholic cardiomyopathy)
- Ischaemic damage (ischaemic dilated cardiomyopathy)
- Pregnancy (peripartum cardiomyopathy)

Treatment is essentially the same as for the management of heart failure. In very severe cases patients may require the implantation of a mechanical ventricular assist device or heart transplantation.

The microcirculation

Most of this chapter has been devoted to the systemic circulation. However, earlier we identified one of the key functions of the cardiovascular system is the exchange of gases and nutrients between the blood and tissues thus supporting cellular metabolism. This exchange is supported by a microcirculation of capillary networks and is of equal importance.

The capillary beds (see Figure 18.10) consists of arterioles, small muscular arteries which lead to metarterioles which subsequently form an interconnected network of capillaries which criss-cross through the tissues in close proximity to the cells and eventually drain into venules and then back into the venous circulation. Blood flow through the capillary beds is regulated by the vasoconstriction of arterioles and the precapillary sphincters. In addition, the capillary beds contain thoroughfare channels which allows blood to bypass through the capillary beds in response to constriction of the pre capillaries sphincter.

6Cs: Courage

Caring for critically ill patient can often be frightening; you must have courage to care for your patients in these difficult situations

A key feature of the capillaries beds is the ability to autoregulate blood flow through each bed to match metabolic demand. This is achieved by changes in the diameter of the arterioles and precapillary sphincters in response to various stimuli. Capillary arterioles demonstrate a

242

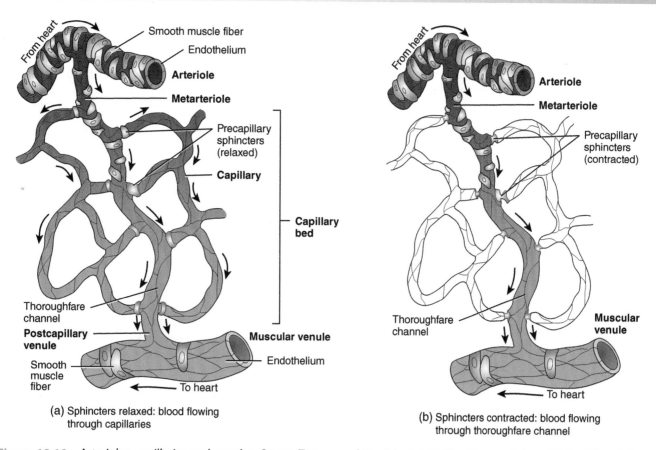

Figure 18.10   Arterioles, capillaries and venules. *Source:* Tortora and Derrickson (2017) with permission of John Wiley & Sons.

myogenic response, that is, they can dilate or constrict in response to blood pressure. For example, as blood pressure falls the arteriole's walls are less stretched, which triggers vasodilation to improve blood flow through the capillary bed. Conversely, if blood pressure increases and the arteriole wall is stretched, vasoconstriction is triggered. This type of myogenic response serves to maintain a relatively constant capillary blood flow over a range of systemic pressures. We see examples of this type of regulation in organs where perfusion is critical such as the brain and kidney.

In addition to this myogenic response the vascular endothelium plays a crucial role in regulating the degree of vasoconstriction (vasomotor tone). The endothelium is a thin layer of cells which lines all vessels. It was once thought to be little more than a barrier but has now been shown to be fundamental in the regulation of vascular tone, coagulation and the inflammatory response. The endothelium secretes various substances which regulate vascular tone including nitric oxide (vasodilation) and endothelin (vasoconstriction). Loss of endothelial regulation, in particular an increase in the production of nitric oxide, is a key reason for the profound vasodilation seen in sepsis.

Medications management: norepinephrine

Norepinephrine is a potent vasoconstrictor commonly used in hypotensive patients. Its mode of action is to stimulate adrenoreceptors in the heart and vasculature, resulting in a slight increase in cardiac output and profound vasoconstriction. It has a very short half-life (wears off quickly) and is therefore administered as a continuous infusion. It must never be stopped abruptly as this could lead to life-threatening hypotension (BNF, 2020, Neal, 2016).

The Surviving Sepsis Campaign guidelines recommend norepinephrine as the first-line vasopressor for patients with severe sepsis and septic shock (Rhodes et al., 2017).

Capillary exchange

Gas exchange across the capillary membranes into the cells is driven by diffusion, just as we see in the alveoli, gases 'flow' down a concentration gradient. High levels of oxygen in the capillary blood force diffusion across the capillary membrane into the cells and carbon dioxide diffuses from the cells into the capillary blood.

The movement of fluid and therefore the nutrients and waste products dissolved within is largely determined by two forces, hydrostatic and oncotic pressure (see Figure 18.11). At the arterial side of the capillary bed the pressure within the capillary (capillary hydrostatic pressure) is greater than the pressure of the fluid surrounding the cells (interstitial hydrostatic pressure) so fluid is forced across the capillary membrane through microscopic pores. At the venous side of the capillary bed, capillary hydrostatic pressure is reduced so the oncotic pressure of the blood can 'suck' the fluid back into the capillary. This oncotic pressure is created largely by proteins within the blood, such as albumin. In health this exchange is not quite perfect, with some fluid left in the interstitial tissues. One of the important functions of the lymphatic system is to drain this excess interstitial fluid and return it to the venous circulation. Alterations in either hydrostatic or oncotic pressure can lead to the accumulation of interstitial fluid, leading to oedema.

Condition: pitting oedema

Oedema is the excessive accumulation of fluid within the interstitial space and often accumulates in the legs resulting in swelling. This can be caused by several mechanisms which commonly occur in critically ill patients.

1. Increase in the size of the capillary pores because of inflammation allows more fluid to leak into the tissues. This is often seen in patients with septic shock.
2. Blood proteins such as albumin are important as they 'suck' fluid from the tissues (osmotic potential) back into the blood. If blood protein levels fall because of reduced production (liver dysfunction) or excessive loss (renal dysfunction), oedema can occur.
3. An increase in venous pressure due to occlusion (deep vein thrombus) or heart failure (increased preload) can reduced the amount of fluid reabsorbed at the venous side of the capillary bed as the increased venous pressure forces fluid into the tissues resulting in oedema.

244

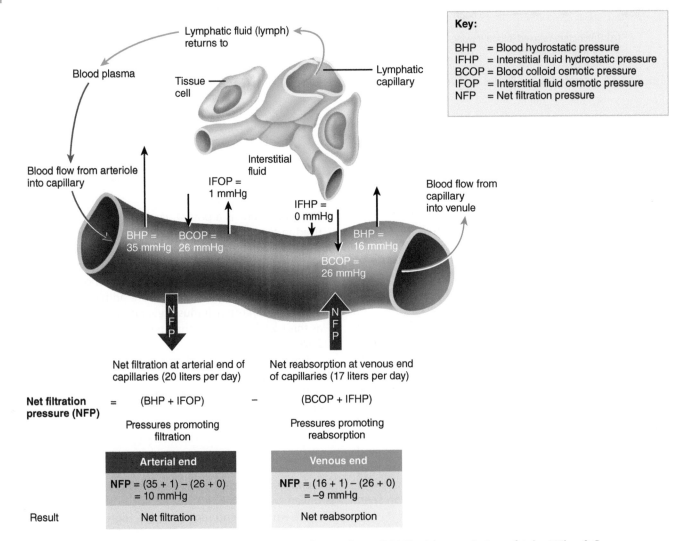

Key:

BHP = Blood hydrostatic pressure
IFHP = Interstitial fluid hydrostatic pressure
BCOP = Blood colloid osmotic pressure
IFOP = Interstitial fluid osmotic pressure
NFP = Net filtration pressure

Arterial end	Venous end
NFP = (35 + 1) − (26 + 0) = 10 mmHg	**NFP** = (16 + 1) − (26 + 0) = −9 mmHg
Net filtration	Net reabsorption

Figure 18.11 Capillary exchange. *Source*: Tortora and Derrickson (2017) with permission of John Wiley & Sons.

Effects of ventilation on the cardiovascular system

You will have discovered in previous chapters that the process of breathing is driven by changes in intrathoracic pressure. During inspiration, expansion of the chest wall and flattening of the diaphragm leads a reduction in intrathoracic pressure and air is drawn into the lungs. At the start of expiration, the elastic recoil of the chest wall then increases intrathoracic pressure, forcing air out of the lungs. As such, pressure within the thoracic cavity cycles between negative and positive with respiration. With this in mind, it is important to remember that the heart also sits within the thoracic cavity and is therefore affected by these changes in pressure. This relationship can be beneficial to cardiovascular function, in particular venous return, which is augmented by the negative intrathoracic pressure during inspiration, drawing blood from the abdomen and limbs.

Learning event: reflection

Before reading, on think about how positive pressure ventilation may affect cardiac function.

During positive pressure ventilation the changes in intrathoracic pressure are essentially reversed as pressure now increases during inspiration. This has numerous effects on heart lung interactions but the two most relevant are a reduction in venous return during inspiration, thus reducing ventricular preload, and a decrease in left ventricular afterload (the increased pressure in the thorax can be thought to support the ventricle contracting). The changes in preload however dominate leading to a reduction in cardiac output in most patients because of positive pressure ventilation (Pinsky, 2018)

However, these changes may not always be detrimental. In patients with decompensated heart failure, who are often fluid-overloaded with ventricular distension (remember Frank–Starlings Law) the changes associated with positive pressure ventilation, a reduction in venous return and afterload can be beneficial. This accounts for why patients in heart failure often respond well to CPAP (Continuous Positive Airway Pressure).

Orange Flag: depression and heart disease

There is a clear, if not fully understood, link between mental health and cardiovascular disease. Patients suffering from depression are twice as likely to have a myocardial infarction when compared to the general population (Chauvert-Gelinier & Bonin, 2017).

It is important that critical care nurses consider both the psychological and physical health needs of their patients

6Cs: Compassion

The compassion you show to both patients and their loved ones will be their overriding memory of the critical care unit.

Conclusion

Cardiovascular function is crucial for the maintenance of heath with cardiovascular disease a leading cause of both mortality and morbidity with critical care. In this chapter we have reviewed some important physiological concepts such as cardiac output and the regulation of blood pressure. We have explored how disease can impact on cardiovascular function and finally we have identified that common critical care therapies such a positive pressure ventilation can impact normal cardiovascular function. In the next chapter we will go on to review cardiovascular assessment, monitoring and support, to enable practitioners to monitor cardiovascular function and care for patient with cardiovascular disease.

Take home points

1. The cardiovascular system has many vital functions.
2. Cardiovascular disease is an important cause of both mortality and morbidity in critically ill adults.
3. The heart supports two interconnected circulations, the pulmonary and systemic.
4. Blood flow through the heart is dependant on the coordinated contraction of the four chambers and the function of the heart valves.
5. Cardiac output is determined by heart rate and stroke volume.
6. Stroke volume is determined by preload, contractility and afterload.
7. Blood pressure is determined by cardiac output, blood viscosity and systemic vascular resistance.
8. Cardiac output and blood pressure are regulated by the cardiovascular centre in response to many stimuli, including baroreceptors and chemoreceptors.

References

British Heart Foundation (2020). British Heart Foundation UK Factsheet. https://www.bhf.org.uk/what-we-do/our-research/heart-statistics (accessed 2 November 2020).

Braunwald, Eugene (2017). Cardiomyopathies: An overview. *Circulation Research* 121(7): 711–721.

Chauvet-Gelinier, Jean-Christophe and Bonin, Bernard (2017). Stress, anxiety and depression in heart disease patients: A major challenge for cardiac rehabilitation. *Annals of Physical and Rehabilitation Medicine* 60(1): 6–12.

Chen, Z.M., Pan, H.C., Chen, Y.P., COMMIT (ClOpidogrel and Metoprolol in Myocardial Infarction Trial) collaborative group et al. (2005). Early intravenous then oral metoprolol in 45,852 patients with acute myocardial infarction: randomised placebo-controlled trial. *Lancet* 5:366(9497): 1622–1632. doi: 10.1016/S0140-6736(05)67661-1.

Critical Care Networks-National Nurse Leads (CC3N) (2015a). National Competency Framework for Registered Nurses in Adult Critical Care Step 1 Competencies.

Critical Care Networks-National Nurse Leads (CC3N) (2015b). National Competency Framework for Registered Nurses in Adult Critical Care Step 2 Competencies.

Gurbel, P.A., Tantry, U.S., and Huber, K. (2014). *Acute Coronary Syndromes*, 1e. Fast Facts.

Intensive Care National Audit and Research Centre. (2019). Case mix programme summary statistics 2018–19. https://www.icnarc.org/DataServices/Attachments/Download/fca008ac-9216-ea11-911e-00505601089b (accessed March 2022).

Joint Formulary Committee. British National Formulary (online). London: BMJ Group and Pharmaceutical Press. https://bnf.nice.org.uk (accessed 15 November 2020).

Kumar, Amit and Cannon, Christopher P. (2009). Acute coronary syndromes: Diagnosis and management, Part I. *Mayo Clinic Proceedings* 84(10): 917–938.

McCance, Kathryn L. and Huether, Sue E. (2014). *Pathophysiology: The Biologic Basis for Disease in Adults and Children*, 7e. Mosby.

Marieb, Elaine N. and Hoehn, Katja N. *Human Anatomy and Physiology*, 10e. Pearson Education.

Minet, Clémence, Potton, Leila, Bonadona, Agnès et al. (2015). Venous thromboembolism in the ICU: Main characteristics, diagnosis and thromboprophylaxis. *Critical Care* 19(1): 287.

Neal, M.J. (2016). *Medical Pharmacology at a Glance*, 8e. At a Glance.

NICE (2018). *Chronic Heart Failure in Adults: Diagnosis and Management*. National Institute for Health and Care Excellence.

NICE (2014). *Acute Heart Failure: Diagnosis and Management*. National Institute for Health and Care Excellence.

Oremus, M., McKelvie, R., Don-Wauchope, A. et al. (2014). A systematic review of BNP and NT-proBNP in the management of heart failure: Overview and methods. *Heart Failure Reviews* 19(4): 413–419.

Pinsky, Michael R. (2018). Cardiopulmonary interactions: Physiologic basis and clinical applications. *Annals of the American Thoracic Society* 15(Supp 1): S45–S48.

Rhodes, A., Evans, L.E., Alhazzani, W. et al. (2017). Surviving Sepsis Campaign: International Guidelines for Management of Sepsis and Septic Shock: 2016. *Intensive Care Medicine* 43(3): 304–377.

Robertson, Colin, Douglas, Graham, and Nicol, Fiona (2013). *Macleod's Clinical Examination*. Churchill Livingstone, 2013.

Tortora, G.J. and Derrickson, B. (2017). *Principles of Anatomy and Physiology*, 15e. Singapore: Wiley.

Wallentin, L., Becker, R.C., Budaj, A. et al. (2009). Ticagrelor versus clopidogrel in patients with acute coronary syndromes. *N Engl J Med* 361(11): 1045–1057. doi: 10.1056/NEJMoa0904327.

WHO (2017). Cardiovascular diseases (CVDs). https://www.who.int/news-room/fact-sheets/detail/cardiovascular-diseases-(cvds) (accessed 2 November 2020).

Wilmer, Amanda, Louie, Kimberley, Dodek, Peter et al. (2010). Incidence of medication errors and adverse drug events in the ICU: A systematic review. *Quality & Safety in Health Care* 19(5): E7.

Yusuf, S., Zhao, F., Mehta, S.R. et al. (2001). Effects of clopidogrel in addition to aspirin in patients with acute coronary syndromes without ST-segment elevation. *N Engl J Med* 345(7): 494–502. doi: 10.1056/NEJMoa010746. Erratum in: *N Engl J Med* 345(23): 1716. Erratum in: *N Engl J Med* 345(20): 1506.

Chapter 19

Cardiovascular critical care

Alice Shaw and Paul Sinnott

Aim

The aim of this chapter is to provide the reader with evidence-based knowledge to support the assessment and management of the critically ill adult with cardiovascular disease or dysfunction.

Learning outcomes

After reading this chapter the reader will be able to:

- Describe how to perform a comprehensive cardiovascular assessment of the critically ill patient.
- Recognise common cardiac arrhythmias and be aware of evidence-based interventions.
- Discuss the rationale, nursing care and management of invasive and non-invasive haemodynamic monitoring applied within the critical care environment.
- Demonstrate an awareness of different advanced cardiac monitoring devices and describe the advantages and disadvantages of each.
- Understand the different types of cardiac pacing and the indications for use.

Test your prior knowledge

- How can we use cardiovascular assessment to assess fluid status in a patient showing signs of cardiac dysfunction?
- Describe an arterial waveform, and the significance of any changes to waveform.
- What classification of medication is amiodarone, and why might it be used? Consider the nursing care associated with its use.
- Discuss the evidence base underpinning the care of a person with a Central Venous Catheter (CVC).
- What are the different methods of advanced haemodynamic monitoring? Discuss how and why they might be used in critical illness.

Fundamentals of Critical Care: A Textbook for Nursing and Healthcare Students, First Edition. Edited by Ian Peate and Barry Hill.
© 2023 John Wiley & Sons Ltd. Published 2023 by John Wiley & Sons Ltd.
Companion website: www.wiley.com/go/peate/criticalcare

Introduction

Cardiovascular dysfunction is the leading cause for admission into critical care units in the UK (Intensive Care Society (ICS), 2019). It is essential that nurses working in critical care are competent in undertaking a comprehensive cardiovascular assessment and responding to any abnormalities they may find.

Step 2 competencies: National standards

2:2.1 Assessment Monitoring and Observation (Critical Care Networks-National Nurse Leads (CC3N), 2015)

Demonstrate your knowledge using a rationale through discussion, and the application to practice.

Comprehensive cardiovascular assessment, recording findings, optimising treatment within prescribed limits and escalating problems to appropriate team members.

Cardiovascular assessment

There are many components to a comprehensive cardiac assessment of which the fundamental aspects will be discussed within this chapter.

To gain a full understanding of a patient's condition all components should be considered in the context of the patient's past medical history, baseline observations and the treatment they are receiving. It is important to utilise an Inspection, Palpation, Percussion, Auscultation (IPPA) approach to clinical assessment (Bickley, 2016).

Cardiovascular assessment

Inspection: Pallor, cyanosis, jugular vein distension, haemorrhage, cardiovascular devices (i.e. pacemaker), supportive therapies (i.e. vasopressors), drains (and output), arterial and central pressure waveforms, signs of distress or discomfort, reduced level of consciousness, echocardiogram, passive leg raise.

Palpation: Pulse, capillary refill, limb temperature, skin turgor.

Percussion: Not needed.

Auscultation: Heart sounds.

Record: Past Medical History (PMH), current therapies, Heart Rate (HR) and rhythm, Blood Pressure (BP), Central Venous Pressure (CVP), urine output, temperature, blood results, advanced cardiac output (CO) studies.

Heart rate and rhythm

Cardiac arrhythmias are a major cause of increased length of hospital stay, poor clinical outcomes, and increased mortality (Senaratne et al., 2020; Tarditi and Hollenberg, 2006). The incidence of cardiac arrhythmias is estimated to be up to 90% of all critical care admissions (Senaratne et al., 2020). Although less common than the atrial arrhythmias, ventricular arrhythmias have a mortality of up to 73% (Annane et al., 2008). Consequently, it is therefore vital that all nursing and medical staff in critical care units are able to recognise cardiac arrhythmias and are aware of the evidence base behind the interventions used in the critical care unit (Badhwar et al., 2011).

An electrocardiogram (ECG) will assess electrical activity in the heart using either 3-5 leads or 12-leads. Continuous 3-5 lead monitoring should be used in all critically ill patients (Figure 19.1). This will ensure early detection of changes and allow for assessment of treatments.

As identified in the 2014 National Patient Safety Goal, alarm limits should be checked and be clinically appropriate (Joint Commission, 2013). Inappropriate settings will have serious implications for patient safety.

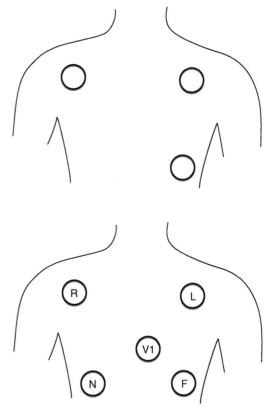

Figure 19.1   3- and 5-lead ECG electrode placement. *Source:* Mallet et al. (2013) with permission of John Wiley & Sons.

Orange Flag

Inappropriate alarm settings will lead to sensory overload for the patient and will affect their overall recovery and memory of critical care.

To detect arrhythmias, nurses must first be able to identify the components that characterise normal sinus rhythm. We have defined normal sinus rhythm using the United Kingdom Resuscitation Council's (UKRC) 6-point approach (UKRC, 2021a).

Sinus rhythm

- Step 1 – Is there electrical activity? *Yes*
- Step 2 – What is the ventricular (QRS) rate? *60–100 beats per minute (bpm)*
- Step 3 – Is the QRS rhythm regular or irregular? *Regular*
- Step 4 – Is the QRS complex width normal or broad? *Normal (<0.12 seconds)*
- Step 5 – Is atrial activity present? *Yes, P waves*
- Step 6 – Is atrial activity related to ventricular activity and, if so how? *Every P wave is followed by a QRS complex, and the P-R interval is <0.2 seconds*

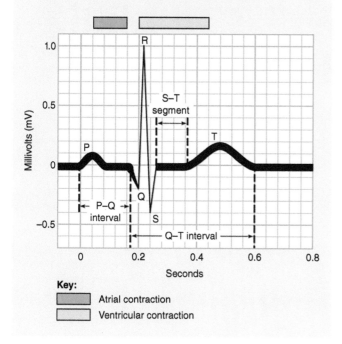

Arrhythmias can be slow in nature – bradyarrhythmia (<60 bpm), of a normal rate – sinus arrhythmia (60–100 bpm), or fast – tachyarrhythmia (>100 bpm). Tachyarrhythmias can be divided into supraventricular (originating from the atrioventricular node or above) or ventricular (originating from the ventricles).

A standardised approach to interpretation alongside pathology guided treatment will help to improve patient outcomes (Senaratne et al., 2020). Table 19.1 uses the 6-point approach to identify the characteristics of common arrhythmias, as well as the possible causes and treatments. It has been designed to give nurses confidence in this approach to rhythm recognition.

For further information on the treatment of cardiac arrest rhythms, please refer to Chapter 21.

Medications management: adenosine

Adenosine is primarily used to treat SVT as part of the UKRC (2021) tachycardia algorithm, and its mechanism of action is based on the blockage of neurotransmission through the AV node. Initially it is administered as a 6 mg bolus dose, but a further 12 mg and later 18 mg dose, may be given if the desired affects are not seen. The half-life is short being approximately 10 seconds.

ECG should be monitored throughout and the resuscitation trolley should be nearby and available.

Side effects include nausea, chest discomfort and flushing. It is contraindicated in people with asthma.

Although not immediately life-threatening nurses should also be able to identify ectopic beats, as they may be an indication of an underlying pathology such as electrolyte imbalance, ischaemia or heart disease.

Atrial ectopic beats

Premature beat arising from somewhere in the atrium but not from the sino-atrial node.

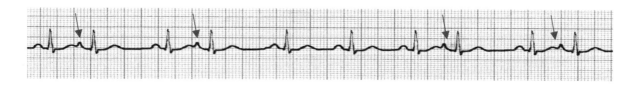

Possible causes: Stimulants such as caffeine, electrolyte disturbance, infections, drug toxicity, heart disease.

Treatment: Correction of underlying cause.

Table 19.1 Characteristic components of common cardiac arrhythmias, possible causes and treatments.

Rhythm	Is there electrical activity?	What is the ventricular QRS rate?	Is the QRS rhythm regular or irregular	Is the QRS width normal or prolonged	Is atrial activity present?	How is atrial activity related to ventricular activity	Causes include	Treatments
Sinus bradycardia *Figure 19.2*	Yes	<60 bpm	Regular	Normal	Yes	P wave followed by QRS PR interval <0.2 s	Physiological Hypothermia Hyperkalaemia Beta-blocker toxicity Drugs (e.g. amiodarone)	If adverse features present may include: Atropine Transcutaneous pacing. Follow UKRC 2021 Bradycardia algorithm
Sinus tachycardia *Figure 19.3*	Yes	>100 bpm	Regular	Normal	Yes	P wave followed by QRS PR interval <0.2 s	Normal physiological response to: Exercise Stress Pain Infection Hypovolaemia Heart failure	Dependent on the underlying cause. For example, intravenous fluids (hypovolaemia) or analgesia (pain).
Supraventricular tachycardia (SVT) *Figure 19.4*	Yes	140–250 bpm	Regular	Normal	Often obscured by rate	If P wave visible, each is followed by QRS	Peri-arrest Wolff–Parkinson–White (WPW) syndrome	May include: A vagal manoeuvre Adenosine Synchronised DC shock Follow UKRC 2021 Tachycardia algorithm
Atrial fibrillation *Figure 19.5*	Yes	Usually >100 bpm	Irregular	Normal	No discernible P wave		Heart disease Chronic obstructive pulmonary disease (COPD) Asthma Diabetes mellitus Surgery Metabolic disorders.	First consider if patient's 'norm' If adverse features present may include: Beta-blocker (to control rate) Amiodarone or digoxin (to control rhythm) Synchronised DC cardioversion Anticoagulation Follow UKRC 2021 tachycardia algorithm
Atrial flutter *Figure 19.6*	Yes	75–150 bpm dependent on flutter ratio	Regular	Normal	Yes	Atrial rate often 250–300 bpm Number of P waves to every QRS often 2:1 or 3:1	COPD Pulmonary embolism (PE) Chronic congestive heart failure Complex congenital heart disease	May include: A vagal manoeuvre Adenosine Beta-blocker Synchronised DC shock Follow UKRC 2021 Tachycardia algorithm

Rhythm	Pulse	Rate	Regularity	QRS	P wave	P–QRS relationship	Causes	Treatment
Complete heart block *Figure 19.7*	Yes	Often 30–50 bpm	Irregular	Narrow or broad depending on origin	Yes	No relationship between P wave and QRS	• Underlying heart condition e.g. cardiomyopathy • Electrolyte imbalance • Age	• Transcutaneous pacing • Follow UKRC 2021 Bradycardia algorithm
Ventricular fibrillation (VF) *Figure 19.8*	Yes	Often >300 bpm	Irregular	Broad	No	N/A	• Heart failure • Cardiomyopathies • Myocardial infarction • Sepsis • 4 Hs and 4 Ts (see Chapter 21)	Adult Advanced Life Support (ALS) Algorithm for shockable rhythms (UKRC 2021)
Ventricular Tachycardia (VT) *Figure 19.9*	Yes	100–300 bpm	Regular	Broad	May continue independently of ventricular activity	Disassociated	• Myocardial infarction • 4 Hs and 4 Ts	Adult ALS Algorithm for shockable rhythms (UKRC 2021)
Asystole *Figure 19.10*	No	No electrical activity					• Untreated VF/VT arrest • 4 Hs and 4 Ts	Adult ALS Algorithm for non-shockable rhythms (UKRC 2021)
Pulseless electrical activity	Yes, but with no identified pulse	Will present like any other rhythm normally associated with a pulse.					• 4 Hs and 4 Ts	Adult ALS Algorithm for non-shockable rhythms (UKRC 2021)

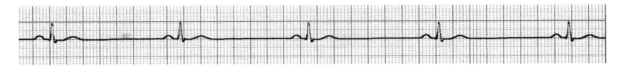

Figure 19.2   Sinus bradycardia.

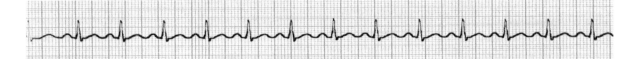

Figure 19.3   Sinus tachycardia.

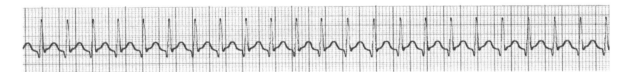

Figure 19.4   Supraventricular tachycardia.

252

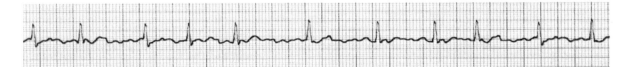

Figure 19.5   Atrial fibrillation.

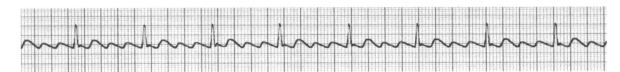

Figure 19.6   Atrial flutter.

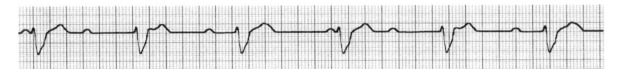

Figure 19.7   Complete heart block.

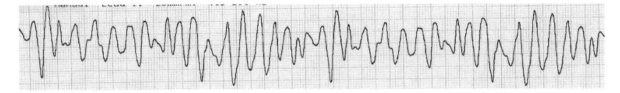

Figure 19.8   Ventricular fibrillation.

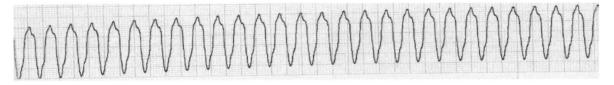

Figure 19.9   Ventricular tachycardia.

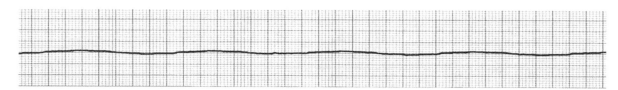

Figure 19.10   Asystole.

Ventricular ectopic beats

Premature beat arising from the Purkinje fibre network in the ventricles. No P wave prior to a widened QRS complex

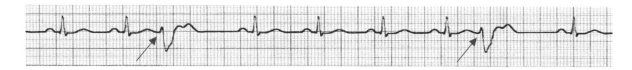

Possible causes: Electrolyte disturbance, hypoxia, drug toxicity, heart disease.

Treatment: Correction of underlying cause.

253

Clinical investigations: manual pulse

When assessing heart rate and rhythm in critically ill people, a manual pulse should be taken, and the patient should receive cardiovascular monitoring. A manual pulse will provide information on rate, regularity, and quality. A weak pulse suggests poor cardiac output, whilst a bounding pulse can denote sepsis (UKRC, 2021).

It is important to remember that prior to any procedure, health care professionals should introduce themselves to the patient. In an environment compounded by alarms and wires, some patients may experience a loss of humanity. By ensuring effective communication, nurses are helping to protect the patients sense of identity (Wilson et al., 2019).

Hand hygiene should be performed, and appropriate personal protective equipment (PPE) donned. The first and second fingers should be placed along the chosen artery, and light pressure applied until a pulse is felt. The pulse should be taken for 60 seconds. It is important to note that placing too much pressure will occlude the vessel and the pulse will be absent. Radial, carotid, femoral and brachial are key arterial pulse points. The pulse will be felt strongest in those arteries as they are closer to the heart (Dougherty and Lister, 2020). After taking the pulse, PPE should be removed and hand hygiene performed. Results should be documented in

the patients notes, and any abnormalities reported to an appropriate health care professional (Figure 19.11).

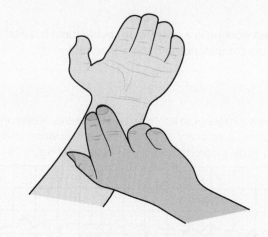

Figure 19.11   Radial pulse. *Source:* Peate and Wild (2018) with permission of John Wiley & Sons.

When changes to a patient's heart rate are detected, a 12-lead ECG will offer a more comprehensive view of the electrical activity in the heart to support diagnosis and guide management. It will allow the clinician to identify which part of the heart is affected by infarction or ischaemia, and allow timely and appropriate interventions to be implemented. It can also help to diagnose differential causes of breathlessness, syncope and dizziness (Hampton, 2013).

Red Flag: peaked T waves

Peaked 'T waves' on an ECG can be indicative of hyper-kalaemia (increased blood potassium levels) (UKRC, 2021). If peaked T waves are detected, patients should continue to have continuous ECG monitoring and urgent blood samples should be taken to measure blood potassium levels. An arterial or venous blood gas will provide quick results if the patient has venous or arterial access. When available, the results of the blood test should be reviewed by a senior practitioner immediately.

If a blood test result reveals a high potassium level, this should be treated according to local hyperkalaemia protocols. The UKRC (2021) outlines the treatment of severe hyperkalaemia with ECG changes (typically >6.5 mmols/L). This may include the following:

10 mL10% calcium chloride
10 units of insulin with 25g dextrose
Urgent referral for renal replacement therapy
Continuous cardiac monitoring
50 mmol of sodium bicarbonate if cardiopulmonary resuscitation is in progress and acidosis present

More information around the use of insulin and dextrose is found later in this chapter.

6Cs: Competence

When working in a critical care environment it is vital to ensure competence in rhythm analysis.

Snapshot

Renu is a 70-year-old lady admitted to the critical care unit, following a coronary artery bypass graft. Postoperatively she has developed the arrhythmia depicted in Figure 19.12.

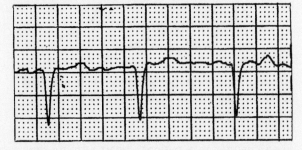

Figure 19.12 ECG demonstrating atrial fibrillation. *Source:* Mallet et al. (2013) with permission of John Wiley & Sons.

Use the UKRC (2021) 6-point approach to determine the arrhythmia.

What rhythm is Renu in? What defines this?

Are you able to develop an individualised care plan for Renu based on your findings?

Further reading: Resuscitation Council (UK) Guidelines: Peri-arrest rhythms (UKRC, 2021b).

Medications management: amiodarone

Amiodarone is a membrane-stabilising anti-arrhythmic drug used to treat arrhythmias such as atrial fibrillation, atrial flutter and ventricular arrhythmias such as ventricular tachycardia and ventricular fibrillation. It can be given orally or by intravenous injection. In a non-cardiac arrest rhythm, an intravenous (IV) dose of 5 mg/kg is initially given over 20–120 minutes with continuous ECG monitoring. Subsequent infusions are given if necessary.

Common side effects include arrhythmias, hypotension, hepatic disorders, hyperthyroidism, respiratory disorders, nausea and skin reactions.

Orange Flag

Patients who have been assessed as having capacity have the right to refuse treatment.

Blood pressure

A normal Blood Pressure (BP) is essential for adequate organ perfusion. Whilst the NEWS2 score specifically looks at systolic blood pressure to determine an appropriate clinical response (Royal College of Physicians (RCP), 2017), in critical care mean arterial blood pressure (MAP) is often used as a more reliable indication of organ perfusion (blood flow).

MAP is the average pressure throughout one cardiac cycle and is calculated using the following equation:

$$\text{MAP (mmHg)} = \text{diastolic pressure (mmHg)} + 1/3 \text{ (systolic pressure} - \text{diastolic pressure) (mmHg)}$$

Although MAP targets should be individualised to the patient, >65 mmHg was widely accepted following the publication of the 2016 Surviving Sepsis Guidelines (Rhodes et al., 2017). More recently Lamontagne et al. (2020) have found targeting a MAP of 60–65 mmHg in patients over the age of 65 years did not worsen 90-day mortality in vasodilatory shock compared to a target MAP of >65 mmHg. Regardless of the chosen target, it is important that nurses caring for patients achieve the target aim, but do not exceed it without clinical reasoning. This is highlighted by Lamontagne et al. (2017), who found that bedside clinicians often aim for a MAP >10 mmHg above the intended target, using unnecessary amounts of vasopressor drugs to achieve this.

The causes and treatments of hypotension can be found in Chapter 8.

Blood pressure can be measured invasively or non-invasively. Although a syphgmomanometer and cuff is one method of non-invasive measurement, it is unlikely to be used in critical care, and instead favoured for the DINAMAP (device for indirect non-invasive automatic mean arterial pressure). The DINAMAP detects changes in amplitude of pressure oscillations, known as oscillometry. Although widely used in hospital and outpatient settings, its accuracy in assessing blood pressure in critically ill patients has been questioned (Lehman et al., 2013, Rhodes et al., 2017).

Learning event

Reflect on how much you understand arterial and central venous pressure waveforms.

Invasive blood pressure monitoring

Monitoring of blood pressure via arterial lines tends to be the gold standard in critical care (Mallett et al., 2013) and although bleeding and infection risks should be considered, these have been found to be <1% (Scheer et al., 2002).

Arterial blood pressure monitoring requires a catheter to be inserted into an artery. It provides a continuous measurement of blood pressure and is essential when patients require inotropic or vasopressor support. It is also indicated when patients have significant changes to circulating blood volume, or require frequent arterial blood gas analysis. As well as providing continuous blood pressure monitoring, the arterial waveform can also give an indication of myocardial contractility and vasoconstriction.

Arterial lines are most frequently inserted into the radial artery due to its good collateral circulation, proximity to the skins surface and visibility (Adam et al., 2017). Less commonly it can also be inserted into brachial, femoral, posterior tibial and axillary arteries (Loveday et al., 2014).

Prior to insertion, the circulation to the hand should be checked. If available, ultrasound analysis will assess blood flow, whilst allowing for identification of the artery and reducing the risk of first attempt failure (Adam et al., 2017). The 'Allen test' is an alternative method which requires both the radial and ulnar arteries to be occluded, followed by the release of the radial artery to assess collateral circulation. It is the colour of the hand during this test which indicates whether there is adequate blood supply. Despite it being simple to perform, its reliability has been questioned (Adam and Osborne, 2013).

Once adequate perfusion has been established, the practitioner will clean the skin using 2% chlorhexidine in 70% alcohol swab (Dougherty and Lister, 2020). A sterile field should be maintained with strict aseptic non-touch technique (ANTT). The patient will be given local anaesthetic and once inserted flash back should be observed. If a guidewire is used, the assisting practitioner should witness its removal. The cannula is then attached to a pressure system which consists of a bag of 0.9% sodium chloride, a pressure transducer and infusion set, and a pressure bag (Dougherty and Lister, 2020). Pressure is transmitted from the cannula to the transducer, where it is relayed to the monitor via an electrical cable. Here it appears as a waveform, with systolic, diastolic and MAP readings (Figure 19.13). The pressure transducer should be calibrated ('zeroed') at the height of

255

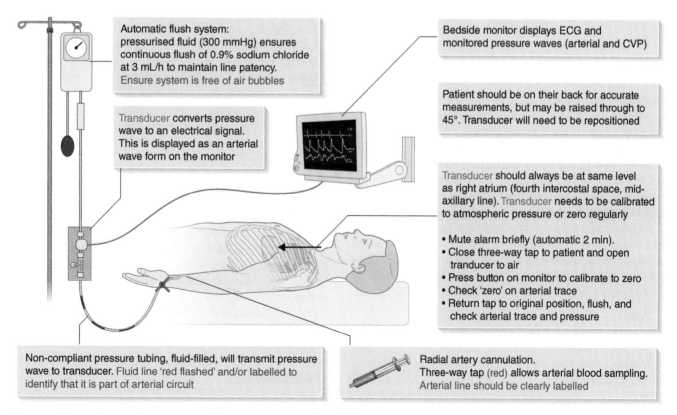

Automatic flush system: pressurised fluid (300 mmHg) ensures continuous flush of 0.9% sodium chloride at 3 mL/h to maintain line patency. Ensure system is free of air bubbles

Transducer converts pressure wave to an electrical signal. This is displayed as an arterial wave form on the monitor

Bedside monitor displays ECG and monitored pressure waves (arterial and CVP)

Patient should be on their back for accurate measurements, but may be raised through to 45°. Transducer will need to be repositioned

Transducer should always be at same level as right atrium (fourth intercostal space, midaxillary line). Transducer needs to be calibrated to atmospheric pressure or zero regularly

- Mute alarm briefly (automatic 2 min).
- Close three-way tap to patient and open tranducer to air
- Press button on monitor to calibrate to zero
- Check 'zero' on arterial trace
- Return tap to original position, flush, and check arterial trace and pressure

Non-compliant pressure tubing, fluid-filled, will transmit pressure wave to transducer. Fluid line 'red flashed' and/or labelled to identify that it is part of arterial circuit

Radial artery cannulation. Three-way tap (red) allows arterial blood sampling. Arterial line should be clearly labelled

Figure 19.13 A transducer system. *Source:* Dutton and Finch (2018) with permission of John Wiley & Sons.

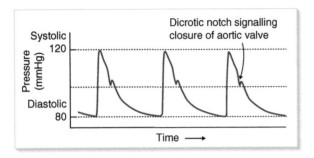

Figure 19.14   Arterial waveform. *Source:* Dutton and Finch (2018) with permission of John Wiley & Sons.

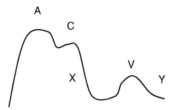

Figure 19.15   Central venous pressure waveform. *Source:* Mallet et al. (2013) with permission of John Wiley & Sons.

the patient's right atrium. This requires the tap to be turned off to the patient and opened to air. A button on the patient's monitor reading 'zero' is pressed and when this figure is achieved, the transducer system is turned off to air and open to the patient. Local policies and procedures should be followed throughout.

The peak of the arterial waveform represents the maximum systolic pressure. Following this, the pressure starts to decrease and the diacrotic notch signifies the closure of the aortic valve. This marks the end of systole and the beginning of diastole (Figure 19.14).

6Cs: Compassion

It is important to recognise the anxieties patients may be facing when undergoing procedures.

Central venous catheters (CVCs) and central venous pressure (CVP)

There are many indications for CVC insertion, they include infusion of multiple and vesicant drugs (such as inotropes, vasopressors and concentrated potassium), CVP monitoring, blood sampling including central venous oxygen saturation readings (ScVO$_2$) and advanced cardiac monitoring.

CVCs are inserted into large veins, most commonly the internal jugular vein, but can also be inserted into the subclavian and femoral veins (Loveday et al., 2014).

A CVC is inserted using the Seldinger technique. This is a technique used to allow safe access to the blood vessels using a needle, guidewire and the relevant catheter. Once inserted it is attached to a transducer system as earlier described and a CVP waveform will appear (Figure 19.15).

1. A wave – Right atrial contraction
2. C wave – Closure of the tricuspid valve
3. X – Atrial relaxation
4. V wave – Right ventricular contraction
5. Y – Atrial emptying

Alongside chest x-ray confirmation, the CVP waveform can provide reassurance that the CVC has been correctly placed into a vein.

Red Flag

A guidewire is used to assist the insertion of a CVC. This should be removed as soon as the line is placed (Dougherty and Lister, 2020). A guidewire is a foreign object and retained guidewires are identified as a 'never event' (NHS Improvement, 2018). Any CVC insertion should follow the National Safety Standards for Invasive Procedures (NatSSIPS) (NHS England, 2020). A sign-out should be performed at the end of the procedure. All members present during the procedure should be present at sign-out and a witness should confirm that the guidewire has been removed.

6Cs: Courage

It is important to have the courage to ensure that the correct processes are followed. If you believe something has been forgotten or is being done incorrectly, you must speak up and act as an advocate for the patient (NMC, 2018).

CVP is a measure of the pressure in the superior vena cava and therefore an estimate of right atrial pressure. Normal CVP is between 3–8 mmHg. An increase in CVP could be indicative of right-sided heart failure, pulmonary hypertension or cardiac tamponade. Historically it was also thought to be a good indication of fluid responsiveness due to the assumption that it was reflective of right ventricular end-diastolic volume or preload. However, evidence now shows that there is little correlation between CVP and preload and therefore if used in isolation, it may not be an accurate measure of fluid responsiveness (Marik et al., 2008; Marik and Cavallazzi, 2013). (More information on measures of fluid responsiveness can be found in Chapter 20.)

Red Flag

Catheter-related blood stream infections (CRBSIs) associated with CVCs are among the most dangerous complications associated with healthcare (Loveday et al., 2014). They are estimated to increase mortality by up to 25% (Bion et al., 2013). It is essential that all healthcare professionals responsible for the care and management are educated in appropriate infection control practices (Loveday et al., 2014). A combination of technical and non-technical interventions has been shown to reduce CVC CRBSIs by up to 60% (Bion et al., 2013).

Nurses should be aware of the signs of infection and familiarise themselves with the most up-to-date sepsis guidelines so that quick identification and treatment can be implemented if required.

Further reading

Loveday et al. (2014) National evidence-based guidelines for preventing healthcare-associated infections in NHS Hospitals in England. Available at https://improvement. nhs.uk/documents/847/epic3_National_Evidence-Based_Guidelines_for_Preventing_HCAI_in_NHSE.pdf (Accessed 06.11.2020).

National Institute for Health and Care Excellence (NICE) (2014). Sepsis: Recognition, Diagnosis and Early Management. Available at https://www.nice.org.uk/guidance/ng51/resources/sepsis-recognition-diagnosis-and-early-management-pdf-1837508256709 (Accessed: 17.10.2020).

EPIC 3 recommendations (Loveday et al., 2014)

- Decontamination of hands before and after any contact with the line.
- Appropriate catheter selection.
- Use of an antimicrobial-impregnated central venous access device for those expected to be in >5 days, where local infection rates are higher than the agreed benchmark.
- Use of maximal sterile barrier precautions for the insertion of CVCs.
- Decontamination of skin prior to insertion with 2% chlorhexidine gluconate in 70% isopropyl alcohol.
- Use of a sterile transparent semi-permeable polyurethane dressing, changing at least every 7 days or sooner if no longer dry and intact.
- Consider use of chlorhexidine-impregnated dressings.
- Single-use application of 2% chlorhexidine gluconate in 70% isoproplyl alcohol to clean the site.
- Arterial and central line catheter duration 7–10 days.

As well as the risk of retained guidewires and infections, there are other risks associated with arterial and central lines. These are summarised in Table 19.2.

Table 19.2   Risks associated with arterial and central lines.

Risk	Line (s)	Cause	Prevention
Infection	Arterial and central lines	· Poor insertion technique · Poor care · Specific location (i.e. femoral)	· Practice in line with EPIC 3 guidelines (Loveday et al., 2014)
Haemorrhage	Arterial and central lines	· Not stitched · Transducer connections loose · Catheter displacement (by staff or patient)	· Stitching · Occlusive dressing · Tighten transducer connections · Ensure visible · Ensure patient nursed safely and any delirium or agitation addressed
Air embolus	Arterial and central lines	· System not primed properly · Empty transducer fluid	· Appropriate priming · Regular inspection of transducer bag to ensure correct pressure and fluid availability
Thrombus formation	Arterial and central lines	· Pressure bag not inflated to 300 mmHg · No priming solution	· Regular inspection of transducer bag to ensure correct pressure and availability of fluid
Accidental injection of drugs	Arterial lines	· Nursing knowledge · Nursing workload	· Appropriate training and competency assessment of staff · Use of colour-coded transducer systems and needle-free bungs · Clear labelling of line
Limb ischaemia	Arterial lines	· Poor collateral supply	· Ultrasound assessment of blood flow prior to insertion · Allen test · Regular observation of limb

257

Examination scenario: removal of CVC

Prior to any clean or aseptic procedure, hand hygiene should be performed (World Health Organisation, 2009) and appropriate PPE should be available and donned. Due to the risk of blood splash, at minimum this should include gloves, apron and visor or goggles.

To avoid the risk of air embolus patients should be nursed in the Trendelenburg position when removing the CVC (Dougherty and Lister, 2020) if their condition allows. The Trendelenburg position involves lying supine, with the level of the patient's head being lower than the level of the feet. If the patient is ventilated the CVC should be removed at the end of inspiration. If self-ventilating the patient should breathe in and hold their breath, at which point the catheter is withdrawn. Whilst being withdrawn, direct pressure should be applied with sterile gauze. Once bleeding has ceased, an occlusive dressing should be applied and the sight should be observed for further signs of bleeding.

After removal of the CVC, PPE should be removed and hand hygiene performed. The procedure should then be documented in the patients notes.

Markers of organ and tissue perfusion

In the absence of adequate circulating volume, organs and tissues will not be sufficiently perfused. There are several markers which can be used to assess this. These are identified below.

Lactate

As a consequence of both anaerobic respiration and high levels of circulating epinephrine, an elevated blood lactate level is a frequently used indicator of critical illness. It is easily measured by taking an arterial or venous blood sample. Although there are several reasons for an increased blood lactate level (>2 mmol/l), poor cardiac output reducing oxygen delivery to the tissues is a potential cause.

Mixed venous oxygen saturation (SvO_2) and central venous oxygen saturation ($ScVO_2$)

SvO_2 and $ScVO_2$ consider the relationship between oxygen supply and demand. To ensure oxygen supply, the body requires an adequate cardiac output and the ability to carry oxygen – as determined by the haemoglobin concen-

tration and oxygen saturations. Even when the tissues have extracted oxygen, an oxygen reserve should remain. However, if demand increases or supply falls, more of the reserve will be used and a lower residual supply would be expected. To obtain a SvO_2, blood is taken from the pulmonary artery. In the pulmonary artery, blood has returned from the superior vena cava, inferior vena cava and coronary veins. Normal SvO_2 should be between 60–80%. However, with the decline of Pulmonary Artery (PA) catheter use, a $ScVO_2$ is more commonly seen in non-cardiac critical care units. This sample is taken from a jugular or subclavian central line. It reflects the oxygen level in the right atrium and therefore includes blood returning via the inferior and superior vena cava, but not the coronary veins. We would therefore expect it to be slightly higher – an $ScVO_2$ of >70% is regarded as normal.

Examination scenario

Capillary Refill Time (CRT) is the time taken for the distal capillary bed to retain its perfusion and its red colour after blanching has been applied. It can be an indication of cardiac output.

When taking peripheral CRT, the fingertip should be held at heart level and cutaneous pressure applied for 5 seconds, causing blanching. The time taken for the skin to return to normal colour is known as CRT. Normal CRT is <2 seconds (UKRC 2021). An increased CRT indicates poor cardiac output.

Age, lighting, cold surroundings, vasoconstrictive and vasodilator drugs and pressure application can all affect peripheral CRT. For these reasons, central CRT can provide a more accurate measurement in the critically ill patient. Cutaneous pressure is applied for 5 seconds at the top of the sternum causing blanching. As with peripheral CRT, it would be expected that the colour returns to normal in <2 seconds.

Neurological status

To achieve a sufficient cerebral perfusion pressure and therefore supply of oxygen and glucose, the brain needs an adequate MAP. Alterations to cardiac function may cause the MAP to fall below the required threshold and as a result conscious level may be reduced (for more information on the importance of blood pressure in maintaining conscious levels, refer to Chapter 14).

Urine output

The kidneys receive around 20% of cardiac output. Any significant drop in cardiac output or blood pressure will result in a reduction in urine output and can lead to the development of an Acute Kidney Injury (AKI). As such the monitoring of urine output and function offers a useful indicator of cardiovascular dysfunction.

Blood results

Snapshot

Beatrice is a 42--year-old female admitted to hospital with pneumonia. She has developed an AKI and the laboratory have just rung through a potassium level of 6.6 mmols/L. As the nurse looking after her that day, you should do the following:

- Depending on the area the patient is critically unwell, you may need to contact the medical team, critical care outreach, or ICU registrar.
- If able to, gain informed consent from the patient for any interventions carried out.
- Ensure continuous ECG monitoring is attached to the patient.
- Record a 12-lead ECG to show the reviewer.
- Commence the hyperkalaemia protocol or policy in accordance with hospital guidelines.
- Provide support and reassurance to the patient throughout.
- Document all interventions in the patient's notes.

There are many blood tests that can be carried out as part of the cardiovascular assessment. Table 19.3 identifies some of these, alongside the normal limits and rationale. The table is not conclusive and it should be ensured that appropriate clinical decision making is used to ensure patients receive the correct tests.

Medications management: potassium

Potassium is used to treat hypokalaemia (potassium level <3.5 mmol/L). The amount given will depend on how low the patient's potassium level is.

When infused peripherally doses must not exceed 40 mmol/L to avoid the risk of extravasation. When infused centrally, higher concentrations can be given, but the patient must have continuous ECG monitoring. In both circumstances, ready-mixed solutions are preferred.

Following infusion, there should be repeat sampling of plasma-potassium concentration to determine the need for repeat doses.

It should be given with caution in people with renal impairment.

Medications management: insulin dextrose

Insulin dextrose works by shifting potassium into the cells to reduce serum potassium concentration. It has a maximal effect up to-60 minutes and can be repeated if necessary. Potassium levels should continue to be monitored after its administration. The recommended dose is 10 international units (iu) of insulin mixed with 25g of glucose (UKRC, 2021).

Blood glucose levels should be closely monitored after administration aiming for normoglycaemia (4–8 mmols/L). For most people without diabetes, normal blood glucose levels are between 4 and to 6 mmol/L before meals and less than 8 mmol/L two hours after eating (British Heart Foundation (BHF), 2020).

259

Table 19.3 Relevant blood tests as part of a cardiovascular assessment.

Investigation	Normal limits	Rationale	Minimum frequency
Haemoglobin	- 120–160g/L (women) - 130–170g/L (men)	- Assess for bleeding	Daily
Clotting studies	- Activated partial thromboplastin time (APTT): 27.4–40.3s - International Normalised Ratio (INR): 1–1.2 - Platelets: 150–400 × 10⁹/L	- Assess risk of excessive bleeding - Assess risk of clot formation - Assess response to treatment	Daily
Urea and electrolytes	- Sodium 135–145 mmol/L - Potassium 3.5–5.3 mmol/L - Calcium 2.2–2.6 mmol/L - Magnesium 0.7–1.0 mmol/L - Urea - 2.5-6.5 mmol/L - Creatinine 70–120 µmol/L	- Derangements in electrolytes can lead to cardiac arrhythmias - Creatinine is used to diagnose acute kidney injury (AKI), which can be caused by reduced cardiac output	Daily
Cardiac biomarkers	- Troponins - Creatinine kinase (CK), aspartate transaminase (AST) and lactate dehydrogenase (LDH) - Brain natriuretic peptide (BNP)	- Rise after myocardial injury, can help exclude myocardial infarction - Indication of myocardial injury - High levels associate with heart failure	- Sensitivity good 12 hours after injury - Peaks 24 hours after injury
Relevant drug levels	- Digoxin 0.5–1.0 µg/L in heart failure and 0.5–2.0 µg/L in AF	- To prevent unwanted side effects associated with toxicity	- At least weekly

Snapshot

Roy is a 36-year-old who was admitted to hospital following an abdominal stabbing. He lost large amounts of blood and required surgery. He was extubated post-operatively and admitted to the critical care unit 4 hours ago. Roy is showing signs of hypovolaemia. At 0900 a Registered Nurse (RN) records the following information on his observation chart:

Airway (A): Patent

Breathing (B): Oxygen saturations 92% (NEWS2 = 2), on 40% humidified oxygen via facemask (NEWS2 = 2), respiratory rate (RR) 28 breaths per minute (NEWS2 = 3).

Cardiovascular System (C): Blood Pressure (BP) is 91/60 (NEWS2 = 2), Heart Rate (HR) 115 beats per minute (NEWS2 = 2), capillary refill time (CRT) 4 seconds, he is cool to touch.

Disability (D): Patient is alert (NEWS2 = 0) under the physiological parameter 'consciousness', Body temperature (T) 35.8°C (NEWS2 = 1).

Exposure (E): Abdomen soft but guarded and painful to touch.

Total NEWS2 score: 12.

Nursing actions:

- Urgent or emergency response to include staff with critical care skills including airway management skills (RCP, 2017).
- A full head-to-toe assessment and diagnostic tests including blood tests and blood cultures.

Findings:

- Roy was not actively bleeding.
- Roy was hypovolemic requiring further fluid resuscitation.
- He was also in pain post-op, requiring review and administration of further analgesia.
- This hypovolaemia lead to his hypotension, and compensatory increase in heart rate.
- Roy received fluid resuscitation, whilst being continuously monitored. His urine output was measured closely and arterial blood gases (ABG) were taken.
- Roy was prescribed an opioid via patient-controlled analgesia (PCA) for his pain control.

Clinical investigations: dynamic measurements (passive leg raise)

Dynamic measurements such as passive leg raises, stroke volume, variations in systolic and pulse pressure have been shown to have better diagnostic accuracy in assessing fluid responsiveness (Rhodes et al., 2017). Fluid boluses are given as long as improvements are seen (more on fluid balance and circulation can be found in Chapter 20).

Passive leg raises involve lying the patient in supine position and then raising the legs to 45°. This will shift the fluid from the legs to the central circulatory system as if a fluid bolus had just been given. Changes in the BP would indicate available space in the circulating volume for fluid administration. More information on these dynamic measurements and fluid responsiveness can be found in Chapter 20 (Fluid balance/circulation).

6Cs: Communication

When changes in a patient's condition are identified, it is essential that these are communicated to the appropriate people in a timely manner. Both the change, as well as the communication should be documented in the patients notes.

Advanced haemodynamic monitoring

The exact indications for advanced haemodynamic monitoring are debated in the literature due to the inability to show a clear reduction in mortality associated with its use (Harvey et al., 2005; Pearse et al., 2014). The European Society of Intensive Care Medicine (Cecconi et al., 2014) concluded that advanced haemodynamic monitoring is indicated when a patient has not responded to initial therapy, and the use of fluid therapy and inotropes is being considered (Cecconi et al., 2014). There are multiple devices available, each with their own advantages and disadvantages. Any decision to start advanced monitoring should include consideration of the risks involved and the potential benefits gained (ICS, 2019).

The Guidelines for the Provision of Intensive Care Services (ICS, 2019), state that transthoracic echocardiography (ECHO) should be available to all critical care patients, and that the PA catheter is the gold standard method of advanced haemodynamic monitoring which all other methods are compared to.

Transthoracic ECHO will provide a rapid, bedside, non-invasive assessment of the patient's heart, giving the clinician information on cardiac contractility, fluid status and the presence of any underlying pathologies such as valvular defects, thrombus and pericardial effusion. It is the favoured method to decipher the cause of shock (Cecconi et al., 2014; NICE, 2014). Nevertheless, transthoracic ECHO will only provide information at the given time and therefore other devices which provide continuous readings are often used. These devices and some of the measurements they provide are explored in Tables 19.4 and 19.5.

6Cs: Care

It is essential to provide holistic care to the critically ill patient. This care has to take into account the person's individual needs ensuring they are at the centre of all that is done.

Table 19.4 Different methods of advanced haemodynamic monitoring.

Device	Invasive or non-invasive	Requires calibration	Additional measurements provided by device include	Advantages	Disadvantages
Pulmonary artery catheter (Pulmonary thermodilution method)	Invasive.	Yes	- Pulmonary artery wedge pressure (PAWP) - Pulmonary artery pressure (PAP) - Right atrial (RA) pressure - Right ventricular (RV) pressure - Mixed venous oxygen saturations	- Provides direct measurements from right atrium, right ventricle and pulmonary artery - Regarded as gold standard	- CRBSIs - Arrhythmias - Thrombosis - Catheter migration - Risk of pulmonary artery rupture - Complex device, requires high level of training and regular use to maintain competence - PAC-MAN study (2008) did not identify clear reduction in mortality associated with its use (Harvey et al., 2005)
Transpulmonary thermodilution (PiCCO)	Invasive but less so than PA catheter – no additional lines needed.	Yes	- Extravascular lung water index (EVLWI) - Global end-diastolic volume (GEDV) - Intrathoracic blood volume (ITBV) - Stroke volume variation (SVV) %	- No additional lines needed. - Provides continuous measurements of cardiac output (CO) and systemic vascular resistance (SVR).	- Refer to complications associated with arterial lines and central lines. - Can provide inaccurate measurements if CVC located in femoral vein and arterial line trace dampened.
Transpulmonary dye dilution (LiDCO)	Invasive but less so than PA catheter as no additional lines needed.	Yes	- SVV % - Pulse pressure variation (PPV) (%) - Systolic pressure variation (SPV) (%)	- No additional lines needed. - Provides continuous measurement of CO and SVR.	- Please refer to complications associated with arterial lines and central lines. - Cannot be used on patients receiving lithium.
Oesophageal Doppler	Non-invasive – ultrasound probe inserted into oesophagus. Blood flow in the descending aorta is measured to establish cardiac output	No	- Flow time corrected (FTc) – duration of blood flow during systole corrected to heart rate - Peak velocity (PV) – highest blood velocity in systole	- Continuous measurements - Easy to insert - Decreased risk of infection compared to other devices	- Dislodgement of probe - Can cause damage to oesophagus - Cannot be used in certain patients i.e. facial trauma, oesophageal damage, <16 years of age.

261

Table 19.5 Advanced haemodynamic readings and normal values.

Cardiac reading	Definition	Normal values	Increased in	Decreased in
Cardiac output (CO)	Amount of blood ejected from the left ventricle in one minute.	4–6 L/min	- Hyperdynamic state – a result of a normal physiological response e.g. anxiety and stress, or linked to a pathological condition such as sepsis.	- Bradycardia - Hypovolaemia - Decreased contractility - Increased afterload
Stroke volume (SV)	Amount of blood ejected from the left ventricle in one beat.	70–100 mL	- Increased pre-load - Increased contractility (use of positive inotropes)	- Hypovolaemia - Tachycardia (reduced filling time) - Decreased contractility - Increased afterload

(Continued)

Table 19.5   (Continued)

Cardiac reading	Definition	Normal values	Increased in	Decreased in
Systemic vascular resistance (SVR)	The resistance in the circulatory system. The pressure the left ventricle has to overcome to eject blood from the heart.	960–1400 dynes.s/cm⁵	Indicates vasoconstriction · Vasopressors e.g. Noradrenaline · Cardiogenic shock	Indicates vasodilation · Sepsis · Anaphylaxis · Vasodilatory drugs such as GTN and labetalol · Side effect of drugs e.g. propofol.
Pulmonary vascular resistance (PVR)	The pressure the right ventricle must overcome to eject blood from the heart	25–125 dynes.s/cm⁵	· Vasoconstriction · Left ventricular heart failure · Acute respiratory distress syndrome (ARDS) · Pulmonary embolism	· Vasodilation · Sepsis · Anaphylaxis · Vasodilatory drugs such as GTN and labetalol · Side effect of drugs e.g. propofol.
Stroke volume variance (SVV) %	Difference between minimum and maximum stroke volumes	<10%	· Likely to need fluid * will be high in arrhythmias i.e. atrial fibrillation	· Normovolemia
Extravascular lung water index (EVLW)	Amount of water in the lungs	3–7ml/kg	· Pulmonary oedema · Acute Respiratory Distress Syndrome (ARDS)	
Right atrial (RA) pressure	Pressure in the right atrium	0–5 mmHg	· Right-sided heart failure · Tamponade · Volume overload	· Hypovolaemia
Pulmonary artery pressure (PAP)	Systolic and diastolic pulmonary artery pressures	20–25/10–15 mmHg	· Pulmonary hypertension · Left-sided heart failure · Chronic lung disease	· Hypovolaemia
Pulmonary artery wedge pressure (PAWP)	Reflection of left ventricular end-diastolic pressure	6–12 mmHg	· Left-sided heart failure · Tamponade	· Hypovolaemia
Mixed venous oxygen saturation (SvO₂)	% of saturated haemoglobin in blood returning to the pulmonary artery.	70–75%	· Decreased oxygen demand · Increased oxygen supply	· Increased oxygen demand – i.e. sepsis · Decreased oxygen supply i.e. heart failure

Definitions and normal values adapted from Mallet et al., 2013

* Many measurements can be 'indexed', this means that the measurement is indexed to the patient's body size, thus providing a more accurate indication of cardiac function, i.e. cardiac output is 4–6 L/min, cardiac index would be expected to be between 2.5–4.0 L/min/m².

Cardiac pacing

When the electrical activity of the heart is insufficient and it fails to generate adequate cardiac output, pacing may be used. This could be the case in persistent bradycardias and heart blocks associated with haemodynamic compromise. It can also be used to suppress tachycardias. This is known as 'overdrive pacing' (Adam and Osborne, 2013). During pacing a small electrical current is delivered to stimulate myocardial contraction. It can be temporary or permanent.

Temporary pacing is available via transcutaneous, transvenous and epicardial routes.

Transcutaneous pacing forms part of the UKRC bradycardia algorithm (2021). It is non-invasive, easy to perform and can be used to maintain cardiac output in an emergency whilst waiting for expert help (UKRC, 2021). Large adhesive pads are placed over the chest and connected to the device where voltage and rate is set to achieve the desired outcome. Transcutaneous pacing is uncomfortable for the patient so their pain should be regularly assessed and analgesia and sedation administered according to prescription. Due to the discomfort experienced and the unreliable ventricular stimulation it provides, it should only be used in an emergency when there is no other option (Brignole et al., 2013).

Transvenous pacing involves the insertion of a wire through a large vein which is advanced through the right atrium to the right ventricle where it sits against the septal wall. Like transcutaneous pacing, it should only be used in an emergency, and if chronotropic drugs such as atropine, have failed (Brignole et al., 2013). Due to the complications associated with its insertion and positioning it is recommended that this option be avoided wherever possible. Where the need for permanent pacing is apparent, every effort should be made to insert it in a timely manner (Brignole et al., 2013).

Epicardial pacing wires may be electively sutured to the pericardial surface of the heart during cardiac surgery. Pacing can be delivered to either the atria, ventricles or both. Various settings are available and set to achieve the desired outcome. Recent research has found that rather than routinely inserting epicardial wires, it may be appropriate to selectively insert them into patients who are more at risk of arrhythmias due to the complications associated with their use – tamponade, infection (Cote et al., 2020).

Regardless of the type of temporary pacing, all patients should have strict ECG monitoring to ensure appropriate capture is maintained. Any invasive lines should be secured in place or removed if not being used. Strict infection control procedures should be maintained in accordance with EPIC 3 guidelines (Loveday et al., 2014). Nursing staff caring for patients receiving pacing should be appropriately trained and competent.

Nursing considerations and recommendations for practice

The Nursing and Midwifery Council (NMC) (2018) requires Registered Nurses and Nursing Associates to preserve safety; this applies to the patient and those you work with.

The nurse must be able to accurately assess needs and where appropriate refer to other practitioners. Nurses are required to act in the best interests of the individual seeking assistance from a suitably qualified and experienced health-care professional if required.

6Cs: Commitment

Nurses must be committed to providing high-quality, evidence-based, safe patient care.

Conclusion

A thorough and timely cardiovascular assessment of the critically ill patient allows for appropriate treatment to be implemented to improve patient outcomes and reduce mortality. There are many elements to a comprehensive cardiovascular assessment. Clinical decisions should not be made because of one of these elements, but on the all assessment findings including the patient's history, physical examination and results of investigations such as blood tests and scans. When the patient has capacity, every effort should be made to involve them in decision making, ensuring they have a clear understanding of any treatments being considered.

Take home points

1. Cardiovascular status should be assessed as part of the head-to-toe assessment provided by critical care nurses and healthcare professionals, and even more frequently when there are changes to a patient's condition.
2. Patients in critical care settings should have continuous 3–5 lead ECG monitoring.
3. Nurses and healthcare professionals working in critical care environments should be able to recognise and respond appropriately to common cardiac arrhythmias.
4. Invasive blood pressure monitoring rather than non-invasive blood pressure monitoring is the gold standard method in critical care units.
5. Catheter-related blood stream infections associated with central venous catheters are amongst some of the most dangerous complications associated with admissions to critical care and can lead to sepsis and death. Nurses must be familiar with the EPIC 3 guidance (Loveday et al., 2014).
6. CVP is not a reliable indicator of fluid responsiveness when used in isolation, but does provide an accurate estimate of right atrial pressure.
7. Lactate and central or mixed venous oxygen saturations are indicators of tissue perfusion.
8. Advanced haemodynamic monitoring is indicated when a patient fails to respond to initial fluid therapy.
9. The pulmonary artery catheter remains the gold standard method of advanced haemodynamic monitoring despite a lack of evidence around reduction in mortality.
10. Within critical care, temporary or permanent pacing can be used to treat arrhythmias and improve cardiac output.

References

Adam, S. and Osborne, S. (2013). *Oxford Handbook of Critical Care Nursing*. Oxford University Press: New York.

Adam, S., Osborne, S., and Welch, J. (2017). *Critical Care Nursing: Science and Practice*, 3e. Oxford: Oxford University Press.

Annane, D., Sebile, V., Duboc, D. et al. (2008). Incidence and prognosis of sustained arrhythmias in critically ill patients. *American Journal of Respiratory and Critical Care Medicine* 178: 20–25.

Badhwar, N., Kusomoto, F., and Goldschlager, N. (2011). Arrhythmias in the coronary care unit. *Journal of Intensive Care Medicine* 27(5): 267–289. doi.org/10.1177%2F0885066611402165.

Bickley, L. (2016). *Bates' Guide to Physical Examination and History Taking*, 12e. Wolters Kluwer.

British Heart Foundation (BHF) (2020). Heart Matters. https://www.bhf.org.uk/informationsupport/heart-matters-magazine/medical/tests/blood-sugar#:~:text=For%20most%20people%20without%20diabetes,L%20two%20hours%20after%20eating (accessed 22 December 2020).

Bion, J., Richardson, A., Hibbert P. et al. (2013). 'Matching Michegan': a 2-year stepped interventional programme to minimise central venous catheter – blood stream infections in intensive care units in England. *BMJ Quality and Safety*. 22: 110–123. doi.10.1136/bmjqs-2012-001325.

BNF (2020). British National Formulary online: Fluids and electrolytes. https://bnf.nice.org.uk/treatment-summary/fluids-and-electrolytes.html (accessed 20 November 2020).

Brignole, M., Auricchio, A., Baron-Esquivias G. et al. (2013). ESC Guidelines on cardiac pacing and cardiac resynchronisation therapy. *European Heart Journal* 34: 2281–2329. doi:10.1093/eurheartj/eht150.

Cecconi, M., Backer, D., and Antonelli, M. (2014). Consensus on circulatory shock and haemodynamic monitoring. *Taskforce of the European Society or Intensive Care Medicine* 40(12): 1795–1815. doi: 10.1007/s00134-014-3525-z.

Cote, C., Bahaffar, A., Tremblay, P., and Herman, C. (2020). Prediction of temporary epicardial pacing wire use in cardiac surgery. *Journal of Cardiac Surgery*. 35: 1933–1940. doi:10.1111/jocs.14870.

Critical Care Networks-National Nurse Leads (CC3N) (2015). National Competency Framework for Registered Nurses in Adult Critical Care. Step 2 Competencies. https://www.cc3n.org.uk/uploads/9/8/4/2/98425184/02_new_step_2_final.pdf (accessed 15 October 2020).

Dougherty, L. and Lister, S. (2020). *The Royal Marsden Manual of Clinical Nursing Procedures*, professional edition, 10e. Oxford: Wiley Blackwell.

Dutton, H. and Finch, J. (2018). *Acute and Critical Care Nursing at a Glance*. Oxford: Wiley Blackwell.

Hampton, J. (2013). *The ECG Made Easy*, 8e. London: Churchill Livingstone Elsevier.

Harvey, S., Harrison, D., Singer M. et al. (2005). Assessment of the clinical effectiveness of pulmonary artery catheters in management of patients in intensive care (PAC-Man): a randomised controlled trial. *Lancet* 366 (9484): 472–477. doi.org/10.1016/S0140-6736(05)67061-4.

Intensive Care Society (ICS) (2019). Guidelines for the Provision of Intensive Care Services , 2e. https://ics.ac.uk/ICS/ICS/GuidelinesAndStandards/GPICS_2nd_Edition.aspx (accessed 7 October 2020).

Intensive Care Society (2020). Safety checklists for invasive procedures. https://www.ficm.ac.uk/safety-and-clinical-quality/safety-checklists-invasive-procedures (accessed 19 November 2020).

Joint Commission (2013). National patient safety goal on alarm management. https://www.jointcommission.org/-/media/tjc/documents/standards/r3-reports/r3_report_issue_5_12_2_13_final.pdf (accessed 8 November 2020).

Lamontagne, F., Cook, D., Meade M. et al. (2017). Vasopressor use for sever hypotension: A multicentre prospective observational study. *PloSone* 12(1). doi.10.1371/journal.pone.0167840.

Lamontagne, F., Richards-Belle, A., and Thomas, K. (2020). Effect of reduced exposure to vasopressors on 90-day mortality in older critically ill patients with vasodilatory hypotension: A randomised clinical trial. *JAMA* 323 (10): 938–949. doi:10.1001/jama2020.0903.

Lehman, L., Mohammed, S., and Talmor, D. (2013). Methods of blood pressure management. *Critical Care Medicine* 41(1): 34–40. doi.10.1097/ccm.0b013e318265ea46.

Loveday, H., Wilson, J., Pratt R. et al. (2014). Epic3: National evidence-based guidelines for preventing healthcare-associated infections in NHS hospitals in England. *Journal of Hospital Infection* 86: S1–S70. doi: 10.1016/s0195-6701(13)60012-2.

Mallet, J., Albarran, J., and Richardson, A. (eds) (2013). *Critical Care Manual of Clinical Procedures and Competencies*. Chichester: Wiley Blackwell.

Marieb, E. (2015). *Essentials of Human Anatomy and Physiology*, 11e. Harlow: Pearson Education Limited.

Marik, P., Baram, M., and Vahid, B. (2008). Does central venous pressure predict fluid responsiveness? A systematic review of the literature and the tale of seven mares. *Chest* 134(1): 172–178. doi:10.1378/chest.07-2331.

Marik, P. and Cavallazzi, R. (2013). Does the central venous pressure predict fluid responsiveness? An updated meta-analysis and a plea for some common sense. *Critical Care Medicine* 41(7): 1774–1781.

NHS England (2015). National Safety Standards for Invasive Procedure (NatSSIPs). https://www.england.nhs.uk/wp-content/uploads/2015/09/natssips-safety-standards.pdf (accessed 15 October 2020).

NHS Improvement (2018). Never Events list 2018. https://improvement.nhs.uk/documents/2266/Never_Events_list_2018_FINAL_v5.pdf (accessed 15 October 2020).

NICE (2014). Sepsis: Recognition diagnosis and early management. https://www.nice.org.uk/guidance/ng51/resources/sepsis-recognition-diagnosis-and-early-management-pdf-1837508256709 (accessed 17 October 2020).

NMC (2018). The Code. Professional Standards of Practice and Behaviour for Nurses, Midwives and Nursing Associates https://www.nmc.org.uk/globalassets/sitedocuments/nmc-publications/nmc-code.pdf (accessed 20 November 2020).

Pearse, R., Harrison, D., MacDonald N. et al. (2014). Effect of a perioperative, cardiac output guided haemodynamic therapy algorithm on outcomes following major gastrointestinal surgery a randomised clinical trial and systematic review. *JAMA*. 311 (21): 2181–2190. doi:.10.1001/jama.2014.5305.

Rhodes, A., Evans, L., Alhazzani, W. et al. (2017). Surviving sepsis campaign: International guidelines for management of sepsis and septic shock: 2016. *Intensive Care Medicine*. 43: 304–377. doi: 10.1007/s00134-017-4683-6.

Royal College of Physicians. (2017). National Early Warning Score (NEWS) 2: Standardising the assessment of acute-illness severity in the NHS. https://www.rcplondon.ac.uk/projects/outputs/national-early-warning-score-news-2 (accessed 15 December 2020).

Scheer, B., Perel, A., and Pfeiffer, U. (2002). Clinical review: Complications and risk factors of peripheral arterial catheters used for haemodynamic monitoring in anaesthesia and intensive care medicine. *Critical Care*. 6(3): 198–204.

Senaratne, J., Sandhu, R., and Barnett, C. (2020). Approach to ventricular arrhythmias in the intensive care unit. *Journal of Intensive Care Medicine*. https://journals.sagepub.com/doi/full/10.1177/0885066620912701 (accessed 7 November 2020).

Tarditi, D. and Hollenberg, S. (2006). Cardiac arrhythmias in the intensive care unit. *Seminars in Respiratory and Critical Care Medicine* 27(3): 221–229. doi:1.1055/s-2006-945525.

UK Resuscitation Council (2021a). The ABCDE approach. https://www.resus.org.uk/library/abcde-approach (accessed 11 September 2020).

UK Resuscitation Council (UK) (2021b). *Advanced Life Support*, 8e. Resuscitation Council: London.

Wilson, M., Beesley, S., Grow A. et al. (2019). Humanzing the intensive care unit. *Critical Care*. https://ccforum.biomedcentral.com/articles/10.1186/s13054-019-2327-7 (accessed 24 January 2021).

World Health Organisation (2009). WHO Guidelines on Hand Hygiene in Health Care: First Global Patient Safety Challenge Clean Care is Safer Care. https://www.who.int/publications/i/item/9789241597906 (accessed 9 January 2021).

Chapter 20

Fluids and electrolytes in critically ill patients

Barry Hill

Aim

This aim of this chapter is to provide the reader with an evidence-based understanding of the importance of fluids and electrolytes in the context of patients who are cared for in critical care settings.

Learning outcomes

After reading this chapter the reader will be able to:

- Understand the complexities of critical care and addressing needs regarding fluids and electrolytes in critically unwell people.
- Gain knowledge about the different fluids and electrolytes in the context of critical illness.
- Explore the complications, investigations, and contemporary clinical management of fluid and electrolyte disorders including the 5 Rs of intravenous (IV) fluid therapy.
- Appreciate the differences between crystalloids and colloids.
- Gain knowledge about fluid and electrolyte management.

Test your prior knowledge

- Can you name the most common types of electrolytes?
- What crystalloids and colloids can you name, and can you identify the differences between them?
- What are the 5 Rs of IV fluid therapy?
- What ECG changes would you expect to see in a patient with hyperkalaemia?
- What does third spacing mean?
- What is the calculation of IV fluid administration for a person who is nil by mouth who requires fluid before surgery?

Fundamentals of Critical Care: A Textbook for Nursing and Healthcare Students, First Edition. Edited by Ian Peate and Barry Hill.
© 2023 John Wiley & Sons Ltd. Published 2023 by John Wiley & Sons Ltd.
Companion website: www.wiley.com/go/peate/criticalcare

Introduction

Chapter 20 establishes the fundamental knowledge critical care nurses and healthcare professionals must have regarding fluids and electrolytes in patients who are critically unwell. Fluid and electrolyte disorders are among the most common clinical problems encountered in people with critical illness. Critical disorders such as severe burns, trauma, sepsis, traumatic brain injuries, and heart failure lead to disturbances in fluid and electrolyte homeostasis. In the context of critical illness, it is imperative that critical care nurses and healthcare professionals can relate multi-organ failure and understand the applied pathophysiology. An excellent book that can support acquisition of knowledge regarding pathophysiology is *Fundamentals of Applied Pathophysiology: An Essential Guide for Nursing and Healthcare Students* (Peate, 2021). In brief, for effective tissue and organ perfusion, maintenance of finely balanced levels of oxygen, fluid and electrolytes (homoeostasis) is essential. Fluid volumes need to be distributed into the intracellular and extracellular spaces (the latter being further divided into the interstitial and intravascular compartments). The movement of fluid between these spaces is continual. This enables cells to receive their necessary supply of electrolytes such as sodium, potassium and carbon. Along with oxygen, these are fundamental for cell performance (Peate and Evans, 2020). Homoeostasis is easily affected by any insult to the body, be it from illness, injury, trauma or medication. This imbalance can quickly lead to worsening illness and/or impede recovery. Hypovolaemia will reduce the circulating fluid volumes, resulting in reduced electrolyte and oxygen supply to the cells. A large reduction in fluid volume can result in hypovolaemic shock. Patients who go into hypovolaemic shock need fluid resuscitation to maintain their cardiac output and organ perfusion.

The possible mechanisms that lead to disturbances in fluid and electrolyte homeostasis include reduced perfusion to the kidney due to hypovolemia or hypotension; activation of hormonal systems such as renin-angiotensin-aldosterone system and vasopressin; and tubular damage caused by ischaemic or nephrotoxic kidney damage, including renal insult caused by a myriad of medications used in intensive care. In addition, inappropriate administration of fluid and electrolytes should be considered in the diagnosis and treatment of fluid and electrolyte disturbances.

The role of the critical care nurse

Critical care nurses play a vital role in caring for critically ill patients. They are well educated and competent in providing continuous monitoring and advanced care for different critical conditions. The nurse:patient ratio in the CCU is mostly 1:1 or 1:2 based on the acuity of a patient's needs. Therefore, critical care nurses can continually monitor and detect any changes in the patient's condition at an early stage that requires prompt management, such as fluid and electrolyte imbalances. Critical care nurses must have knowledge and clinical skills required for optimal maintenance of patients' hydration status and electrolyte balance. They should also have critical thinking and advanced problem-solving skills, and practice based upon evidence-based research to provide high-quality patient care.

Step 2 competencies: National standards

2:2.2 Fluid Management

This chapter will support the critical care student to demonstrate appropriate knowledge. Use this book as well as other chapters such as blood transfusions to enable you to develop competence in formulating a rationale through discussion, and the application to your practice.

- Fluid compartments within the body
- Osmosis and diffusion in relation to fluid movement
- Identify the clinical indications that necessitate fluid intervention
- Identify key differences between colloids, crystalloids and blood products
- Rationalise the choice of colloids, crystalloids and blood products in relation to the cardiac compromised patient
- Rationalise the choice of colloids, crystalloids and blood products in relation to the patient with pre-existing cardiac disease
- Adjust fluid management to the patient's physiological condition

Intravenous fluids

The human body is approximately 80% water that is distributed unevenly between extracellular and intracellular compartments, with extracellular fluid further divided between intravascular and interstitial compartments (Woodrow, 2018). Fluid and electrolyte disturbances among critically ill patients are common in people with critical illness. The use of intravenous fluids is challenging in critically ill patients because of predisposing factors that result in altered fluid distribution and accelerated volume losses. These complexities are perpetuated by the dynamic nature of critical illness, in which fluid requirements can change frequently and rapidly. Critical care nurses must be able to navigate these challenges because uncorrected fluid disturbances are associated with increased morbidity and mortality. Optimal fluid management requires a thorough understanding of fluid homeostasis, composition, and impact on haemodynamic stability.

266

Snapshot

Orange Flag

Health care professionals regard the use of needles as routine; yet for patients, needles can arouse anxiety. Needle phobia is a fear of medical procedures that involve needles or injections. It is very common and is nothing to be ashamed of. Many patients with needle phobia may have had a lot of blood tests or procedures as a child. A fear of needles and injections often, but not always, results from bad memories of needles earlier in life.

There are ways in which the nurse can comfort the patient and minimise the anxiety and pain they are experiencing.

The intravenous fluids available for use can be broadly classified as crystalloids or colloids (Table 20.1). Indications for fluid therapy include replacement of insensible fluid losses, replacement of volume deficits, and restoration of intravascular volume depletion. The selection of fluid composition, dose, and duration should be tailored to meet the goal of fluid therapy. For example, intravenous fluid resuscitation to rapidly restore systemic circulation is a fundamental component of treating critically ill patients with sepsis. Although intravenous fluids can be life-saving, risks associated with treatment also have the potential to influence patient outcomes.

Medicines management

The management of intravenous fluids is a common activity, safe and unambiguous fluid prescribing is a key safety requirement. Errors in intravenous fluid management are common and have been attributed to inadequate training and knowledge. When there is poor fluid management this can result in serious morbidity, including pulmonary oedema and dangerous hyponatraemia due to excessive fluid administration and acute kidney injury.

Always remember the 5 Rs when prescribing and administrating of intravenous fluids. Intravenous fluids must be recognised as drugs with individualised prescriptions and vigilant monitoring for each patient. At all times adhere to local policy and procedure and this includes the correct procedure for documenting the administration of the fluids and the completion of fluid balance charts

Table 20.1 Crystalloid and colloids.

Crystalloid	Colloid
Sodium chloride NaCl Glucose Compound sodium lactate (Hartmann's)	Blood and blood components (see Chapter 8 for more information on blood transfusions) Gelatins Dextrans Starches

Crystalloids versus colloids critical care

Crystalloids and colloids are plasma volume expanders used to increase a depleted circulating volume. Over the years they have been used separately or together to manage haemodynamic instability. Both are suitable in fluid resuscitation, hypovolaemia, trauma, sepsis and burns, and in the pre-, post- and peri-operative period. On occasion, they are used together. Colloids carry an increased risk of anaphylaxis, are more expensive and come with an added complication for vegetarian or vegan patients, as some preparations contain gelatin (Joint Formulary Committee, 2021). However, colloid solutions are less likely to cause oedema than crystalloid solutions. Crystalloids are less expensive, carry little or no risk of anaphylaxis, and pose no problem for vegetarian or vegan patients. However, evidence on any potential harmful effects of crystalloids is inconclusive. Table 20.2 summarises the main characteristics of crystalloid and colloid solutions.

The question of which plasma volume expander to use has long been controversial, resulting in several studies and systematic reviews. In recent years, numerous research studies have been performed in different clinical situations

Table 20.2 A summary of the main characteristics of crystalloid and colloid solutions. *Source:* Smith, 2017.

Crystalloid solution	Colloid sollution
Half-life of 30-60 minutes	Half-life of several hours or days
Three times the volume needed for replacernent	Replaces fluid volume for volume
Excessive use can cause peripheral and pulmonary oedema	Excessive use can precipitate cardiac failure
Molecules small enough to freely cross capillary walls, so less fluid remains in the intravascular spaces	Molecules too large to cross capillary walls, so fluid remains in intravascular spaces for longer
Inexpensive	More expensive than crystalloids
Non-allergenic	Risk of anaphylactic reactions
Suitable for vegetarian or vegan patients	Some preparations unsuitable for vegetarian or vegan patients

to compare crystalloids and colloids and consider their advantages and disadvantages. In 2021, Lewis et al's systematic review 'Colloids versus crystalloids for fluid resuscitation in critically ill people' found that using colloids (starches; dextrans; or albumin or fresh frozen plasma (FFP)) compared to crystalloids for fluid replacement probably makes little or no difference to the number of critically ill people who die. They noted that it may make little or no difference to the number of people who die if gelatins or crystalloids are used for fluid replacement. Their research (Lewis et al., 2021) found that starches probably increase the need for blood transfusion and renal replacement therapy slightly within CCU patients. Using albumin or FFP may make little or no difference to the need for renal replacement therapy. They were uncertain whether using dextrans, albumin or FFP, or crystalloids affects the need for blood transfusion. Similarly, they were uncertain if colloids or crystalloids

increase the number of adverse events. However, the National Institute for Health and Care Excellence (NICE, 2021a) makes evidence-based recommendations alongside the British National Formulary and advocates specific fluid types to help guide clinicians in their clinical decision-making processes.

Fluid management

Volume resuscitation of a patient with hypovolaemic shock or sepsis is an essential component of patient care. Vast amounts of intravenous fluid are usually administered to replace intravascular volume deficit and to minimise complications attributed to hypovolaemia such as tachycardia (a heart rate (HR) above 100 beats per minute), hypotension (blood pressure (BP) systolic less than 90 mmHg), acute kidney injury (AKI) and multi-organ failure (MOF). Goal-directed therapies focus on restoration of normal blood pressure and organ perfusion have been advocated in the management of critically ill patients. Early goal-directed therapy, which is instituted in the initial phase of management of patients with fluid status altering pathology, such as severe sepsis or septic shock improves overall survival. Clinicians should bear in mind that assessment of haemodynamic response to volume resuscitation and vasopressors (vasopressin and phenylephrine) and inopressors (norepinephrine, epinephrine, and dopamine) should be based on specific haemodynamic and oxygenation parameters such as mean arterial pressure (MAP), central venous pressure (CVP) and central venous oxygen saturation, not solely on symptoms and physical findings.

In contrast to the notion of aggressive and liberal volume resuscitation, it is important to consider that fluid overload may be detrimental to critically ill patients. Relatively little attention has been paid to the consequences of fluid overload such as respiratory failure, increased cardiac demand, and peripheral oedema. Fluid overload is noted to be associated with adverse outcomes. Although uniform definitions of fluid overload and well-designed randomised clinical trials are lacking, there seems to be a need to avoid overenthusiastic fluid resuscitation in a subset of patients.

Examination scenario

Pitting oedema is a physical examination finding that occurs when you press on a patient's skin, usually in the lower limbs, for example, ankles or feet, and a 'pit' forms at the site of pressure.

Pitting oedema can be graded on a scale from 0 to 4, which is based on both the depth the 'pit' leaves and how long the pit remains.

A patient with a score of 0 has no pitting oedema.
A patient with a score of 1 has oedema that is slight (roughly 2 mm in depth) and disappears rapidly.
A score of 2 is somewhat deeper (4 mm) and disappears within 10–15 seconds.
A score of 3, the pit is notably deeper (6 mm), and can last longer than a minute; in stage 3 pitting oedema the extremity also looks grossly swollen.
Stage 4 is the most severe, with deep pitting (8 mm or greater in depth) that may last more than 2 minutes. The dependent extremity is noticeably distorted.

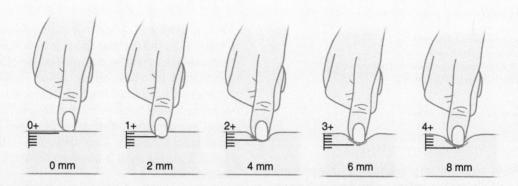

1. Explain to the patient what it is that you are going to do and why, seek their consent
2. Provide privacy
3. Wash hands
4. Gently, but firmly press with your thumb for at least 2 seconds on each extremity
5. Take note of the indention recovery time in seconds
6. Ensure patient is comfortable and discuss findings
7. Wash hands
8. Report and record finding as per local policy and procedure

Generally, daily input and output of fluid should be closely monitored for all patients who are acutely unwell, and loss into 'third spaces' should be considered. In a healthy adult, nearly all fluid is contained in the intracellular, intravascular, or interstitial spaces, with the intracellular space holding about two thirds of total body water. Normally, fluid moves freely between these three spaces to maintain fluid balance. An example overview of fluid management strategies can be seen in Table 20.3.

Table 20.3   IV Fluid management strategies. *Source:* AMBOSS, 2021; Finfer at el, 2018; Malbrin et al., 2020; Stroud et al., 2018.

Clinical scenario	Fluid management strategy	Goal
Hypovolaemic shock	Immediate haemodynamic support with aggressive IV fluid resuscitation	Patient rescue
Hypovolaemia or dehydration without shock	Judicious fluid replacement (e.g. with IV fluid challenge)	Organ rescue
Ongoing fluid loss greater than oral intake	Replacement of ongoing fluid loss	Organ support
Hyponatraemia	Correction of free water deficit	
Inability to meet daily fluid requirements enterally	Maintenance fluid therapy	
Recovering patients	De-escalation of IV fluid therapy	Organ recovery

Third spacing

Third spacing occurs when too much fluid moves from the intravascular space (blood vessels) into the interstitial or 'third' space, which is the non-functional area between cells. This can cause potentially serious problems such as oedema, reduced cardiac output, and hypotension.

Third spacing has two distinct phases being (1) loss and (2) reabsorption. In the loss phase, increased capillary permeability leads to a loss of proteins and fluids from the intravascular space to the interstitial space. This phase lasts 24 to 72 hours after the initial insult that led to the increased capillary permeability (for example, surgery, trauma, burns, sepsis or systemic inflammatory response syndrome (SIRS)). Fluid loss from diarrhoea, vomiting, or bleeding can be measured, but fluid loss from third spacing is not so easy to quantify. Signs and symptoms include weight gain, decreased urinary output, and signs of hypovolaemia, such as tachycardia and hypotension. During the reabsorption phase, tissues begin to heal, and fluid is transported back into the intravascular space. Signs of hypovolaemia resolve, urine output increases, the patient's weight stabilises, and signs of shock (if any) begin to reverse. If the patient was given fluid resuscitation during the loss phase, monitor for fluid overload as interstitial fluid shifts back to the intravascular space.

Assessment and monitoring

NICE's 2017 guidance on IV fluid therapy indicates that the assessment of patients should include physical examination, observation of vital signs over time, and clinical presentation. It also provides a set of parameters that may indicate that a patient needs fluid resuscitation (Table 20.4).

Table 20.4   Parameters for fluid resuscitation. *Source:* Based on NICE, 2017.

- Systolic blood pressure: <100 mmHg
- Heart rate: >90 beats per minute
- Capillary refill: >2 seconds or peripheries cool to touch
- Respiratory rate: >20 breaths per minute
- NEWS2: ≥5

NEWS2 = National Early Warning Score2

The parameters highlight the importance of assessing patients' fluid and electrolyte balance. This involves ascertaining the person's history of fluid intake and any complaints of thirst. Consideration should also be given to the likelihood of insensible fluid loss – for example, from altered bowel function such as diarrhoea, or injuries such as burns. Comorbidities such as diabetes and cardiovascular disease can also lead to fluid and electrolyte imbalances.

The monitoring of vital signs, along with the assessment of jugular venous pressure and observation for possible oedema and postural hypotension, can help identify abnormalities in patients' fluid and electrolyte balance. The National Early Warning Score2 (NEWS2) and fluid balance and weight charts are essential tools. Additional tests such as full blood count and urea and electrolytes can confirm the need for IV fluid therapy (NICE, 2017).

6Cs: Communication

Effective communication is a key requisite when undertaking assessment of needs.

Vital signs, findings from physical examination, and chest radiographs are of great importance in assessing the volume status of the patient. Invasive monitoring of central venous pressure or pulmonary capillary wedge pressure may be useful. Novel techniques involving invasive monitoring of extracellular fluid volume have been proposed, but none of them have been rigorously validated in clinical care.

Assess the patient's likely fluid and electrolyte needs from their history, clinical examination, current medications, clinical monitoring and laboratory investigations. History should include any previous limited intake, thirst, the quantity and composition of abnormal losses (see Figure 20.1) and any comorbidities, including patients who are malnourished and at risk of refeeding syndrome (see nutrition support in adults (NICE Clinical Guideline 32)). Clinical examination should include an assessment of the patient's fluid status, including pulse, blood pressure, capillary refill and jugular venous pressure; presence of pulmonary or peripheral oedema; and presence of postural hypotension. Clinical monitoring should include current status and trends in: NEWS2 score, fluid balance charts and weight.

Clinical investigations

There are a range of clinical investigations that will need to be undertaken in order to assist with fluid management. Laboratory studies are an extension of the physical examination in which tissue, blood, urine or other specimens are obtained from patients and subjected to microscopic, biochemical, microbiological or immunological examination. Information obtained from these investigations help in identifying the nature of the disease. Blood analysis is the most common laboratory investigation.

Laboratory investigations should include current status and trends in full blood count and urea, creatinine and electrolytes. Appropriate documentation of the investigation being undertaken must be kept. It is important to monitor trends in results, comparing and contrasting. Patient management should be adapted to any developing trends that emerge.

All patients continuing to receive IV fluids need regular monitoring. This should initially include at least daily reassessments of clinical fluid status, laboratory values (urea, creatinine, and electrolytes) and fluid balance charts, along with weight measurement twice weekly. Be aware that patients receiving IV fluid therapy to address replacement or redistribution problems may need more frequent monitoring. Additional monitoring of urinary sodium may be helpful in patients with high-volume gastrointestinal losses. Reduced urinary sodium excretion (less than 30 mmol/L) may indicate total body sodium depletion even if plasma sodium levels are normal (NICE, 2017). Urinary sodium may also indicate the cause of hyponatraemia and guide the achievement of a negative sodium balance in patients with oedema. However, urinary sodium values may be misleading in the presence of renal impairment or diuretic therapy. Patients on longer-term IV fluid therapy whose condition is stable may be monitored less frequently, although decisions to reduce monitoring frequency should be detailed in their IV fluid management plan. Clear incidents of fluid mismanagement (for example, unnecessarily prolonged dehydration or inadvertent fluid overload due to IV fluid therapy) should be reported through standard critical incident reporting to encourage improved training and practice (see consequences of fluid mismanagement to be reported as critical incidents).

Red Flag: Resuscitation

If patients need IV fluid resuscitation, use crystalloids that contain sodium in the range 130–154 mmol/L, with a bolus of 500 mL over less than 15 minutes (NICE, 2017).

Training and education

Hospitals should establish systems to ensure that all healthcare professionals involved in prescribing and delivering IV fluid therapy are trained on the principles covered in guidance, and are then formally assessed and reassessed at regular intervals to demonstrate competence in the physiology of fluid and electrolyte balance in patients with normal physiology and during illness assessing patients' fluid and electrolyte needs (the 5 Rs: Resuscitation, Routine maintenance, Replacement, Redistribution and Reassessment) (see Table 20.5); assessing the risks, benefits and harms of IV fluids; prescribing and administering IV fluids; monitoring the patient response; evaluating and documenting changes and taking appropriate action as required. Hospitals should have an IV fluids lead, responsible for training, clinical governance, audit and review of IV fluid prescribing and patient outcomes. It is noted by NICE (2017) that weight-based potassium prescriptions should be rounded to the nearest common fluids available (for example, a 67 kg person should have fluids containing 20 mmol and 40 mmol of potassium in a 24-hour period). Potassium should not be added to intravenous fluid bags as this is dangerous.

6Cs: Competence

A competent practitioner has insight and knowledge of the key issues enabling them with the patient, where appropriate, to make clinical decisions.

Learning event: reflection

Reflect on how the critical care team use the 5R approach and discuss this with the critical care clinical practice educator.

Electrolyte replacement therapy

The following information on oral and parental preparations for fluid and electrolyte imbalance have been taken directly from NICE (2021a) and have not be altered due to the prescriptive nature of this treatment summary.

Oral preparations

Sodium and potassium salts may be given by mouth to prevent deficiencies or to treat established deficiencies of mild or moderate degree.

Oral potassium

Compensation for potassium loss is especially necessary:

- In those taking digoxin or anti-arrhythmic drugs, where potassium depletion may induce arrhythmias

Table 20.5 The 5 Rs of IV fluid therapy. *Source:* Based on NICE, 2017.

Resuscitation: This is for patients needing IV fluids urgently to restore circulation to vital organs following loss of plasma in the blood (intravascular volume). This can be caused by excessive external fluid and electrolyte loss as well as bleeding or plasma loss, usually from the gastrointestinal tract, or severe internal losses.

Routine maintenance: Patients may need IV fluid therapy because they are unable to maintain normal fluid levels orally or by another enteral route. These patients are otherwise well in terms of fluid and electrolyte balance and are haemodynamically stable. Some patients with routine maintenance requirements may not be able to eat properly as well as being unable to drink and may therefore need electrolyte supplementation; the maintenance prescription should be adjusted for this. Estimates of routine maintenance requirements are essential for all patients on continuing IV fluid therapy; this is calculated by the patient's weight, oral intake and any other IV input (outlined in the routine maintenance algorithm).

Replacement: This is for patients needing fluids to correct water and/or electrolyte deficits or ongoing abnormal losses, such as high-output ileostomies, diarrhoea or vomiting.

Redistribution: Some hospital patients have complex fluid and electrolyte balance problems, due to the shift – or lack of shift – of fluid between different body compartments. This is seen particularly in those who are septic, otherwise critically ill, following major surgery or with major cardiac, liver or renal comorbidities. Health professionals should consider whether patients need IV fluids for their fluids to be redistributed correctly. Expert help should be sought to manage IV fluid therapy in patients with complex redistribution needs.

Reassessment: Health professionals should reassess patients at regular intervals, as part of their monitoring of IV fluid therapy.

- In patients in whom secondary hyperaldosteronism occurs, e.g. renal artery stenosis, cirrhosis of the liver, the nephrotic syndrome, and severe heart failure
- In patients with excessive losses of potassium in the faeces, e.g. chronic diarrhoea associated with intestinal malabsorption or laxative abuse

Measures to compensate for potassium loss may also be required in the elderly since they frequently take inadequate amounts of potassium in the diet (but see warning on renal insufficiency). Measures may also be required during long-term administration of drugs known to induce potassium loss (e.g. corticosteroids). Potassium supplements are seldom required with the small doses of diuretics given to treat hypertension; potassium-sparing diuretics (rather than potassium supplements) are recommended for prevention of hypokalaemia due to diuretics such as furosemide or the thiazides when these are given to eliminate oedema.

If potassium salts are used for the prevention of hypokalaemia, then doses of potassium chloride daily (in divided doses) by mouth are suitable in patients taking a normal diet. Smaller doses must be used if there is renal insufficiency (common in the elderly) to reduce the risk of hyperkalaemia.

271

Potassium salts cause nausea and vomiting and poor compliance is a major limitation to their effectiveness; when appropriate, potassium-sparing diuretics are preferable.

When there is established potassium depletion, larger doses may be necessary, the quantity depending on the severity of any continuing potassium loss (monitoring of plasma-potassium concentration and specialist advice would be required). Potassium depletion is frequently associated with chloride depletion and with metabolic alkalosis, and these disorders require correction.

Management of hyperkalaemia

Acute severe hyperkalaemia (plasma-potassium concentration above 6.5 mmol/L or in the presence of ECG changes) calls for urgent treatment with calcium gluconate 10% by slow intravenous injection, titrated and adjusted to ECG improvement, to temporarily protect against myocardial excitability. An intravenous injection of soluble insulin (5–10 units) with 50 mL glucose 50% given over 5–15 minutes, reduces serum potassium concentration; this is repeated if necessary or a continuous infusion instituted. Salbutamol (unlicensed indication), by nebulisation or slow intravenous injection may also reduce plasma-potassium concentration; it should be used with caution in patients with cardiovascular disease. The correction of causal or compounding acidosis with sodium bicarbonate infusion should be considered (important: preparations of sodium bicarbonate and calcium salts should not be administered in the same intravenous line – risk of precipitation). Drugs exacerbating hyperkalaemia should be reviewed and stopped as appropriate; occasionally haemodialysis is needed.

Ion-exchange resins may be used to remove excess potassium in *mild hyperkalaemia* or in *moderate hyperkalaemia* when there are no ECG changes.

Oral sodium and water

Sodium chloride is indicated in states of sodium depletion and usually needs to be given intravenously. In chronic conditions associated with mild or moderate degrees of sodium depletion, e.g. in salt-losing bowel or renal disease, oral supplements of sodium chloride or sodium bicarbonate, according to the acid-base status of the patient, may be sufficient.

Oral rehydration therapy (ORT)

As a worldwide problem diarrhoea is by far the most important indication for fluid and electrolyte replacement. Intestinal absorption of sodium and water is enhanced by glucose (and other carbohydrates). Replacement of fluid and electrolytes lost through diarrhoea can

therefore be achieved by giving solutions containing sodium, potassium, and glucose or another carbohydrate such as rice starch.

Oral rehydration solutions should:

- enhance the absorption of water and electrolytes;
- replace the electrolyte deficit adequately and safely;
- contain an alkalinising agent to counter acidosis;
- be slightly hypo-osmolar (about 250 mmol/L) to prevent the possible induction of osmotic diarrhoea;
- be simple to use in hospital and at home;
- be palatable and acceptable
- be readily available.
- It is the policy of the World Health Organization (WHO) to promote a single oral rehydration solution but to use it flexibly.

Examination scenario

Skin turgor refers to the elasticity of the skin. The skin normally returns to its original state quickly when stretched.

To check for skin turgor where dehydration is suspected:

1. Explain to the patient what is going to be done and why, gain consent.
2. Provide privacy.
3. Wash hands.
4. Gently grasp the patient's skin between two fingers so that it is tented up. Usually this on the dorsum of the hand, the lower arm or abdomen. The skin is held for a few seconds then released. Skin with normal turgor will snap rapidly back to its normal position. Skin with poor turgor takes time to return to its normal position.
5. Ensure patient is comfortable, explain findings.
6. Wash hands.
7. Report and record finds aligned with local policy and procedure.

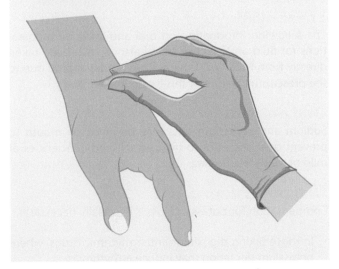

Oral rehydration solutions used in the UK are lower in sodium (50–60 mmol/L) than the WHO formulation since, in general, patients suffer less severe sodium loss.

Rehydration should be rapid over 3 to 4 hours (except in hypernatraemic dehydration in which case rehydration should occur more slowly over 12 hours). The patient should be reassessed after initial rehydration and if still dehydrated rapid fluid replacement should continue.

Once rehydration is complete, further dehydration is prevented by encouraging the patient to drink normal volumes of an appropriate fluid and by replacing continuing losses with an oral rehydration solution; in infants, breast-feeding or formula feeds should be offered between oral rehydration drinks.

Oral bicarbonate

Sodium bicarbonate is given by mouth for *chronic acidotic states* such as uraemic acidosis or renal tubular acidosis. The dose for correction of metabolic acidosis is not predictable and the response must be assessed. For severe *metabolic acidosis*, sodium bicarbonate can be given intravenously.

Sodium bicarbonate may also be used to increase the pH of the urine; it is also used in dyspepsia.

Sodium supplements may increase blood pressure or cause fluid retention and pulmonary oedema in those at risk; hypokalaemia may be exacerbated.

Where *hyperchloraemic acidosis* is associated with potassium deficiency, as in some renal tubular and gastrointestinal disorders it may be appropriate to give oral potassium bicarbonate, although acute or severe deficiency should be managed by intravenous therapy.

Parenteral preparations for fluid and electrolyte imbalance
Electrolytes and water

Solutions of electrolytes are given intravenously, to meet normal fluid and electrolyte requirements or to replenish substantial deficits or continuing losses, when the patient is nauseated or vomiting and is unable to take adequate amounts by mouth. When intravenous administration is not possible, fluid (as sodium chloride 0.9% or glucose 5%) can also be given by subcutaneous infusion (hypodermoclysis). The nature and severity of the electrolyte imbalance must be assessed from the history and clinical and biochemical investigations. Sodium, potassium, chloride, magnesium, phosphate and water depletion can occur singly and in combination with or without disturbances of acid-base balance. Isotonic solutions may be infused safely into a peripheral vein. Solutions more concentrated than plasma, e.g. 20% glucose, are best given through an indwelling intravenous catheter positioned in a large vein. The problems leading to fluid and electrolyte imbalance and the consequences of electrolyte imbalance can be seen in Figures 20.1. and 20.2

273

Ion (normal range SI units)	Abnormality	Consequences
Sodium (132–144 mmol/L)	Hypernatraemia Na^+ ↑ Dehydration, excessive IV NaCl	Thirst, confusion, lethargy. If severe, coma, twitching and convulsions
	Hyponatraemia Na^+ ↓ Excessive loss Burns, diuretics, excess H_2O ingestion	If due to excessive water: brain swelling, mental confusion, giddiness, coma. If due to water and Na^+ loss, then circulatory shock
Potassium (3.6–5.1 mmol/L)	Hyperkalaemia K^+ ↑ Renal failure IV KCL	Bradycardia, peaked T waves on ECG, arrhythmias, cardiac arrest Nausea, muscle weakness
	Hypokalaemia K^+ ↓ GI disturbance Diuretic therapy	Cardiac arrhythmias, muscle weakness, confusion
Calcium (2.12–2.62 mmol/L)	Hypercalcaemia Ca^{2+} ↑ Hyperparathyroidism	Cardiac arrhythmias, muscle weakness, confusion, nausea
	Hypocalcaemia Ca^{2+} ↓ Renal failure diarrhoea	Tingling fingers, cramps, tetany, convulsions
Magnesium (0.75–1.00 mmol/L)	Hypermagnesaemia Mg^{2+} ↑ Rare	Lethargy, respiratory depression, cardiac arrest
	Hypomagnesaemia Mg^{2+} ↓ Alcoholism, chronic diarrhoea, diuretic therapy	Tremors, tetany convulsions

Figure 20.1   The consequences of electrolyte imbalance. *Source:* Dutton and Finch (2018) with permission of John Wiley & Sons.

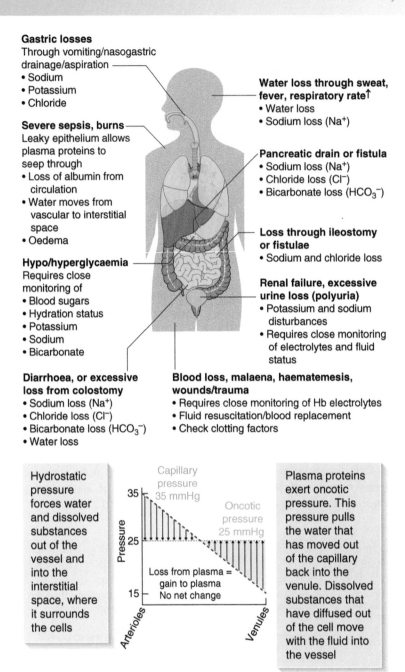

Gastric losses
Through vomiting/nasogastric drainage/aspiration
• Sodium
• Potassium
• Chloride

Severe sepsis, burns
Leaky epithelium allows plasma proteins to seep through
• Loss of albumin from circulation
• Water moves from vascular to interstitial space
• Oedema

Hypo/hyperglycaemia
Requires close monitoring of
• Blood sugars
• Hydration status
• Potassium
• Sodium
• Bicarbonate

Diarrhoea, or excessive loss from colostomy
• Sodium loss (Na⁺)
• Chloride loss (Cl⁻)
• Bicarbonate loss (HCO₃⁻)
• Water loss

Water loss through sweat, fever, respiratory rate↑
• Water loss
• Sodium loss (Na⁺)

Pancreatic drain or fistula
• Sodium loss (Na⁺)
• Chloride loss (Cl⁻)
• Bicarbonate loss (HCO₃⁻)

Loss through ileostomy or fistulae
• Sodium and chloride loss

Renal failure, excessive urine loss (polyuria)
• Potassium and sodium disturbances
• Requires close monitoring of electrolytes and fluid status

Blood loss, malaena, haematemesis, wounds/trauma
• Requires close monitoring of Hb electrolytes
• Fluid resuscitation/blood replacement
• Check clotting factors

Hydrostatic pressure forces water and dissolved substances out of the vessel and into the interstitial space, where it surrounds the cells

Capillary pressure 35 mmHg
Oncotic pressure 25 mmHg
Loss from plasma = gain to plasma No net change

Plasma proteins exert oncotic pressure. This pressure pulls the water that has moved out of the capillary back into the venule. Dissolved substances that have diffused out of the cell move with the fluid into the vessel

Figure 20.2   The problems leading to fluid and electrolyte imbalance. *Source:* Dutton and Finch (2018) with permission of John Wiley & Sons.

Intravenous sodium

Sodium chloride in isotonic solution provides the most important extracellular ions in near physiological concentrations and is indicated in *sodium depletion*, which can arise from such conditions as gastro-enteritis, diabetic ketoacidosis, ileus, and ascites. In a severe deficit of 4 to 8 litres, 2 to 3 litres of isotonic sodium chloride may be given over 2 to 3 hours; thereafter the infusion can usually be at a slower rate.

Chronic hyponatraemia arising from inappropriate secretion of antidiuretic hormone should ideally be corrected by fluid restriction. However, if sodium chloride is required for acute or chronic hyponatraemia, regardless of the cause,

the deficit should be corrected slowly to avoid the risk of osmotic demyelination syndrome and the rise in plasma-sodium concentration should not exceed 10 mmol/L in 24 hours. In severe hyponatraemia, sodium chloride 1.8% may be used cautiously.

Compound sodium lactate (Hartmann's solution) can be used instead of isotonic sodium chloride solution during or after surgery, or in the initial management of the injured or wounded; it may reduce the risk of hyperchloraemic acidosis.

Sodium chloride with glucose solutions are indicated when there is combined *water and sodium depletion*. A 1:1 mixture of isotonic sodium chloride and 5% glucose allows some of the water (free of sodium) to enter body cells which suffer most from dehydration while the sodium salt with a volume of water determined by the normal plasma Na+ remains extracellular.

Combined sodium, potassium, chloride and water depletion may occur, for example, with severe diarrhoea or persistent vomiting; replacement is carried out with sodium chloride intravenous infusion 0.9% and glucose intravenous infusion 5% with potassium as appropriate.

Intravenous glucose

Glucose solutions (5%) are used mainly to replace water deficit. Average water requirements in a healthy adult are 1.5 to 2.5 litres daily and this is needed to balance unavoidable losses of water through the skin and lungs and to provide sufficient for urinary excretion. Water depletion (dehydration) tends to occur when these losses are not matched by a comparable intake, as may occur in coma or dysphagia or in the elderly or apathetic who may not drink enough water on their own initiative.

Excessive loss of water without loss of electrolytes is uncommon, occurring in fevers, hyperthyroidism and in uncommon water-losing renal states such as diabetes insipidus or hypercalcaemia. The volume of glucose solution needed to replace deficits varies with the severity of the disorder, but usually lies within the range of 2 to 6 litres.

Glucose solutions are also used to correct and prevent hypoglycaemia and to provide a source of energy in those too ill to be fed adequately by mouth; glucose solutions are a key component of parenteral nutrition.

Glucose solutions are given in regimens with calcium and insulin for the emergency management of *hyperkalaemia*. They are also given, after correction of hyperglycaemia, during treatment of diabetic ketoacidosis, when they must be accompanied by continuing insulin infusion.

Intravenous potassium

Potassium chloride with sodium chloride intravenous infusion is the initial treatment for the correction of *severe hypokalaemia* and when sufficient potassium cannot be taken by mouth.

Repeated measurement of plasma-potassium concentration is necessary to determine whether further infusions are required and to avoid the development of hyperkalaemia, which is especially likely in renal impairment.

Initial potassium replacement therapy should not involve glucose infusions, because glucose may cause a further decrease in the plasma-potassium concentration.

Bicarbonate and lactate

Sodium bicarbonate is used to control severe *metabolic acidosis* (pH<7.1) particularly that caused by loss of bicarbonate (as in renal tubular acidosis or from excessive gastro-intestinal losses). Mild metabolic acidosis associated with volume depletion should first be managed by appropriate fluid replacement because acidosis usually resolves as tissue and renal perfusion are restored. In more severe metabolic acidosis or when the acidosis remains unresponsive to correction of anoxia or hypovolaemia, sodium bicarbonate (1.26%) can be infused over 3–4 hours with plasma-pH and electrolyte monitoring. In severe shock, metabolic acidosis can develop without sodium or volume depletion; in these circumstances sodium bicarbonate is best given as a small volume of hypertonic solution, such as 50 mL of 8.4% solution intravenously (see Box 20.1 and Box 20.2).

Sodium lactate intravenous infusion is no longer used in metabolic acidosis because of the risk of producing lactic acidosis, particularly in seriously ill patients with poor tissue perfusion or impaired hepatic function.

For *chronic acidotic states*, sodium bicarbonate can be given by mouth.

Box 20.1   Hypertonic saline.

Hypertonic saline is a crystalloid intravenous fluid composed of NaCl dissolved in water with a higher sodium concentration than normal blood serum. Hypertonic saline (HS) is currently used in hyponatraemia and increased intracranial pressure (ICP). Patients with hyponatraemia with severe features should have their serum sodium gradually corrected with boluses of hypertonic saline. Patients should have their serum sodium monitored at regular intervals. Patients with traumatic brain injury (TBI) should be administered hypertonic solution with caution due to prevent secondary brain injury.

Box 20.2   Mannitol.

Mannitol is a crystalloid intravenous fluid composed of a six-carbon simple sugar dissolved in water. It is for use in decreasing intracranial pressure and brain mass and decreasing intraocular pressure when other interventions have failed to do so. When needed, 15 to 25% mannitol can be given as a bolus to reduce intracranial pressure and intraocular pressure. Mannitol is solely confined to the intravascular space when administered intravenously, unlike hypertonic saline, which can have some movement of electrolytes into the interstitial space. Patients with TBI should be administered hypertonic solution with caution due to prevent secondary brain injury.

Plasma and plasma substitutes

Plasma and plasma substitutes ('colloids') contain large molecules that do not readily leave the intravascular space where they exert osmotic pressure to maintain circulatory volume. Compared to fluids containing electrolytes such as sodium chloride and glucose ('crystalloids'), a smaller volume of colloid is required to produce the same expansion of blood volume, thereby shifting salt and water from the extravascular space. If resuscitation requires a volume of fluid that exceeds the maximum dose of the colloid, then crystalloids can be given; packed red cells may also be required.

Albumin solution, prepared from whole blood, contain soluble proteins and electrolytes but no clotting factors, blood group antibodies, or plasma cholinesterases; they may be given without regard to the recipient's blood group. Albumin is usually used after the acute phase of illness, to correct a plasma-volume deficit; hypoalbuminaemia itself is not an appropriate indication. The use of albumin solution in acute plasma or blood loss may be wasteful; plasma substitutes are more appropriate. Concentrated albumin solution (20%) can be used under specialist supervision in patients with an intravascular fluid deficit and oedema because of interstitial fluid overload, to restore intravascular plasma volume with less exacerbation of the salt and water overload than isotonic solutions. Concentrated albumin solution may also be used to obtain a diuresis in hypoalbuminaemic patients (e.g. in hepatic cirrhosis). Recent evidence does not support the previous view that the use of albumin increases mortality (NICE, 2021a).

Plasma substitutes

Dextran, gelatin and the hydroxyethyl starch, tetrastarch, are macromolecular substances which are metabolised slowly. Dextran and gelatin may be used at the outset to expand and maintain blood volume in shock arising from conditions such as burns or septicaemia; they may also be used as an immediate short-term measure to treat haemorrhage until blood is available. Dextran and gelatin are rarely needed when shock is due to sodium and water depletion because, in these circumstances, the shock responds to water and electrolyte repletion.

Hydroxyethyl starches should only be used for the treatment of hypovolaemia due to acute blood loss when crystalloids alone are not sufficient; they should be used at the lowest effective dose for the first 24 hours of fluid resuscitation. Plasma substitutes should not be used to maintain plasma volume in conditions such as burns or peritonitis where there is loss of plasma protein, water, and electrolytes over periods of several days or weeks. In these situations, plasma or plasma protein fractions containing large amounts of albumin should be given. Large volumes of some plasma substitutes can increase the risk of bleeding through depletion of coagulation factors.

NICE guidelines (2017) recommend best evidence-based practice regrading intravenous fluid therapy in adults in hospital. This clinical evidence is helpful regarding the selection of fluid and the fluid resuscitation process. These can be seen in algorithms (https://www.nice.org.uk/guidance/cg174/resources/intravenous-fluid-therapy-in-adults-in-hospital-algorithm-poster-set-191627821).

Fluid overload

Administering too much IV fluid inevitably results in some degree of salt and water overload. First and foremost, this is the result of the initial fluid resuscitation with the aim of restoring intravascular volume, increasing cardiac output, augmenting oxygen delivery, and improving tissue oxygenation. Salt and water overload can also result from the administration of large volumes of fluid as drug diluents, artificial nutrition and maintenance fluids. Critically unwell patients with multi-organ failure are at risk of capillary leak, particularly if they have acute pyrexia, sepsis or SIRS causing extravasation of large amounts of fluid, inducing relative central hypovolemia that often requires further fluid administration, despite interstitial oedema. Capillary leak represents the maladaptive, often excessive, and undesirable loss of fluid and electrolytes with or without protein into the interstitium that generates anasarca and end-organ oedema causing organ dysfunction and eventually failure.

The four Ds of fluid management

Drug

Fluids are drugs with indications, contraindications and side effects. Different indications need different types of fluids, e.g., resuscitation fluids should focus on rapid restoration of circulating volume; replacement fluids must mimic the fluid that has been lost; maintenance fluids must deliver basic electrolytes and glucose for metabolic needs.

Dosing

Dosing of fluids and electrolytes must be determined using national and local guidelines and formularies as well as hospital policy and procedures.

Duration

The duration of fluid therapy is crucial, and volume must be tapered when shock is resolved. However, while 'starting triggers' for fluid resuscitation are quite clear, clinicians are less aware of 'stopping triggers' of fluid resuscitation.

276

De-escalation

The final step in fluid therapy is to withhold/withdraw fluids when they are no longer required, thus reducing the risk of fluid overload and related deleterious effects.

Hyponatraemia

NICE (2020) define hyponatraemia as a serum sodium concentration of less than 135 mmol/L. It is the most common electrolyte disorder encountered in clinical practice and is usually an incidental finding on routine blood tests. The severity of hyponatraemia can be classified as mild, with a serum sodium concentration 130–135 mmol/L. Moderate, with a serum sodium concentration of 125–129 mmol/L, and severe, with a serum sodium concentration less than 125 mmol/L (NICE, 2020). The rate of onset of hyponatraemia can be classified as acute, with the duration of less than 48 hours, or chronic, with a duration of 48 hours or more. The cause of hyponatraemia is often multifactorial. Common causes include medications (most commonly thiazide diuretics), syndrome of inappropriate antidiuresis, and any underlying medical conditions (such as heart failure, kidney disease, and liver disease).

Most people with hyponatraemia are asymptomatic, particularly if it is mild and has developed slowly. When symptoms are present, they are often non-specific and are related to both the severity of the hyponatraemia and its rate of onset. Rapid changes in serum sodium levels or severe hyponatraemia can cause symptoms of vomiting, headache, drowsiness, seizures, coma and cardiorespiratory arrest.

Chronic hyponatraemia can lead to increased risk of falls, bone fractures, osteoporosis, gait instability, and concentration and cognitive deficits. Assessment of a person with hyponatraemia involves taking a focused history, determining the person's volume status, and arranging appropriate investigations (including serum and urine osmolality, and urinary sodium concentration) to help identify the cause of hyponatraemia and guide management. After the initial identification of hyponatraemia, serum sodium measurement should be repeated (timescale dependant on clinical judgement) to exclude a rapidly decreasing serum sodium concentration, which will require admission to hospital. If the person has severe or symptomatic hyponatraemia, admission to hospital for urgent treatment should be arranged. If the person has asymptomatic, moderate hyponatraemia, specialist advice from an endocrinologist should be sought regarding the need for admission or referral. If the person has asymptomatic, mild hyponatraemia, the underlying cause of hyponatraemia should be sought in primary care (if possible and appropriate). If the person has an acute illness that may be contributing to the hyponatraemia, it should be treated, and the serum sodium concentration rechecked after 2 weeks. Medications that may be contributing to the hyponatraemia should be stopped if appropriate and the serum sodium concentration rechecked after 2 weeks (NICE, 2020).

Hypernatraemia

Hypernatraemia is defined as a serum sodium concentration exceeding 145 mmol/L. Serum sodium concentration, and hence osmolality, is normally kept from rising significantly by the release of antidiuretic hormone (ADH) or vasopressin which limits water losses, and the stimulation of thirst which increases water intake. Hypernatraemia from free water loss causes dehydration as intracellular water is drawn out of cells into the extracellular fluid (ECF) preserving the latter to a large extent; however, if sodium is lost as well as water then significant hypovolaemia (reduction in ECF volume) can also occur. Severe symptoms are usually only found with acute and large rises in sodium plasma concentration above 160 mmol/L.

Hypokalaemia

Hypokalaemia is usually defined as a serum concentration of potassium <3.5 mmol/L. It can be classified as Mild – 3.1–3.5 mmol/L, Moderate – 2.5–3.0 mmol/L or Severe – <2.5 mmol/L. It is probably the most common electrolyte abnormality affecting hospitalised patients. Most cases are mild but in 5% of cases the potassium level it is <3.0 mmol/L. Severe hypokalaemia is even rarer. Importantly, even mild hypokalaemia can increase the incidence of cardiac arrhythmias. Therefore, ECGs are an important diagnostic at this point. All critically unwell patients with moderate or severe hypokalaemia should have an ECG to determine whether the hypokalaemia is affecting cardiac function and/or to detect digoxin toxicity. Mild hypokalaemia in high-risk individuals should also prompt an ECG, particularly if of recent onset. Typical ECG findings when potassium is <3.0 mmol/L are flat T waves, ST depression, prominent U waves. Additionally the QT interval may appear prolonged, but this is usually a pseudo-prolongation as the flattened T waves merge into the U waves. Ventricular arrhythmias such as premature ventricular contractions, torsades de pointes, ventricular tachycardia and ventricular fibrillation can also occur.

Hyperkalaemia

Hyperkalaemia is a plasma potassium more than 5.5 mmol/L. Hyperkalaemia has three stages including Mild – 5.5–5.9 mmol/L, Moderate – 6.0–6.4 mmol/L or Severe – >6.5 mmol/L. Potassium is the most abundant intracellular cation – 98% of it being located intracellularly. Hyperkalaemia has four broad causes including, renal causes – eg, due to decreased excretion or drugs; increased circulation of potassium – can be exogenous or endogenous; a shift from the intracellular to the extracellular space, and pseudohyperkalaemia.

Hypophosphataemia

Hypophosphataemia is low phosphate. The normal range in adults is generally considered to be 0.8–1.5 mmol/L (Abbott, 2015). Significant hypophosphataemia (below 0.4 mmol/L) may occur due to redistribution into cells, renal losses, or decreased intake. Patients with low phosphate often also have other electrolyte deficiencies. The aetiology of hypophosphataemia includes inadequate intake, increased renal excretion, movement of fluid and electrolytes from extracellular to intracellular compartments, for example in DKA insulin drives phosphate into cells.

Hypocalcaemia

Hypocalcaemia is low calcium. The normal range for serum calcium is 2.25–2.5 mmol/L. However, in hypercalcaemia, just over half the circulating calcium is protein-bound and therefore the level of circulating protein, principally albumin, must also be taken into consideration in making this measurement. The level for serum calcium is frequently given by laboratories as both an uncorrected level and a corrected level which has allowed for changes in albumin levels. It is only the ionised (unbound) calcium, which is physiologically important, taking part in cellular activities such as neuromuscular contraction, coagulation and other cellular activities.

Hypomagnesaemia

Magnesium is an essential constituent of many enzyme systems, particularly those involved in energy generation; the largest stores are in the skeleton. Magnesium salts are not well absorbed from the gastro-intestinal tract, which explains the use of magnesium sulphate as an osmotic laxative. Magnesium is excreted mainly by the kidneys and is therefore retained in renal failure, which can result in hypermagnesaemia (causing muscle weakness and arrhythmias). Calcium gluconate injection is used for the management of magnesium toxicity. Since magnesium is secreted in large amounts in the gastro-intestinal fluid, excessive losses in diarrhoea, stoma or fistula can cause hypomagnesaemia; deficiency may also occur in alcoholism or because of treatment with certain drugs. Hypomagnesaemia often causes secondary hypocalcaemia, and also hypokalaemia. Symptomatic hypomagnesaemia is usually associated with severe magnesium depletion. Magnesium can be given by intravenous infusion or by intramuscular injection of magnesium sulphate; the intramuscular injection is painful. Patients with mild magnesium depletion are usually asymptomatic. Oral magnesium glycerophosphate is licensed for hypomagnesaemia. Oral magnesium aspartate is licensed for the treatment and prevention of magnesium deficiency (NICE, 2021b).

Table 20.6 identifies electrolyte concentrations in intravenous fluids that will support the understanding of why an IV fluid maybe chosen.

Table 20.6   Electrolyte concentrations in intravenous fluids. *Source:* NICE, 2021a.

Normal plasma values	Sodium 142 mmol/L Potassium 4.5 mmol/L Bicarbonate 26 mmol/L Chloride 103 mmol/L Calcium 2.5 mmol/L
Sodium chloride 0.9%	Sodium 150 mmol/L Chloride 150 mmol/L
Compound sodium lactate (Hartmann's)	Sodium 131 mmol/L Potassium 5 mmol/L Bicarbonate 29 mmol/L Chloride 111 mmol/L Calcium 2 mmol/L
Sodium chloride 0.18% and glucose 4% (Adults only)	Sodium 30 mmol/L Chloride 30 mmol/L
Potassium chloride 0.3% and glucose 5%	Potassium 40 mmol/L Chloride 40 mmol/L
Potassium chloride 0.3% and sodium chloride 0.9%	Sodium 150 mmol/L Potassium 40 mmol/L Chloride 190 mmol/L
Sodium bicarbonate 1.26%	Sodium 150 mmol/L Bicarbonate 150 mmol/L To correct metabolic acidosis
Sodium bicarbonate 8.4%	Sodium 1000 mmol/L Bicarbonate 1000 mmol/L To correct metabolic acidosis
Sodium lactate (m/6)	Sodium 167 mmol/L Bicarbonate 167 mmol/L To correct metabolic acidosis
Electrolyte content – gastro-intestinal secretions	
Gastric	Hydrogen 40–60 mmol/L Sodium 20–80 mmol/L Potassium 5–20 mmol/L Chloride 100–150 mmol/L
Biliary	Sodium 120–140 mmol/L Potassium 5–15 mmol/L Bicarbonate 30–50 mmol/L Chloride 80–120 mmol/L
Pancreatic	Sodium 120–140 mmol/L Potassium 5–15 mmol/L Bicarbonate 70–110 mmol/L Chloride 40–80 mmol/L
Small bowel	Sodium 120–140 mmol/L Potassium 5–15 mmol/L Bicarbonate 20–40 mmol/L Chloride 90–130 mmol/L

278

Conclusion

Adequate hydration is essential for the body to maintain organ perfusion and cell metabolism, key to maintaining homeostasis. This chapter has provided an overview of fluid and electrolyte management in critically ill patients. Fluid management for adults, particularly in hospitals, addresses replacement during resuscitation, the management of malnourished patients and the need for fluids after large electrolyte losses have occurred, for example in the case of burns.

Take home points

1. Intravenous fluid therapy involves the intravenous administration of crystalloid solutions and, less commonly, colloidal solutions.

2. The type, amount and infusion rates of fluids are determined based on the indication for fluid therapy and specific patient needs.

3. Crystalloid solutions are used to resuscitate patients who are hypovolaemic or dehydrated, correct free water deficits, replace ongoing fluid losses and meet the fluid requirements of patients who cannot take fluids enterally.

4. The use of colloidal solutions is controversial and should be reserved for special situations (e.g. severe cases of low oncotic pressure). All patients should be closely monitored using a combination of clinical parameters and laboratory tests to determine therapeutic endpoints, and fluid therapy should be appropriately de-escalated for patients in recovery to avoid fluid overload.

5. The loss of circulating fluid volume can lead to imbalances in homoeostasis

6. Recognising, assessing and monitoring patients' need for fluid therapy is crucial

7. The '5Rs' of intravenous fluid administration are resuscitation, routine maintenance, replacement, redistribution and reassessment

8. Crystalloids and colloids, both plasma volume expanders, are used to increase depleted circulating volumes

9. To administer intravenous fluids, health professionals must understand what crystalloids and colloids do and when to use them

References

Abbott, D. (2015). How is acute hypophosphataemia treated in adults? https://www.sps.nhs.uk/articles/how-is-acute-hypophosphataemia-treated-in-adults/ (accessed March 2022).

AMBOSS (2021). Intravenous fluid therapy. https://www.amboss.com/us/knowledge/Intravenous_fluid_therapy/ (accessed March 2022).

Finfer, S., Myburgh, J., and Bellomo R. (2018) Intravenous fluid therapy in critically ill adults. *Nat Rev Nephrol* 14(9): 541–557. doi: 10.1038/s41581-018-0044-0.

Joint Formulary Committee (2021) *British National Formulary*, 82e. London: BMJ Group and Pharmaceutical Press.

Lewis, S.R., Pritchard, M.W., Evans DJW et al. (2021). Colloids versus crystalloids for fluid resuscitation in critically ill people. *Cochrane Database of Systematic Reviews* Issue 8 (Art. No.: CD000567). doi: 10.1002/14651858.CD000567.pub7.

Malbrain, M.L.N.G., Langer, T., Annane, D. et al. (2020). Intravenous fluid therapy in the perioperative and critical care setting: Executive summary of the International Fluid Academy (IFA). *Ann. Intensive Care* 10(1). doi: 10.1186/s13613-020-00679-3.

NICE (2017). Intravenous fluid therapy in adults in hospital Clinical guideline [CG174]. https://www.nice.org.uk/guidance/cg174/chapter/key-priorities-for-implementation.

NICE (2020). Hyponatraemia. https://cks.nice.org.uk/topics/hyponatraemia/ (accessed March 2022).

NICE (2021a). Fluids and electrolytes. https://bnf.nice.org.uk/treatment-summary/fluids-and-electrolytes.html (accessed March 2022).

NICE (2021b). Magnesium, imbalance. https://bnf.nice.org.uk/treatment-summary/magnesium-imbalance.html (accessed March 2022).

Peate I. (2021). *Fundamentals of Applied Pathophysiology: An Essential Guide for Nursing and Healthcare Students*, 4e. Chichester: Wiley.

Peate I. and Evans, S. (2020). *Fundamentals of Anatomy and Physiology for Nursing and Healthcare Students*, 3e. Chichester: Wiley Blackwell.

Smith, L. (2017). Choosing between colloids and crystalloids for IV infusion. *Nursing Times* 113(12): 20–23.

Stroud M. (2017). Intravenous fluid therapy in adults in hospital. https://www.nice.org.uk/guidance/cg174/chapter/recommendations#routine-maintenance-2 (accessed 15 February 2018).

Woodrow, P. (2018). *Intensive Care Nursing: A Framework for Practice*, 4e. Routledge.

Chapter 21

Critical care emergencies

Alexandra Gatehouse and Sadie Diamond-Fox

Aim

The aim of this chapter is to provide the reader with an introduction to some of the common time-critical emergency situations that may be encountered within the critical care environment (CCE).

Learning outcomes

After reading this chapter the reader will be able to:

- Have gained an understanding of the key life-threatening emergencies within critical care.
- Discuss the algorithm for adult in-hospital resuscitation and key elements of advanced life support.
- Appreciate clinical signs and potential causes and associations leading to life-threatening emergencies.
- Consider the relevant and current guidance available with regards to cardiopulmonary resuscitation (CPR) and life-threatening emergencies.
- Understand the key principles of management of CPR and life-threatening emergencies.

Test your prior knowledge

- Describe the initial sequence for the management of a collapsed patient in-hospital in cardiac arrest.
- Name two causes of life-threatening emergencies for airway, breathing, circulation, disability and exposure.
- Differentiate between respiratory and cardiac arrest.
- Based upon current evidence, critically discuss two drugs that may be used in the treatment of cardiac arrest.
- Discuss the importance of team working and human factors during cardiac arrest.

Fundamentals of Critical Care: A Textbook for Nursing and Healthcare Students, First Edition. Edited by Ian Peate and Barry Hill.
© 2023 John Wiley & Sons Ltd. Published 2023 by John Wiley & Sons Ltd.
Companion website: www.wiley.com/go/peate/criticalcare

Introduction

Emergencies can be a common occurrence within the CCE. The following chapter outlines some of the common emergencies that may be encountered within the CCE and provides an overview as to their recognition, potential causes, potential treatments and relevant evidence-based guidance. There are a plethora of scenarios which may encountered by the healthcare student, and some of these scenarios are outlined within Figure 21.1. It is beyond the scope of this chapter to explore this subject in depth. Further information on this subject can be found in Dutton and Finch (2018), Leach (2014) and Beed et al. (2013). The reader is also encouraged to consider utilising e-learning modules 'e-ICM' that map directly to CC3N competencies (Health Education England & Faculty of Intensive Care Medicine, 2021) and the 'Further reading' material detailed on the companion website.

As with any emergency scenario, regardless of the clinical area, assessment and immediate management by a suitably trained healthcare professional should follow the well-established A to E approach (Figures 21.1 and 21.2) Chapter 6 discusses the A–E approach in more detail.

Life-threatening emergencies may require interventions such as those detailed within the Adult in-hospital resuscitation algorithm (RCUK, 2021a) (Figure 21.3) and advanced life support (ALS) algorithms (Figures 21.4 and 21.5) may need to be performed by appropriately trained members of the team. The ALS interventions performed within critical care may differ slightly compared to that of other clinical areas that do not routinely care for critically ill patients due to the rapid availability of diagnostic tools such as ultrasound, point-of-care testing, invasive monitoring and alternative drugs not commonly used in areas outside of the CCE.

Step 2 competencies: National standards

Elements of the following Critical Care Networks-National Nurse Leads (CC3N) (2015) competencies are covered within this chapter:

2.1.2 – Respiratory Assessment, Monitoring and Observation
2.1.4 – Endotracheal Intubation
2.1.7 – Tracheostomy Care
2.2.2 – Fluid Management
2.5.2 – Neurological Assessment, Monitoring and Observation
2.10.1 – Leadership

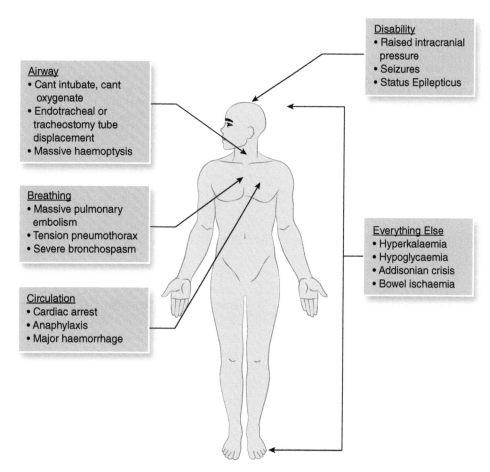

Airway
• Cant intubate, cant oxygenate
• Endotracheal or tracheostomy tube displacement
• Massive haemoptysis

Breathing
• Massive pulmonary embolism
• Tension pneumothorax
• Severe bronchospasm

Circulation
• Cardiac arrest
• Anaphylaxis
• Major haemorrhage

Disability
• Raised intracranial pressure
• Seizures
• Status Epilepticus

Everything Else
• Hyperkalaemia
• Hypoglycaemia
• Addisonian crisis
• Bowel ischaemia

Figure 21.1   Overview of emergencies The ABCDE approach.

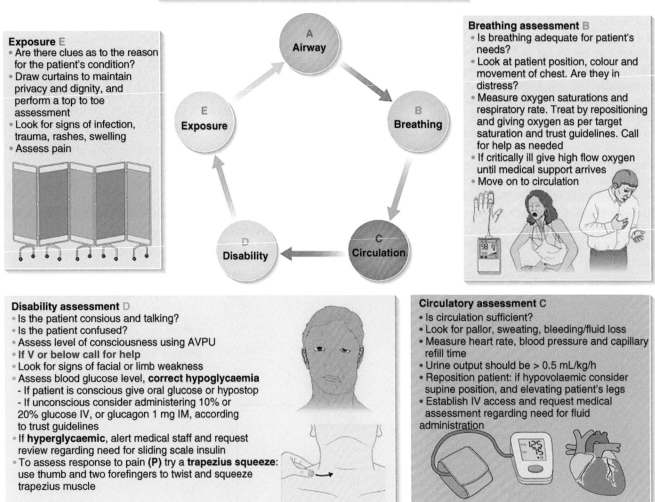

Airway assessment A
• Is the airway patent?
• Are there any signs of partial airway obstruction? (listen for stridor, snoring)
  If YES: then **call for help** and establish a clear airway
• Is the patient talking?
• Can they cough effectively?
• If **YES** move on to breathing assessment

Exposure E
• Are there clues as to the reason for the patient's condition?
• Draw curtains to maintain privacy and dignity, and perform a top to toe assessment
• Look for signs of infection, trauma, rashes, swelling
• Assess pain

Breathing assessment B
• Is breathing adequate for patient's needs?
• Look at patient position, colour and movement of chest. Are they in distress?
• Measure oxygen saturations and respiratory rate. Treat by repositioning and giving oxygen as per target saturation and trust guidelines. Call for help as needed
• If critically ill give high flow oxygen until medical support arrives
• Move on to circulation

Disability assessment D
• Is the patient consious and talking?
• Is the patient confused?
• Assess level of consciousness using AVPU
• If V or below call for help
• Look for signs of facial or limb weakness
• Assess blood glucose level, **correct hypoglycaemia**
  - If patient is conscious give oral glucose or hypostop
  - If unconscious consider administering 10% or 20% glucose IV, or glucagon 1 mg IM, according to trust guidelines
• If **hyperglycaemic**, alert medical staff and request review regarding need for sliding scale insulin
• To assess response to pain (P) try a **trapezius squeeze**: use thumb and two forefingers to twist and squeeze trapezius muscle

Circulatory assessment C
• Is circulation sufficient?
• Look for pallor, sweating, bleeding/fluid loss
• Measure heart rate, blood pressure and capillary refill time
• Urine output should be > 0.5 mL/kg/h
• Reposition patient: if hypovolaemic consider supine position, and elevating patient's legs
• Establish IV access and request medical assessment regarding need for fluid administration

A — Airway

B — Breathing

C — Circulation

D — Disability

E — Exposure

Figure 21.2   The ABCDE approach to patient assessment. *Source:* Dutton and Finch (2018) with permission of John Wiley & Sons.

6Cs: Communication

Good communication is critical to ensuring effective management of emergencies within the critical care environment.

A – Airway

Airway emergencies cover a wide spectrum of presentations within the CCE that include airway obstruction, complications with endotracheal intubation as well as endotracheal tube and tracheostomy difficulties. Chapter 16 explores the respiratory system pathologies associated with THE CCE in more depth, however, Table 21.1 describes some of the common airway emergencies that may be encountered.

Within the UK, the Difficult Airway Society (DAS) in conjunction with the Royal College of Anaesthetists (RCoA), the Faculty of Intensive Care Medicine (FICM) and the Intensive Care Society (ICS) formulated guidelines for the management of tracheal intubation in critically ill adults (Higgs et al., 2017). They were based upon the findings of the 4th National Audit Project which reported higher rates of major complications and avoidable deaths due to deficient airway management, in this group of patients (Cook et al., 2011). One of the most used algorithms is tracheal intubation of critically ill adults, which may be found in Figure 21.6.

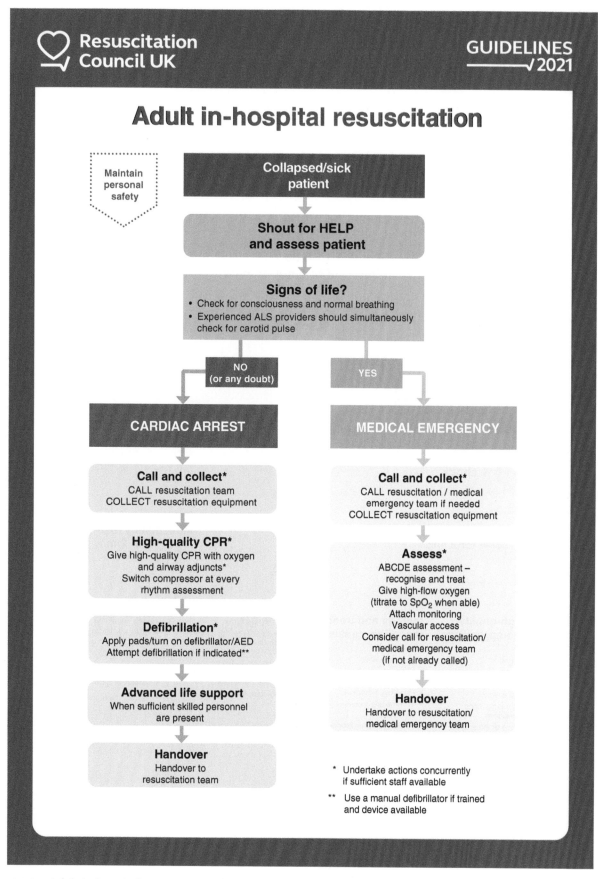

Figure 21.3 Adult in-hospital resuscitation algorithm. *Source:* Resuscitation Council UK, 2021a. Reproduced with the kind permission of Resuscitation Council UK.

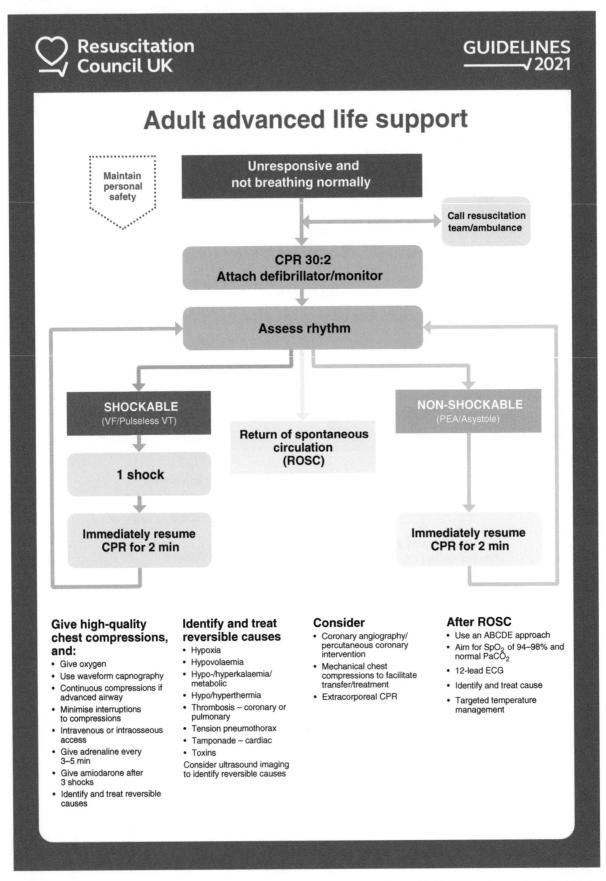

Figure 21.4 Adult advanced life support algorithm. *Source:* Resuscitation Council UK, 2021a. Reproduced with the kind permission of Resuscitation Council UK.

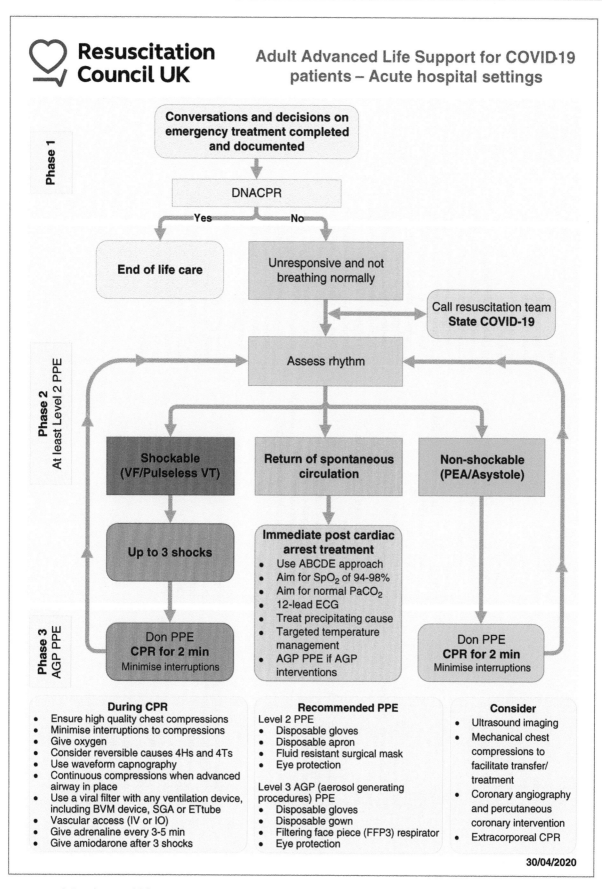

Figure 21.5   Adult advanced life support algorithm for COVID19 positive patients. *Source:* Resuscitation Council UK, 2020. Reproduced with the kind permission of Resuscitation Council UK.

Table 21.1 Airway emergencies that may be encountered within critical care.

Scenario	Recognition	Potential causes and/or associations	Potential treatments	Relevant guidance
Airway obstruction	◦ Grunting ◦ Snoring ◦ Coughing, choking, drooling ◦ Stridor ◦ Voice change ◦ Paradoxical breathing pattern ◦ Neck swelling ◦ Difficulty swallowing ◦ Respiratory distress ◦ Cyanosis ◦ Epistaxis, haemoptysis ◦ Trismus ◦ Fever ◦ Hypotension ◦ Bradycardia ◦ Poor or absent air entry and chest expansion ◦ Anxiety ◦ Soot in airway ◦ Facial burns and/or swelling ◦ Decreased level of consciousness ◦ Cardiac arrest	◦ Intrinsic – – Tumour – Foreign body – Bleeding – Vomit – Infection – Laryngospasm – Oedema – burns, inhalation injury, upper airway manipulation or instrumentation, surgery, angio-oedema ◦ Extrinsic – – Haematoma – neck surgery or trauma, central venous catheter insertion, – Neck trauma – Tumour or mass ◦ Neurological – – Head injury – Intracerebral bleed or thrombosis – Drug overdose – Alcohol intoxication – Neurological pathology - Guillain–Barré, myaesthenia gravis – Recurrent laryngeal nerve palsy or damage – Inadequate muscle relaxant reversal	◦ Open airway – manual in-line stabilisation in suspected cervical spine injury ◦ Airway clearance ◦ Airway adjuncts ◦ Bag mask ventilation ◦ Intubation ◦ Specialist considerations – – Bleeding – correct coagulopathy, transfuse, blood products – Laryngospasm – low dose propofol 0.25mg/kg intravenous (IV), suxamethonium 1mg/kg IV, positive end-expiratory pressure, Larson's manoeuvre – Oedema – IV steroids – Swelling, physical obstruction or infection - Nebulised adrenaline 5 mg/5ml 1:1000 – Surgical haematoma – open sutures – Drug overdose – reversal agent as appropriate – Muscle relaxant reversal – neostigmine 2.5 mg with glycopyronium bromide 0.5 mg intravenous (non-depolarising muscle agent), sugammadex 2-4 mg/kg intravenous (rocuronium)	Adult Basic Life Support Guidelines, 2021d Adult Advanced Life Support Guidelines, 2021a Difficult Airway Society Guidelines, 2012
Anaphylaxis	◦ Skin and/or mucosal changes – urticaria, flushing, angioedema ◦ Airway swelling ◦ Hoarse voice ◦ Stridor ◦ Bronchospasm ◦ Hypoxia ◦ Respiratory distress ◦ Respiratory arrest ◦ Cardiovascular shock ◦ Confusion or decreased level of consciousness ◦ Cardiac arrest	◦ Food ◦ Medication ◦ Sting or bite ◦ Latex	◦ Remove trigger ◦ Intramuscular adrenaline 500 micrograms (0.5 millilitres 1:1000), up to two doses ◦ Intravenous fluid challenge 500–1000 millilitres of crystalloid ◦ Oxygen	Adult Advanced Life Support Guidelines, 2021a

Intubation complications	- Oesophageal intubation
	  – Hypoxaemia
	  – No chest wall movement
	  – No endotracheal tube misting
	  – Absence or diminishing end-tidal carbon dioxide waveform
	- Bronchial intubation
	  – Hypoxia
	  – Unilateral chest wall movement
	  – High airway pressures
	  – Length of endotracheal tube at the lips
	- Vocal cords not visualised on intubation
	- Difficult grade of intubation
	- Endotracheal tube dislodgement on patient positioning, loose tube ties
		- Follow 'Tracheal intubation of critically ill adults' algorithm (Higgs et al., 2017)
		- Remove endotracheal tube and reintubate
		- Reposition endotracheal tube
		- Secure tube ties
		- Anticipate complications – checklist including preparation of patient, equipment, team and difficulties
			Difficult Airway Society Guidelines, 2012
			Difficult Airway Society ICU intubation guidelines, 2017
			4th National Audit Project, 2011

Can't Intubate, Can't Oxygenate (CICO)	- Profound hypoxaemia - Failed intubation – maximum three attempts - Failed rescue oxygenation with second-generation supraglottic airway – maximum three attempts - Airway obstruction - Poor mouth opening, dentition and neck mobility - Reduced thyro-mental distance and sternomental distance - Distorted anatomy due to tumour, trauma, airway oedema, radiotherapy, previous tracheostomy and surgery - Body habitus - Pregnancy - Craniofacial pathology - Documented previous difficult intubation - Airway assessment indicative of difficult intubation – high Mallampati score	- Follow 'Can't Intubate, Can't Oxygenate' algorithm (Higgs et al., 2017) - Front of neck airway – scalpel cricothyroidotomy	Difficult Airway Society ICU intubation guidelines, 2017
Endotracheal complications	- Respiratory distress - Hypoxaemia - Cyanosis - Increasing ventilatory setting requirements - Poor tidal volumes associated with high ventilator pressures - Loss of end-tidal carbon dioxide waveform - Audible leak associated with ventilator leak alarm and loss of airway pressures - Decreased air entry or widespread crackles on auscultation - Accidental extubation due to mobile, awake or delirious patient - Obstruction due to sputum, blood or foreign body - Cuff leak or herniation - Trachea mucosal ulceration or granulation due to high cuff pressures - Vocal cord damage - Aspiration of gastric contents	- Follow 'Tracheal intubation of critically ill adults' algorithm (Higgs et al., 2017) - Give 100% oxygen - Check endotracheal tube position - Pass suction catheter via the endotracheal tube - Manually ventilate with a waters circuit - Check cuff pressure and inflate as required - Bronchoscopy - Assisted ventilation with airway adjuncts as required in accidental extubation - Consider removing endotracheal tube and re-intubating	Difficult Airway Society ICU intubation guidelines, 2017 4th National Audit Project, 2011

(Continued)

Table 21.1 (Continued)

Scenario	Recognition	Potential causes and/or associations	Potential treatments	Relevant guidance

Tracheostomy complications	• As for endotracheal complications
	• Haemoptysis, bleeding from airway or around tracheostomy
	• Cellulitis, erythema or pus from or around the tracheostomy
	• Subcutaneous surgical emphysema
	• Ability to vocalise with cuff inflated
		• On insertion –
		  – bleeding
		  – loss of airway
		  – misplacement
		  – damage to neck structures
		• Post insertion -
		  – Accidental dislodgement due to mobile, awake or delirious patient
		  – Obstruction due to sputum, blood or foreign body
		  – Cuff leak or herniation
		  – Trachea mucosal ulceration or granulation due to high cuff pressures
		  – Bleeding
		  – Skin breakdown or infection
		  – Fistulae
		  – Aspiration of gastric contents
			• Follow 'Emergency tracheostomy management – patent upper airway' (McGrath et al, 2012)
			• Give 100% oxygen via face and tracheostomy
			• Check tracheostomy position
			• Pass suction catheter via the tracheostomy
			• Attach waters circuit, gentle manual ventilation if no spontaneous breathing
			• Remove and check inner tube
			• Extremis or obstruction – deflate cuff, remove tracheostomy, apply occlusive dressing, bag mask ventilate with airway adjuncts as required, re-intubate with oral endotracheal tube or consider re-siting tracheostomy
			• Follow 'Emergency laryngectomy management' (McGrath et al, 2012) if no patent upper airway, ventilate via stoma and consider intubating via the stoma
			• Bleeding –
			  – Minor – apply pressure, haemostatic dressing
			  – Major – intubate orally cuff below tracheostomy stoma, digital pressure to stoma, fluid resuscitation and blood product transfusion
			  – Sputum plugging – suction and chest physiotherapy
			  – Infection - antibiotics
				National Tracheostomy Safety Project, 2012
				4th National Audit Project, 2011
				The Faculty of Intensive Care Medicine, 2020

288

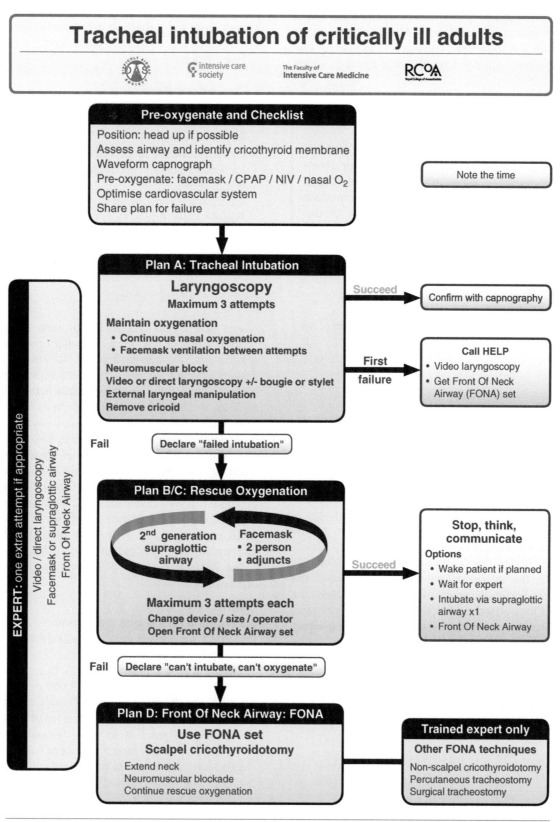

Figure 21.6 Difficult airway tracheal intubation of critically ill adults. *Source:* Higgs et al., 2017. Reproduced with permission from Elsevier.

In addition, the National Tracheostomy Project (2012) produced guidance regarding the emergency management of tracheostomies and laryngectomies. All guidelines provide clinicians with a standardised approach to managing life-threatening airway emergencies, the algorithms of which are utilised within the CCE.

Red Flag

End-tidal carbon dioxide is used to monitor patients ventilatory status within critical care. Loss of, or diminishing, capnography waveform may indicate several life-threatening emergencies and warrants immediate attention. These include airway obstruction or dislodgement, detached airway circuit, inadequate ventilation, pneumothorax, respiratory or cardiac arrest.

6Cs: Care

High-quality care should always be at the centre of all work practices when caring for patients.

B – Breathing

Breathing emergencies cover a wide spectrum of presentations within the CCE. The overarching presentation is that of respiratory failure which encompasses severe bronchospasm, tension pneumothorax and pulmonary embolus. Chapter 16 explores respiratory system pathologies in more depth; however, Table 21.2 describes some of the common breathing emergencies that may be encountered.

The Resuscitation Council (2021a), in addition to the British Thoracic Society (BTS) (2019), Difficult Airway Society (2011: 2015a, 2015b), the Faculty of Intensive Care Medicine (2016, 2020), the Intensive Care Society (2019) and the Intensive Care Society & Faculty of Intensive Care Medicine (2019), have formulated evidence-based guidance regarding the management of life-threatening breathing emergencies. These guidelines are utilised within the CCE. The British Medical Journal (BMJ) Best Practice online series (www.bestpractice.bmj.com) also provides quality-assessed evidence that informs clinical decision making, giving a structured approach to diagnosis and treatment.

Examination scenario: tension pneumothorax

Tension pneumothorax is a life-threatening emergency and requires time-critical treatment. Prompt needle decompression, and subsequent chest drain insertion, may prevent progressive intrathoracic air accumulation, haemodynamic compromise, and cardiac arrest. Recognition of tension pneumothorax is based upon clinical

signs, unless cardiovascular stability allows for an urgent chest X-ray, chest ultrasound or a computerised tomography (CT) scan to be performed.

Signs include:

- Tracheal deviation
- Diminished or absent unilateral air entry on auscultation
- Respiratory distress
- Hyper-resonance on percussion
- Increasing oxygen requirements
- Hypoxaemia
- Cardiovascular compromise
- Pulseless electrical activity cardiac arrest

Snapshot

Martin is a 56-year-old gentleman who presented to hospital having felt faint and light-headed whilst playing golf. He had laparotomy for resection of an adenocarcinoma 10 weeks ago with a protracted stay on critical care due to post-operative hypotension and an ileus. He has noticed that his right calf has become more swollen over the preceding few days.

On presentation to the Emergency Department (ED), he complains of acute shortness of breath and 'sharp' chest pain on the right side, which worsens on deep inspiration. A computerised tomography pulmonary angiogram (CTPA) demonstrated a large saddle pulmonary embolus with evidence of right ventricle strain and reflux of contrast into the inferior vena cava. Martin is admitted to the High Dependency Unit for monitoring.

The Registered Nurse (RN) finds the following on assessment:

Airway (A): Patent.
Breathing (B): Oxygen saturations of 92% (NEWS2 = 2) 4 L oxygen via nasal cannula (NEWS2 = 2), respiratory rate 22 (NEWS2 = 2).
Circulation (C): Heart rate 114 beats per minute (NEWS2 = 2) Blood pressure 98/65 mmHg (NEWS2 = 2) peripherally he has cool hands and feet.
Disability (D): Alert on AVPU scale (NEWS2 = 0). Pupils equal and reactive to light. Temperature 38.2°C (NEWS2 = 2) and blood glucose of 6.8 mmol/L.
Exposure (E): Tender swollen right calf, 4 cm larger than the left in diameter. Urine output adequate for weight.
Total NEWS2: 11

Nursing actions:
- Request urgent medical review of patient.
- Perform A–E assessment – recognise and treat concerns as appropriate to experience.

- Supplementary oxygen increased to maintain SpO2 94–98%.
- Ensure adequate venous access and that it is patent.
- Communicate findings to senior team using SBAR framework.

Diagnosis:
- Martin has a sub-massive pulmonary embolus as demonstrated by systemic hypotension, evidence of right ventricular failure and confirmation on a CTPA.
- He requires an increased oxygen concentration and high flow oxygen would be beneficial to optimise ventilation perfusion mismatch.
- An arterial line should be inserted to guide monitoring of haemodynamic stability and gas exchange.
- Anticoagulation in the form of low molecular weight heparin should be commenced.
- Martin requires monitoring within a critical care environment as in the event of haemodynamic instability he may require initially inotropic support and then subsequent thrombolysis with alteplase.

6Cs: Commitment

Quality of care and patient experience is improved through clinicians high level of commitment.

C – Circulation/ Cardiovascular

Circulatory emergencies within the CCE cover a large spectrum of presentations that may be due to a primary cardiac disorder such as acute coronary syndrome with associated acute heart failure, or due to a secondary problem such as circulatory collapse because of major haemorrhage. Chapters 8 and 19 cover cardiovascular system (CVS) pathologies in more depth, however, Table 21.3 describes some of the common CVS emergencies which may be encountered.

The Resuscitation Council UK (2021a) produce evidence-based guidance and standardised training for the provision of resuscitation in the adult, paediatric and neonatal population. Said guidance is based upon recommendations from the European Resuscitation Council (ERC, 2021). The algorithms that are produced as part of said guidance provide clinicians with a standardised way in which to approach and subsequently treat life-threatening emergencies. These algorithms are utilised within the CCE. Two common cardiovascular emergencies that may be encountered are tachycardia and bradycardia. Their respective algorithms can be found in Figures 21.7 and 21.8

Snapshot 1

Pierre is a 51-year-old male who has been admitted to hospital with chest pain whilst attending a social event. He is currently in monitoring in the Emergency Department (ED). He has a history of recreational cocaine usage, but otherwise no other documented medical history. Pierre comments that he had been engaging in 'heavy' cocaine usage during the social event. Shortly after arriving in the ED, Pierre comments that he is feeling more unwell. The Registered Nurse (RN) finds the following on assessment:

Airway (A): Patent, but Pierre is only able to speak in short, broken sentences.
Breathing (B): Oxygen saturations of 82% on room air (NEWS2 =3), respiratory rate 30 (NEWS2 = 3) and audible crackles on approach.
Circulation (C): Heart rate 140 (NEWS2 = 3), wide-complex tachycardia, blood pressure 225/130 mmHg (NEWS2 = 3), diaphoretic and peripherally warm.
Disability (D): Pierre presents with new-onset confusion, or 'C', on the ACVPU scale (NEWS2 = 3). He rapidly became combative and his pupils were found to be dilated bilaterally, but equal and reactive to light. Blood glucose is 10, temperature 38.1°C (NEWS2 = 1).
Exposure (E): There is nothing else to find on full body examination. One 20gauge cannula in the right antecubital fossa. There is no urinary catheter.
Total NEWS2: 16.

Nursing actions:
- Request urgent medical review of patient.
- Contact critical care outreach team.
- Perform A–E assessment – recognise and treat concerns as appropriate to experience.
- Supplementary oxygen increased to maintain SpO$_2$ 94–98%.
- Ensure adequate venous access and that it is patent.
- Communicate findings to senior team using SBAR framework.

Diagnosis
- Pierre has several symptoms consistent with sympathomimetic stimulation (high heart rate, high blood pressure, diaphoresis and dilated pupils) which are likely due to recent cocaine usage.
- His blood pressure is dangerously high and he has signs of end-organ dysfunction as evidenced by symptoms consistent with heart failure (low oxygen saturations, high respiratory rate and audible crackles), chest pain and new-onset confusion.
- An arterial blood gas was taken and results were as follows pH 7.31 pCO$_2$ 2.8 pO$_2$ 12 HCO$_3$ 18 BXS -8.
- Pierre was intubated and ventilated, received vasodilator agents to stabilise his blood pressure whilst further investigations were performed to assess whether a myocardial infarction or aortic dissection had occurred because of the cocaine usage.

Table 21.2   Breathing emergencies that may be encountered within critical care.

Scenario	Recognition	Potential causes and/or associations	Potential treatments	Relevant guidance
Respiratory failure – Type I respiratory failure – hypoxaemia Type II respiratory failure – hypoxaemia and hypercarbia	• Respiratory distress • Cyanosis • Hypoxaemia and or hypercarbia on arterial blood gas • Reduced air entry on auscultation • Altered percussion note • Poor chest expansion • Decreased respiratory rate • Decreased level of consciousness • Cardiovascular compromise • Ventilator alarms	• Airway obstruction • Lung parenchymal pathology – adult respiratory distress syndrome, lung fibrosis, pneumonia, pulmonary oedema, lung contusion, inhalation injury haemorrhage, chronic lung disease • Pulmonary circulation pathology – pulmonary embolus, cardiac failure, vascular disease • Neurological compromise – head injury, intra-cranial bleed or ischaemia • Neuromuscular weakness or paralysis • Respiratory mechanical compromise – chest wall deformity, pleural effusion, fractured ribs, heamothorax, pneumothorax, ascites	• Oxygen • Airway clearance • Non-invasive ventilation • Bag mask ventilation • Direct laryngoscopy • Bronchoscopy • Intubation and mechanical ventilation • Cricothyroidotomy • Tracheostomy • Review of mechanical ventilator settings • Treatment of underlying cause	Adult Basic Life Support Guidelines, 2021d BTS/ICS Guidelines, 2017 Adult Advanced Life Support Guidelines, 2021a Difficult Airway Society Guidelines, 2012 The Faculty of Intensive Care Medicine, 2016 British Medical Journal (BMJ) Best Practice, 2020b
Severe bronchospasm	• Respiratory distress • Bilateral wheeze • Reduced peak expiratory flow rate • Cyanosis • Silent chest on auscultation • Altered conscious state • Cardiovascularly compromise • Normal or rising arterial carbon dioxide • Mechanical ventilation – increasing peak inspiratory pressures, decreasing tidal volumes, 'gas trapping'	• Asthma • Chronic obstructive pulmonary disease • Hay fever • Eczema	• Oxygen • Nebulised salbutamol (5 mg every 15–30 minutes) and ipratropium bromide (500 mcg 4–6 hourly) • Corticosteroids • Intravenous magnesium sulphate • Additional specialist treatment – ketamine, salbutamol and aminophylline infusions • Intubation and ventilation • Ventilator – remove positive end-expiratory pressure (PEEP), disconnect from ventilator circuit allowing chest to decompress, 'permissive' hypercapnia	Adult Advanced Life Support Guidelines, 2021a BTS/SIGN, 2019 BMJ Best Practice, 2020a
Tension pneumothorax	• Tracheal deviation • Diminished or absent unilateral air entry on auscultation • Respiratory distress • Hyper-resonance on percussion • Increasing oxygen requirements • Chest pain • Hypoxaemia • Cardiovascular compromise • Cardiac arrest	• Trauma to chest • High ventilator pressures • Central line insertion • Underlying lung disease – asthma, chronic obstructive pulmonary disease • Chest or abdominal surgery • Blocked chest drain	• Oxygen • Needle decompression • Chest drain	Adult Advanced Life Support Guidelines, 2021a British Thoracic Society, 2010 BMJ Best Practice, 2020c
Pulmonary embolism (PE)	• Dyspnoea • Hypoxaemia • Pleuritic hest pain • Haemoptysis • Syncope • Features of a deep vein thrombosis (DVT) • Cardiovascular compromise • Right ventricle heave • Raised jugular venous pressure • Cardiac arrest	• DVT or history of thromboembolic disease • Malignancy • Recent major surgery • Reduced mobility • Pregnancy • Orthopaedic pelvic or lower limb fractures • Coagulation disorders	• Oxygen • Thrombolysis for unstable massive PE – alteplase • Anticoagulation for stable patient with a PE – therapeutic low molecular weight heparin	Adult Advanced Life Support Guidelines, 2021a BMJ Best Practice, 2020d

Table 21.3 Circulatory emergencies that may be encountered within critical care.

Scenario	Recognition	Potential causes and/or associations	Potential treatments	Relevant guidance
Cardiac arrest (CA)	• Unexpected CA are rare in CC due, in part, to access to extensive monitoring and diagnostics • ECG trace change, e.g. VT or VF • Sudden loss of consciousness • Sudden loss of arterial trace, and/or impalpable pulse • Sudden loss of end-trial CO_2 trace	Hypoxia	• Airway adjuncts • Oxygen therapy	• RCUK, 2021a, 2021b • National Poisons Information Service, 2020
		Hypovolaemia	• Intravenous (IV) fluid • Blood products	
		Hypokalaemia	• Intravenous potassium infusion	
		Hyperkalaemia	• Intravenous calcium • Insulin/glucose infusion	
		Hypothermia	• Active internal re-warming via cardiopulmonary bypass • Forced air warming • Warm IV fluids	
		Hyperthermia (e.g serotonin syndrome)	• Stop triggering agent • Dantrolene IV	
		Tamponade	• Sternotomy • Pericardiocentesis	
		Tension pneumothorax	• Needle decompression • Chest drain insertion	
		Thrombosis – coronary or pulmonary	• Thrombolytic "clot busting" therapy	
		Toxins	• Reversal agents (e.g. naloxone for opioid overdose) • Support therapies (e.g. renal replacement therapy in metformin overdose)	
Cardiogenic shock	• Hypotension • ECG trace change, e.g. ST segment elevation • Sudden change in conscious level	'Pump failure' – acute coronary syndrome (ACS)	• Primary coronary intervention (PCI)	• NICE, 2020a • NICE, 2019
		Outflow obstruction – malignant hypertension	• Vasodilator medications	
		Valvular pathology – valvular rupture	• Valve replacement surgery	

(Continued)

Table 21.3 (Continued)

Scenario	Recognition	Potential causes and/or associations	Potential treatments	Relevant guidance
Hypovolaemic shock	• Hypotension • Increased lactate • Metabolic acidosis	Major haemorrhage secondary to upper gastrointestinal bleed	• Massive transfusion – red cells, platelets, cryoprecipitate, etc. • IV calcium • Sengstaken tube placement	• JPAC, 2020
Bradycardia with haemodynamic instability/ symptomatic bradycardia	• Heart rate <60 beats/min • Systolic blood pressure (<90 mmHg) • Signs of ischaemia on ECG trace, e.g. ST segment depression	• ACS • Medications (e.g. beta-blockers) • Raised intracranial pressure	• PCI for ACS • Atropine IV • Glycopyrrolate IV • Isoprenaline IV • Transcutaneous pacing	• RCUK, 2021
Tachycardia with haemodynamic instability/ symptomatic tachycardia	• Heart rate >100 beats/min • Systolic blood pressure (<90 mmHg) • Signs of ischaemia on ECG trace, e.g. ST segment depression	• ACS • Pulmonary embolism • Haemorrhage • Electrolyte abnormalities	• PCI for ACS • Thrombolysis • Blood products • Rapid correction of electrolyte abnormalities	• RCUK, 2021
Hypertensive crisis	• Blood pressure (BP) ≥220/120 mmHg or high BP with 'emergency symptoms', also referred to as end-organ damage (i.e. retinal haemorrhage, papilloedema, new-onset confusion, chest pain, heart failure, or acute kidney injury)	• Drugs (e.g. amphetamines, cocaine) • Endocrine emergencies (e.g. Cushing's syndrome) • Renal disease • Aortic dissection • Raised ICP • Preeclampsia/eclampsia	• Systemic vasodilators • Beta-blockers • Calcium channel blockers	• NICE, 2019 • International Society of Hypertension, 2020

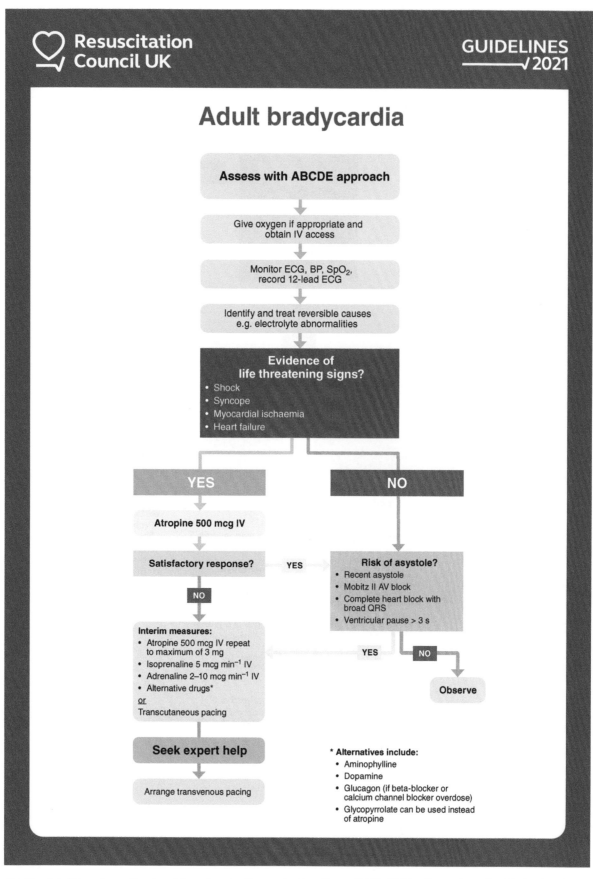

Figure 21.7 Adult bradycardia algorithm. *Source:* Resuscitation Council UK, 2021a. Reproduced with the kind permission of Resuscitation Council UK.

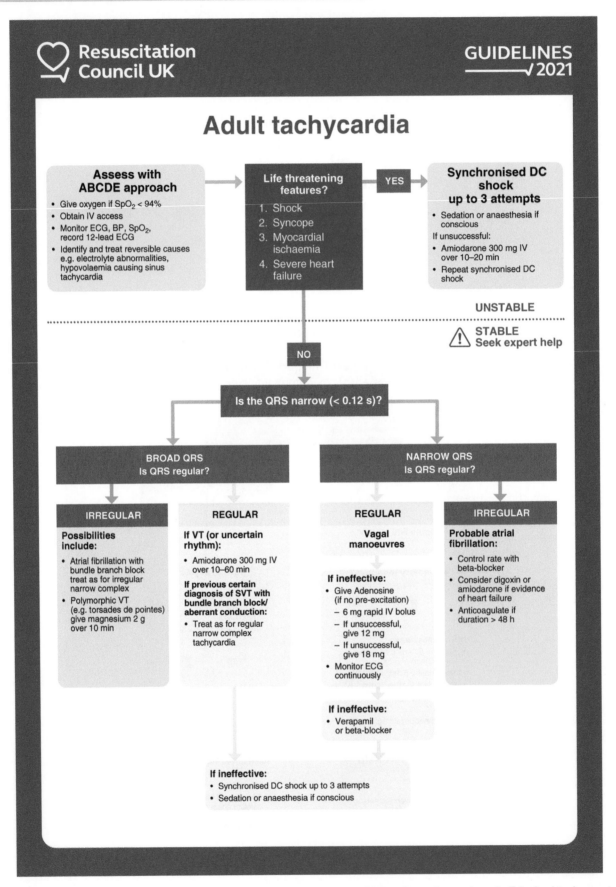

Figure 21.8 Adult tachycardia algorithm. *Source:* Resuscitation Council UK, 2021a. Reproduced with the kind permission of Resuscitation Council UK.

Clinical investigations: 12-lead ECG

An electrocardiogram (ECG) is a tracing of the electrical activity of the heart. An ECG is a common clinical investigation that provides vital information about pathological processes that may be affecting the heart. Figure 21.9 details the standard positioning of ECG electrodes, a normal 12-lead ECG and the coronary artery territories that each of the areas of the ECG relates to.

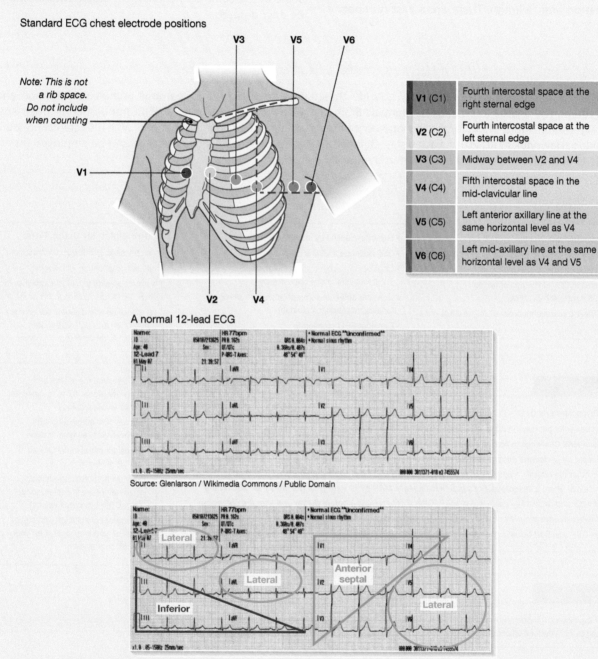

Figure 21.9 12-lead ECG Standard ECG electrode positions, a normal 12-lead ECG and 12-lead ECG territories. *Source:* Holbery and Newcombe (2016) with permission of John Wiley & Sons.

Learning event: reflection

Reflect upon the complications you have observed within your own practice for patients who have suffered a cardio-vascular event (e.g. myocardial infarction).

D – Disability

Neurological emergencies cover a wide spectrum of presentations within the CCE, including decreased level of consciousness, seizures, meningitis, encephalitis, raised intracranial pressure (ICP), neuromuscular weakness, as well agitation and delirium. There are a vast number of European and International clinical guidelines available and these are utilised for management of specific life-threatening neurological emergencies, within the CCE. Chapters 14 and 15 explore the neurological system pathologies in more depth, however Table 21.4 describes some of the common neurological emergencies that may be encountered.

Examination scenario: raised intra-cranial pressure (ICP)

Raised ICP and 'critical neuroworsening' is a life-threatening emergency and warrants immediate attention and management. The Seattle International Traumatic Brain Injury Consensus Conference (SIBICC) published a consensus-based algorithm (Figure 21.10) for the management of severe traumatic brain injury patients with intracranial pressure monitoring (Hawryluk et al., 2019). Each tier (1–3) incorporates treatments, the lower tiers should be employed first as the side effects have preferential and less detrimental side effects.

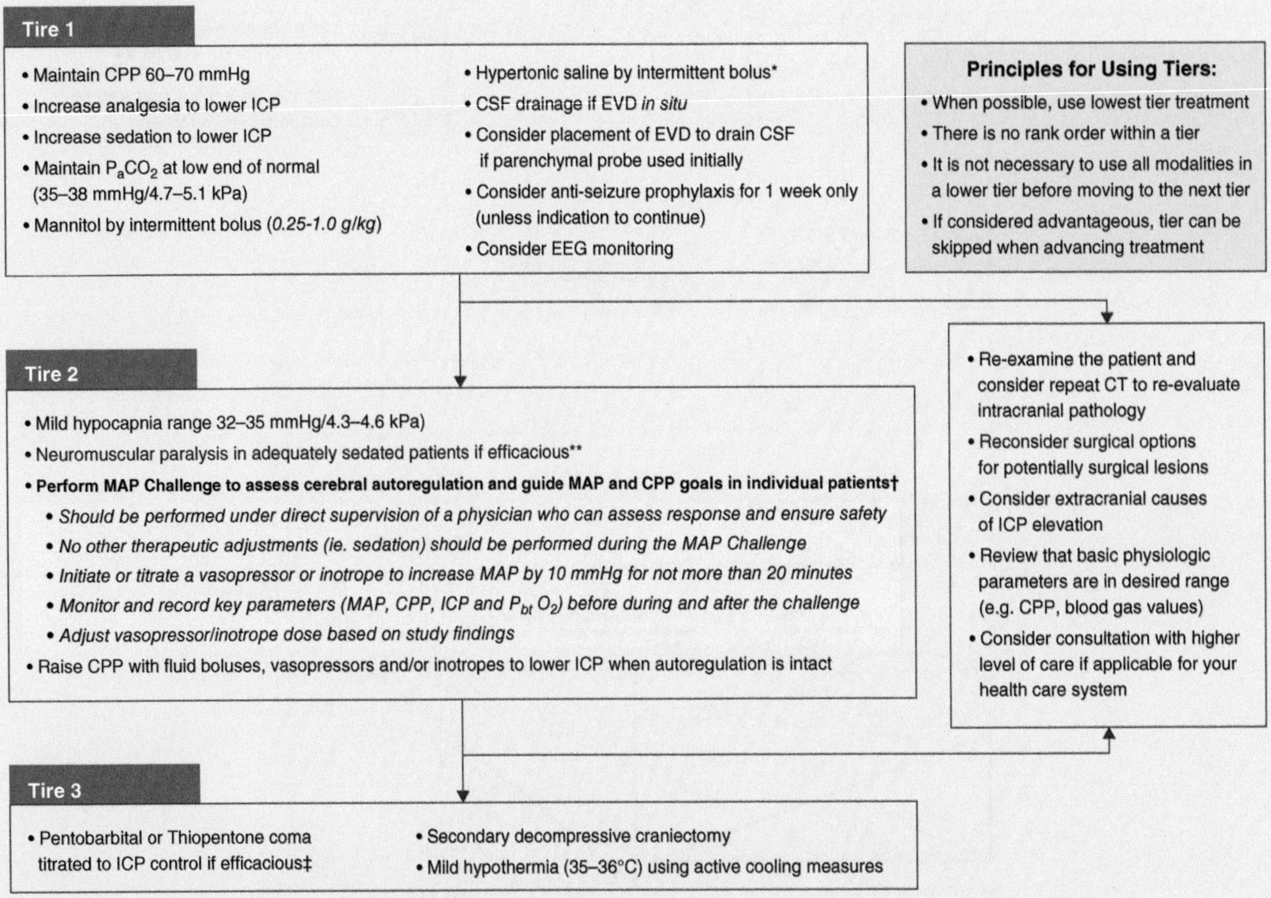

Tire 1

- Maintain CPP 60–70 mmHg
- Increase analgesia to lower ICP
- Increase sedation to lower ICP
- Maintain P_aCO_2 at low end of normal (35–38 mmHg/4.7–5.1 kPa)
- Mannitol by intermittent bolus (0.25-1.0 g/kg)

- Hypertonic saline by intermittent bolus*
- CSF drainage if EVD *in situ*
- Consider placement of EVD to drain CSF if parenchymal probe used initially
- Consider anti-seizure prophylaxis for 1 week only (unless indication to continue)
- Consider EEG monitoring

Principles for Using Tiers:
- When possible, use lowest tier treatment
- There is no rank order within a tier
- It is not necessary to use all modalities in a lower tier before moving to the next tier
- If considered advantageous, tier can be skipped when advancing treatment

Tire 2

- Mild hypocapnia range 32–35 mmHg/4.3–4.6 kPa)
- Neuromuscular paralysis in adequately sedated patients if efficacious**
- **Perform MAP Challenge to assess cerebral autoregulation and guide MAP and CPP goals in individual patients†**
  - *Should be performed under direct supervision of a physician who can assess response and ensure safety*
  - *No other therapeutic adjustments (ie. sedation) should be performed during the MAP Challenge*
  - *Initiate or titrate a vasopressor or inotrope to increase MAP by 10 mmHg for not more than 20 minutes*
  - *Monitor and record key parameters (MAP, CPP, ICP and $P_{bt}O_2$) before during and after the challenge*
  - *Adjust vasopressor/inotrope dose based on study findings*
- Raise CPP with fluid boluses, vasopressors and/or inotropes to lower ICP when autoregulation is intact

- Re-examine the patient and consider repeat CT to re-evaluate intracranial pathology
- Reconsider surgical options for potentially surgical lesions
- Consider extracranial causes of ICP elevation
- Review that basic physiologic parameters are in desired range (e.g. CPP, blood gas values)
- Consider consultation with higher level of care if applicable for your health care system

Tire 3

- Pentobarbital or Thiopentone coma titrated to ICP control if efficacious‡
- Secondary decompressive craniectomy
- Mild hypothermia (35–36°C) using active cooling measures

* We recommend using sodium and osmolality limits of 155 mEq/L and of 320 mEq/L respectively as administration limits for both mannitol and hypertonic saline.

** We recommend a trial dose of neuromuscular paralysis and only proceeding to a continuous infusion when efficacy is demonstrated.

† Rosenthal G. et al 2011

‡ Barbiturate administration should only be continued when a beneficial effect on ICP is demonstrated.
 Titrate barbiturate to achieve ICP control but do not exceed the dose which achieves burst suppression.
 Hypotension must be avoided when barbiturates are administered.

Figure 21.10 Consensus-based algorithm for the management of severe traumatic brain injury guided by intracranial pressure measurements. Author: Hawryluk et al., 2019 with permission of Springer Nature.

Recognition of the *Cushings Triad* is essential as this is a late sign of raised ICP and represents imminent brain herniation followed by death. The three physiological signs include:

1. Hypertension
2. Bradycardia
3. Irregular breathing or Cheyne–Stokes respiration

Immediate response to suspected herniation includes:

1. Hyperventilation (*not* limited to $PaCO_2$ 30 mmHg/4.0 kPa)
2. Bolus hypertonic solution

(Hawryluk et al., 2019)

Definitive treatment requires management of the underlying cause of the raised ICP.

Table 21.4   Neurological emergencies that may be encountered within critical care.

Scenario	Recognition	Potential causes and/or associations	Potential treatments	Relevant guidance
Decreased consciousness	· Falling Glasgow Coma Score (GCS) or Alert Voice Pain Unconscious (AVPU) score · Patient history – including loss of consciousness, mechanism of injury · Headache · Vomiting · Agitation · Incontinence · Loss of sensation, co-ordination, motor power, balance, gait · Abnormal reflexes · Seizures · Altered speech or vision · Abnormal pupil size or reaction · Partial or complete airway obstruction · Abnormal breathing pattern or rate · Cardiovascular compromise or cardiac arrest	· Seizures · Central nervous or systemic infection · Traumatic brain injury (TBI) · Intra-cranial haemorrhage including subarachnoid haemorrhage (SAH) · Thromboembolic stroke · Tumour · Agitation and delirium · Neuromuscular weakness · Drugs · Alcohol · Respiratory failure · Cardiovascular compromise · Liver or renal failure · Metabolic derangement including hypo- or hyperglycaemia	· Oxygen · ABCDE approach · Intubation for compromised airway, GCS ≤ 8 or rapidly falling GCS · Sedation for management of seizures, significant TBI, stroke, intra-cranial haemorrhage, neurological weakness · Hypertonic saline or mannitol for raised intra-cranial pressure (ICP) · Stroke – thromboembolic – aspirin if haemorrhage has been ruled out, thrombolysis (tissue plasminogen activator) · Neurosurgical management – clot evacuation, decompressive craniotomy, external ventricular drain, clipping or coiling of cerebral aneurysm · SAH – enteral nimodipine · Intravenous (IV) glucose or glucose gel for hypoglycaemia · Drug reversal agents · Treat the underlying cause	American Heart Association/ American Stroke Association, 2012 Brain Trauma Foundation, 2016 British Infection Association, 2016 NICE, 2019a NICE, 2019b NICE, 2021 SIGN, 2018 The Association of British Neurologists British Infection Association, 2012
Status epilepticus and seizures	· Loss of consciousness · Vacant episode · Abnormal eye movements · Mydriasis · Tonic-clonic movements · Urinary incontinence · Teeth clenching · Tongue biting · Facial twitching · Hallucinations · Autonomic symptoms · Physiological manifestations – increased respiratory rate, tachycardia, hypertension, sweating, hyperthermia	· History of seizures · Intra-cerebral tumour · TBI · Stroke or intracranial haemorrhage · Hypoxia · Central nervous system infection · Metabolic or electrolyte derangement · Alcohol withdrawal · Eclampsia in pregnancy	· Oxygen · ABCDE approach · First-line treatment – rectal, buccal, intramuscular or IV benzodiazepines · Second line treatment – IV anti-epileptic drugs including levetiracetam, phenytoin or sodium valproate · Hypoglycaemia – give glucose · Alcohol withdrawal – give high potency thiamine	NICE, 2021 SIGN, 2018

(Continued)

299

Table 21.4 (Continued)

Scenario	Recognition	Potential causes and/or associations	Potential treatments	Relevant guidance
Meningitis and encephalitis	• Headache • Vomiting • Neck stiffness • Photophobia • Decreased GCS • Altered mental state • Seizures • Focal neurological signs • Physiological signs of infection or sepsis • Rash • Respiratory or cardiovascular compromise	• Infection secondary to bacterial, viruses, tuberculosis or fungal • Head injury • Sinus or ear infection • Neurosurgery • Immunocompromised patients • Autoimmune disease • Malignancy	• Oxygen • ABCDE approach • Antibiotics • Antivirals • Steroids for meningitis	The Association of British Neurologists British Infection Association, 2012 British Infection Association, 2016
Raised intra-cranial pressure	• As for decreased consciousness • Late signs – bradycardia, hypertension, irregular breathing pattern • Increasing pressure as evidenced on ICP monitor or via an intraventricular drain	• TBI • Intra-cerebral haemorrhage • Space occupying lesions (SOLs) – tumour, abscess • Hydrocephalus • Cerebral oedema – hyponatraemia, eclampsia, infection, encephalopathy (hepatic/hypertensive), altitude • Intra-cranial hypertension	• Oxygen • ABCDE approach • Intubation and ventilation • Ventilated patient – adequate sedation and analgesia, IV paralysing agent, head up 30°, strict control of arterial oxygen and carbon dioxide levels, minimal obstruction of neck veins, cerebral perfusion pressure ≥ 60 mmHg, • IV mannitol or hypertonic saline • Avoid pyrexia • Treatment of underlying precipitant	Brain Trauma Foundation, 2016 NICE, 2019a
Neuromuscular weakness	• Inability to maintain airway • Respiratory failure or failure to wean from ventilation • Limb weakness • Loss of sensation, reflexes, co-ordination • Poor cough • Inadequate swallow • Presentation will be dependent upon cause	• TBI • Stroke or intra-cranial haemorrhage • SOLs • Spinal cord injury • Motor neuron disease • Gullain-Barré syndrome (GBS) • Myaesthenia gravis • Poliomyelitis • Critical illness polyneuropathy or myopathy • Electrolyte disorders • Metabolic disorders • Autoimmune disease • Congenital – muscular dystrophy	• Oxygen • ABCDE approach • Intubation and ventilation • Correction of electrolytes • Treatment of the underlying cause • GBS – IV immunoglobulins, plasmaphoresis • Myaesthenia gravis – acetylcholinesterase inhibitor, IV immunoglobulins, plasmaphoresis	NICE, 2016 NICE, 2019b NICE, 2021 SIGN, 2018
Agitation and delirium	• Shouting out • Confusion • Pulling off or pulling out non-invasive or invasive monitoring • Inattention • Disorganised thinking • Fluctuating mental status • Assessment according to Richmond Agitation Scale, Confusion Assessment Method for the Intensive Care Unit, Clinical Institute Withdrawal Assessment for alcohol	• Drugs • Respiratory failure • Infection • Sleep or sensory deprivation • Elderly • Poor nutritional state • Surgery • Visual, cognitive or hearing impairment • Constipation • Urinary retention • Neurological insult • Metabolic or electrolyte derangement • Drug or alcohol withdrawal	• Oxygen • ABCDE approach • Antipsychotics – haloperidol, olanzapine, clonidine • Benzodiazepines – withdrawal or rescue therapy • Electrolyte replacement • Sleep hygiene	NICE, 2019c American College of Critical Care Medicine, 2018

E – Everything else (exposure, endocrine, electrolytes and environmental)

The 'E' section of an A–E clinical assessment can be referred to as 'everything else', this then encourages the clinician to use a 'top-to-toe' approach after undertaking a detailed assessment of body systems encompassed within the A-D sections of the examination. Emergencies within this section include immediately life-threatening endocrine and electrolyte abnormalities. Other considerations include intra-abdominal catastrophes such as: bowel perforation due to ulcers, diverticulitis and tumours; bowel ischaemia and intra-abdominal compartment syndrome. Chapters 22, 25 and 28 cover pathologies associated with these body systems in more depth. Table 21.5 describes some of the common emergencies which may be encountered.

Clinical investigation: blood glucose monitoring

Essential equipment
- Personal protective equipment
- Blood glucose monitor
- Test strips
- Control solution
- Single-use safety lancets
- Cotton wool or low-linting gauze
- Sharps box

Action	Rationale
Pre-procedure	
1 Turn the machine on and ensure the correct date and time are presented on screen, and that there is adequate battery life. Where applicable, enter or scan operator number and/or password.	To ensure accuracy in the record and patient safety (Roche Diagnostics 2017, **C**).
2 Ensure that the device is reading in mmol/L prior to each use.	Units of measure may change from mmol/L to mg/dL, which could result in an incorrect result (MHRA 2013a, **C**).
3 Before taking the device to the patient, calibrate the monitor and test strips (where applicable) using the relevant steps below (always follow the manufacturer's instructions in case of any difference): · Ensure the testing strips are in date and have not been left exposed to air. · Calibrate the monitor and test strips together. · Carry out a quality control test using both high and low or level 1 and 2 solutions (in accordance with trust and manufacturer's guidelines). Ensure the LOT number is recorded, either manually or via a bar code scanning system. · Record the result (pass or fail) in the equipment log book and sign it. · Where an automated device is used, ensure the device is docked in its base unit to enable the centrally held electronic records to be updated. · Ensure the meter has been decontaminated per local guidelines and is fit for use. · Ensure the meter service record is in date according to local policy. · Ensure the screen or display is intact and the 'screen safety check' has been completed in accordance with the manufacturer's guidelines (Roche Diagnostics 2017).	To ensure the device can be used under safe conditions (MHRA 2013a, **E**). Some machines will self-calibrate; check the manufacturer's instructions.
4 Identify the patient, introduce yourself, explain and discuss the procedure with them, and gain their consent to proceed.	To ensure that the patient feels at ease, understands the procedure and gives their valid consent (NMC 2018, **C**).
5 Select a site that is warm, well perfused and free of any skin damage. The ideal site for lancing is the palmar surface of the distal segment of the third or fourth finger (**Action figure 5**) of the non-dominant hand, avoiding the thumb and the index finger. Also avoid sites that have recently been punctured.	Fingers on the non-dominant hand are generally less callused and the index finger is potentially more sensitive to pain due to additional nerve endings (Marini and Dries 2016, **C**). The thumb also may be callused and has a pulse, indicating arterial presence, and the distance between the skin surface and the bone in the fifth finger makes it unsuitable for puncture (WHO 2010, **C**). Tips and pads of fingers should be avoided as they have a denser nerve supply and can be more painful (WHO 2010, **C**). Rotating puncture sites avoids fingertip soreness and reduces callus formation (WHO 2010, **C**).

Procedure

6	Ask the patient to wash their hands with soap and water and dry them thoroughly.	To avoid sample contamination (Adam et al. 2017, **C**). Not washing hands can lead to inaccurate results, especially with fingers exposed to fruit or a sugar-containing product (Pickering and Marsden 2014, **R**).
7	Ask patient to sit or lie down.	To ensure the patient's safety and minimize the risks if they feel faint when blood is taken (Roche Diagnostics 2017, **C**).
8	Wash and dry hands and/or use an alcohol-based handrub and apply personal protective equipment.	To minimize the risk of cross-infection and contamination (NHS England and NHSI 2019, **C**).
9	Turn on the device (where applicable and if not automated) and insert a testing strip.	Some devices will turn on automatically once the strip has been inserted. The manufacturer's guidelines should be followed to ensure accurate results (MHRA 2013a, **C**).
10	Take a single-use lancet and set the appropriate depth (if applicable).	To minimize the risk of cross-infection and accidental needle stick injury (NICE 2015a, **C**; Pickering and Marsden 2014, **E**; Weston 2013, **E**). The correct depth setting will minimise patient pain (Roche Diagnostics 2017, **C**).
11	Using the lancet, puncture the chosen site (see step 5). If necessary, 'milk' the fingertip from the palm of the hand towards the finger to gain a large enough droplet of blood.	Reusable lancet devices may be used in the patient's own environment; they should never be used for more than one person due to the risk of blood-borne viruses (Weston 2013, **C**). Milking the finger only (and not from the palm) can cause tissue fluid contamination and a false low reading (WHO 2010, **R**).
12	Dispose of the lancet in a sharps container.	To minimize the risk of cross-infection and accidental needle stick injury (Pickering and Marsden 2014, **E**; Weston 2013, **E**).
13	Apply the drop of blood to the testing strip (some strips are hydrophilic and are dosed/filled from the side, whereas others require a drop of blood to be placed directly onto the strip). Ensure that the window on the test strip is entirely covered with blood (**Action figure 13**).	To ensure the result is accurate, the window on the test strip needs to be adequately filled as per the manufacturer's guidelines (Roche Diagnostics 2017, **C**).
14	Immediately read and make note of the result on the display screen (**Action figure 14**). Document the result.	To interpret the results of the test. Some devices will turn off automatically after the result has been displayed for a short while. **E** To ensure accuracy in record keeping (NMC 2018, **C**).
15	Dispose of the testing strip in a sharps container.	To minimize the risk of sharps injury and cross-infection (Weston 2013, **E**).
16	Place gauze over the puncture site, apply firm pressure and monitor for excess bleeding.	To ensure patient safety (Walden et al. 2018, **E**) and to stop the bleeding (WHO 2010, **C**).
17	Once the bleeding has subsided, the site can be left exposed. It is not necessary to dress the site unless bleeding persists.	To allow the site to heal effectively. **E**
18	Remove gloves, place them in the clinical waste and perform hand hygiene again.	To prevent cross-infection (NHS England and NHSI 2019, **C**).

Post-procedure

19	Where applicable, dock the machine.	To ensure centralized records are maintained and the machine is charged (Roche 2017, **C**).
20	Report and/or act on any unexpected results.	To ensure appropriate treatment and obtain an optimal blood glucose range (Adam et al. 2017, **E**).

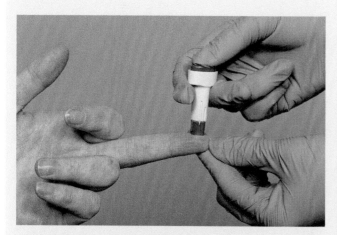

Action Figure 5 Take a blood sample from the side of the finger using a lancet, ensuring that the site of piercing is rotated.

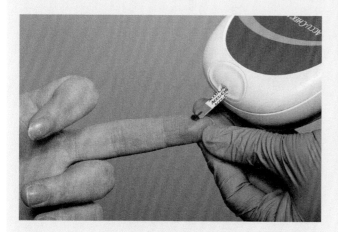

Action Figure 13 Insert the test strip into the blood glucose monitor and apply the blood to the test strip. Ensure that the window on the test strip is entirely covered with blood.

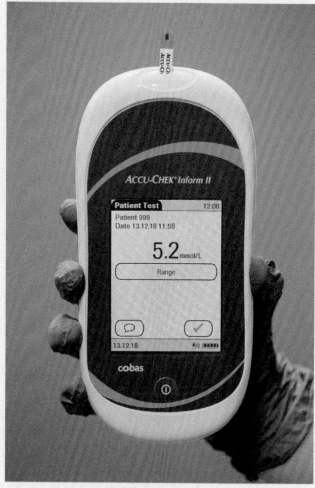

Action Figure 14 Read the result.

Table 21.5 Emergencies concerning exposure, endocrine, electrolyte and environmental aspects that may be encountered within critical care. *Source:* Sadie Diamond-Fox, 2021.

Scenario	Recognition	Potential Causes &/or Associations	Potential Treatments	Relevant Guidance
Cardiac Arrest (CA)	• Unexpected CA are rare in CC due, in part, to access to extensive monitoring and diagnostics • ECG trace change, e.g. VT or VF • Sudden loss of consciousness • Sudden loss of arterial trace, and/or impalpable pulse • Sudden loss of end-trial CO_2 trace	Hypoxia	• Airway adjuncts • Oxygen therapy	• RCUK, 2021[a,b] • National Poisons Information Service, 2020
		Hypovolaemia	• Intravenous (IV) fluid • Blood products	
		Hypokalaemia	• Intravenous potassium infusion	
		Hyperkalaemia	• Intravenous calcium • Insulin/glucose infusion	
		Hypothermia	• Active internal re-warming via cardiopulmonary bypass • Forced air warming • Warm IV fluids	
		Hyperthermia (e.g Serotonin syndrome)	• Stop triggering agent • Dantrolene IV	
		Tamponade	• Sternotomy • Pericardiocentesis	
		Tension pneumothorax	• Needle decompression • Chest drain insertion	
		Thrombosis – coronary or pulmonary	• Thrombolytic "clot busting" therapy	
		Toxins	• Reversal agents (e.g. naloxone for opioid overdose) • Support therapies (e.g. renal replacement therapy in metformin overdose)	

Condition	Signs/Criteria	Causes	Management	Guidelines
Cardiogenic Shock	• Hypotension • ECG trace change, e.g. ST segment elevation • Sudden change in conscious level	• "Pump failure" – Acute Coronary Syndrome (ACS) • Outflow obstruction - Malignant hypertension • Valvular pathology - Valvular rupture	• Primary coronary intervention (PCI) • Vasodilator medications • Valve replacement surgery	• NICE, 2020 • NICE, 2019
Hypovolaemic Shock	• Hypotension • Increased lactate • Metabolic acidosis	• Major haemorrhage secondary to upper-gastrointestinal bleed	• Massive transfusion – red cells, platelets, cryoprecipitate, etc. • IV calcium • Sengstaken tube placement	• JPAC, 2020
Bradycardia with haemodynamic instability/ Symptomatic bradycardia	• Heart rate <60 beats/min • Systolic blood pressure <90mmHg • Signs of ischaemia on ECG trace, e.g. ST segment depression	• ACS • Medications (e.g. beta blockers) • Raised intracranial pressure	• PCI for ACS • Atropine IV • Glycopyrrolate IV • Isoprenaline IV • Transcutaneous pacing	• RCUK, 2021
Tachycardia with haemodynamic instability/ Symptomatic tachycardia	• Heart rate >100 beats/min • Systolic blood pressure <90mmHg • Signs of ischaemia on ECG trace, e.g. ST segment depression	• ACS • Pulmonary embolism • Haemorrhage • Electrolyte abnormalities	• PCI for ACS • Thrombolysis • Blood products • Rapid correction of electrolyte abnormalities	• RCUK, 2021
Hypertensive crisis	• Blood pressure (BP) ≥220/120 mmHg or high BP with "emergency symptoms", also referred to as end-organ damage (i.e. retinal haemorrhage, papilloedema, new onset confusion, chest pain, heart failure, or acute kidney injury)	• Drugs (e.g. amphetamines, cocaine) • Endocrine emergencies (e.g. Cushing's syndrome) • Renal disease • Aortic dissection • Raised ICP • Pre-eclampsia/Eclampsia	• Systemic vasodilators • Beta blockers • Calcium channel blockers	• NICE, 2019 • International Society of Hypertension, 2020

Snapshot

Adanna is a 41-year-old female who has been admitted to hospital with a week long history of non-specific symptoms of fatigue, weakness and back pain following gastroenteritis. She was recently diagnosed with Addison's disease and commenced on hydrocortisone and fludrocortisone. She has been admitted to the high dependency unit (HDU) for vasopressor therapy as she has hypotension refractory to fluid resuscitation. Shortly after arriving on the HDU, Adanna is noted to be unresponsive. The Registered Nurse (RN) finds the following on assessment:

Airway (A): Semi-obstructed. Snoring sounds audible on approach.°

Breathing (B): Oxygen saturations of 88% (NEWS2 = 3) on 2 L oxygen via nasal cannula (NEWS2 = 2), respiratory rate 28 (NEWS2 = 3) with a deep, rapid breathing pattern (Kussmaul breathing).

Circulation (C): Heart rate 38 (NEWS2 = 3), wide-complex bradycardia with peaked T waves. Blood pressure 68/42 mmHg (NEWS2 = 3), peripherally warm. Phenylephrine infusion at 10 ml/hr via peripheral cannula in left antecubital fossa.

Disability (D): Responsive to pain, or 'P', on ACVPU scale (NEWS2 = 3). Pupils were found to be unequal (*anisocoria*), but equal and reactive to light. Blood glucose is 3.8 mmol/L, temperature 39.1°C (NEWS2 = 2).

Exposure (E): There is nothing else to find on full body examination. One 20 gauge cannula in the right anticubital fossa. Urine output in the last hour was 20 mls. An arterial blood gas shows the following:

pH	7.25
pCO_2 (mmHg)	35.3
pO_2 (mmHg)	89.0
HCO_3 (mmol/L)	14.9
Base (mmol/L)	−11.1
Na+ (mmol/L)	125
K+ (mmol/L)	7.1
Glucose (mmol/L)	2.8

Total NEWS2: 19.

Nursing actions:
- Emergency bedside alarm activated to summon immediate help from critical care colleagues.
- Senior critical care medical team review requested.
- Jaw thrust.
- 15 L oxygen applied via bag-valve mask.
- Supplementary oxygen increased to maintain SpO_2 94–98%.
- Vascular accesses checked for patency.
- Communicate findings to senior team using SBAR framework.

Diagnosis
- Adanna has several indicators within her history, physical assessment and arterial blood gas results that are consistent with Addisonian crisis:
  - **History:** Recent diagnosis of Addison's disease. Recent gastroenteritis means she was unlikely to absorb her prescribed hydrocortisone and fludrocortisone. Nausea, vomiting, fatigue, weakness and back pain and are also non-specific symptoms of adrenal crisis.
  - **Physical assessment:** Kussmaul breathing due to metabolic acidosis, Hypotension, bradycardia, peaked T waves due to hyperkalaemia, reduced conscious level, low blood glucose level and anisocoria
  - **Arterial blood gas:** Metabolic acidosis, hyperkalaemia, hyponatraemia and hypoglycaemia.
- Adanna was intubated and ventilated. She also received vasoconstrictor agents and high dose intravenous hydrocortisone to stabilise her blood pressure.
- Fluid resuscitation and careful correction of electrolyte abnormalities was conducted.

Red Flag: hypoglycaemia

Rapid recognition and correction of hypoglycaemia is vital to prevent seizures and coma which can lead to permanent brain damage. There are several cardinal symptoms of hypoglycaemia that may proceed seizures and coma; diaphoresis, tachycardia, confusion, visual changes, slurred speech and dizziness.

6Cs: Competence

All healthcare professionals must have the ability to understand an individual's health and social needs and the expertise, clinical and technical knowledge to deliver competent care and treatments based on research and evidence.

Care of the patient post return of spontaneous circulation (ROSC)

The Resuscitation Council UK (2021b) have produced evidence-based guidance regarding post-resuscitation care. This is underpinned by recommendations for the European Resuscitation Council (2021) and the ILCOR. It begins immediately following sustained ROSC and can impact significantly upon patient outcome. An algorithm has been produced as part of this guidance which provides a standardised approach to post-resuscitation care, and this is utilised within the CCE. This can be found in Figure 21.11.

Initial management includes assessment and management of airway, breathing, circulation and temperature control. The cause of cardiac arrest needs to be established due to the time-critical nature of subsequent treatment such as percutaneous coronary intervention. Respiratory or neurological causes, such as PE or stroke, will require further investigation including CT or CTPA. Physiological derangement is expected following cardiac arrest and other tests are required such as full blood count, biochemistry, arterial blood gas, 12-lead ECG, chest X-ray, and echocardiography.

Optimisation of organ function is critical following stabilisation and transfer to a CCE, in order to prevent further secondary organ injury. This includes targeted temperature management, treatment of myocardial dysfunction and neurological protective strategies such as normoxia, normocapnia, haemodynamic optimisation, normoglycaemia and seizure control.

Prognostication following cardiac arrest is complex, multimodal and tends not to be reliable until 72 hours following ROSC. It is dependent upon clinical examination, electroencephalography, biomarkers and further imaging including CT and magnetic resonance imaging and assists in guiding targeted treatments in order to achieve a neurological meaningful recovery for the patient. Evidence of significant hypoxic brain injury with poor neurological recovery may lead to withdrawal of life-sustaining treatment and subsequent death. Organ donation should be considered.

In cardiac arrest survivors, screening for cognitive, emotional and fatigue problems following hospital discharge is standard and early rehabilitation may be indicated as a result of hospital functional assessments.

6Cs: Courage

Courage is important to ensure that patients receive the care that they deserve.

Orange Flag: Communication with relatives during resuscitation

Communication and providing support to patient's relatives during resuscitation is crucial and allows healthcare professionals to establish the wishes of both the patient and their relatives in terms of their presence during resuscitation. The advantages of relatives witnessing resuscitation includes being able to speak to their relative, reduced distress at being separated, observing optimal treatment given to the patient and the reality of the patient's death. Disadvantages include distress if the relatives are not fully informed, or their expectations or cultural beliefs have not been considered and relatives emotional or physical hinderance of resuscitation.

Critical care emergencies and human factors

The CCE is one of the highest risk environments within the healthcare setting. Managing time-critical emergencies requires multiple team members managing often unrehearsed and complex situations. Acknowledgement of the way in which non-technical skills such as teamworking, communication, leadership and decision making have been acknowledged as a potential impact upon patient safety for over a decade (Odell, 2011). The application of these non-technical skills is often referred to as 'human factors'. Human factors are key to all aspects of clinical practice and providing safe and

308

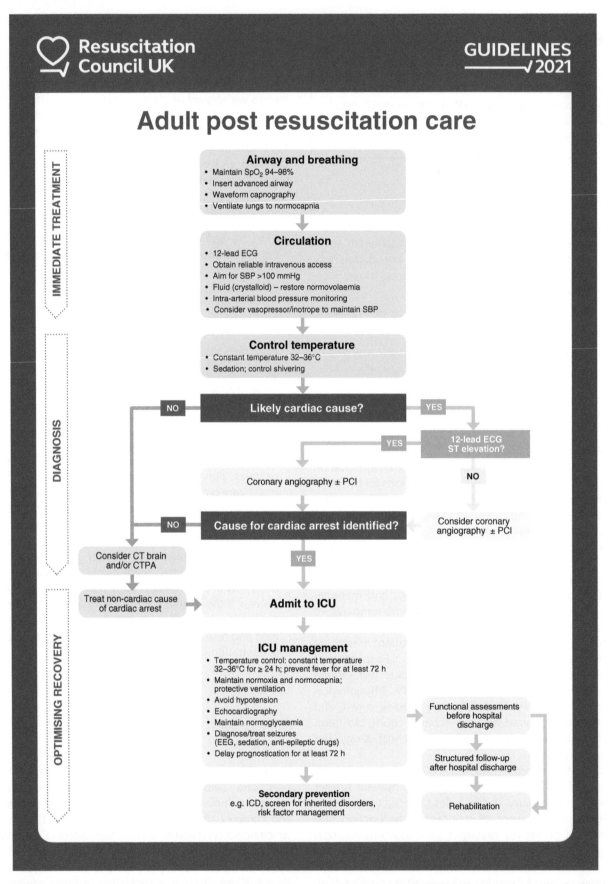

Figure 21.11   Post-resuscitation care algorithm. *Source:* Resuscitation Council UK, 2021b. Reproduced with the kind permission of Resuscitation Council UK.

effective care. Consequently, these are core strands of health-care training and ongoing professional development.

Effective team working, communication, leadership and decision making (all human factors) can lead to improvement in both treatment quality and safety metrics (Brock et al., 2013; Krug, 2008; Scalise, 2006); conversely, poor communication, leadership and teamwork has been highlighted as one of the main concerns that lead to complaints to the Parliamentary and Health Service Ombudsman (2020a, 2020b).

Human factors should always be a consideration during any high-stress, time-sensitive situation, particularly in the CCE where the cognitive load is high and there are multiple team members and multiple decibels being emitted from an array of devices. Concepts applied in the combat field are often applied to the resuscitation scenario, a concept which is now widely taught within resuscitation courses and has rather neatly been coined by Reid (2016) as speaking 'Resuscitese'. Communication is 'Directive, descriptive and informative' with a focus upon limiting non-essential communication to promote a 'sterile cockpit' (Lauria, 2020). 'Resuscitese' also focuses upon loops of communication being closed, with communication between team members being reinforced, for example, 'Mark, please administer 300 mg of amiodarone IV' followed by a response from the person administering the medication, '300 mg of amiodarone administered' (Lauria, 2020).

Several structured communication tools exist that can be used during time-critical emergency and resuscitation scenarios. The 'SBAR' tool is advocated by the Resuscitation Council UK (2021) (see Table 21.6) Further, extensive information can be found here: https://www.england.nhs.uk/improvement-hub/publication/safer-care-sbar-situation-background-assessment-recommendation-implementation-and-training-guide/.

The Department of Defense (DoD) and the Agency for Healthcare Research and Quality (AHRQ) have developed a comprehensive evidence-based teamwork system (TeamSTEPPS® 2.0) to improve communication and teamwork skills. TeamSTEPPS® 2.0 'Module 4: Leading Teams' is particularly useful when considering the intricacies of effective leadership and teamworking. Further details regarding the online training course may be found here: https://www.ahrq.gov/teamstepps/index.html.

Debriefing

Dealing with emergency situations within the CCE can be emotional and stressful. Debriefing is considered a powerful learning tool after emergency situations in the context of clinical education, quality improvement, systems learning and team wellbeing (Kessler et al., 2014). It can prove to be a useful tool in all cases; where things went well, near misses and where adverse events occurred. TeamSTEPPS® 2.0 advocates the use of an after-action review using a debrief for critical team events which focuses upon the evaluation of the following:

1. Communication
2. Roles and responsibilities
3. Situational awareness
4. Workload distribution
5. Asking for or offering assistance (cross-monitoring)
6. Errors: made or avoided
7. What went well, what should change and what could be improved

Do-not-attempt-cardiopulmonary-resuscitation (DNACPR) and Recommended Summary Plan for Emergency Care and Treatment (ReSPECT)

A DNACPR order is a sensitive advanced decision. Instituting DNACPR orders has been shown to be sub-optimal (Hawkes et al., 2020), as such the Recommended Summary Plan for Emergency Care and Treatment (ReSPECT) was developed (RCUK, 2021c). It details a summary of recommendations tailored to the patient regarding care provision during an emergency. The document is completed through conversations between the patient and their healthcare team, at a time when the patient has mental capacity to make such decisions. It aims to respect both patient preferences and clinical judgement (RCUK, 2021). An interactive learning web-application has been designed so that both healthcare professionals and patients can learn about the ReSPECT tool. This can be accessed via https://learning.respectprocess.org.uk/. Not all healthcare providers within the UK utilise the ReSPECT tool, therefore it is advised that healthcare professionals familiarise themselves with local practice and policy.

Table 21.6   The SBAR tool. *Source:* Holbery and Newcombe, 2016; Lindsey et al., 2018.

SBAR	Overview
Situation	· Identify yourself · State the site or unit you are calling from · Identify the patient by name and the reason for your call · Briefly describe your concern.
Background	· Give the patient's reason for admission · Explain significant medical history · Briefly describe relevant recent events.
Assessment	· Provide key vital signs · Use ABCDE and NEWS · Suggest your clinical impression.
Recommendation	· Explain what you need · Be specific about request and time frame · Make suggestions · Clarify expectations.

Conclusion

As a student healthcare practitioner working with critically ill patients, you will undoubtedly encounter and be involved in CPR and life-threatening emergencies with critically ill patients. These situations are often complex, multi-factorial and require prompt recognition, in order to try and prevent cardiac arrest. However, this is not always possible and once cardiac arrest has occurred interventions, such as CPR, high-quality chest compressions and early defibrillation if appropriate, will categorically improve survival. Therefore it is crucial that healthcare professionals involved in providing care in emergencies, life-threatening situations and cardiac arrest have a sound understanding of the evidence base and guidelines that underpin the management of these patients.

Take home points

1. Emergencies can be a common occurrence within the CCE and may require interventions such as those detailed within the adult in-hospital resuscitation and ALS algorithms (RCUK, 2021a). They ensure that patients receive standardised, evidence-based, good-quality care.
2. The ABCDE approach is essential to assessment and management of emergency situations facilitating timely recognition and prompt treatment.
3. Following CPR, patients require post-resuscitation care to prevent secondary organ injury.
4. Team working, human factors, debriefing and team wellbeing are essential, creating learning opportunities, allowing constructive reflection, with recognition of the delivery of excellent care.

References

Association of Anaesthetists. (2020). Guidelines: Malignant hyperthermia 2020. https://anaesthetists.org/Home/Resources-publications/Guidelines/Malignant-hyperthermia-2020 (accessed June 2021).

Beed, M. Sherman, R. & Mahajann, B. (2013). *Emergencies in Critical Care*, 2e. Oxford: OUP.

Brain Trauma Foundation (2016). *Guidelines for the Management of Severe Traumatic Brain Injury*, 4e. https://www.braintrauma.org/uploads/13/06/Guidelines_for_Management_of_Severe_TBI_4th_Edition.pdf (accessed June 2021).

British Thoracic Society/ Scottish Intercollegiate Guidelines Network (2019). British Guideline on the management of asthma. https://www.brit-thoracic.org.uk/quality-improvement/guidelines/asthma/ (accessed June 2021).

Connolly, E.S. Rabstein, A.A. Carhuapoma, J.R. et al. (2012). Guidelines for the management of aneurysmal subarachnoid haemorrhage. A guideline for healthcare professionals from the American Heart Association/American Stroke Association. doi: 10.1161/STR.0b013e3182587839 (accessed June 2021).

Cook, T.M. Woodall, N. Harper, J. et al. (2011). Major complications of airway management in the UK: results of the Fourth National Audit Project of the Royal college of Anaesthetist and the Difficult Airway Society. Part 2: Intensive care and emergency departments. https://bjanaesthesia.org/article/S0007-0912(17)33210-5/pdf (accessed June 2021).

Davidson, C. Banham S. Elliot, M. et al. (2017). BTS/ICS Guidelines for the ventilatory management of acute hypercapnic respiratory failure in adults. https://thorax. bmj.com/content/thoraxjnl/71/Suppl_2/ii1.full.pdf (accessed June 2021).

Devlin, J.W. Skrobik, Y. Gelinas, C. et al. American College of Critical Care Medicine (2018). Clinical Practice Guidelines for the prevention and management of pain, agitation/sedation, delirium, immobility, and sleep disruption in adult patients in the ICU. https://journals.lww.com/ccmjournal/Fulltext/2018/09000/Clinical_Practice_Guidelines_for_the_Prevention.29.aspx (accessed June 2021),

Difficult Airway Society (2011). DAS extubation guidelines. https://das.uk.com/guidelines/das-extubation-guidelines1 (accessed June 2021).

Difficult Airway Society (2015a). DAS guidelines for management of unanticipated difficult intubation in adults 2015. https://das.uk.com/guidelines/das_intubation_guidelines (accessed June 2021).

Difficult Airway Society (2015b). Guidelines for the management of difficult and failed tracheal intubation in obstetrics – 2015. https://das.uk.com/guidelines/obstetric_airway_guidelines_2015 (accessed June 2021).

Dutton, H. and Finch, J. (2018). *Acute and Critical Care Nursing at a Glance*. Hoboken, NJ: John Wiley & Sons.

Faculty of Intensive Care Medicine (2016). Guidelines on the management of acute respiratory distress syndrome. https://www.ficm.ac.uk/sites/default/files/ficm_ics_ards_guideline_-_july_2018.pdf. (accessed June 2021).

Faculty of Intensive Care Medicine (2020). Guidance for: Tracheostomy Care. https://www.ficm.ac.uk/sites/default/files/2020-08-tracheostomy_care_guidance_final.pdf. (accessed June 2021).

Hawkes, C.A., Fritz, Z., Deas, G. et al. (2020). Development of the Recommended Summary Plan for eEmergency Care and Treatment (ReSPECT). *Resuscitation*. doi: 10.1016/j. resuscitation.2020.01.003.

Hawryluk, G.W. J Aguilera, S. Buki, A. (2019). A management algorithm for patients with intracranial pressure monitoring: the Seattle International Severe Traumatic Brain Injury Consensus Conference (SIBCC). https://www.ncbi.nlm.nih. gov/pmc/articles/PMC6863785/ (accessed June 2021).

Higgs, A. McGrath, B.A. Goddard, C. et al. (2017). Guidelines for the management of tracheal intubation in critically ill adults. https://bjanaesthesia.org/article/S0007-0912(17)54060-X/ fulltext (accessed June 2021).

Holbery, N. & Newcombe, P. (2016). *Emergency Nursing at a Glance*. John Wiley & Sons.

Health Education England & The Faculty of Intensive Care Medicine (2021). e-Learning for Intensive Care Medicine. https:// www.e-lfh.org.uk/programmes/intensive-care-medicine/ (accessed June 2021).

Intensive Care Society & Faculty of Intensive Care Medicine (2019). Guidance For:Prone Positioning in Adult Critical Care. https://www.ics.ac.uk/Society/Guidance/PDFs/Prone_ Position_Guidance_in_Adult_Critical_Care (accessed June 2021).

Intensive Care Society (2019). Management of Patients With Gas Embolism: Guidance For Intensive Care And Resuscitation Teams. https://www.ics.ac.uk/Society/Guidance/PDFs/Gas_ Embolism_guidance (accessed June 2021).

International Society of Hypertension (2020). ISH Global Hypertension Practice Guidelines. https://ish-world.com/global-hypertension-practice-guidelines/ (accessed June 2021).

JPAC: Joint United Kingdom (UK) Blood Transfusion and Tissue Transplantation Services Professional Advisory Committee (2020). Transfusion Handbook – 7.3: Transfusion management of major haemorrhage. https://www.transfusionguidelines. org/transfusion-handbook/7-effective-transfusion-in-surgery-and-critical-care/7-3-transfusion-management-of-major-haemorrhage (accessed June 2021).

Kessler, D.O. Cheng, A. & Mullen, P.C. (2014). Debriefing in the emergency department after clinical events: a practical guide. *Annals of Emergency Medicine* 65(6): 690–698.

Leach, R. (2014). *Critical Care Medicine at a Glance*, 3e. Chichester: John Wiley & Sons.

Lindsey, P. Bagness, C. & Peate, I. (2018). *Midwifery Skills at a Glance*. John Wiley & Sons, Incorporated.

MacDuff, A. Arnold, A. Harvey, J. et al. (2010). Management of spontaneous pneumothorax: British Thoracic Society pleural disease guideline 2010. https://thorax.bmj.com/ content/thoraxjnl/65/Suppl_2/ii18.full.pdf (accessed June 2021).

McGill, F. Heyderman, R.S. Michael, B.D. et al. on behalf of The British Infection Association (2016). The UK joint specialist societies guideline on the diagnosis and management of acute meningitis and meningiococcal sepsis in immunocompetent adults. https://www.journalofinfection. com/action/showPdf?pii=S0163-4453%2816%2900024-4 (accessed June 2021).

McGrath, B.A. Bates, L. Atkinson, D. et al. (2012). Multidiscplinary guidelines for the management of tracheostomy and laryngectomy airway emergencies. doi: 10.1111/j.1365-2044.2012.07217.x (accessed June 2021).

National Poisons Information Service (2020). Healthcare Professionals. https://www.npis.org/Healthcare.html (accessed June 2021).

NICE: National Institute for Health and Care Excellence (2021). Hypoglycaemia. https://bnf.nice.org.uk/treatment-summary/ hypoglycaemia.html (accessed June 2021).

NICE: National Institute for Health and Care Excellence (2021). Epilepsies: diagnosis and management (Clinical Guideline 137). https://www.nice.org.uk/guidance/CG137 (accessed June 2021).

NICE: National Institute for Health and Care Excellence (2020a). Acute Coronary Syndromes. NICE guideline [NG185]. https://www.nice.org.uk/guidance/ng185 (accessed June 2021).

NICE: National Institute for Health and Care Excellence (2020b). Hyponatraemia. https://cks.nice.org.uk/topics/hyponatraemia/ (accessed June 2021).

NICE: National Institute for Health and Care Excellence (2019). Hypertension in adults: diagnosis and management. NICE guideline [NG136]. https://www.nice.org. uk/guidance/ng136/chapter/recommendations (accessed June 2021).

NICE: National Institute for Health and Care Excellence (2019a). Head Injury: assessment and early management (Clinical Guideline 176). https://www.nice.org.uk/guidance/cg176 (accessed June 2021).

NICE: National Institute for Health and Care Excellence (2019b). Stroke and transient ischaemic attack in over 16s: diagnosis and initial management (NICE Guideline 128). https://www. nice.org.uk/guidance/ng128 (accessed June 2021).

NICE: National Institute for Health and Care Excellence (2019c). Delirium: prevention, diagnosis and management (Clinical Guideline 103). https://www.nice.org.uk/Guidance/CG103 (accessed June 2021).

NICE: National Institute for Health and Care Excellence (2017). NICE guideline [NG71] Parkinson's disease in adults. https://www. nice.org.uk/guidance/ng71 (accessed June 2021).

NICE: National Institute for Health and Care Excellence (2016). Spinal injury: assessment and initial management (NICE guideline 41). https://www.nice.org.uk/guidance/ng41 (accessed June 2021).

RCUK: Resuscitation Council UK Guidelines (2020). Statements on COVID-19: In-hospital Settings. https://www.resus.org.uk/ covid-19-resources/statements-covid-19-hospital-settings (accessed June 2021).

RCUK: Resuscitation Council UK Guidelines (2021a). Adult advanced life support Guidelines. https://www.resus.org.uk/ library/2021-resuscitation-guidelines/adult-advanced-life-support-guidelines (accessed June 2021).

RCUK: Resuscitation Council UK Guidelines (2021b). Post-resuscitation care Guidelines. https://www.resus.org.uk/ library/2021-resuscitation-guidelines/post-resuscitation-care-guidelines (accessed June 2021).

RCUK: Resuscitation Council UK Guidelines (2021c). ReSPECT for healthcare professionals. https://www.resus.org.uk/respect/ respect-healthcare-professionals (accessed June 2021).

RCUK: Resuscitation Council UK Guidelines (2021d). Adult Basic Life Support Guidelines. https://www.resus.org.uk/library/2021-resuscitation-guidelines/adult-basic-life-support-guidelines (accessed June 2021).

Society for Endocrinology (2021). Adrenal Crisis Information. https://www.endocrinology.org/adrenal-crisis (accessed June 2021).

Scottish Intercollegiate Guidelines Network (2018). Diagnosis and management of epilepsy in adults. https://www.sign.ac.uk/ our-guidelines/diagnosis-and-management-of-epilepsy-in-adults (accessed June 2021).

Solomon, T. Michael, B.D. Smith, P.E. et al. on behalf of The Association of British Neurologists and British Infection Association National Guidelines (2012). Management of suspected viral encephalitis in adults. https://www.journalofinfection.com/article/S0163-4453%2811%2900563-9/fulltext (accessed June 2021).

The Renal Association (2020). Renal Association Clinical Practice Guidelines – Treatment of Acute Hyperkalaemia in Adults. https://renal.org/health-professionals/guidelines/guidelines-commentaries (accessed June 2021).

The Royal College of Anaesthetists and The Difficult Airway Society (2011). 4th National Audit Project of The Royal College of Anaesthetists and The Difficult Airway Society (2011). Major complications of airway management in the United Kingdom. https://www.nationalauditprojects.org.uk/downloads/NAP4%20Full%20Report.pdf (accessed June 2021).

WSACS: World Society of the Abdominal Compartment Syndrome (2021). WSACS Consensus Guidelines Summary. https://www.wsacs.org/education/436/wsacs-consensus-guidelines-summary/ (accessed June 2021).

Chapter 22

Gastrointestinal critical care

Anna Riley, Joe Box, and Aileen Aherne

Aim

This aim of this chapter is to equip the student with an understanding of the function and anatomy of the gastrointestinal system, common GI conditions and their relevant considerations, and an ability to recognise dysfunction in the context of patients cared for in a critical care setting.

Learning outcomes

After reading this chapter the reader will be able to:

- Draw on a knowledge base of GI anatomy and physiology to best inform their practice in a critical care setting.
- Identify both normal and abnormal GI function.
- Understand the appropriate investigations used to monitor and evaluate GI function.
- Have an awareness of common GI conditions that either require the patient to be cared for in a critical care area, or indeed develop as a result of the patient being admitted to a critical care area.
- Recognise common medications used in the critical care clinical area to support or improve GI function.

Test your prior knowledge

- Can you describe the key functions of the GI tract and discuss how and why these functions may be affected in a critical care environment?
- Are you able to recognise when a patient's GI function is deteriorating and describe what signs or symptoms the patient may display?
- Can you discuss the main modalities used to investigate and assess for intra-abdominal pathologies and critically evaluate the available evidence base surrounding their use?
- Can you identify two nursing interventions that can help in preserving normal GI function, and critically discuss their use with reference to the relevant evidence?

Fundamentals of Critical Care: A Textbook for Nursing and Healthcare Students, First Edition. Edited by Ian Peate and Barry Hill.
© 2023 John Wiley & Sons Ltd. Published 2023 by John Wiley & Sons Ltd.
Companion website: www.wiley.com/go/peate/criticalcare

Introduction

Digestion and the absorption of fluids and nutrients are the primary functions of the GI system, whereby food is absorbed and converted into energy. However, the GI system also performs an essential role in endocrine and immune function in addition to affecting fluid, electrolyte and acid-base balance. These functions are performed by the associated organs that collectively make up the GI system in addition to the GI tract through which food and then faeces pass.

Structurally, the GI tract comprises of a hollow muscular tube – starting at the mouth, it continues down the oesophagus and into the stomach, the small intestines, the large bowel and finally the rectum. All mammals have complimentary organs that support the GI tract; for example, organs such as the salivary glands, the liver, the pancreas and gallbladder that all secrete enzymes to aid the breakdown of food. Contents of the GI tract are moved along its length by its muscular walls in a motion called 'peristalsis'.

Food and fluids are ingested via the mouth, where they are chewed and moistened before digestion occurs in the stomach and small intestine. Here, enzymes help to break down carbohydrates, fats and proteins into smaller molecules, which can be absorbed across the epithelium to enter circulation. The large bowel absorbs surplus water before unabsorbed matter and metabolic waste products are formed into faeces and excreted.

During GI disorder or disease, these functions are disrupted. This can result in diarrhoea and vomiting, malabsorption or even loss of peristalsis (ileus). Common and benign symptoms of GI distress include heartburn, indigestion or nausea but can range up to more serious pathologies such as complete obstruction.

Step 2 Competencies: National Standards

2:4.1 Gastrointestinal Assessment and Management and Associated Pharmacology (Critical Care Networks, CC3N, 2015)

Demonstrate your knowledge using a rationale through discussion, and the application to practice:

Surgical procedures and common reasons for intervention:

- Hartmann's procedure
- Oesophagectomy
- Colectomy
- Toxic mega-colon
- Paralytic ileus – causes and effects

Acute GI conditions, signs, symptoms and common causes:

- Pancreatitis
- GI bleed
- Oesophageal varices
- Peptic/duodenal ulcers

Physiological changes associated with chronic and acute liver disease and how a patient may present in critical care depending on the cause:

- Acute liver and biliary impairment; signs, symptoms and common causes specifying how a patient may present to critical care depending on the cause
- Process of bacterial translocation

Drain management associated with abdominal disorders. Risk of sepsis associated with GI disorders. Indication for the following medications in relation to specific GI disorders:

- Prokinetics and motility
- Laxatives
- Anti-stimulants
- Anti-diarrhoea drugs
- Anti-secretory drugs

Anatomy and physiology
Anatomy and physiology of the GI system

The GI system performs several functions essential to life; primarily energy intake, acting as a physical barrier, immunological defence and endocrine function. The anatomy of the gastrointestinal system can be seen in Figure 22.1.

Ingestion, digestion and then absorption of the resulting nutrients is the GI system's primary function. In the critically ill, however, ingestion is commonly bypassed with insertion of nasogastric tubes, for example. To facilitate the absorption of nutrients across the lumen of the intestines, foods require digestion.

Following manual breakdown of food in the oral cavity, secretions in the stomach and small intestines, plus pancreatic enzymes and bile salts (produced in the liver and stored in the gallbladder) play an important role in the breakdown of food into its constituent parts.

The lining of the GI tract, known as the mucosa, acts as a physical barrier to pathogens entering the body, while a series of sphincter muscles prevent back-flow of oral intake or gastric and intestinal contents. The gastrointestinal tract lining can be seen in Figure 22.2.

There are many peptides (amino acid chains) released along the GI tract that have a chemical messenger action and regulate motility, secretions, absorption and immune response. Cholecystokinin (CCK) is of particular importance. CCK is secreted in response to the presence of nutrients in the small intestine and is a stimulant of gallbladder emptying, slowing gastric emptying and suppressing appetite. Insulin, secreted by the pancreas, is another important hormone implicit in regulating gastrointestinal function, responsible for lowering blood glucose levels and stimulating the storage of carbohydrates.

314

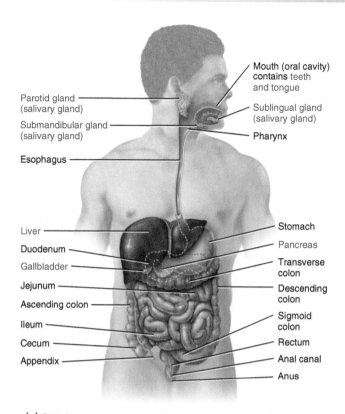

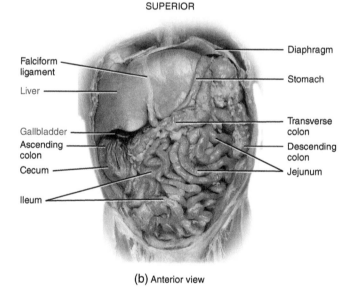

Figure 22.1 The anatomy of the gastrointestinal system. *Source:* Tortora and Derrickson (2009) with permission of John Wiley and Sons.

Normal GI function requires harmonious working of multiple complex systems controlled by the autonomic nervous system. These include vascular perfusion, muscle motility, synchronous action of the oro-pharynx, oesophagus, stomach, small intestine and large intestine in addition to salivary, gastric, pancreatic and intestinal secretions. This complex interplay is precisely controlled by neural and myogenic mechanisms. Gut motility changes dependent on whether the patient is recently fed or fasting and is profoundly disturbed during critical illness with delayed gastric emptying, reflux and aspiration being of particular concern in the acutely unwell, bed-bound patient.

The coeliac artery supplies blood to the stomach and pancreas while the small and large intestine has a complex system of mesenteric arteries. The portal vein provides return blood flow from the stomach, pancreas and intestines. In homeostasis, GI blood supply is increased several-fold after nutrient intake, although this is thought to be vastly reduced in the critically ill (Reintam et al., 2020).

The neural regulation of the GI system is via the vagus nerve which provides parasympathetic motor supply to the GI system whilst the enteric nerves convey information both to and from the central nervous system.

Anatomy and physiology of the hepatic system

Located in the right upper quadrant of the abdominal cavity, the liver is the largest internal organ and delivers a myriad of functions including metabolism and detoxification. Classified as a right and left lobe, the liver is further subdivided into eight smaller lobes based on their vascular supply. The portal vein supplies 75% of the blood received by the liver, carrying deoxygenated blood that has passed the gallbladder and pancreas with the remainder made up via the hepatic artery. Each lobe of the liver has an independent vascular supply via a branch of the portal vein and hepatic artery, as well as separate biliary drainage. The liver receives around 25% of cardiac output and is the only organ that has the capacity to regenerate lost tissue from its remaining tissue, therefore being able to regenerate after surgical intervention or chemical injury. The anatomy of the hepatic system can be seen in Figure 22.3.

The liver is the body's largest store of numerous substances such as vitamins, minerals and carbohydrates. It acts as the source of blood coagulation factors and changes in its functional ability can often be assessed early in deranged clotting factors via a simple blood test.

Detoxification is the primary function of the liver, being able to process and dispose of metabolites and toxic compounds. It is the principal site of drug metabolism and excretion, and as a result it also plays a role in adverse drug reactions. Therefore, when considering the dose of prescribed medications, liver function should be assessed simultaneously. Liver function may be affected by factors such as age, gender and previous hepatic disease. These factors can all affect the metabolism of drugs with variable therapeutic significance (Kortgen et al., 2010).

Bile is produced in the liver at the rate of around 500 ml per day, then stored in the gallbladder to be used in digestive and excretory functions. Evidence of cholestasis (reduced bile flow) is a common finding in critical illness and can result from changes in normal biliary action due to sepsis, medications and biliary obstruction (Jenniskens et al., 2018). Hepatic function can therefore be quickly altered in response to systemic inflammation and critical illness.

315

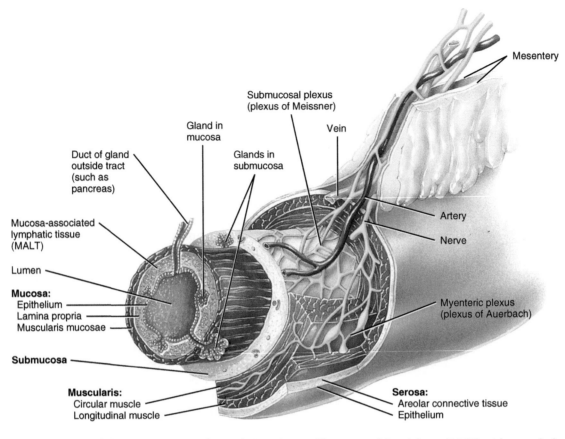

Figure 22.2   The layers of the gastrointestinal tract lining. *Source:* Tortora and Derrickson (2009) with permission of John Wiley & Sons.

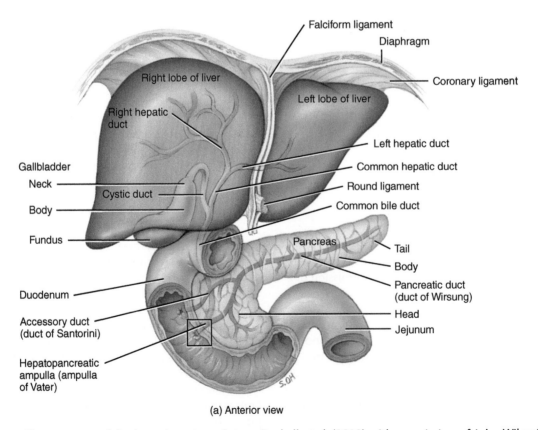

(a) Anterior view

Figure 22.3   The anatomy of the hepatic system. *Source:* Rockall et al. (2013) with permission of John Wiley & Sons.

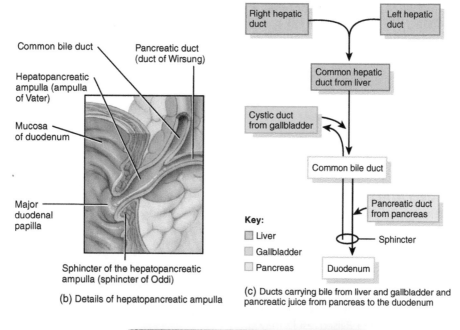

(b) Details of hepatopancreatic ampulla

Right hepatic duct

Left hepatic duct

Common hepatic duct from liver

Cystic duct from gallbladder

Common bile duct

Pancreatic duct from pancreas

Key:
- Liver
- Gallbladder
- Pancreas

Sphincter

Duodenum

(c) Ducts carrying bile from liver and gallbladder and pancreatic juice from pancreas to the duodenum

Common bile duct

Pancreatic duct (duct of Wirsung)

Hepatopancreatic ampulla (ampulla of Vater)

Mucosa of duodenum

Major duodenal papilla

Sphincter of the hepatopancreatic ampulla (sphincter of Oddi)

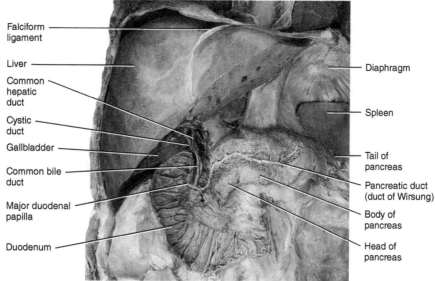

Falciform ligament

Liver

Common hepatic duct

Cystic duct

Gallbladder

Common bile duct

Major duodenal papilla

Duodenum

Diaphragm

Spleen

Tail of pancreas

Pancreatic duct (duct of Wirsung)

Body of pancreas

Head of pancreas

(d) Anterior view

Figure 22.3 (Continued)

GI monitoring and investigation in the critically ill

- GI and hepatic dysfunction is a common problem in the critically ill.
- Some degree of hepatic dysfunction is noted in over 50% of critical care patients (Webb et al., 2016).

Blood tests

The complex and varied roles of the liver mean no single test can determine hepatic function. This is further complicated by sepsis, ischaemia,or a hepatic stress response cause by tissue damage in surgery or trauma (Horvatits et al., 2019). Conventional laboratory tests of, for example, enzyme levels in venous blood can be useful tools for the monitoring of hepatic function and diagnosis of disease. Cholestasis as a result of sepsis is the leading cause of jaundice in hospital inpatients and the critically ill. Deranged liver function and damage to hepatic tissue is largely reversible. However, damage to the biliary drainage system is not and may result in lifelong effects – hence the importance of routine monitoring of hepatic function and early intervention. Altered or reduced hepatic function is under investigated in critical care patients (Kramer et al., 2007) and it has been suggested that over 50% of

317

patients in critical care experience a degree of hepatic dysfunction (Barrett, 2006).

Clinical investigations: hepatic function blood tests

Liver Function Test (LFT): A routine blood test that is sent for biochemical analysis. It has several components and serial repeated LFTs can be very useful tool for monitoring hepatic function in the critically ill patient for whom hepatic disease/dysfunction will be a dynamic process.

Alanine aminotransferase (ALT): Raised results indicate hepatocellular damage. A very sensitive test. It is, however, not specific to any one cause of liver damage. Mild elevation is a common finding in routine blood testing, often due to prolonged alcohol consumption even in moderate amounts.

Alkaline phosphatase (ALP): An enzyme used to break down proteins, produced predominantly in the liver but also in the bones, kidneys and placenta. Raised results may indicate liver or gallbladder disease such as hepatitis, cirrhosis or blocked bile duct due to gallstone or cancer.

Bilirubin: Bilirubin is produced from the breakdown of red cells and a raised level indicates jaundice (often before it is visible in your patient's skin or sclera) (Kumar and Clark, 2011). It is often elevated in the instance of biliary obstruction; again, due to a stone or malignancy.

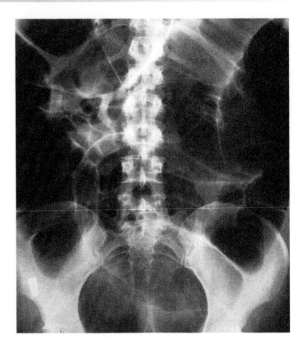

Figure 22.4 Paralytic ileus, showing both large and small bowel dilatation. *Source:* Rockall et al. (2013) with permission of John Wiley & Sons.

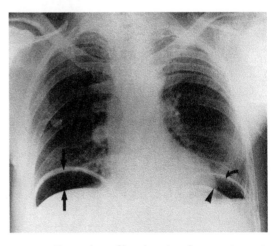

Figure 22.5 Erect chest film showing free gas in peritoneal cavity *Source:* Rockall et al. (2013) with permission of John Wiley & Sons.

Imaging and endoscopy

X-ray and ultrasound (USS) are first-line, easily accessible and cost-effective imaging modalities in the bedside assessment of stable patients with suspected GI pathology; however, a CT (Computerised Tomography) scan is the gold standard for investigating symptoms in an unstable, clinically unwell patient.

Diagnosing abdominal pathology is challenging due to conflicting differential diagnoses and often poorly defined symptoms. This is further complicated by multi-organ involvement, comorbidities and a ventilated, sedated patient. Often resuscitation, mechanical ventilation and haemofiltration are needed before detailed investigations can be undertaken and formal diagnosis can be made. These challenges reinforce the importance of imaging in the correct care planning of critically ill patients.

X-ray

A plain abdominal film or erect chest film are often the initial imaging investigations ordered in diagnosing abdominal pathology. They are of particular use when assessing for evidence of dilated bowel in intestinal obstruction (Figure 22.4) and subdiaphragmatic free air in the detection of stomach or bowel perforation (Figure 22.5). An X-ray is a relatively cheap, readily available and low-risk investigation; however, they do not provide a detailed picture of abdominal

pathology and due to its increased sensitivity, most patients will go on to be assessed via CT.

Ultrasound (USS)

An ultrasound is of particular use in the assessment of a critically unwell patient as it is portable and safe. In fact, a Focused Assessment with Sonography for Trauma (FAST) scan is becoming an increasingly common routine investigation for the detection of free fluid in the abdomen and is often performed by Critical Care and Emergency Department clinicians to rule out abdominal aortic aneurysm rupture (Figure 22.6). USS is also of particular use in examining the biliary system for signs of occluded hepatic veins,

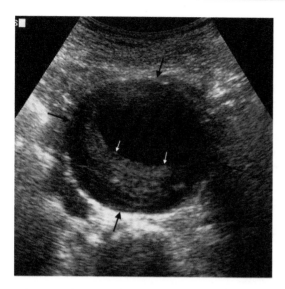

Figure 22.6 Ultrasound appearances of an abdominal aortic aneurysm. The blood clot lines the wall (white arrows) within the aneurysm (black arrows). *Source:* Rockall et al. (2013) with permission of John Wiley & Sons.

cirrhosis, biliary tract obstruction and biliary sepsis. It is, however, limited by factors including operator proficiency (Ziesmann et al., 2015) and patient body habitus (Rajapakse and Chang, 2014).

Snapshot

Francesca is a 47-year-old female and is brought to the Emergency Department by the local ambulance service. She was found collapsed at home by her daughter and is reporting severe, colicky upper abdominal pain. She is vomiting bilious content.

Her observations are documented as follows:

Airway: Airway is patent, able to speak.

Breathing: Oxygen saturations 97% (NEWS2 = 0), on 2 litres via nasal cannula (NEWS2 = 2), RR 28 breaths per minute (NEWS2 = 3).

Circulation: Blood pressure (BP) is 86/57 (NEWS2 = 3), heart rate (HR) 126 beats per minute (NEWS2 = 2), capillary refill time 3 seconds, cool to touch.

Disability: Alert (NEWS2 = 0) on the AVPU scale (see Chapter 14), body temperature (T) is 38.6 degrees C (NEWS2 = 1).

Exposure: Yellow sclera and skin. Reporting widespread itching.

Total NEWS2 score: 11

A bedside FAST scan is performed as per local sepsis escalation policy. The scan reveals biliary duct dilatation and a possible stone in the common duct.

Outcome: Francesca is treated for biliary obstruction and sepsis and is admitted to Critical Care, under joint care with the surgical team who refer her for specialist intervention to clear the obstruction.

Computer tomography (CT)

CT remains the imaging of choice for a comprehensive assessment of abdominal pathology. CT can be performed with or without iodinated contrast to enhance the resulting images and the decision on whether to use contrast is dependent on the patient's renal function and allergy status. Bowel pathology such as appendicitis, diverticulitis and inflammatory bowel conditions, as well as pancreatitis, necrosis and fluid collections, are identified with a high sensitivity on CT imaging (Figure 22.7). CT, however, administers a substantial dose of radiation and should be used with caution and not repeatedly performed.

> # 6Cs: Compassion
>
> Compassion is demonstrated through developing therapeutic and professional relationships with patients that are based on respect, understanding and dignity.

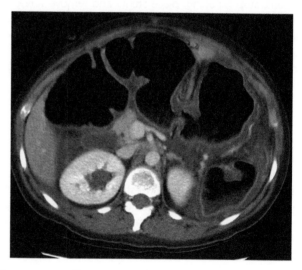

Figure 22.7 Toxic megacolon demonstrated on CT abdomen. *Source:* Rockall et al. (2013) with permission of John Wiley & Sons.

Endoscopy

Oesophago-Gastro-Duodenoscopy (OGD) and colonoscopy are endoscopic procedures frequently performed on critically ill patients either in critical care, theatre or in the endoscopy department. They have both a diagnostic and a therapeutic role, allowing direct visual examination and biopsy in addition to administration of treatments such as injections and ligation of varices. Caution must be used when both deciding to perform and during an endoscopic procedure, and the potential benefits must be weighed against risk. The critically ill patient may present with many signs which could indicate the need for an endoscopy that could be caused by other complex pathologies such as sepsis, acute kidney injury and bleeding of unknown origin. Incidental findings of GI tract mucosal lesions that do not

319

require endoscopic or pharmacological treatment such as gastritis or nasogastric tube associated ulcers are also common (Jean-Baptiste et al., 2018).

Clinical Investigations: Endoscopy

As an invasive procedure all endoscopic procedures requires comparable nursing considerations, preparation and post-procedure monitoring to those performed for a minor surgical intervention.

It is essential for the critical care nurse to have a good understanding of these procedures with their similarities and differences to achieve the best patient outcomes. Not only is endoscopy used for the detection and monitoring of GI tract disease, but increasingly endoscopic treatments are also routinely performed.

During the procedure it is possible to take tissue for biopsies, remove potential pre-cancerous or cancerous lesions, stop bleeding, place stents and remove foreign bodies. Individual procedures have various levels of sedation and varying levels of risk for post-procedure complications which include aspiration, perforation, and bleeding. These factors all affect both pre-procedure nursing care and post-procedure monitoring (Scholten, 2010).

320

Orange Flag

For a patient, the critical care environment alone can be terrifying, but when invasive investigations and procedures are required, this can further add to their fear. Patients may or may not be able to communicate these fears to you, as their nurse, but offering them reassurance and ensuring that all interventions are in their best interest is vital.

Bowel charts and abnormal GI motility

Bowel care is a fundamental area of patient care in any clinical setting that is frequently overlooked, yet it is of paramount importance. The aim of accurately recording bowel function is to promote and maintain normal bowel function, which allows early recognition and treatment of bowel dysfunction (Vincent and Preiser, 2015). The importance of accurate bowel charting and an appropriate response to changes in bowels cannot therefore be underestimated in the critical care setting and should form part of the daily nursing observational routine.

Constipation

Constipation is defined as the difficult passage of stool due to impaired peristalsis and or paralysis of the lower GI tract

(Sharma and Rao, 2016). Constipation is a common problem in the critical care patient population, which, in extreme cases can affect length of stay and mortality rates (Mostafa et al., 2003) and if left untreated, can result in abdominal pain and distension, nausea and vomiting, failure to tolerate enteral feeding and bowel obstruction or perforation. Laxatives can be administered to treat constipation effectively, although in the mechanically ventilated patient, early introduction of enteral feeding is known to improve bowel function (Nassa et al., 2009).

Causes of constipation in critical care

- Immobility
- Opiates
- Dehydration
- Vasoconstrictors (e.g. noradrenaline)
- Hypoperfusion of the gastrointestinal tract

Red Flag

Approximately one in five patients are diagnosed with bowel cancer after presenting as an emergency (Mayor, 2016).

Early symptoms of rectal bleeding, change in bowel habit, abdominal pain and iron-deficiency anaemia are concerning for colon or rectal malignancy and require specialist input. When presenting as an emergency, patients may present with symptoms of partial or complete bowel obstruction, or GI haemorrhage.

Diarrhoea

Diarrhoea is also common in critically ill patients. It is defined as greater than 300ml or 3 liquid bowel motions in a 24-hour period (Urden et al., 2013) and can be characterised as either acute or chronic according to its onset and duration. Causes are listed in Table 22.1. Untreated diarrhoea can lead to dehydration with resulting electrolyte

Table 22.1   Causes of diarrhoea. Source: adapted from Baid et al., 2016.

Non-infective	Infective
Enteral feeding	Clostridium difficile
Medications, including antibiotic therapy	E. Coli
Inflammatory bowel conditions and disease	Salmonella/campylobacter
Malabsorption	Tropical diseases
Overflow in faecal impaction	

imbalance, skin damage and of course loss of privacy and dignity. Caution should be taken prior to commencing treatment. Loperamide, for example, a medication which can help regulate peristalsis, slowing the passage of digestive matter and affording the bowel more time to absorb key nutrients and fluid, also comes with common adverse effects such as abdominal distension and constipation. Historically, many clinicians avoided the use of loperamide due to these potential adverse effects, although more recent studies and indeed current NICE guidance advocate its use (NICE, 2013).

Faecal management systems

Faecal management systems (FMS) are rectal catheters, held in place with a balloon seal and attached to a drainage bag. They are commonly used in the critical care environment for the temporary containment of liquid faeces in bed ridden, incontinent adults. It is important that you understand when they are indicated, and indeed when they are contraindicated. They should only ever be used once a discussion has been held with the multidisciplinary team and a holistic assessment has been completed.

6Cs: Care

Care is at the heart of every nursing intervention and drives our professional practice.

For indications and contraindications, please see Figure 22.8.

Red Flag

Scott is a 56-year-old admitted to hospital with severe abdominal pain. A CT scan performed whilst he was in the Emergency Department reported free gas in the abdomen, likely secondary to a perforated duodenal ulcer. Scott was taken to theatre for an emergency laparotomy and repair of the perforation in his duodenum and comes to intensive care post-operatively.

His operation was now 4 days ago, and he has not yet opened his bowels. Bowel sounds have been documented as present since yesterday however, and the surgical team have agreed to start enteral feeding. His abdomen feels firm and slightly distended.

Nursing actions:
- Daily assessment and documentation of bowel function.
- A full set of baseline blood tests inclusive of renal, hepatic and bone profiles.
- Assess fluid balance and correct any imbalance.
- Consider switching enteral feed to one that contains fibre, only after discussion with critical care medical team and dieticians.
- Perform digital rectal examination to check for presence of stool in the rectum.
- Review current medications for any that may be contribute to constipation as a side effect.
- Look to local policy and guidance and consider seeking prescription of laxatives.

Indications:
Four or more episodes of watery diarrhoea in a 24-hour-period, in order to:
- Help protect the skin from breaking down
- Protect surgical wounds, burns and other wounds
- Prevent the spread of infection
- Improve patient comfort and dignity
- **Contraindications:**
- If a patient deemed as having capacity refuses the intervention
- If a patient has either faecal loading or impaction (with the watery stool representing 'overflow diarrhoea'
- Patient has inflammatory bowel condition; rectal or anal injury; severe haemorrhoids; recent low rectal or anal surgery (necessitating a conversation with the surgical team as a priority); suspected or confirmed rectal or anal malignancy; anal stricture; proctitis; perianal Crohn's disease; established spinal cord lesion; sensitivity or allergy to any of the materials used in the product.

Removal of the device should be considered when:
- Stool becomes semi-formed or formed
- Your patient spends prolonged periods of time sitting out of bed in a chair.
- The existing device has been in for 29 days. If still indicated, the device should then be changed.

Figure 22.8   Indications and contraindications for use of faecal management systems.

Conclusion:

- Scott's fluid balance was reviewed, and it was noted that he was in a three-litre deficit. Intravenous fluids were prescribed, and the deficit corrected.
- Hard stool was present in the rectum. A phosphate enema was prescribed and administered with good effect.
- The medical team reviewed his medication and discontinued codeine phosphate.
- Stimulant laxatives were prescribed on a regular, daily basis to prevent further constipation.
- The dietetics team reviewed his enteral feed prescription and added fibre.

6Cs: Competence

Being aware of your own scope of practice, level of competence and seeking support when needed is paramount in safe nursing practice and optimal patient care.

Examination scenario: abdominal examination

As part of core critical care nursing duties, an abdominal examination with comprehensive documentation of findings should be undertaken at the start of each shift and then again in the afternoon (Urden et al., 2013). This is dependent on local area policy and individual clinical competence in clinical examination.

	Normal	Abnormal
Inspection	Pink, moist mucous membranes White sclera Non-distended, symmetrical abdomen	Pallor Jaundice Dry mucous membranes Abdominal asymmetry Wounds Drains Bruising Scars
Palpation	Soft, non-tender abdomen	Painful, firm Mass Faeces
Percussion	Tympanic abdominal percussion note	Dullness on percussion
Auscultation	Bowel sounds present	Bowel sounds absent, hypoactive, high-pitched or tinkling

Source: Baid et al. (2016)

The acute abdomen in critical care

The clinical presentation of an acute abdomen encompasses a broad spectrum of disease. These patients can be very unwell, or rapidly deteriorate and often require early input from the critical care team. The abdominal cavity itself hosts vast potential for catastrophe, predominantly through haemorrhage, sepsis or ischaemia (Buczacki and Davies, 2018). The prompt assessment of patients reporting or illustrating signs an acute onset of abdominal symptoms is crucial in establishing an early diagnosis, facilitated by a systematic approach to history, clinical examination findings, imaging and laboratory results. This need for early detection of abnormal abdominal pathology is further added to by the associated increase in mortality and prevalence of multi-organ failure faced by patients requiring critical care admission. The intra-abdominal conditions described below are the most common gastrointestinal pathologies encountered in the critical care environment.

Perforation

A hole in the GI tract at any point (oesophagus, stomach, small or large intestines) is a medical emergency, with patient quickly experiencing pain and sepsis due to the contamination of the peritoneal cavity with gastric content (peritonitis). Common causes include inflammation, trauma, cancers, ulcers and medical or surgical procedures, and additionally mechanical ventilation is strongly associated with gastrointestinal stress ulceration (Granholm et al., 2019), posing additional risk of perforation and haemorrhage. CT imaging is often required, followed by surgical repair.

Patients with a gastrointestinal perforation may experience severe abdominal pain, distension, vomiting and signs of sepsis. In the mechanically ventilated and sedated patient, however, signs may be subtle at first and reflected primarily in clinical observations (e.g., tachycardia, pyrexia) and raised inflammatory biochemistry markers). Small diverticulae perforations may occasionally be treated conservatively but most bowel perforations are repaired surgically.

The most common cause of oesophageal perforation is endoscopic dilation of strictures, although it can occur following persistent vomiting, trauma or in the presence of a foreign body. Patients may present following collapse and in shock. The treatment options are limited and will almost always require surgical intervention.

Nursing considerations

- Assess vital observations and blood results and monitor trends for signs of sepsis.
- Monitor drain output if drains present (e.g., post-surgery).
- Patients should be nil by mouth and considered for nasogastric tube insertion.
- Provide adequate IV fluid and analgesia.
- Broad-spectrum antibiotics.
- Stress ulcer prophylaxis as per local policy.
- Elevating head of bed at 30-degree position.

Gastrointestinal haemorrhage

Gastrointestinal (GI) bleeding is common among critical care patients and can originate from either the upper or lower portion of the GI tract, delineated by the ligament of Treitz (Figure 22.9).

Upper GI bleeding most frequently stems from existing peptic or duodenal ulcers, iatrogenic stress ulceration, or oesophageal varices in advanced liver disease (Booker, 2015). Diverticular disease or vascular abnormalities, including ischaemic bowel, are often responsible for lower gastrointestinal bleeding. Additionally, patients on intensive care units are at increased risk of GI haemorrhage with invasive mechanical ventilation, hepatic or renal dysfunction and coagulopathies (Krag et al., 2018).

Haematemesis is the vomiting of blood caused by a bleeding point higher than the duodenum. Maleana is the passing of black, tar like stools as a result of blood passing through the intestines, suggestive of an upper GI bleed. More subtle symptoms can include dizziness, abdominal pain and signs of hypovolemic shock, notably hypotension and tachycardia.

Treatment is dictated by the patient's clinical condition. In haemodynamically unstable patients, invasive circulatory volume monitoring is indicated and volume repletion paramount, achievable with colloid or crystalloid intravenous fluids or alternatively transfusion of blood products. Endoscopy, CT and interventional radiological procedures have a role in treating the source of bleeding, as an alternative to invasive surgery which is sometimes unavoidable.

Red Flag

Chronic gastrointestinal bleeding can be indicative of underlying established peptic ulcer disease. If patients report symptoms of maleana, previous known peptic ulcer, severe or persistent dyspepsia or gastritis, and have a history of long-term non-steroidal anti-inflammatory (NSAID) use (even aspirin), you should alert the medical team and ensure that a proton pump inhibitor (PPI) is prescribed.

Ischaemic colitis

Ischaemic colitis refers to inflammation of the large bowel resulting from reduced blood flow, due to occluded branches of the mesenteric arteries that supply the large bowel or extreme hypotension and subsequent hypoperfusion in acutely unwell patients. Predominantly seen in older patients, who present with sudden onset abdominal pain and fresh rectal bleeding without stool, it is difficult to diagnose due to the overlapping symptoms of several pathologies which often leads to delays in treatment. Mild to moderate cases require no intervention but supportive intravenous fluids and antibiotics, however severe cases may require surgical intervention in the form of bowel resection, or interventional radiology input.

6Cs: Courage

To act as a true advocate for patients under our care and ensuring that we speak up on their behalf, especially when you have any concerns, takes courage.

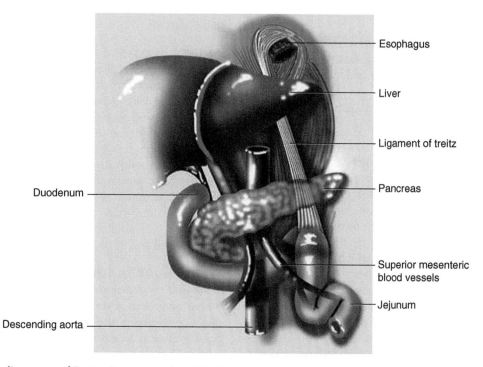

Figure 22.9   The ligament of Treitz. *Source:* Booker (2015) with permission of John Wiley & Sons.

Acute pancreatitis

Acute inflammation of the pancreas is predominantly caused by gallstones, alcohol or cancer, although other, less common causes include medications, viral and autoimmune conditions. Pancreatitis can range from mild, self-limiting episodes to prolonged, severe, acute, life-threatening episodes resulting in extensive pancreatic necrosis. It is this cohort of patients that you will care for in the critical care environment. Patients with pancreatic necrosis are at risk of necrotic bacterial colonisation and once infected, antibiotic therapy is indicated (Siriwardena et al., 2019). There is little evidence to support prophylactic antibiotic use in acute pancreatitis and studies have found it to be potentially detrimental (IAP/APA, 2013). There is increasing evidence in support of serum procalcitonin level monitoring to predict both the risk of severe acute pancreatitis and infected pancreatic necrosis (Siriwardena et al., 2019).

Serum amylase or lipase levels can also aid in determining disease severity with ultrasound and CT imaging playing an essential role in identifying the potential cause and percentage of pancreatic tissue death. Treatment modalities are dependent on the cause, e.g., cholecystectomy during admission to remove the gallbladder and stones within instances of gallstone pancreatitis. Early resuscitation with targeted intravenous fluid therapy and close monitoring greatly alters patient outcomes (IAP/APA, 2013). Complications can include necrotising pancreatitis and multi-organ failure, with life-long effects that are both physical and psychosocial. Pancreatitis is exquisitely painful, and patients often require opioid analgesia with regular pain score assessment to evaluate efficacy. Local policy and validated assessment tools will guide you in assessing pain scores in the sedated patient where there may be difficulties in communication.

> # 6Cs: Communication
> Utilisation of non-verbal and visual assessment and communication tools ensures equality and inclusiveness of patient care.

Bowel obstruction

The passage of food content, fluid and gas through the GI tract can become partially or totally obstructed due to a physical blockage – 'mechanical' obstruction – or temporary cessation of normal peristalsis and bowel function, known as 'functional' obstruction. Mechanical obstructions are most commonly caused by adhesions or by fibrous tissue that forms post abdominal or pelvic surgery (Ten Broek et al., 2018) but can also be caused by tumours, hernias, stricture or tortuosity of the bowel (volvulus or intussception). Conversely, in functional bowel obstruction there are symptoms of obstruction in the absence of a physical structure as a cause and is most frequently referred to as 'paralytic ileus' or 'pseudo-obstruction'. Ileus is common following abdominal or pelvic surgery due to intraoperative handling of the gut. Patients

may present with abdominal pain, distension, vomiting and with large bowel obstruction particularly, absolute constipation or inability to pass flatus. Patients may, however, continue to pass stool and flatus, and this does not exclude obstruction (Ten Broek et al., 2018). Bowel sounds may be high-pitched and 'tinkling' on auscultation. Patients require gastric decompression with a large-bore 'Ryles' nasogastric tube, symptom control with analgesia and anti-emetics, close monitoring of urinary output and a surgical review, with subsequent CT imaging likely to ascertain the aetiology. Endoscopic or surgical intervention may be indicated.

Peritonitis

Acute inflammation of the peritoneum is known as peritonitis and is the second most prevalent cause of sepsis in intensive care units internationally (Ross et al., 2018). Peritonitis can develop as a result of gastrointestinal perforation, where GI content contaminates the peritoneum or secondary to other medical interventions such as peritoneal dialysis. GI perforation causing peritonitis requires supportive resuscitative management initially, followed by emergency surgical repair.

Bacterial translocation – 'leaky gut'

An intact and healthy luminal wall acts as a barrier between gastrointestinal content and the peritoneal cavity, but its strength can be weakened by acute inflammatory conditions, medications or toxin exposure (Nagpal and Yadav, 2017). The luminal tissues become more permeable allowing for the transmission of microbes into the circulation, eliciting an acute inflammatory response. Promoting optimum gut health and considering the use of probiotics should be considered (Nagpal and Yadav, 2017), with input from critical care dieticians.

Biliary sepsis

Obstruction of the biliary system can cause disturbance to normal function or structure of the biliary system and increases the risk of biliary sepsis (Liu et al., 2020). Additionally, medical and surgical procedures that instrumentalise the biliary system such as endoscopic retrograde cholangiopancreatography (ERCP) further promote the opportunity for microbes to migrate into the systemic circulation. Management ranges from conservative treatment with sepsis resuscitative measures, to percutaneous drainage, endoscopic intervention and surgery. In addition to symptoms of systemic inflammatory response and sepsis, patients may be jaundiced and in pain.

Acute liver failure

Acute and new-onset hepatic dysfunction with associated altered conscious state, confusion and coagulopathy is a clinical emergency and patients often require critical care input, ideally in a centre that has a liver transplant service or close links with one nearby. Patients can present in shock, with acutely deranged hepatic function blood tests, jaundice, decreased conscious level and confusion due to hepatic encephalopathy and abnormal serum coagulation profiles (INR > 1.5) (Cardoso, 2017). Acute liver failure can develop rapidly as a result of drug toxicity (commonly acetaminophen and non-acetaminophen and as a result of recreational drug use), and viral infections such as hepatitis, cytomegalovirus, Eppstein-Barr, with the subsequent liver injury affecting the liver's ability to regulate primary and secondary haemostasis, excrete waste product and metabolise drugs. A plethora of investigations in the form of serum laboratory tests and imaging will be performed to illicit both the cause and severity of the acute liver failure and during this, patients may require multi-organ support.

Hepatic encephalopathy ensues as a result of excess ammonia, causing confusion and reduced conscious level. All potential causes of confusion should be investigated prior to commencing treatment for acute liver failure associated encephalopathy, specifically sepsis screen and CT head to exclude intracranial pathology (Wendon et al., 2017). Lactulose is often administered regularly to aid ammonia excretion but should be done so with consideration of potential abdominal side effects (Williams and Wendon, 2013).

Learning event: reflection

Reflect on what you have learned about the common intra-abdominal conditions that usually require critical care input. What do you understand about the acute abdomen and how will your new knowledge enhance the care that you give to your patients?

Snapshot

Sariya is a 59-year-old female admitted to hospital with abdominal pain and jaundice. She is known to have gallstones and was waiting to have elective surgery, in the form of laparoscopic cholecystectomy (keyhole surgery to remove the gallbladder).

Bloods taken in the Emergency Department report deranged hepatic function, with ALP 489, ALT 256, and a bilirubin of 67. An ultrasound confirms the presence of multiple stones in the common duct and an ERCP with sphincterotomy is scheduled.

Following the ERCP, Sariya becomes unwell and reports worsening upper abdominal pain. Her liver function is now normalising but her serum lipase level is now 3573.

Sariya develops severe acute pancreatitis post ERCP, which is confirmed on a CT scan and is admitted to the High Dependency Unit for both resuscitation and monitoring. The following nursing interventions need to be completed:

- Complete regular pain assessments and administer analgesia accordingly.
- Targeted intravenous fluid therapy.

- A nutritional assessment and early nutritional support. Consider NG tube placement and the commencement of enteral feed. Patients do not need to be kept nil by mouth.
- Site a urinary catheter and closely monitor fluid input and output.
- Monitor vital signs and inflammatory markers closely. New pyrexia and raised inflammatory markers may indicate pancreatic necrosis that is becoming infected.
- Provide explanation and reassurance to Sariya and her relatives regarding nursing and medical procedures.
- Report and document findings.

Common surgical procedures cared for in critical care

- **Colectomy** is a surgical procedure to remove all or part of the large bowel.
- **Total colectomy** involves removing the entire colon.
- **Partial colectomy** involves removing part of the colon and may also be called subtotal colectomy.
- **Hemicolectomy** involves removing the right or left portion of the colon.
- **Proctocolectomy** involves removing both the colon and rectum
- **Hartmann's procedure** (proctosigmoidectomy) is resection of the colon whereby an end colostomy is formed and the remaining downstream section of bowel is closed.
- **Oesophagectomy** involves removal of some or all of the oesophagus with reconstruction usually using the stomach.

Orange Flag

Patients undergoing abdominal surgery may require a stoma to be formed. Many patients with a newly formed stoma struggle with their new perceived body image, self-confidence and maintaining their dignity. Referring patients for early specialist nurse input and acknowledging this life-changing event and how it may affect them psychologically, will greatly aid in facilitating truly holistic care.

Post-operative monitoring

To provide comprehensive, holistic and safe post-operative care, good monitoring, assessment and observation skills are needed. Early warning systems are widely used in a variety of acute settings to assist in the early identification of deteriorating patients – in the post-operative and critical care setting there are numerous other observations that should be checked and recorded some specific to the surgical intervention. These include pain assessment, capillary refill time, central venous pressure, infusion rates, drain out puts and hourly urine output. Vital signs should be taken in line with local area policy or as dictated by the surgical or critical care team but should not be taken in isolation, and the nurse should perform a thorough visual check for signs such as blood-soaked dressings or new-onset abdominal distension (Liddle, 2013). NCEPOD (2011) found in 30% of patient data reviewed, there was insufficient recording of post-operative fluid balance.

Examination Scenario

Intra-abdominal pressure (IAP) monitoring is indicated in patients that are at risk of abdominal compartment syndrome, or who develop new abdominal distension. Causes of abdominal compartment syndrome include but are not limited to; increased abdominal content (through haemorrhage, ascites, inflammation or mass); capillary leakage following fluid resuscitation (through sepsis, burns, trauma, SIRS response); increased intra-luminal content (bowel obstruction, ileus); and decreased compliance of the abdominal wall (following abdominal surgery, due to prone positioning, high PEEP) (Baid et al., 2016).

IAP readings are acquired from the bladder and can be monitored by connecting a Foley manometer to a Foley indwelling urinary catheter, which is then attached to a transducer (see Figure 22.10):

IAP value

5–7 mmHg: Normal
  < 12 mmHg: Not significant (COPD, ascites, obesity)
  Constant > 12 mmHg: Intra-abdominal hypertension, increased risk of abdominal compartment syndrome
  Constant > 20 mmHg w/ new organ dysfunction: Abdominal compartment syndrome
  (adapted from Baid et al., 2016)
  Treatment of abdominal compartment syndrome varies according to the cause but include; drainage of abdominal contents (e.g. nasogastric tube on free drainage) or ascites; surgical decompression; strategies to improve abdominal wall compliance (adjusting ventilator settings, patient positioning); and renal replacement therapy to remove excess fluid overload (Baid et al., 2016).

Abdominal surgical drains

Surgical drains are tubes placed near surgical incisions during surgery to allow the drainage of fluids such as blood, pus or surgical irrigation. There are many types of drains in use that are used dependant on the procedure, the fluid it will

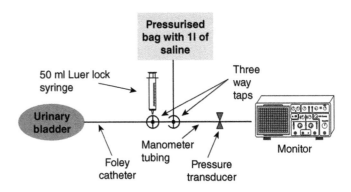

Figure 22.10   An intra-abdominal pressure monitoring transducer set. *Source:* Hunter and Damani, 2004 with permission of John Wiley & Sons.

drain and surgeon preference. Drains should be proactively and thoroughly monitored while in situ. Observing for signs of leakage, infection or skin irritation at the site of insertion should be performed routinely. The drain itself should not be blocked or kinked and should be securely fastened with the collection device below the insertion site. Documentation of output should be accurate with prompt recognition and escalation of changes in content or volume. Pain assessments and documentation should include the drain site and additional analgesia offered prior to drain removal.

Anaesthetics

Anaesthetic required for surgery can be administered in a variety of ways including local anaesthetic or nerve block; spinal anaesthetic for high-risk patients; sedation for procedures such as endoscopy and general anaesthetic which uses drugs to cause unconsciousness. These drugs have complex effects on the lungs and heart requiring careful monitoring by an anaesthetist. An understanding of how these drugs work, common side effects or interactions and common combinations used intra-operatively will benefit your practice in the post-operative critical care setting.

Post-operative complications

Any assessment of post-operative complications such as infection should include a structured holistic assessment using a systems-based approach. The '5 Ws' mnemonic has long been used in surgical settings to aid clinical reasoning in the instance of post-operative fever (Table 22.2):

Complications relevant to gastrointestinal surgery are outlined in the sections below.

Ileus

Defined as hypomotility of the GI tract in the absence of obstruction, the exact cause of ileus is often multi-factorial and complex and causes full or partial paralysis of the muscles controlling the intestines. Paralysis does not have to be total to cause an ileus, but only enough to stop the passage of bowel contents which leads to symptoms of obstruction.

Table 22.2 The Five Ws mnemonic for post-operative fever.

W	Consideration
Wind	Is this atelectasis, pneumonia, or aspiration?
Water	Is this a urinary tract infection?
Wound	Check the wound(s). Is there evidence of surgical site infection?
Walking	Is there evidence of deep vein thrombosis or pulmonary embolism?
'Wonder drugs'	Has the patient had a blood transfusion? Review all of the medications that the patient has received. Consider anaesthetic medications.

Ileus that persists for 3 days post-operatively is termed paralytic ileus. An expected coincidence of colorectal surgery, it can also be caused be medications, spinal injury or intrabdominal inflammation. When an ileus occurs in the stomach it is termed gastroparesis or delayed gastric emptying.

Anastomotic leak

Intestinal anastomosis is the site where two ends of resected bowel are joined together, either by hand-sewing or staples. The decision to create an anastomosis, as opposed to forming a stoma, is dependent on site, surgical skill and a number of patient factors. An anastomotic leak is considered a serious complication associated with very high mortality rates. Breakdown of the newly formed anastomosis generally occurs on day 1–2 post-operatively, or day 7–8 dependent on the cause of the leak as to whether it is related to technical or procedural factors, or abnormal healing. The risk of leak is reduced with robust pre-operative workup only achievable in elective surgery, and the nature of emergency surgical interventions prevents pre-operative optimisation from being attained. Optimising nutritional status pre-operatively, if possible, greatly reduces the risk of anastomotic breakdown (Xu and Kong, 2020). Intraoperatively and immediately post-operatively preventing hypothermia and hypovolemia can reduce the risk. Careful monitoring, nutritional optimisation and fluid replacement are essential roles of the critical care nurse in this setting.

6Cs: Commitment

Being committed to our patients is a cornerstone of nursing practice and allows for innovative ways of working to be developed, to improve the care we provide and the patient experience.

Wound dehiscence

Wound breakdown, or 'dehiscence', is a distressing but common occurrence and one that causes significant delay to overall recovery. Although the primary cause is infection, multiple patient factors (high BMI, diabetes and smoking), surgical site, activity levels and surgical skill all contribute to increased risk of dehiscence. In most cases it is accidental but can be done intentionally if the wound becomes infected and is reopened to be debrided or washed out. A dehisced wound is rarely reclosed but allowed to heal by secondary intent, resulting in increased pain, delayed recovery and scarring.

Red Flag

Necrotising fasciitis is a severe, but thankfully rare bacterial infection of the subcutaneous tissues below the skin known as the 'fascia' and is often referred to as the 'flesh-eating disease'. Most predominantly affecting the perineum, it is also seen in the toes, abdomen, post-surgical wounds and the urogenital area, where it is known as 'Fournier's gangrene' (Diab et al., 2020). Infection spreads rapidly, engulfing muscle tissue and leading to sepsis with high associated morbidity and mortality (Diab et al., 2020).

Patients who are diabetic, of old age, immunosuppressed, obese or malnourished are more at risk (Wilson, 1952). Skin may appear purple, dusky, with spreading erythema and often blisters, with early symptoms including pain and clinical deterioration that is disproportionate to skin findings. Patients quickly progress into shock and show signs of multi-organ failure (Lee Spark NF Foundation, 2020).

Early referral for a surgical opinion is vital and surgical debridement is very common, with often multiple procedures required. Sepsis treatment, microbiology specialist input and serial skin assessments are imperative.

GI pharmacology

Medications management: antiemetics

There are several classes of medications prescribed for nausea and vomiting dependent on the cause (aetiology) if known.

Phenothiazines are a class of antiemetic that act on the central nervous system and are of particular use in prophylactic treatment of nausea and vomiting, for example in a post-operative patient.

Ondansetron (4–16 mg orally or IV) is often prescribed as first-line treatment due in part to its low interaction and side effect profile.

Medications management: protein pump inhibitors (PPI)

PPIs reduce gastric acid secretion by blocking the 'proton pump' of the gastric parietal cells.

Omeprazole is one of the most commonly prescribed PPI. You may see a 20 mg OD or BD oral dose or a higher dose prescribed as an infusion. PPIs are used to treat a number of GI pathologies, such as reflux and gastric ulcers as well as acute upper GI haemorrhage.

Medications management: laxatives

There are four main types of laxatives which are often used in tandem (docusate sodium is believed to have two actions): bulk-forming laxatives, faecal softeners, stimulant laxatives and osmotic laxatives. Understanding the cause of a patient's constipation will inform choice of laxatives.

In addition to this you will see bowel cleansing preparations prescribed to patients in critical care prior to investigations such as colonoscopy and before some colorectal surgical interventions.

It is important to note other causes of intestinal dysmotility should be considered prior to commencing a patient on laxatives and if able adequate oral fluid intake should be encouraged to prevent intestinal obstruction.

Medications management: insulin and hypoglycaemic agents

Insulin is a hormone made in the pancreas that allows the body to utilise glucose in the production of energy. Close monitoring of blood sugar levels is of particular importance in a patient with a GI presentation.

Generally given via subcutaneous injection, in critical care settings it is often administered intravenously and is prescribed as a 'sliding scale' whereby the rate/dose is adjusted in line with changes in the patient's blood sugar.

Dose adjustments are often made due to both hepatic and renal impairment in critically unwell patients. There is often great variability in prescribing protocols across critical care settings even with in the same hospital.

Conclusion

The human GI tract is a complex body system essential to life, consisting of multiple organs involved in many functions. It is mediated by an unknown number of microbes and bacteria which make up healthy gut flora and play a diverse role in absorption of nutrients, metabolism and immune response to pathogens. Critical care admission can result from a myriad of GI pathologies and critical care nurses play a key role within the multidisciplinary team in monitoring the function of the GI tract and adverse effects resulting from disease or trauma.

Take home points

1. The gastrointestinal system carries out digestive, endocrine, immune and barrier functions.
2. The gastrointestinal system protects against pathogens using physical, non-immune and immune-mediated mechanisms.
3. Hepatic function can be quickly altered in response to systemic inflammation and critical illness.
4. Assessment and monitoring of gastrointestinal tract function is achievable with the monitoring of vital signs, serial blood tests and various imaging modalities.
5. Procedures to rectify abnormal gastrointestinal function range from simple but skilled nursing interventions to invasive endoscopic and surgical procedures.
6. Acute abdominal catastrophe can necessitate an admission to the critical care environment or develop during a critical care admission due to other iatrogenic factors.
7. There are several major surgical procedures that require critical care input post-operatively.
8. Post-operative monitoring is crucial in aiding early recognition of complications.
9. There are multiple medications that can be administered to treat or prevent gastrointestinal dysfunction.
10. Although not well defined, critical illness can have profound effects on GI function.

References

Ziesmann, M.T., Park, J., Unger, B.J., Kirkpatrick, A.W., Vergis, A., Logsetty, S., Pham, C., Kirschner, D. and Gillman, L.M., 2015. Validation of the quality of ultrasound imaging and competence (QUICk) score as an objective assessment tool for the FAST examination. Journal of Trauma and Acute Care Surgery, 78(5), pp.1008–1013.

Baid, H., Creed, F., and Hargreaves, J. (2016). Systematic assessment. In: *Oxford Handbook of Critical Care Nursing* (ed. S. Adam and S. Osborne), 15–40. Oxford: Oxford University Press.

Barrett, K. E. (2006). *Gastrointestinal Physiology*. New York, NY: Lange Medical.

Booker, K. (2015). *Critical Care Nursing: Monitoring and Treatment for Advanced Nursing Practice*. Wiley Blackwell.

Buczacki, S.J. and Davies, J. (2018). The acute abdomen in the cardiac intensive care unit. *Core Topics in Cardiothoracic Critical Care* (ed. K. Valchanov, N. Jones, and C.W. Hogue), 294–300. Cambridge: Cambridge University Press.

Cardoso, F.S., Marcelino, P., Bagulho, L., and Karvellas, C.J., (2017). Acute liver failure: an up-to-date approach. *Journal of Critical Care* 39: 25–30.

Critical Care Networks-National Nurse Leads (CC3N) (2015). National Competency Framework for Registered Nurses in Adult Critical Care. Step 2 Competencies. https://www.cc3n.org.uk/uploads/9/8/4/2/98425184/02_new_step_2_final.pdf (accessed 21 December 2020).

Diab, J., Bannan, A., and Pollitt, T. (2020). Necrotising fasciitis. *BMJ* 369. doi: 10.1136/bmj.m1428.

Granholm, A., Zeng, L., Dionne, J., Perner, A., Marker, S., Krag, M., MacLaren, R., Ye, Z., Møller, M., Alhazzani, W., and the GUIDE group. (2019). Predictors of gastrointestinal bleeding in adult ICU patients: a systematic review and meta-analysis. *Intensive Care Medicine* 45: 1347–1359.

Horvatits, T., Drolz, A., Trauner, M., and Fuhrmann, V. (2019). Liver injury and failure in critical illness. *Hepatology* 70(6): 2204–2215.

Hunter, J. and Damani, Z. (2004). Intra-abdominal hypertension and the abdominal compartment syndrome. *Anaesthesia* 59(9:) 899–907.

IAP/APA (2013). Evidence-based guidelines for the management of acute pancreatitis. *Pancreatology* 13(4supp2): e1–e15.

Jean-Baptiste, S., Messika, J., Hajage, D. et al. (2018). Clinical impact of upper gastrointestinal endoscopy in critically ill patients with suspected bleeding. *Annals of Intensive Care* 8(1): 1–5.

Jenniskens, M., Langouche, L. and Van den Berghe, G. (2018). Cholestatic alterations in the critically ill: some new light on an old problem. *Chest* 153(3): 733–743.

Kortgen, A., Recknagel, P., and Bauer M. (2010). How to assess liver function? *Current Opinions in Critical Care* 16: 136–41.

Krag, M., Marker, S., Perner, A. et al. (2018). Pantoprazole in patients at risk for gastrointestinal bleeding in the ICU. *New England Journal of Medicine* 379(23): 2199–2208.

Kramer, L., Jordan, B., Druml, W. et al. (2007). Incidence and prognosis of early hepatic dysfunction in critically ill patients – a prospective multicenter study. *Critical Care Medicine* 35(4): 1099–e7.

Kumar, P. and Clark, M. (2011). *Medical Management & Therapeutics*. Elsevier.

Lee Spark NF Foundation (2020). https://nfsuk.org.uk (accessed 13 March 2021).

Liddle, C. (2013). Postoperative care 1: principles of monitoring postoperative patients. *Nursing Times* 109(22): 24–26.

Liu, Q., Zhou, Q., Song, M. et al. (2020). A nomogram for predicting the risk of sepsis in patients with acute cholangitis. *Journal of International Medical Research* 48(1). doi: 10.1177/0300060519866100.

Mayor, S. (2016). One in five with bowel cancer diagnosed as emergency had previous 'red flag' symptoms. *BMJ* 354. doi: 10.1136/bmj.i5277.

Mostafa, S.M., Bhandari, S., Richie, G. et al. (2003). Constipation and its implications in the critically ill patients. *Br J Anaesth* 91:815–819.

Nagpal, R., and Yadav, H. (2017). Bacterial translocation from the fut to the distant organs: an overview. *Annals of Nutrition and Metabolism* 71(S1): 11–16.

Nassa, A., da Silva, F., and de Cleva, R. (2009). Constipation in intensive care unit: Incidence and risk factors. *Journal of Critical Care* 24(4): 630.e9–12.

National Confidential Enquiry into Patient Outcome and Death (NCEPOD) (2011) *Knowing the Risk. A Review of the Peri-Operative Care of Surgical Patients*. https://www.ncepod.org.uk/2011poc.html (accessed March 2022).

National Institute of Health and Care Excellence (NICE) (2013) *Acute Diarrhoea in Adults: Racecadotril*. ESNM11. https://www.nice.org.uk/advice/esnm11/chapter/Overview (accessed 12 January 2021).

Rajapakse, C.S. and Chang, G., 2014. Impact of body habitus on radiologic interpretations. *Academic Radiology* 21(1): 1–2.

Reintam Blaser, A., Preiser, J.C., Fruhwald, S. et al. (2020). Gastrointestinal dysfunction in the critically ill: a systematic scoping review and research agenda proposed by the Section of Metabolism, Endocrinology and Nutrition of the European Society of Intensive Care Medicine. *Critical Care* 24: 1–17.

Ross, J., Matthay, M., and Harris, H. (2018). Secondary peritonitis: principles of diagnosis and intervention. *BMJ* 361: k1407.

Scholten, S.R. (2010). Endoscopy: a guide for the registered nurse. *Crit Care Nurs Clin North Am* 22(1): 19–32. doi: 10.1016/j.ccell.2009.10.002.

Sharma, A. and Rao, S., 2016. Constipation: pathophysiology and current therapeutic approaches. *Gastrointestinal Pharmacology* 239: 59–74.

Siriwardena, A., Jegatheeswaran, S., Mason, J. et al. (2019). PROCalcitonin-based algorithm for antibiotic use in Acute Pancreatitis (PROCAP): study protocol for a randomised controlled trial. *Trials* 20: 463. doi: 10.1186/s13063-019-3549-3.

Ten Broek, R.P., Krielen, P., Di Saverio, S. et al. (2018). Bologna guidelines for diagnosis and management of adhesive small bowel obstruction (ASBO): 2017 update of the evidence-based guidelines from the world society of emergency surgery ASBO working group. *World Journal of Emergency Surgery* 13(1): 1–13.

Urden, L.D., Stacy, K.M., and Lough, M.E. (2013). Gastrointestinal anatomy and physiology. In: *Critical Care Nursing: Diagnosis and Management*, 7e (ed. L.D. Urden, K.M. Stacy, and M.E. Lough), 737–749. St. Louis: Mosby.

Vincent, J., Preiser, J. (2015). Getting critical about constipation. *Practical Gastroenterology*, 14–25.

Webb, A., Angus, D., Finer, S. et al. (2016). *Oxford Textbook of Critical Care*, 2e. Oxford: Oxford University Press.

Wendon, J., Cordoba, J., Dhawan, A. et al. (2017). EASL clinical practical guidelines on the management of acute (fulminant) liver failure. *Journal of Hepatology* 66(5): 1047–1081.

Williams, R. and Wendon, J. (2013). *Critical Care in Acute Liver Failure*. London: Future Medicine.

Wilson, B. (1952). Necrotising fasciitis. *Am Surg* 18: 416–431.

Xu, H. and Kong, F. (2020). Malnutrition-related factors increased the risk of anastomotic leak for rectal cancer patients undergoing surgery. *BioMed Research International*. doi: 10.1155/2020/5059670.

329

Chapter 23

Nutrition in critical care

Barry Hill and Lorraine Mutrie

Aim

This aim of this chapter is to provide the reader with an evidence-based understanding of contemporary nutrition requirements for patients who are cared for in critical care settings.

Learning outcomes

After reading this chapter the reader will be able to:

- Gain an appreciation of the complexities critical care patients encounter with their nutritional needs.
- Understand the pathophysiology of nutrition.
- Describe how to assess the nutritional risk of the critically ill patient.
- Discuss the risks and benefits of starting enteral nutrition (EN) in critical illness.
- Recall the indications for supplemental or total parenteral nutrition (PN).

Test your prior knowledge

- In relation to nutrition, define stress response and its three phases, and discuss how it impacts homeostasis for patients who are critically unwell.
- When screening a critically unwell patients' nutritional status, are you able to define and give a rationale for the use of the Malnutrition Universal Screening Tool (MUST)?
- Can you name the different methods of delivering nutrition to critically unwell patients and give a rationale for their use?
- Are you able to critically discuss the evidence base that supports the care of people with feeding tubes?
- Can you identify when feed should be discontinued, and critically evaluate the reasons behind your choices?

Fundamentals of Critical Care: A Textbook for Nursing and Healthcare Students, First Edition. Edited by Ian Peate and Barry Hill.
© 2023 John Wiley & Sons Ltd. Published 2023 by John Wiley & Sons Ltd.
Companion website: www.wiley.com/go/peate/criticalcare

Introduction

Chapter 23 explores contemporary nutritional recommendations for patients who are critically unwell. The aim of nutritional support is to attenuate the detrimental effects of critical illness on nutritional state, such as increased energy deficit and catabolism; it may favourably influence outcomes and prevent or reverse malnutrition. Currently, it is unknown how long starvation in critical illness can last without harmful consequences, but most guidance agrees that nutritional therapy should be started as soon as possible and certainly within the first week of critical illness (Chowdhury and Lobaz, 2019).

Nutritional support for critical care patients is complex and multifaceted and is highly debated due to the variety and complexity of clinical presentations, routes of administration and available research studies. Nutritional support is so significant for critically ill patients that in contemporary healthcare, it is recognised as a definitive therapy in its own right (Ramprasad and Kapoor, 2012) and initiating and maintaining appropriate nutrition for patients suffering from critical illness continues to be challenging due to a variety of reasons, including: acute clinical presentations, level of organ failure/s, injuries and disease processes (Casaer and Van den Berghe, 2014; Desai et al., 2013). Woodrow (2018) suggests that nutrition is a fundamental component of critical care therapy, with Singer et al. (2019), adding that it aids medical treatment and fuels improved recovery. Faculty of Intensive Care Medicine (FICM) (2019) identify that up to 55% of patients are malnourished on admission to critical care. The number at nutritional risk subsequently rises due to a prevalent hypercatabolic state and barriers that impair adequate conventional oral intake. Adequate nutritional support is vital and is safe when delivered either enterally (EN) or parenterally (PN). Defining the 'optimal dose' of nutrition support, however, remains contentious. An initial period of protocolised feeding (e.g. less than 72 hours), with subsequent individualising of intake in response to the changing metabolic demands, clinical condition and nutritional risk of each patient, is generally advocated. A multi-professional approach is required and there should be a dietitian as part of the critical care multidisciplinary team

Step 2 competencies: National standards

2:4.2 Nutrition in Critical Illness (Critical Care Networks-National Nurse Leads (CC3N) 2015)

Demonstrate your knowledge using a rationale through discussion, and the application to practice

- Refer to patients past medical history, outline how this may affect gastrointestinal function
- Determine monitoring needs for the individual at risk of deterioration related to gastrointestinal function
- Report abnormalities to appropriate MDT member

- Correctly review a patient's biochemistry and haematology results, interpret findings in relation to gastrointestinal function
- Evaluate effectiveness of therapeutic interventions, adjusting care accordingly
- Alter nutritional regimes in line with MDT recommendations and local policy
- Recognise the patient at risk of deteriorating from sepsis

Pathophysiology

Nutrition is essential for cellular function. The intake of micronutrients and macronutrients is essential for the metabolic processes (the breakdown and synthesis of nutrients) that maintain homeostasis within the human body. In health, this is normally achieved by maintaining a balanced diet (World Health Organization (WHO), 2015), consisting of enough nutrients to fulfil basal metabolic requirements (energy required at rest) and daily activity. For adequate nutrition, the human body depends on the availability of energy substrates; these include carbohydrates, proteins, and lipids, with glucose from carbohydrates being the preferred source for slow release energy (Galgani and Ravussin, 2008). During illness, the metabolic requirements of the body changes because of the stress response.

The stress response is the body's natural response to a stimulus or stressor to try to maintain homeostasis. Examples of stressors in illness are raised temperature, infection, or bleeding. The response is triggered after a distress signal has been sent to the hypothalamus (Marieb, 2015; Yancey, 2016) and can be divided into three phases: the fight-or-flight response, resistance and exhaustion (Tortora and Derrickson, 2017). A simplified explanation of each is below.

331

Snapshot

Jaden is a 32-year-old admitted to hospital followed an out-of-hospital cardiac arrest. Jaden was discharged from the intensive care unit 10 days ago and admitted for step-down care on a cardiac high dependency unit (HDU). Jaden was sedated and mechanically ventilated for 7 days, he has developed muscle weakness and continues to require nasogastric feeding over night to ensure he maintains his nutrition and calorific intake. Jaden's body is in final phase of stress response identified as exhaustion (Tortora and Derrickson, 2017). At 0600 a Registered Nurse (RN) records the following information on his observation chart:

Airway (A): Airway is patent, patient is speaking.
Breathing (B): oxygen saturation 96% (NEWS2 = 0), on 3 litres nasal cannula (NEWS2 = 2), respiratory rate (RR) 26 breaths per minute (NEWS2 = 3). Cardiovascular System (C): Blood Pressure (BP) is 90/65 (NEWS2 = 0), Heart Rate (HR) is 106 beats

per minute (NEWS2 = 1), capillary refill time (CRT) is 4 seconds, he is cool to touch.

Disability (D) (neurological system), Patient is Alert (NEWS2 = 0), on the AVPU scale (see Chapter 14), Body Temperature (T) is 38.0°C

Exposure (E) no abnormal findings.

Total NEW2 Score: 6.

Nursing actions:
- RN contacts the critical care outreach team on call.
- A full head-to-toe assessment and diagnostic tests including blood test and blood cultures were taken.

Diagnosis:
- Concluded Jaden did not have an infection as initially indicated.
- Jaden was fatigued due to muscle loss and weakness, muscle breakdown led to increased metabolic demand
- Significant weight loss, had reduced his blood glucose, increased his body temperature and compensated his blood pressure and heart rate.
- Jaden continued on hourly observations
- Prescribed a new EN prescription form the dietitian and intravenous fluids
- Additional physiotherapy to aid his rehabilitation.

Fight or flight

In response to a distress signal, the hypothalamus activates the adrenal glands (one located on top of each kidney) by sending nerve impulses via the sympathetic nervous system. The adrenal medulla releases the catecholamine hormones epinephrine (adrenaline) and norepinephrine (noradrenaline) which lead to physiological changes to help the body deal with extreme situations. The catecholamine release leads to an increased heart rate, increased blood pressure, dilation of the small airways in the lungs (bronchioles) and a rise in glucose levels as the liver converts its stores of glycogen into glucose (glycogenolysis) in order to increase oxygen delivery to the essential body systems (heart, brain and muscles) that provide energy to either fight or flee the stressor (Marieb, 2015; Tortora and Derrickson, 2017). Because of this mechanism, blood flow to the kidneys is restricted, which triggers the release of renin and in turn, aldosterone and antidiuretic hormone activation helping to regulate fluid balance and maintain blood pressure. This fight-or-flight response is mounted to deal with short-term stressors (Marieb, 2015).

Resistance

To maintain energy levels and repair cellular function, the hypothalamus excretes hormones that prompt further endocrine responses from the anterior pituitary gland that help the body to deal with prolonged stressors. The hormones released from the anterior pituitary gland stimulate hormone responses from the adrenal cortex (cortisol), the

liver (growth hormone) and the thyroid gland (thyroid hormones). This regulates metabolism and glucose supply in the body, helping to generate new sources of glucose from other sources e.g. proteins and fats via the process of gluconeogenesis, which can then be used for energy or cell repair (Tortora and Derrickson, 2017). In addition to glucose regulation, cortisol also acts to reduce and terminate the inflammatory response (Hinson et al., 2010). Further information about glucose control and the role of insulin is in the glycaemic control section of this chapter.

Exhaustion

If the body is unable to deal with the initial stressor via the resistance phase of the stress response glucose reserves will soon be depleted, leading to exhaustion of energy supply. With the continued attempt to deal with the stressor, the high levels of hormone release during the resistance phase continues, and this can lead to further breakdown of tissue for example muscle leading to muscle wastage (Tortora and Derrickson, 2017). The continued presence of cortisol to try to reduce the immune response can lead to suppression of the immune system (Hinson et al., 2010).

During all illnesses, the initial fight-or-flight response ensures that large amounts of oxygen and glucose are quickly available to areas that need it but restricted in non-essential body systems therefore preserving as much energy as possible. In critical illness, this is referred to as the 'ebb' phase of the metabolic response and lasts up to 24 hours (Rutledge and Nesbitt, 2013).

The 'flow' phase of critical illness is associated with increased levels of hormones during prolonged exposure to a stressor as described in the stress response (Rutledge and Nesbitt, 2013). To continue to combat the stressor, the body requires more energy and increased levels of oxygen to meet this increased metabolic demand. This is commonly referred to as a hypermetabolic state (an abnormal increase in the body's basal metabolic rate). To meet this demand, the body uses up its stores of glucose from carbohydrate metabolism so must create a new energy source; derived from breakdown of proteins and fats from muscle and adipose tissue. This is known as a catabolic state (Heyland et al., 2003) and can lead to some of the complications associated with critical illness including rapid weight loss, delayed wound healing, a reduction in immunity and hyperglycaemia (Heyland et al., 2003; Mehanna et al., 2008).

It is well recognised that critically ill patients are frequently unable to feed themselves, and regularly present in a fasting state (Cove and Pinsky, 2011). This, and their disease process, leaves them at risk of undernourishment and malnourishment. Nutritional therapy in critical illness targets the 'flow' phase of critical illness, and if initiated early and correctly, is considered to reduce muscle wastage, reduce hospital length of stay and improve recovery times (Casaer and Van den Berghe, 2014; Desai et al., 2013) as well as providing much needed energy. To provide appropriate nutrition to patients, accurate patient assessment must take place.

6Cs: Communication
Effective communication is a key requisite when undertaking assessment of needs.

6Cs: Care
Listening to people and respecting their unique needs are hallmarks of professional practice.

Nutritional screening and assessment

To guide nutritional support for patients, the National Institute for Health and Care Excellence (NICE) (2017) recommend screening for malnutrition and risk of malnutrition in all hospitalised patients using a recognised tool, for example the Malnutrition Universal Screening Tool (MUST) and those considered 'high risk' should have nutritional intervention (NICE, 2017). Critically ill patients will invariably be considered 'high risk' under the NICE guidelines due to their potential for reduced dietary intake and the resulting catabolic impact of illness, and under current guidance should be screened on a weekly basis. Rahman et al. (2016) have suggested that nutritional risk for critically unwell patients is more complex than for other patients and should therefore have a different approach to routine nutritional screening but until accepted into United Kingdom (UK) guidance (i.e. Intensive Care Society (ICS) or NICE), application of NICE (2017) guidelines and NICE Quality Standards (2012) must be utilised.

Nutritional therapy aims to provide patients with the nutrients that they need to fulfil their basal metabolic requirements. Assessment of nutritional requirements for critically ill patients should include lead dieticians (ICS, 2019) due to the variability of patient needs (Frankenfield and Ashcraft, 2011) and the complexity of condition and assessment (Preiser et al., 2014).

Snapshot

Sally is a 45-year-old patient admitted to hospital on a surgical ward for a gastric bypass procedure. Sally's medical history includes obesity, hypertension, and type two diabetes mellitus. Sally's height is 1.64 m and her weight is 100 kg. Sally's Body Mass Index (BMI) is 38 kg/m². To calculate her Malnutrition Universal Screening Tool (MUST) score the Nurse was required to complete a MUST score using 5 steps.

- **Step 1:** Measure Sally's BMI,
- **Step 2:** Explore any unexplained weight loss in the past 3–6 months.
- **Step 3:** Explore if Sally has had any acute illness or not had nutritional intake in the past 5 days or more.
- **Further reading:** https://www.bapen.org.uk/pdfs/must/must_full.pdf

What MUST Score does Sally have? Step 4 would identify Sally's risk of malnutrition.

Are you able to complete Step 5 by utilising clinical guidelines and local policies to write an individualised care plan for Sally?

Indirect calorimetry (IC)

In practice, indirect calorimetry (IC) is considered to be the most reliable measure of assessing energy utilisation as it provides an accurate measurement of oxygen consumption and carbon dioxide so that energy requirements can be determined but in critically ill patients this technology is inaccurate due to the metabolic disturbances that patients have; the high oxygen concentrations patients often receive; and for patients that require invasive ventilation, the air that can leak from ventilator circuits, therefore restricting its use in the critical care setting (Frankenfield and Ashcraft, 2011). Instead, metabolic equations based on patient weight, gender, age and activity (whether someone is breathing independently/ on a ventilator, whether they are mobile/ bedbound, or severity of illness i.e. raised temperature) are used to determine energy required. Despite these equations also being considered as highly inaccurate in acute and critical illness, they are currently the most used in critical care practice (Berger and Pichard, 2014; Frankenfield and Ashcraft, 2011; Raham et al., 2016).

6Cs: Competence
A competent practitioner has insight and knowledge of the key issues enabling them with the patient where appropriate to make clinical decisions.

Regular review of calorific needs should take place to contend with the changing physiological and activity needs of the patient and Berger and Pichard (2014) recommend that when prescribing nutrition, non-nutritional sources of energy should also be taken into account, to prevent overfeeding i.e. glucose and lipids from drug administration such as Propofol. Dietary review may need to be revised and prescribed by a critical care dietician every 24 hours in the critical care setting depending on the patient's acuity, blood results and absorption (amongst other factors). Rutledge and Nesbitt (2013) propose that nutritional requirements should be at the forefront of management of critically ill patients, considering both short and long-term requirements of the feeding regime, in addition to the route of administration.

Learning event: reflection
Reflect on how much you understand about EN and PN and nutritional prescriptions prescribed by the critical care dietitian.

333

6Cs: Courage

Acknowledging your limitations and seeing support are courageous things to do.

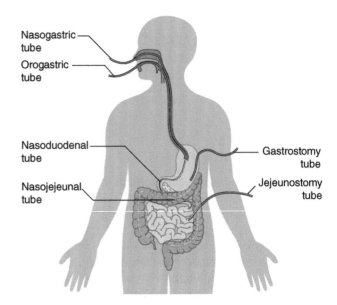

Figure 23.1 Methods of enteral feeding. *Source:* Finch (2018) with permission of John Wiley & Sons.

Routes of administration

Enteral nutrition

Enteral nutrition (EN) consists of feeding directly into the gastrointestinal (GI) tract via a feeding tube. The different placement sites for feeding tubes include the stomach, duodenum and jejunum, and the tube can be passed nasally, orally, or via a gastrostomy or jejunostomy tube (PEG or J-tube) depending on what is most suitable for the patient (see Figure 23.1, methods of enteral feeding). For example, patients with facial traumas may not be suitable for either nasal or oral feeding tubes due to difficult placement and neurological trauma patients would need oral gastric or jejunal feeding tubes until basal skull clearance had been met so that feeding tubes could not penetrate the skull and cause damage to the brain (Dutton and Finch, 2018).

et al., 2013; Schetz et al., 2013). However, when feeding via the enteral route, some patients display signs of enteral nutrition intolerance.

Medications management: omeprazole

Omeprazole is a Protein Pump Inhibitor (PPI). These are used to treat gastric acid-related disorders. These disorders may include gastroesophageal reflux disease, peptic ulcer disease, and other diseases characterised by the over-secretion of gastric acid. PPI's inhibit gastric acid secretion by blocking the hydrogen-potassium adenosine triphosphatase enzyme system (the 'proton pump') of the gastric parietal cell. The dose of omeprazole may need to be reduced in patients with hepatic impairment.

Red Flag

In critically ill patients, Tatsumi (2019) recommends that EN must be discontinued or interrupted, if gastrointestinal complications, particularly vomiting and bowel movement disorders do not resolve with appropriate management. To avoid such complications, EN should be started as soon as possible with a small amount first, gradually increased. Measures to decrease the risk of reflux and aspiration include elevation the head of the bed (30° to 45°), switch to continuous administration, administer prokinetic drugs or narcotic antagonists to promote gastrointestinal motility, and switch to jejunal access (postpyloric route).

Early enteral nutrition (EEN) is the provision of enteral nutrition within the initial 24–48 hours of critical illness presentation (American Society for Parenteral and Enteral Nutrition (ASPEN) 2016) and ICS Standards (ICS, 2019) dictate that nutrition should be commenced on admission to critical care. Providing EN early has been found to reduce mortality in critically ill patients (ASPEN, 2016) and EEN is also considered to preserve gut mucosal integrity, reduce the risk of bacterial translocation and is thought to be beneficial in the early catabolic phase of critical illness. It is worth noting that the benefits of EEN are largely based on historic, poorly designed trials hence the revived interest in the subject (Casaer and Van den Berghe, 2014; Desai

Enteral nutrition intolerance is when the feed administered is not absorbed by the GI tract, and common symptoms including vomiting, oesophageal regurgitation, abdominal distention and diarrhoea (Desai et al., 2013; Ozen et al., 2016; Montejo et al., 2010; Reignier et al., 2013). A common method used to check absorption of feed is to aspirate contents from the gut to measure Gastric Residual Volume (GRV) and the ICS Standard (2019) is to accept up to 500 mL of residual volume if the patient is showing no any other signs of intolerance. Historically it has been thought that if GRV is high, the patient is at more risk of aspiration pneumonia. However, this has recently been contested (Montejo et al., 2010; Ozen et al., 2016; Reignier et al., 2013). ASPEN guidelines (2016) now advise that GRV does not need to be measured in critical care patients, as the risk of aspiration is unfounded. It is noteworthy that their recommendations are based on studies involving patients on mechanical ventilation (i.e. with presumed protected airway) that were nursed in an upright 30-degree angle, minimising the risk of aspiration pneumonia, therefore it may be prudent to continue to monitor GRV in critical care patients without a protected airway. Local policies should always be followed for methods such as this.

6Cs: Compassion

Compassion concerns how care is given through relationships that are funded on empathy, respect and dignity.

Medications management: intestinal motility disorders medication

Drugs used in the management of intestinal motility disorders include cholinergic agonists, prokinetic agents, opioid antagonists, antidiarrheals and antibiotics. The agents that are most useful in the treatment of these disorders are neostigmine, bethanechol, metoclopramide, cisapride and loperamide.

Clinical investigations: bowel sounds

Auscultating for bowel sounds is common nursing practice when patients are being administered EN. Finding no bowel sounds can be indicative of an ileus, or an obstruction above that area of the intestine. Hypoactive bowel sounds are considered as one every three to five minutes, this can indicate diarrhoea, anxiety or gastroenteritis. Hyperactive bowel sounds are often found before a blockage. It is quite common to find one abdominal quadrant with hyperactive bowel sounds and one with none or hypoactive ones. This is because the intestine is attempting to clear the blockage with increased peristalsis.

Enteral nutrition targets either full calorific feeding or trophic feeding (lower than normal calorific content) (Desai et al., 2013). Full calorific feeding in critically ill

patients has been linked to intolerance, which can lead to the under provision of enteral feed and subsequently failure to meet calorific and protein feeding targets. Trophic feeding aims to maintain gut integrity whilst minimising the risk of feeding intolerance, and although ethically questioned by Montejo et al. (2010), if combined with parenteral nutrition, can and does contribute to meeting full calorific need. NICE guidance section 1.4.4 (2017) recommends cautiously introducing feed to seriously ill patients, starting any feed at no more than 50% of target requirement and increasing over 24–48 hrs but this is not a common approach to practice.

Orange Flag

Feeding against the will of the patient should be an intervention of the last resort in the care and management of those with severe eating disorders or other mental illness. It should be considered in the context of the Mental Health Act 1983, the Mental Capacity Act 2005 or the Children Act 1989 (and their respective Codes of Practice).

Parenteral nutrition

Parenteral nutrition (PN) is the provision of nutrients directly into a central vein. PN relies on venous access and is commonly administered into a central vein to avoid venous irritation from the solution, although some solutions can be administered via a peripheral cannula for short-term use. PN can be used as the sole source of nutritional intake but its use over EN has no substantive evidence, i.e. it has not been proven to improve patient outcomes (Desai et al., 2013). Casaer et al. (2014) believes that PN can be used to meet calorific targets when enteral nutrition fails however, evidence is inconclusive as to the risk/benefit to patients, and the optimum time at which PN should be introduced. Harvey et al. (2016) argue that PN is more likely to accurately deliver targeted nutrition than EN, and that the commonly associated risk of infection from the use of PN is now outdated due to better infection control measures. ASPEN (2016) recommends the use of PN as a supplement to EN after 7–10 days if a patient is unable to meet more than 60% of their energy target, and early (as soon after admission to intensive care as possible) PN in patients where EN is not feasible.

PN can be withdrawn once adequate oral or enteral nutrition is tolerated, and the patients' nutritional status is stable. Withdrawal should be planned and stepwise with a daily review of the patient's progress. This being said, Preiser et al. (2014) suggest that it is important to recognise that enteral feed targets are frequently not met in critically ill patients and consequently critically unwell patients either can be under or overfed. Having a clear protocol to follow when establishing feeding has been shown to help reduce this risk (NICE, 2017).

Snapshot

Aruna is a 61-year-old female admitted to hospital with complete bowel obstruction, multiple adhesions and recurrent Crohn's disease. She is 1.65 metres weighing 65 kg (usual weight of 75 kg). Her medical history includes Crohn's disease and type two diabetes mellitus. Exploratory laparotomy is scheduled, lysis of adhesions and small bowel resection to remove diseased bowel are performed. In the meantime, whilst awaiting her procedure nursing actions need to be completed. These include:

- Abdominal girth measured daily.
- Note the colour and character of all vomitus. Test for the presence of occult blood.
- Any stool passed should be tested for the presence of occult blood.
- Monitor vital signs closely. Elevations of temperature and pulse may indicate infection or necrosis.
- Monitor fluid balance input and output very closely. Fluid and electrolyte losses must be replaced.
- Provide explanations to Aruna and her family regarding processes and procedures
- Report and document findings

Nursing considerations and recommendations for practice

The Nursing and Midwifery Council (NMC) (2018) require Registered Nurses and Nursing Associates to preserve safety, this applies to the patient and those you work with. The nurse must be able to accurately assess needs and where appropriate refer to other practitioners. At all time you are required to act in the best interests of the individual seeking assistance from a suitably qualified and experienced healthcare professionals if required. The patient must always be at the centre of all that is done

6Cs: Commitment

Being committed to providing high-quality and safe patient care demonstrates that you are aware of the professional values that underpin practice.

Care of people with feeding tubes

When delivering nutritional treatments to patients, nurses must ensure they follow the correct procedures for care and management of any feeding tubes used (see Figure 23.2).

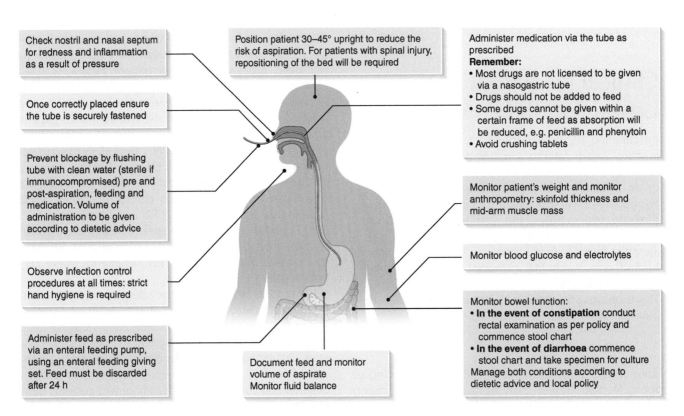

Check nostril and nasal septum for redness and inflammation as a result of pressure

Once correctly placed ensure the tube is securely fastened

Prevent blockage by flushing tube with clean water (sterile if immunocompromised) pre and post-aspiration, feeding and medication. Volume of administration to be given according to dietetic advice

Observe infection control procedures at all times: strict hand hygiene is required

Administer feed as prescribed via an enteral feeding pump, using an enteral feeding giving set. Feed must be discarded after 24 h

Position patient 30–45° upright to reduce the risk of aspiration. For patients with spinal injury, repositioning of the bed will be required

Document feed and monitor volume of aspirate
Monitor fluid balance

Administer medication via the tube as prescribed
Remember:
- Most drugs are not licensed to be given via a nasogastric tube
- Drugs should not be added to feed
- Some drugs cannot be given within a certain frame of feed as absorption will be reduced, e.g. penicillin and phenytoin
- Avoid crushing tablets

Monitor patient's weight and monitor anthropometry: skinfold thickness and mid-arm muscle mass

Monitor blood glucose and electrolytes

Monitor bowel function:
- **In the event of constipation** conduct rectal examination as per policy and commence stool chart
- **In the event of diarrhoea** commence stool chart and take specimen for culture
Manage both conditions according to dietetic advice and local policy

Figure 23.2   Feeding tubes. *Source:* Finch (2018) with permission of John Wiley & Sons.

Before providing any care, it is imperative that registered nurses and nursing associates act in the best interests of patients at all time (see Box 23.1).

Orange Flag

Patients have a fundamental legal and ethical right to determine what happens to their own bodies. Valid consent to treatment is therefore absolutely central in all forms of healthcare

The most used enteral feeding tube in practice is a nasogastric tube (NG) (Dougherty and Lister, 2015). There is high risk of infection associated with central venous access and typically, PN will be administered centrally therefore recognised infection prevention and control guidelines should be used, particularly recognising that a dedicated lumen should be used for PN and any catheter manipulations should be considered a sterile procedure using Aseptic Non-Touch Technique (ANTT) procedures (EPIC3 Guidelines) (Loveday et al., 2014).

Glycaemic control

In health, blood glucose regulation is via the hormone's glucagon and insulin, which help to increase or reduce blood glucose levels, respectively. Hyperglycaemia is common in critical illness due to both the initial 'fight-or-flight' response,

Box 23.1   Acting in the best interest of the patient (*Source*: NMC, 2018).

4.1 balance the need to act in the best interests of people at all times with the requirement to respect a person's right to accept or refuse treatment
4.2 make sure that you get properly informed consent and document it before carrying out any action
4.3 keep to all relevant laws about mental capacity that apply in the country in which you are practising, and make sure that the rights and best interests of those who lack capacity are still at the centre of the decision-making process, and
4.4 tell colleagues, your manager and the person receiving care if you have a conscientious objection to a particular procedure and arrange for a suitably qualified colleague to take over responsibility for that person's care

and because of 'new' glucose formation from protein and fat in the presence of cortisol. Insulin is resistant to this new glucose and therefore secretion is inhibited, leading to a rise in blood glucose levels. Glycaemic control in critically ill patients is complex as blood sugar levels are not only raised a consequence of the stress response, but also as a direct result of the nutritional support received and some of the pharmacological therapies patients receive.

337

Examination scenario

The position of all nasogastric tubes must be confirmed after placement and before each use by aspiration and pH graded paper (with X-ray if necessary) as per the advice from the National Patient Safety Agency (further patient safety alerts for nasogastric tubes have also been issued in 2013 and 2016) (NICE Pathway, 2017) (see Figure 23.3).

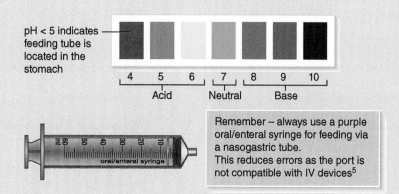

Figure 23.3   Confirmation of tube placement. *Source*: Finch (2018) with permission of John Wiley & Sons.

Medications management: insulin infusion

Elevated blood glucose in critically ill patients is a common clinical finding and is associated with increased mortality and poorer outcomes. The aetiology is multi-factorial occurring in both diabetic and non-diabetic patients. Endogenous cytokines and hormones such as cortisol and adrenaline reduce insulin production, increasing insulin resistance, promoting glycogenolysis and gluconeogenesis whilst impairing peripheral utilisation. Many critical care therapies such as exogenous steroids and catecholamines further exacerbate the situation. The NICE-SUGAR study (2009) indicate that overly aggressive glucose control with intravenous insulin results in worse outcomes than moderate control due to increased tendency to develop hypoglycaemia. Thus, critical care practitioners must be vigilant avoiding harmful hyper and hypoglycaemia.

Prior to a seminal study by Van den Burghe et al. (2001) proving that hyperglycaemia is associated with adverse effects notably increased mortality, a high glucose level was often left untreated. The Van den Burghe study led to the aggressive treatment of hyperglycaemia to maintain blood sugar levels of 80–110 mg/dL (4.4–6.1 mmols/L); however, the outcome of this was a higher incidence of hypoglycaemia. In 2009, the NICE-SUGAR study (NICE-SUGAR Study Investigators, 2009) concluded that a more modest approach to blood sugar control should be adopted. ASPEN (2016) recommend a target blood glucose range of 140–180 mg/dL for critically ill patients and within clinical practice; insulin therapy is usually initiated as a continuous infusion once the patients' glucose readings are above 180 mg/dL (10 mmols/L), in line with the NICE-SUGAR recommendations. Once insulin therapy has commenced, regular blood glucose monitoring should occur as per local trust protocols, with additional monitoring after changes to insulin infusion rate, during periods of nutritional therapy change (increase, decrease or temporary discontinuation), or at mealtimes for patients taking oral diet to allow for safe titration.

Refeeding syndrome

Starved or severely malnourished patients are at risk of refeeding syndrome when re-introducing nutrition to them. Refeeding syndrome is a serious condition that alters the electrolyte balance of cells and can be life-threatening. As nutrition is reintroduced, the body's demand for electrolytes and micronutrients increases therefore the patient might need supplements of potassium, phosphate, and magnesium (Martyn, 2011). NICE (2017) recommend that commencing feed at no more than 50% for the first 2 days of therapy could help to combat this risk.

Clinical investigations: biochemistry monitoring

Biochemical monitoring should be interpreted in a timely manner by health professionals with relevant expertise. Patients at risk of refeeding syndrome should be monitored daily with correction of electrolytes as needed. See Table 23.1.

Table 23.1 Biochemistry Monitoring. *Source: BAPEN, 2016.*

Sodium Urea Creatinine	Daily until stable then as clinically indicated	Assess fluid status Detect electrolyte or metabolic abnormalities Assess renal function
Potassium Phosphate Magnesium Corrected calcium	Daily if refeeding risk; then three times a week until stable; then as clinically indicated.	To detect electrolyte/metabolic abnormalities Monitor for refeeding syndrome
Glucose	Baseline then twice daily if indicated	To ensure optimum glycaemic control
Liver function tests	Baseline then weekly until stable then as needed	To detect overfeeding
C-reactive protein	Twice weekly until stable	To assess acute phase response and assist interpretation of protein and micronutrient results
Albumin	Weekly until stable then as clinical concern	Aids interpretation of minerals. Low albumin reflects disease not protein status

(Continued)

Table 23.1 (Continued)

Full blood count	Twice weekly until stable then as clinically indicated	To monitor for infection and anaemia
Zinc Copper Selenium	When clinically indicated.	Deficiency common with increased losses but results can be difficult to interpret as altered by disease, infection and trauma
Folate B12	Baseline if indicated and if clinical concern	Deficiency common in certain disease states
Vitamin D	6 monthly on long-term nutrition or if deficiency suspected	Often low in housebound patients

---

Medicines management: thiamine (Pabrinex)

Vitamins B and C are important for several bodily functions including releasing energy from food and in the formation of healthy skin, bones and teeth. Pabrinex Intravenous High Potency, Concentrate for Solution for Infusion ('Pabrinex IVHP') provides additional vitamins B and C to correct deficiencies that may have occurred, for example:

- In alcoholism
- After infections
- After operations
- In certain psychiatric states.

The product is also used to maintain levels of vitamins B and C in patients who are on long-term intermittent haemodialysis.

Discontinuing feed

When discontinuing EN or PN, the ability of the patient to consume enough nutrients must be considered. To help with this assessment a multidisciplinary team (MDT) approach (including the patient, where appropriate) should be adopted and review by a dietician should take place. Referral to the Speech and Language Therapy team should be considered for any patient where a concern about their ability to swallow exists. Examples of this are patients that have had an endotracheal or tracheostomy tube in place, those with neurological deficits and patients with muscular dystrophies.

Red Flag

Dysphagia (difficulty in swallowing), refers to the transit of food and liquid as well as oral secretions from the pharynx to the stomach. It may be complicated by aspiration pneumonia. Recurrent or chronic dysphagia may affect nutrition, leading to weight loss. The condition can occur in up to 10% of the general population over the age of 50 years; the incidence is considerably higher in people over 65 years of age (Kochhar, 2018).

It can be useful to leave any feeding tubes in place when a patient first commences oral diet and fluids until you are confident that sufficient calorie and protein intake is achieved. If nutritional intake is inadequate, overnight nutritional support can be used to ensure nutritional goals are met. When discontinuing feed, caution must be used with any glycaemic control measures in place, as continuation of insulin therapy during this period could result in hypoglycaemia.

Nutritional guidance

There is a wide variety of literature surrounding nutrition for the critically ill, however few extensive primary research studies exist. Of the research studies that do exist, variable control and sample size make them difficult to interpret (NICE, 2017; Schetz et al., 2013; Scottish Intensive Care Society (SICS), 2016). Preiser et al., (2014) summarise that the reported consequences of malnutrition in critical illness include impaired immune function; increased length of stay; muscle weakness; prolonged recovery times (approximately 4 additional days); more ventilator-dependent days (up to a 19% increase); and increased morbidity and mortality. This highlights the significance of getting nutritional therapy right.

Critical care practices in the UK are largely influenced by the ICS and the SICS however their recommendations do vary. The nutritional practice guidance from ICS is limited to the Core Standards for ICUs (2019). The Core Standards provide little guidance to management of nutrition within critical care but their recommendations for service provision of dieticians in the management of critically ill patients is underpinned by NICE and ASPEN guidelines; however, both underpinning guidelines have been revised since the publication of the Core Standards. The Scottish Intensive Care Society (SICS, 2016) have produced key recommendations for nutritional management of patients in critical care units in Scotland based on guidelines produced by the Canadian Critical Care Network and the European Society for Parenteral and Enteral Nutrition (ESPEN). Box 23.2 contains the key recommendations from SICS and the latest ASPEN bundle statement as a source of reference.

Box 23.2   Key recommendations for nutritional management of patients in critical care units (*Source:* Adapted ASPEN 2016; Scottish Intensive Care Society 2016).

- Nurses should assess patients for nutrition risk on admission to critical care, and calculate their energy and protein requirements to determine the aims of nutritional support.
- Scottish Intensive Care Society (2016) guidelines state that patients who are critically ill should be fed, preferably enterally, within 24 hours of admission to critical care, while the American Society for Parenteral and Enteral Nutrition (ASPEN) (2016) guidelines state that enteral nutrition should be initiated within 24–48 hours, and that the target nutrition levels should be increased over the first week of their stay.
- Measures to improve the delivery of enteral feed should be employed as soon as possible if nasogastric feeding proves inadequate, for example by using a prokinetic drug (a drug that improves gastric motility) or post-pyloric feeding (enteral feeding but with the tube reaching the small bowel).
- Steps should be taken as required to reduce the risk of aspiration or improve the patient's tolerance to gastric feeding, for example by using a prokinetic drug, continuous infusion or chlorhexidine mouthwash. Patients should be nursed at a 30–45-degree angle with their head elevated, to reduce the risk of aspiration.
- If enteral feeding is not successful or is contraindicated, parenteral nutrition should be considered in patients who are high risk or malnourished.
- Every effort should be made to avoid breaks in the delivery of nutritional support, since achieving calorific targets is challenging even in stable patients in critical care.
- The placement of a patient's nasogastric tube should be checked regularly. Scottish Intensive Care Society (2016) guidelines state that gastric residual volumes (GRVs) of 250 mL should be tolerated as part of a feeding protocol, while the ASPEN (2016) guidelines state that GRV should not be used as part of routine care to monitor patients in critical care who are receiving enteral nutrition

Examination Scenario

The initial placement of post-pyloric tubes should be confirmed with an abdominal X-ray (unless placed radiologically). Agreed protocols setting out the necessary clinical checks need to be in place before this procedure is carried out (NICE Pathway, 2017).

Conclusion

Providing nutritional support for patients who are critically ill can be complex, because of the variety of potential clinical presentations. It is important that screening and assessment of the nutritional status of these patients is undertaken on admission to critical care, then on a weekly basis and/or if there are significant changes to their clinical condition. Early assessment of nutritional status enables appropriate nutritional interventions to be undertaken that provide energy for cell repair, as well as preventing muscle wastage and premature fat breakdown. Nurses must work with other members of the multidisciplinary team, providing appropriate nutritional support for patients who are critically ill, following local policies and practising within their own scope of practice (NMC, 2018).

Take home points

1. Nutritional status and risk should be assessed on admission, and energy, protein and micronutrient needs determined by a clinician with appropriate specialist training or experience.
2. It is recommended that nutrition support (PN if EN is not possible) should be instigated within 48 hours in patients expected not to be on a full oral diet within three days.
3. Nutritional intake targets should be set and compared daily with actual intake.
4. Efforts need not be made to cover full energy targets with EN or PN until clinical stability has been achieved.
5. The energy content from certain drugs (e.g. propofol, IV glucose and citrate anti-coagulation renal replacement therapy) should be accounted for to avoid overfeeding.
6. Feeding plans should be adjusted for those with a BMI greater than 30 kg/m² according to international guidelines.
7. Volume-based or 'catch up' feeding should be used to allow nursing staff to adjust the hourly infusion rate of EN to optimise delivery after interruptions.

8. There should be access to nasal bridles to secure NGTs in agitated patients and guidelines for their use and aftercare.
9. Nutrition support targets should be included in the rehabilitation of critically ill patients.
10. There should be bowel management guidelines which include:
    a. regular monitoring and documentation of bowel habits (frequency and type)
    b. minimising the use of drugs that can cause constipation or diarrhoea
    c. the need for rectal examinations and treating faecal loading/impaction
    d. when to use laxatives, enemas, and suppositories
    e. management of ileus.

References

ASPEN – American Society for Parenteral and Enteral Nutrition. (2016). Guidelines for the Provision and Assessment of Nutrition Support Therapy in the Adult Critically Ill Patient. *Society of Critical Care Medicine (SCCM) and American Society for Parenteral and Enteral Nutrition (A.S.P.E.N.)*. http://www.nutritioncare.org/Guidelines_and_Clinical_Resources/Clinical_Guidelines/ (accessed 20 May 2020).

BAPEN (2016). Enteral Feed Monitoring. https://www.bapen.org.uk/nutrition-support/enteral-nutrition/enteral-feed-monitoring (accessed 20 May 2020).

Berger, M. and Pichard, C. (2014). Development and current use of parenteral nutrition in critical care – an opinion paper. *Critical Care* 18(4). doi: 10.1186/s13054-014-0478-0.

Casaer, M. and Van den Berghe, G. (2014). Nutrition in the acute phase of critical illness. *The New England Journal of Medicine* 370(13): 1227–1236. doi: 10.1056/NEJMra1304623.

Chowdhury, R. and Lobaz, S. (2019). Nutrition in critical care. *BJA* 19(3): 90–95. https://bjaed.org/article/S2058-5349(18)30155-0/fulltext (accessed 19 May 2020).

Cove, M.E. and Pinsky, M.R. (2011). Early or late parenteral nutrition: ASPEN vs. ESPEN. *Critical Care* 15(6): 317. doi: 10.1186/cc10591.

Critical Care Networks-National Nurse Leads (CC3N) (2015). National Competency Framework for Registered Nurses in Adult Critical Care. Step 2 Competencies. https://www.cc3n.org.uk/uploads/9/8/4/2/98425184/02_new_step_2_final.pdf (accessed 20 May 2020).

Desai, S., McClave, S., and Rice, T. (2013). Nutrition in the ICU. An evidence-based approach. *Chest* 145(5): 1148–1157. doi: 10.1378/chest.13-1158.

Dougherty, L. and Lister S. (2015). *The Royal Marsden Manual of Clinical Nursing Procedures*, professional edition, 9e. Oxford: Wiley Blackwell.

Dutton, H. and Finch, J. (2018). *Acute and Critical Care Nursing at a Glance*. Wiley Blackwell.

Faculty of Intensive Care Medicine (FICM) and Intensive Care Society (ICS) (2019). Guidelines for the Provision of Intensive Care Services, 2e. https://www.ficm.ac.uk/sites/default/files/gpics_v2_-_version_for_release_-_final2019.pdf (accessed 20 May 2020).

Frankenfield, D. and Ashcraft, C. (2011). Estimating Energy Needs in Nutrition Support Patients. *Journal of Parenteral and Enteral Nutrition* 35(5): 563–570. doi: 10.1177/0148607111415859.

Galgani, J. and Ravussin, E. (2008). Energy metabolism, fuel selection and body weight regulation. *International Journal of Obesity* 32(S7): 109–119. doi: 10.1038/ijo.2008.246.

Harvey, S., Parrott, F., Harrison, D. et al. (2016). A multicentre, randomised controlled trial comparing the clinical effectiveness and cost-effectiveness of early nutritional support via the parenteral versus the enteral route in critically ill patients (CALORIES). *National Institute for Health Research* doi: https://dx.doi.org/10.3310/hta20280.

Heyland, D., Schroter-Noppe, D., Drover, J. et al. (2003). Nutrition support in the critical care setting: Current practice in canadian ICUs – opportunities for improvement? *JPEN. Journal of Parenteral and Enteral Nutrition* 27(1): 74–83.

Hinson, J., Raven, P., and Chew, S. (2010). *The Endocrine System*, 2e. Edinburgh: Churchill Livingstone Elsevier.

Kochhar, S. (2018). Red Flag Symptoms: *Dysphagia*. https://www.gponline.com/red-flag-symptoms-dysphagia/gi-dyspepsia/article/1319820 (accessed 20 May 2020).

Loveday, H.P., Wilson, J.A., Pratt, R.J. et al. (2014). Epic3: National evidence-based guidelines for preventing healthcare-associated infections in NHS hospitals in England. *Journal of Hospital Infection* 86: S1–S70. doi: 10.1016/s0195-6701(13)60012-2.

Marieb, E. (2015). Essentials of Human Anatomy and Physiology. 11th Edn. Pearson Education Limited: Essex.

Martyn, K. (2011). Gastrointestinal tract. In: *Care of the Acutely Ill Adult: An Essential Guide for Nurses* (ed. F. Creed and C. Spiers), 165–204. Oxford: Oxford University Press.

Mehanna, H.M., Moledina, J., and Travis, J. (2008). Refeeding syndrome: What it is, and how to prevent and treat it. *Clinical Review* 336(7659): 1495–1498. doi: 10.1136/bmj.a301.

Montejo, J., Minambres, E., Bordeje, L. et al. (2010). Gastric residual volume during enteral nutrition in ICU patients: the REGANE study. *Intensive Care Medicine* 36(8): 1386–1393. doi: 10.1007/s00134-010-1856-y.

National Patient Safety Agency (NPSA) (2011). Patient Safety Alert NPSA/2011/PSA002: Reducing the harm caused by misplaced nasogastric feeding tubes in adults, children, and infants. http://www.nrls.npsa.nhs.uk/alerts/?entryid45=129640 (accessed 20 May 2020).

NICE Pathway (2017). *Enteral tube feeding*. http://pathways.nice.org.uk/pathways/nutrition-support-in-adults (accessed 20 May 2020).

NICE (2017). *Nutrition Support for Adults: Oral Nutrition Support, Enteral Tube Feeding and Parenteral Nutrition*. https://www.nice.org.uk/guidance/cg32 (accessed 20 May 2020).

NICE (2012). *Nutrition Support in Adults*. https://www.nice.org.uk/guidance/qs24/chapter/Quality-statement-1-Screening-for-the-risk-of-malnutrition (accessed 20 May 2020).

NICE-SUGAR Study Investigators (2009). Intensive versus conventional glucose control in critically ill patients. *New England Journal of Medicine* 360(13): 1283–1297. doi: 10.1056/nejmoa0810625.

NMC (2018). The Code. Professional Standards of Practice and Behaviour for Nurses, Midwives and Nursing Associates. https://www.nmc.org.uk/globalassets/sitedocuments/nmc-publications/nmc-code.pdf (accessed 23 May 2020).

Ozen, N., Tosun, N., Yamanel, L. et al. (2016). Evaluation of the effect on patient parameters of not monitoring gastric residual volume in intensive care patients on a mechanical ventilator receiving enteral nutrition: A randomized clinical trial. *Journal of Critical Care* 33: 137–144. doi: 10.1016/j.jcrc.2016.01.028.

341

Preiser, J-C., Ichai, C., Orban, J-C and Groeneveld, A. (2014). Metabolic response to the stress of critical illness. *British Journal of Anaesthesia* 14(4): 945–954. doi: 10.1093/bja/aeu187.

Rahman, A., Hasan, R., Agarwala, R. et al. (2016). Identifying critically-ill patients who will benefit most from nutritional therapy: Further validation of the 'modified NUTRIC' nutritional risk tool. *Clinical Nutrition* 35(1): 158–162.

Ramprasad, R. and Kapoor, M.C. (2012). Nutrition in intensive care. *Journal of Anaesthesiology Clinical Pharmacology* 28(1): 1. doi: 10.4103/0970-9185.92401.

Reignier, J., Mercier, E., Le Gouge, A. et al. (2013). Effect of Not Monitoring Residual Gastric Volume on Risk of Ventilator-Associated Pneumonia in Adults Receiving Mechanical Ventilation and Early Enteral Feeding: a randomized controlled trial. *Journal of the American Medical Association* 309(3): 249–256. doi: 10.1001/jama.2012.196377.

Rutledge, K. and Nesbitt, I. (2013). Assessment and support of hydration and nutrition status and care. In: *Critical Care Manual of Clinical Procedures and Competencies* (ed. J. Mallett, J. Albarran, and R. Richardson), 277–307. Chichester: Wiley Blackwell.

Schetz, M., Casaer, M., and Van den Berghe, G. (2013). Does artificial nutrition improve outcome of critical illness? *Critical Care* 14(1) 302. doi: 10.1186/cc11828.

Scottish Intensive Care Society (SICS) (2016). Nutritional Guidelines. http://www.scottishintensivecare.org.uk/quality-improvement/sics-nutrition-group/sics-nutritional-guidelines/ (accessed 20 May 2020).

Singer, P., Reintam, A., Blaser, M. et al. (2019). ESPEN guidelines on enteral nutrition in the intensive care unit. *Clinical Nutrition* 25(2): 210–223. doi: doi: 10.1016/j.clnu.2018.08.037

Tatsumi, H. (2019). Enteral tolerance in critically ill patients. *J Intensive Care* 7: 30. doi: 10.1186/s40560-019-0378-0 (accessed 20 May 2020).

Tortora, G. and Derrickson, B. (2017). *Principles of Anatomy and Physiology. Organization, Support and Movement, and Control Systems of the Human Body*, 15e. Global Edition. Wiley: Asia.

Van den Berghe, G., Wouters, P., Weekers F. et al. (2001). Intensive insulin therapy in critically ill patients. *New England Journal of Medicine* 345:1359–1367.

Woodrow, P. (2018). *Intensive Care Nursing: A Framework for Practice*, 4e. London: Taylor & Francis.

World Health Organization (WHO) (2015). Healthy Diet. http://www.who.int/mediacentre/factsheets/fs394/en/ (accessed 20 May 2020).

Yancey, V. (2016). Psychosocial and spiritual alterations and management. In: *Priorities in Critical Care Nursing*, 7e (ed. L. Urden., K. Stacy, and and M. Lough), 30–40. St. Louis: Elsevier Mosby.

Chapter 24

Renal critical care

Alexandra Gatehouse and Sadie Diamond-Fox

Aim

The aim of this chapter is to provide the reader with an introduction to the anatomy and physiology of the renal system, explore both acute and chronic renal failure with emphasis upon management encountered in critical care clinical practice.

Learning outcomes

After reading this chapter the reader will be able to:

- Have gained an understanding of the key aspects of renal anatomy and physiology.
- Have gained an understanding of the definition, classification, pathophysiology, clinical features and examination, investigations and management of acute kidney injury.
- Have gained an understanding of specific disorders associated with AKI and drug toxicity.
- Have gained an understanding of CKD and its management.
- Understand the key principles, indications, modalities, dosing and safety considerations of renal replacement therapy.

Test your prior knowledge

- Describe the principle anatomy and functions of the renal system.
- Name four causes of AKI.
- Discuss chronic renal failure and its clinical manifestations.
- List the different types of renal replacement therapy and discuss how they differ.

Fundamentals of Critical Care: A Textbook for Nursing and Healthcare Students, First Edition. Edited by Ian Peate and Barry Hill.
© 2023 John Wiley & Sons Ltd. Published 2023 by John Wiley & Sons Ltd.
Companion website: www.wiley.com/go/peate/criticalcare

Introduction

Renal disease encompasses a wide range of reduced kidney function because of an acute or chronic insult and is a general umbrella term that can encompass disease terminology such as acute kidney injury (AKI), chronic kidney disease (CKD) and end-stage renal disease (ESRD). Within the United Kingdom (UK) approximately 1 in 10 of the general population are affected by renal disease, with people from black, Asian and minority ethnic communities five times more likely to experience kidney failure in their lifetime (Kidney Research UK, 2018). Mortality from the subtype of renal disease AKI show that in-hospital deaths have increased in all age groups from 5,107 registered deaths in 2001 (where AKI was either the underlying cause, or a contributory factor toward death) to 12,822 in 2016 (Office for National Statistics, 2018). Critically ill patients who develop AKI are twice as likely to die in hospital (Girling et al., 2020). This chapter will introduce the reader to some of the pertinent anatomy, physiology and pathophysiology of the renal system, along with an introduction to some of the commonly-usedinterventions and relevant clinical considerations,with case studies used to bring together theory and practice.

Step 2 competencies: national standards

Elements of the following Critical Care Networks-National Nurse Leads (CC3N) (2015) competencies are covered within this chapter:

2.3.1 – Anatomy and Physiology (Renal System)
2.3.2 – Renal Replacement Therapy
2:8.1 – Renal disease and patterns of recovery

Anatomy and physiology of the renal tract

Anatomy and physiology of the renal tract is complicated, and as such it is beyond the scope of this chapter to explore this subject in depth. Further information on this subject can be found in O'Callaghan (2017) and Peate and Nair (2017).The reader is also encouraged to consider utilising e-learning modules 'e-ICM' that map directly to CC3N competencies (Health Education England and Faculty of Intensive Care Medicine, 2020).

The main function of the kidneys is maintenance of homeostasis (physiological stability) through excretory, regulatory and metabolic mechanisms. A summary of all functions can be found in Table 24.1. Figure 24.1 also details the multiple factors that influence renal function and the complex and mutual biological communication between the kidney and other distant organs (organ crosstalk).

Table 24.1 Summary of the functions of the kidney (Peate and Nair, 2017, John Wiley & Sons).

Regulation of electrolytes – help to regulate ions such as sodium, potassium, calcium, chloride and phosphate ions
Regulation of blood pH – excrete hydrogen ions into the urine and conserve bicarbonate ions, thus helping to regulate pH of blood
Regulation of blood volume – by conserving or eliminating water in the urine
Secretes renin (regulates blood pressure) and erythropoietin (production of ref blood cells)
Production of calcitriol for the regulation of calcium level
Aids in regulation of blood glucose level by gluconeogenesis
Detoxification of free radicals and drugs
Excrection of waste products, such as urea, uric acid and creatinine

Vascular supply

The renal system comprises the kidneys, the ureters, the urinary bladder and the urethra. Each kidney receives its blood supply via a renal artery arising from the aorta, and filters approximately 1200 mL of blood per minute (~25% cardiac output) which then flows into the renal vein and consequently the inferior vena cava. Vascular resistance is mainly controlled by the afferent and efferent arterioles. Renin-producing granular cells (RPGC) within the afferent arterioles of the juxtaglomerular apparatus release the enzyme renin in response to several physiological responses:

1. ß-1 adrenergic receptor stimulation on granular cells
2. A fall in angiotensin II levels
3. Decreased afferent arteriolar pressure
4. Decreased renal tubular fluid flow rate
5. A fall in tubular sodium and chloride concentration at the macula densa

(see Figure 24.2; O'Callaghan, 2017).

There are multiple other regulatory mechanisms that ensure adequate perfusion of the kidney, these include; the renin-angiotensin-aldosterone system (RASS); myogenic reflex, tubuloglomerular feedback, prostaglandins vasoactive peptides (such as bradykinin, atrial natriuretic peptide and anti-diuretic hormone); sympathetic nervous system innovation and dopamine.

Renin-angiotensin-aldosterone system (RASS)

Under normal physiological circumstances, baroreceptors in the carotid body and aortic arch detect a fall in blood pressure, producing sympathetic stimulation and so vasoconstriction globally, as well as of the glomerular efferent arteriole. The therenin-angiotensin-aldosterone system (RAAS) is activated, and adaptations occur to compensate for changes in renal perfusion, allowing regulation of blood flow and GFR (see Figure 24.3).

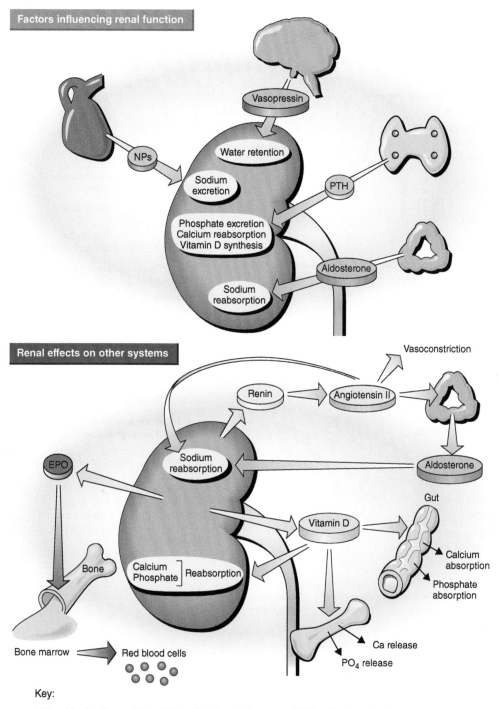

Factors influencing renal function

Renal effects on other systems

Key:

NPs = Natriuretic peptides, PTH = Parathyroid hormone, EPO = Erythropoietin

Figure 24.1 Factors influencing renal function and renal-organ cross talk. *Source:* O'Callaghan (2017) used with permission from John Wiley & Sons.

The nephrons

The nephrons are the functional units of the kidney and they consist of several segments including: the Bowman's capsule, the glomerulus, the proximal convoluted tubule, the Loop of Henle, the distal convoluted tubule, and the collecting ducts. The function of the nephron is filtration, selective reabsorption and excretion through various transport processes. Table 24.2 outlines the functions of the segments of the nephron. Urine formed by the kidney passes from the collecting duct to the renal pelvis via the papillary duct in the renal pyramid, minor calyx, and major calyx. The structure is depicted in Figure 24.4. Peristalsis facilitates the movement of urine along the ureter into the bladder. Each segment of the nephron presents an opportunity for targeted therapies within critical care and this will be discussed in subsequent sections of the chapter.

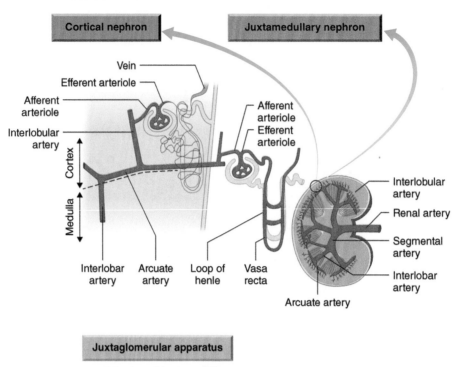

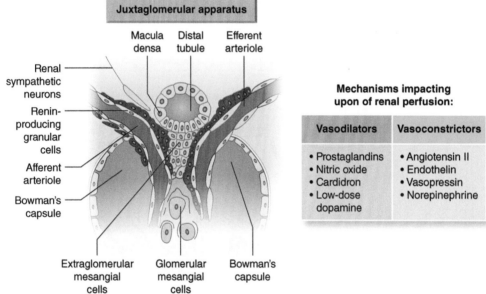

Figure 24.2   The structure of the vascular supply to the kidney and nephron. *Source:* O'Callaghan (2017) used with permission from John Wiley & Sons.

Control of plasma osmolality

Plasma osmolality concerns the solute particles (Na+, K+) present within the blood (a solution) per kilogram of solution. It is maintained within narrow limits (275–295 mOsm/kg) by several mechanisms (see Figure 24.5) and determines the direction of fluid. Water will flow from a fluid compartment with low osmolality to a compartment of high osmolality, if the membrane between the two compartments is permeable to water (Shah and Mandiga, 2020), as is the case across plasma membranes of human cells. A cells permeability to water differs depending upon its lipid bilayer and

presence of aquaporins and other channels and carriers. Optimal osmolality is crucial for the creation of cellular homeostasis, ion gradients between intracellular and interstitial fluid and subsequent action potential generation.

Electrolyte balance

The renal system plays an essential role in maintenance of homeostasis, controlling fluid, electrolyte and acid-base balance. Figure 24.6 details the various points along the nephron in which electrolyte and water exchange occurs and the targets at which various hormones and drugs act. Renal disease, either acute or chronic, may affect all these

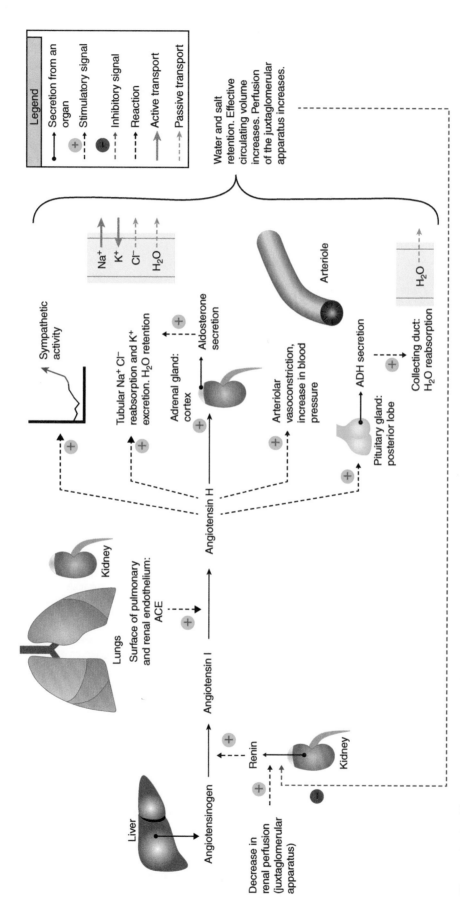

Figure 24.3 The Renin–angiotensin–aldosterone system – the hormones and their effects. *Source:* https://commons.wikimedia.org/wiki/File:Renin-angiotensin-aldosterone_system.svg / Wikipedia / CC BY SA 4.0.

Table 24.2 Functions of the segments of the nephron.

Segment	Function	Types of cell	Transport process
Glomerulus and Bowman's Capsule	Filtration of plasma – allows passage of: • Water • Glucose • Vitamins • Very small plasma proteins • Amino acids • Urea • Ions • Ammonia	• Glomerular capillaries – endothelial cells • Basement membrane – combination of collagen fibres and glycoproteins • Bowman's capsule – podocytes	• Filtration due to high hydrostatic pressure within the afferent and efferent arterioles • Dependent upon molecular size • Glomerular filtration – large fenestrations, passage of all solutes except red blood cells and platelets • Basement membrane – negatively charged, repels negatively charged plasma proteins • Bowman's capsule filtration – filtration slits between foot-like projections of the podocytes
Proximal convoluted tubule (PCT)	• Accounts for approximately 60–70% of all reabsorption • Includes sodium (Na$^+$), potassium (K$^+$), calcium (Ca^{2+}), magnesium (Mg^{2+}), chloride (Cl$^-$), glucose, phosphate (PO^{4-}), urea, water and bicarbonate (HCO$_3^-$) • Excretion of hydrogen ions (H$^+$), ammonium ions, creatinine, uric acid and drug metabolites	Simple cuboidal epithelial cells with microvilli (increased surface area)	• Electrochemical gradient – sodium hydrogen (Na$^+$-H$^+$) antiporter, sodium reabsorbed into the cells from tubular filtrate • Osmosis – PCT highly permeable to water, water moves into the cells from the tubular filtrate due to the movement of Na$^+$ • Passive diffusion – of Cl$^-$, K$^+$, Ca^{2+} and urea from the tubular filtrate into the cell • Cotransport – glucose, phosphate, amino acids with sodium
Loop of Henle	• Reabsorption of approximately 15% of water, 20–30% of sodium, potassium and chloride, 10–20% of bicarbonate, variable amounts of calcium and magnesium	• Descending limb and thin ascending limb – simple squamous epithelial cells • Thick ascending limb – simple cuboidal to low columnar epithelial cells	• Generation of a concentration gradient through: • Descending loop – impermeable to solute but permeable to water, aquaporins • Thick ascending loop: – impermeable to water but permeable to ions – Na$^+$, K$^+$, Ca^{2+}, Mg^{2+} – Na$^=$-K$^+$-Cl$^-$ symporter
Distal convoluted	• Active reabsorption of 4–8% of sodium and chloride • Secretion of potassium • Selectively reabsorbs water • Regulation of calcium ions • Regulates pH by absorbing bicarbonate and secreting hydrogen ions	Simple cuboidal epithelial cells	• Sodium channels in principal cells (ENaC) increase reabsorption • Antidiuretic hormone (ADH) causes insertion of water channels (aquaporins) into the membrane • K$^+$ channels and K$^+$-Cl$^-$ cotransporter with increased tubular flow contribute to potassium excretion • Parathyroid hormone (PTH) activates Ca^{2+} channels, 1,25-dihydroxycholecalciferol triggers an active Ca^{2+} channel
Collecting ducts	• 2–5% of sodium reabsorption coupled with potassium and hydrogen ion secretion	Simple cuboidal epithelial cells – principal cells and intercalated cells	• Sodium channels • Hydrogen ion transporter • Aquaporins

348

processes. Fluid balance refers to the distribution of body fluid within the intracellular and extracellular (interstitial and intravascular) compartments. Total body volume, and therefore total body water, is regulated within a narrow range, through alteration of sodium and water content (O'Callaghan, 2017; Peate and Nair, 2017).

Inappropriate renal handling of sodium may occur due to a primary renal problem or due to an abnormality in the volume regulation mechanism. Renal tubulointerstitial disease and Addison's disease (deficiency of the hormone aldosterone) both cause excessive sodium excretion, whilst primary hyperaldosteronism, renal failure or oedema syndromes (liver disease, congestive heart failure, nephrotic syndrome) result in inadequate sodium excretion (O'Callaghan, 2017). The underlying cause should be identified and treated; however, pharmacotherapy manipulation of renal sodium using diuretics may be useful (see Chapter 11).

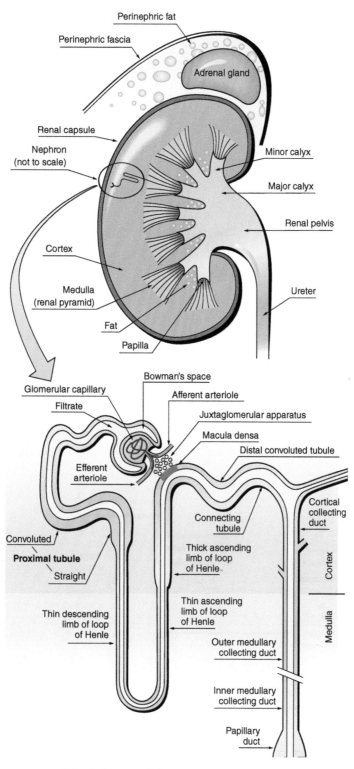

Figure 24.4 The internal structure of the kidney and the nephron. *Source:* O'Callaghan (2009) John Wiley & Sons.

Potassium is integral to the maintenance of an electro-chemical gradient across the cell membrane, and the ability of nerves and muscle to create an action potential. Hypoka-laemia and hyperkalaemia are life-threatening, causing cardiac dysrhythmias and potentially cardiac arrest, and the kidneys and adrenal glands are vital in the maintenance of potassium homeostasis.

Learning event: reflection

Reflect on how much you understand about the electrolyte concentrations of fluid prescriptions prescribed by the medical and non-medical prescriber professionals on critical care.

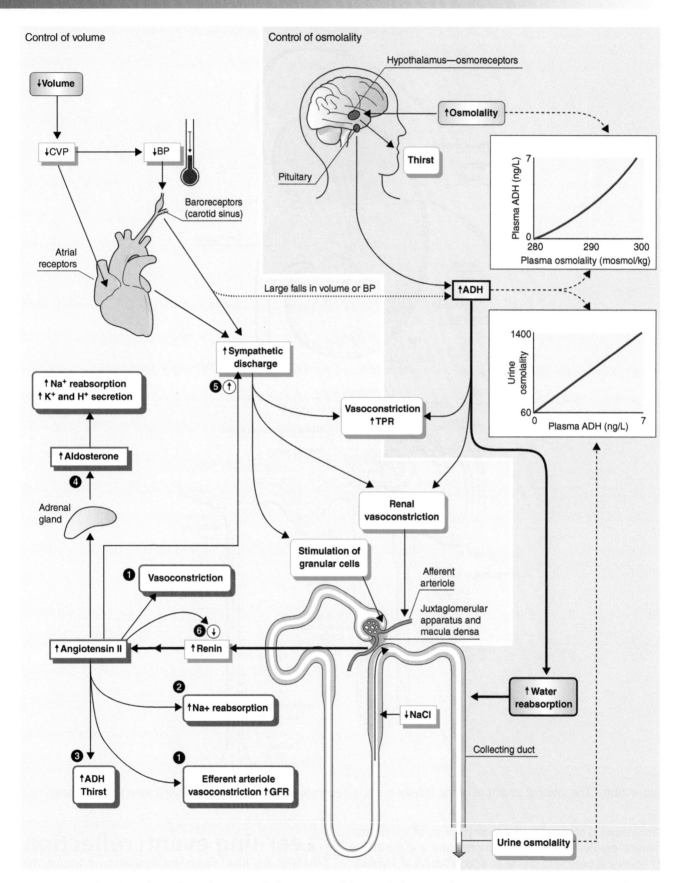

Figure 24.5 The physiological mechanisms of plasma osmolality and plasma volume maintenance. *Source:* Ward and Linden (2017) John Wiley & Sons.

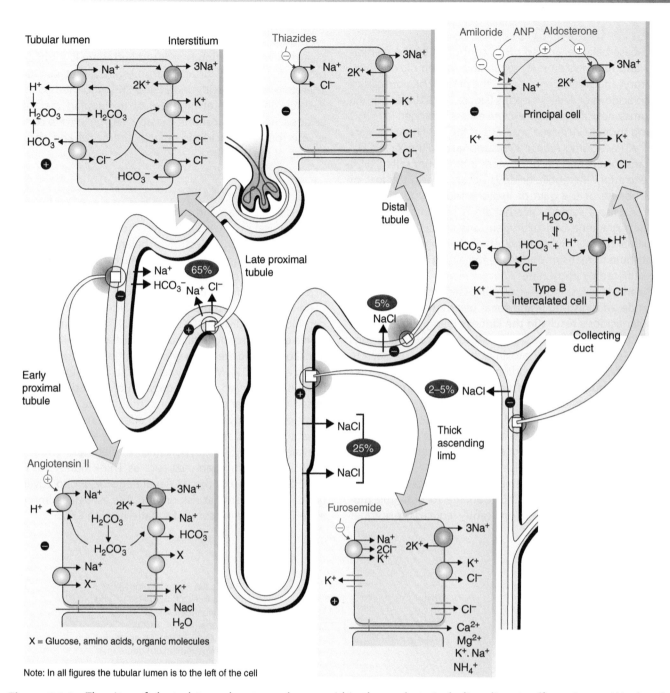

Figure 24.6 The sites of electrolyte and water exchange within the nephron including diuretic effects. *Source:* Ward and Linden (2017) John Wiley & Sons.

Calcium and phosphate are inextricably linked and are essential to the maintenance of bone density. They are regulated by one of several mechanisms including gut reabsorption, bone reabsorption and renal handling. Calcium is regulated by the thyroid gland, and when levels fall, parathyroid hormone (PTH) stimulates bone reabsorption (release of calcium and phosphate from bone), increases Vitamin D synthesis, increases renal phosphate excretion and increases renal calcium reabsorption. Vitamin D is synthesised within the kidney, increasing phosphate and calcium levels via reabsorption through the gut, bones and renal tubules. In renal failure bone disease can be caused by Vitamin D deficiency and renal phosphate retention. Due to lack of gut reabsorption and the formation of calcium phosphate deposits (due to hyperphosphataemia), the fall in calcium stimulates PTH, triggering further bone reabsorption and eventually hyperparathyroidism. Pharmacotherapy aims to maintain normal calcium and phosphate levels, preventing hyperparathyroidism, bone pain, poorly mineralised bone and soft tissue deposits as typically seen in chronic kidney disease.

Acid-base balance

Acid-base balance, and so pH, is controlled by the respiratory and renal systems. By regulating carbon dioxide (respiratory) and bicarbonate (renal) the pH may be normalised when acidosis or alkalosis occurs (Figure 24.7). Under normal circumstances the kidneys excrete excess hydrogen ions (H^+) or acid through increased synthesis of the Na^+-H^+ exchangers or H^+ ATPase pump, reabsorb bicarbonate via the Na^+-HCO_3^- cotransporters and produce more ammonium salts (NH_4^+) for excretion. Metabolic acidosis occurs due to the loss of bicarbonate or the gain of hydrogen ions. Under normal circumstances sodium bicarbonate is reabsorbed, via the sodium gradient, and hydrogen ions are secreted in the proximal tubule. In the distal tubule, hydrogen ions either contribute to reabsorption of the remaining bicarbonate or are buffered by phosphate.

Bicarbonate loss is caused by gut losses, increased sodium chloride administration and renal bicarbonate loss. Renal tubular acidosis results in the kidneys being either unable to excrete hydrogen ions and reabsorb bicarbonate ions due to disorders of the proximal tubule (rare) or secrete hydrogen ions or absorb sodium ions due to secretory, permeability and voltage defects as well as hypoaldosteronism in the distal tubule (O'Callaghan, 2017). The gain of hydrogen ions occurs in lactic acidosis, ketoacidosis, poisoning and renal failure. In renal disease the kidneys are unable to effectively perform these processes and so metabolic acidosis occurs causing hyperkalaemia, due to H^+ moving into cells and driving K^+ out. Metabolic acidosis becomes more common with advancing CKD. Damage to both the glomerulus and renal tubules significantly reduces the number of functioning nephrons and as CKD progresses ammonia excretion is impaired (less hydrogen ions are excreted), bicarbonate absorption is reduced and there is insufficient production of renal bicarbonate (Adamczak et al., 2018). Therefore, patients with underlying CKD who then go on to develop an AKI are at high risk of developing metabolic acidosis. Renal replacement therapy may be used to correct severe metabolic acidosis in both the acute and chronic setting of renal failure.

Renal failure

Renal disease is vast and complex, with the common pathophysiological processes including the inability to maintain fluid, acid-base and electrolyte balance. It is beyond the scope of this chapter to discuss all of these conditions, however, those commonly seen within critical care will be explored in the following sections.

Renal disease encompasses acute kidney injury (AKI) and chronic kidney disease (CKD). In the UK, approximately one in five emergency hospital admissions have an AKI and over 3 million people are living with CKD (Kidney Care UK, 2020; Wang et al., 2012). Mortality rates could be reduced, kidney function preserved, and progression of renal disease minimised with fewer complications through the correct treatment of AKI, early detection and effective management of renal conditions, as well as other diseases implicated in the prevalence of CKD (hypertension, diabetes) (NCEPOD, 2009). National programmes, such as 'Think Kidneys', as well as NHS England and the UK Renal Registry, aim to advance the care of patients at risk or with AKI, as well as improve experiences and outcomes for patients with CKD.

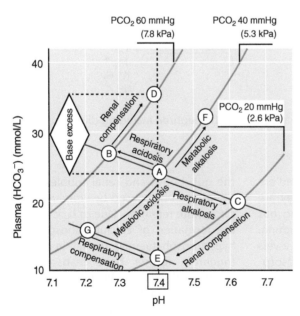

The line BAC is the buffer line for whole blood: changes in PCO_2 alter HCO_3^- and pH along this line. Point A represents normal conditions (pH 7.4. HCO_3^- 24 mmol/L, PCO_2 5.3 kPa). An acute rise in PCO_2 (e.g. hypoventilation) decreases the HCO_3^-; PCO_2 ratio and hence pH. This respiratory acidosis is represented by a move from A to B. A to C represents a respiratory alkalosis (e.g. hyperventilation). Sustained respiratory acidosis (e.g. chronic respiratory failure) is compensated for by renal HCO_3^- reabsorption and H^+ excretion. The HCO_3^-: PCO_2 ratio is restored and pH returns to normal. This renal compensation is described by the arrow B to D. Conversely a respiratory alkalosis may be compensated for by increased renal excretion of HCO_3^- (C to E). Metabolic acidosis (G) may be partially compensated by increased ventilation and a reduction in PCO_2 (G to E). There is little respiratory compensation of metabolic alkalosis (F).

Figure 24.7 Acid base balance, disorders and compensation. *Source:* Leach (2014) John Wiley & Sons.

6Cs: Care

High-quality care should always be at the centre of all work and practices when caring for the community.

Acute kidney injury

AKI is a spectrum of renal impairment, from mild to severe renal failure requiring renal replacement therapy (Davies, 2014; Lafayette, 2019). It occurs when glomerular filtration rate (GFR) falls, leading to a rise in serum creatinine with, or without, a decline in urine output (KDIGO, 2012; O'Callaghan, 2017). Within the UK, AKI is seen in 13–18% of patients admitted to hospital, particularly in older adults, with an incidence of 13–22% in those already hospitalised (NICE, 2013; Wang et al., 2012). AKI affects 26–67% of critically ill patients and is associated with poorer outcomes, such as CKD and end-stage renal disease (ESRD) (Girling et al., 2020; Leach, 2014). Inpatient mortality, due to AKI in the UK, varies considerably but is estimated to be 25–30% or more, with the risk of death in hospital being approximately double for patients in critical care (Girling et al., 2020; NICE, 2013). The need for early intervention through risk assessment, prevention, early recognition, and treatment of AKI is paramount.

Definition

According to KDIGO (2012) the definition of AKI includes any of the following:

- An increase in serum creatinine by ≥25.6 micromol/L within 48 hours
- An increase in serum creatinine to ≥1.5 times baseline, known or presumed within the previous 7 days
- A urine output of <0.5 mL/kg for 6 hours

There are several classification systems that may be employed to determine severity of AKI (Bellomo et al., 2004; KDIGO, 2012; Mehta et al., 2007).

Clinical Investigations

NICE (2013) produced criteria for the detection of AKI, taking into consideration the definitions by Bellomo et al. (2004), KDIGO (2012) and Mehta et al. (2007). The criteria includes:

- A rise in serum creatinine of 26 micromol/L (0.3 mg/dL) or greater within 48 hours; or
- A 50% or greater rise in serum creatinine known or presumed to have occurred within the past 7 days; or
- A fall in urine output to <0.5 mL/kg/hour for more than 6 hours in adults and more than 8 hours in children and young people; or
- A 25% or greater fall in estimated GFR in children and young people within the past 7 days

Red Flag

Early recognition of AKI is critical to prevent progression of renal failure and the associated complications. One of the earliest clinical signs is a fall in urine output which, if left unaddressed, may lead to cardiorespiratory vascular compromise, severe metabolic acidosis, hyperkalaemia, cardiac arrest and death. A urine output of <0.5 ml/kg/hr for more than 2 hours, which equates to 35 mls per hour for a 70 kg adult, requires prompt investigation.

Clinical investigations: estimating glomerular filtration rate

Direct measurement of glomerular filtration rate (GFR) as marker of overall renal function is practically rather difficult. Estimations of renal function are therefore derived from either estimated glomerular filtration rate or creatinine clearance.

Normal eGFR is >90 mL/min/1.73m² but levels >60 mL/min/1.73m² should be interpreted with caution, as estimates of GFR become less accurate with relatively good renal function. If CKD is suspected initial investigations should include a serum creatinine, eGFR and measurement of the urinary albumin:creatinine ratio (ACR) (NICE, 2019). An eGFR should always be interpreted with caution in pregnancy, oedema, extremes of muscle mass, malnourishment, protein supplementation or patients of Asian or Chinese origin (NICE, 2019). Further information regarding prescribing in renal impairment is available via https://bnf.nice.org.uk/guidance/prescribing-in-renal-impairment.html.

Classification of AKI

The aetiology of AKI is classified into pre-renal, intrinsic and post-renal, the causes of which are outlined in Table 24.3. Approximately 50–65% of cases are pre-renal and occur due to impaired renal perfusion.

Pathophysiology

The pathophysiology of AKI is complex, multifactorial, arises from a broad range of aetiologies and occurs essentially due to ischaemia, toxicity, and inflammation. The clinical features and findings in AKI vast and detailed in Figure 24.8. Knowledge of renal physiology is paramount when understanding the pathophysiology of AKI.

The kidney receives approximately 25% of the total cardiac output and is therefore high susceptible to ischaemia, the most common cause of AKI. Acute tubular

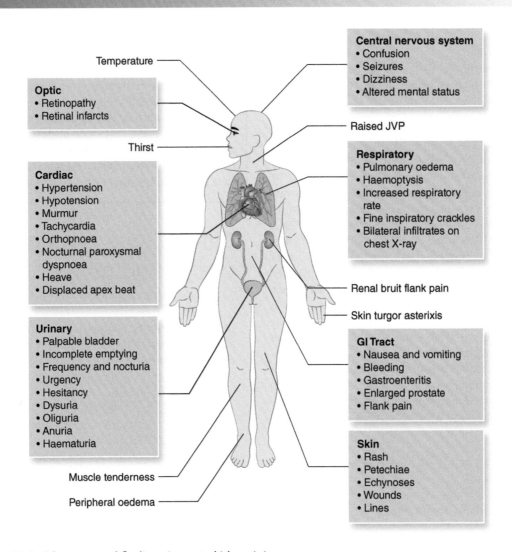

Figure 24.8 Clinical features and findings in acute kidney injury.

necrosis (ATN) occurs when compensatory mechanisms fail due to persistent, prolonged or severe inadequate renal perfusion. The consequences of which include hypoxaemia, inflammation, cellular injury and organ dysfunction. ATN may be classified into phases comprising initiation, maintenance and recovery.

The initiation phase includes onset to renal tubular epithelial cell injury. Structures of the nephron critically dependent upon perfusion include the proximal tubule and the thick ascending Loop of Henle. These cells are metabolically active with a high oxygen requirement of approximately 80% of renal consumption, due to active sodium absorption via intracellular ATP. During the extension or maintenance phase, ongoing hypoxaemia causes increased reactive oxygen species and intracellular acidosis, disruption of cell membranes and subsequent cellular injury and cellular death. Shedding of dead endothelial cells, into the lumen of the tubule, results in tubular blockage and a reduction in GFR. Disruption of the basement membrane in addition to activation of inflammatory mediators and the complement system leads to swelling of the renal tubules, interstitial oedema and further compression of blood vessels. Following this the

recovery phase incorporates cell repair and proliferation to re-establish integrity of the cells and tubules as well as intracellular and intercellular homeostasis (Basile et al., 2012).

6Cs: Compassion

Compassion, also known as 'intelligent kindness', requires the delivering of care to be focused around several key aspects; empathy, respect, dignity, recognising people's emotions, and forming therapeutic relationships with patients based on empathy.

Organ cross-talk

In normal physiology homeostasis is maintained via 'organ cross-talk'. However, when these bi-directional pathways become pathological or cease to exist, organ responses may result in deleterious effects, leading to multi-organ dysfunction, as observed within critical care (Prowle, 2018). The resultant significant morbidity and mortality associated

Table 24.3 Pre-renal, intrinsic and post-renal causes of AKI. *Source:* adapted from Davies, 2014; Lafayette, 2019; Makris and Spanou, 2016.

	Aetiology
Pre-renal	Hypovolaemia: • Haemorrhage • Burns • Gastrointestinal losses • Over diuresis • Severe pancreatitis Vasodilatation: • Sepsis • Anaphylaxis • Anti-hypertensive drugs Cardiovascular: • Heart failure • Cardiac tamponade • Pulmonary embolism • Myocardial infarction Renovascular disease: • Renal artery stenosis Hepatorenal syndrome Increased vascular resistance: • Surgery • Anaesthesia • NSAID drugs • Medications that cause renal vasoconstriction
Intrinsic	Acute tubular necrosis Glomerular nephritis Interstitial nephritis Nephrotoxic drugs: • Non-steroidal anti-inflammatories • Antibiotics • Proton pump inhibitors Hypertension Vasculitis Tubular toxins: • Drugs • Heavy metals • Contrast • Haemoglobin • Myoglobin • Uric acid • Calcium phosphate precipitation • Infection
Post-renal	Mechanical obstruction: • Tumour • Renal calculi • Blood clot • Prostate hyperplasia • Urinary infection • Urinary retention

with pure loss of renal function is disproportionate to the morbidity and mortality observed, with increasing evidence to support the concept of distant organ dysfunction associated. Opinions regarding AKI as single organ failure are changing due to its effects upon the lungs, heart, brain, liver and GI tract.

An understanding of organ cross-talk may facilitate management strategies that are not only specific to the kidneys but also other organs, with the aim to reduce multi-organ dysfunction, and overall mortality associated with AKI.

Risk factors for AKI

% of cases, if recognised early. An understanding and identification of risk factors for AKI is paramount, without which there is progression of renal damage. Table 24.4 identifies potential risk factors implicated in AKI.

Clinical features and examination

Pertinent information, from history taking and past medical history, may allow identification of risk factors for AKI. It is important to have a systematic approach to assessment and the use of airway, breathing, circulation, disability and exposure (ABCDE) is recommended.

> # 6Cs: Competence
>
> Competence in healthcare means the individual must possess the necessary expertise, clinical knowledge, and technical knowledge to deliver treatments that are effective and based on research and evidence.

Investigations

Various investigations are utilised in the presence of renal failure including biochemistry, haematology, urinalysis, urine microscopy and culture, immunology, renal biopsy, as well as radiological investigations such as ultrasound and computerised tomography (CT).

Biochemical investigations include serum urea, creatinine, potassium, pH and creatinine kinase. Knowledge of normal values, as in Table 24.5, in addition to the patient's usual results, is essential for interpretation. Urea and creatinine alone should be interpreted with caution as diet and muscle mass may affect results.

Table 24.4 Risk factors for AKI. *Source:* adapted from Dutton and Finch, 2018; Lafayette, 2019; Leach, 2014.

Risk factor
• Age>65 years • Pre-existing history of AKI • Pre-existing cardiac, renal or liver disease • Hypovolaemia – haemorrhage, GI losses, sweating • Hypertension • Peripheral vascular disease • Diabetes mellitus • Diuretic use and abuse • Drugs known to cause nephrotoxicity • Contrast media or recent intervention • Sepsis, burns, surgery, pancreatitis • Rhabdomyolysis • Hypercalcaemia • Cognitive or neurological impairment • Myeloproliferative disorders • Renal, prostate, cervical or bowel carcinoma

Table 24.5 Biochemistry investigations.

Biochemistry investigation	Normal value
• Urea	• 2.5–6.6 mmol/L
• Creatinine	• 55–120 µmol/L
• Potassium	• 3.6–5.2 mmol/L
• pH	• 7.35–7.45
• Creatinine kinase	• 22–198 units/L

Red Flag

Hyperkalaemia and severe metabolic acidosis may cause cardiac arrest and requires close monitoring in AKI. High levels of creatinine kinase, with history and clinical features, may suggest rhabdomyolysis. This is discussed in a subsequent section of this chapter.

Anaemia, due to significant blood loss, or haemolysis because of haemolytic uremic syndrome, as well as a raised eosinophil count observed with acute interstitial nephritis may be apparent on haematological investigations.

Urine analysis will detect the presence of blood, protein, ketones, glucose, leukocytes, nitrites, pH, bile and urobilinogen. The presence of these substances in the urine may indicate different renal disease should not be interpreted in isolation and prompt further investigations (see Examination scenario box).

Examination scenario: urinalysis

Substance present	Interpretation
Blood	• Haematuria (renal – glomerulonephritis, pyelonephritis, tumour, infarction, polycystic kidney disease), haemoglobinuria (haemolysis of intravascular origin), myoglobinuria (rhabdomyolysis) • If present with more than a trace of protein, blood is renal in origin
Protein	• Test ranges from + to ++++ • Only sensitive to albumin • Causes of proteinuria include renal disease, particularly glomerular in nature, non-renal causes include fever, exercise, burns, congestive cardiac failure, post-operative, blood transfusion and acute alcohol abuse
Ketones	• Presence occurs in diabetic ketoacidosis, starvation and low carbohydrate diets
Glucose	• Small amounts may be present in the urine • Presence may indicate diabetes mellitus or the inability of the renal tubules to reabsorb glucose
Leukocytes	• Presence may indicate urinary Infection, inflammation, carcinoma
Nitrites	• Presence may indicate Gram-negative bacteria
pH	• Normally acidic • Treatment of specific conditions such as myoglobinuria or urinary calculi may include urinary alkalisation • Renal tubular acidosis should be suspected if urine is never acidic • Infection e.g. *Proteus mirabilis* may cause alkaline urine
Bile and urobilinogen	• Presence may indicate hepatobiliary disease or haemolysis

(Cumming and Payne, 2009; Talley and O'Connor, 2010)

Examination scenario: palpation of the bladder

To ascertain if a patient is in urinary retention the bladder may be palpated. If it is empty, it will be impalpable, but in the presence of retention, it will palpable above the pubic symphysis and associated with abdominal distension. The patient should be assessed lying flat, with one pillow under their head, and the abdomen exposed, to inspect, palpate and auscultate. Palpation should be performed with the palmar surface of the fingers, initially it should be light pressure and then deep palpation. If the bladder is full, palpation will indicate an oval shape which is firm, smooth and regular in nature. This may be confirmed with a bladder scanner or with re-palpation following insertion of a urinary catheter.

Specific disorders associated with AKI

Intrinsic renal disease accounts for approximately 30% of AKI and includes glomerular and tubulointerstitial disease in addition to drugs and toxins (Leach, 2014; O'Callaghan, 2016).

Glomerular disease

Glomerular disease occurs because of glomerular injury and is diagnosed according to the clinical syndrome it produces and histopathology. There are five clinical syndromes causing reduced GFR, haematuria, proteinuria, oedema and hypertension. These include asymptomatic haematuria or proteinuria, acute glomerulonephritis (acute nephritic syndrome), chronic glomerulonephritis, rapidly progressive glomerulonephritis and nephrotic syndrome.

Acute glomerulonephritis

Acute glomerulonephritis is a serious condition which, if left untreated, may rapidly progress to irreversible kidney damage. The trigger is usually immunological, causing acute glomerular inflammation with histopathological changes including expansion of the mesangial into the capillaries and diffuse proliferation of the epithelial, endothelial, and mesangial cells, affecting all the glomeruli.

Hepatorenal syndrome (HRS)

HRS is reversible functional renal failure that occurs as a result of advanced liver cirrhosis with ascites or fulminant hepatic failure and is associated with significant morbidity and mortality. Approximately 19–26% of patients with cirrhosis admitted to hospital have acute renal impairment (Simonetto, Gines and Kamath, 2020).

The pathophysiology of HRS is not completely understood but circulatory dysfunction leading to reduced renal perfusion, systemic inflammation, adrenal insufficiency, raised intra-abdominal hypertension and cirrhotic cardiomyopathy have been implicated. Risk factors for the development of HRS-AKI include hyponatraemia, infection, large volume paracentesis with inadequate or no albumin replacement, liver size and high plasma rennin activity (Simonetto et al., 2020).

Rhabdomyolysis

Rhabdomyolysis is a clinical syndrome wherein destruction of skeletal muscle results in the release of breakdown products into the systemic circulation, AKI is one of the most common complications. The causes of rhabdomyolysis may be classified as acquired (muscle ischaemia or compression secondary to trauma or 'crush' injuries, burns, excessive exercise, prolonged surgery, a 'long lie', obesity, anaesthetic, lipid-lowering or recreational drugs, alcohol, infection, hyper- or hypothermia, endocrine disease, or toxins) or inherited (structural or metabolic myopathies, certain genetic diseases) (Chavez et al., 2016).

Clinical features include muscle tenderness or pain, dark urine, oliguria or anuria, fever and electrolyte disturbances. Biochemical markers will demonstrate a raised plasma creatinine kinase and, depending upon the onset and severity, rising serum urea and creatinine with associated hyperkalaemia, in addition to hypocalcaemia. Plasma creatinine kinase concentration is at least five times the normal level in rhabdomyolysis, proportional to the severity of the muscle injury, and if above 5000 units/L, associated with a 50% incidence of AKI (Hunter et al., 2006). Urine analysis will be positive for the presence of myoglobin or haemoglobin. A metabolic acidosis on an arterial blood gas may indicate worsening renal function in addition to an elevated anion gap secondary to the presence of organic acids and lactate.

6Cs: Communication

Effective communication skills involve multiple dimensions: active listening, adapting your communication style to your audience, confidence, offering and taking feedback, empathy, respect, understanding body language and being responsive.

Drug-induced renal damage

There are several sites within the renal system in which pathology can occur, leading to acute or chronic kidney dysfunction. One of the most common, and potentially avoidable causes of acute and chronic renal damage, is pharmacotherapy itself. Drugs can cause renal damage in several ways, including altered renal blood flow, damage to the nephron or damage to the interstitial tissues. Figure 24.9 provides a non-exhaustive list of some of the adverse effects that pharmacotherapies can exert upon the kidneys.

6Cs: Courage

Courage is important to ensure that everyone gets the quality of care that they deserve.

Medicines management

Non-steroidal anti-inflammatories (NSAIDs) have analgesic and anti-inflammatory effects with regular dosage and are used to treat pain associated with inflammation. It inhibits cyclo-oxygenase, preventing the synthesis of prostaglandins which are implicated in the inflammatory response. Prostaglandins cause vasodilatation, therefore inhibition may result in vasoconstriction, decreased renal perfusion and, in the presence of other risk factors of acute renal failure, may cause an AKI and ATN. In longer-term use minimal change glomerulonephropathy and interstitial nephritis may occur secondary to toxicity. NSAIDs should be discontinued or, if prescribed, not administered in the presence of an AKI, following consultation with the prescriber.

Medicines management

Aminoglycosides are a class of antibiotic that inhibit bacterial protein synthesis, examples of which include gentamicin and vancomycin. Gentamicin has a narrow therapeutic range and supra-therapeutic doses may lead to nephrotoxic effects and AKI. In the presence of renal failure serum concentration monitoring is required as gentamicin may accumulate due to reduced renal excretion. Peak and trough levels will determine dosage and administration frequency. Monitoring of renal function prior to and during treatment is essential.

Medicines management

Radiocontrast-induced nephropathy has been long debated within the literature with the most recent evidence suggesting that it has been greatly overstated. Renal injury is thought to be caused due to its direct nephrotoxic effects as well as generation of reactive oxygen species causing vasoconstriction and ischaemia, and increased urine viscosity due to movement of water out of the tubules (Morcos et al., 2019). It is defined as an acute decrease in GFR occurring 48–72 hours after administration. Careful consideration must be given to the risk-benefit ratio of intravenous radiocontrast with vigilance in monitoring of renal function if deemed necessary. Previous treatments have included adequate hydration, intravenous sodium bicarbonate, n-acetylcysteine and statins.

Medicines management

Many opioids are renally excreted (see Chapter 11) and therefore renal failure can lead to reduced clearance and accumulation, resulting in extreme opiod sensitivity and eventually toxicity. Prescribing and subsequentadministration of opiods with in this patient group should be carefully considered on a case-by-case basis, which may require dose adjustmentor complete avoidance.

6Cs: Commitment

Being highly committed to our patients helps to improve their quality of care and experience as well as that of other patients.

358

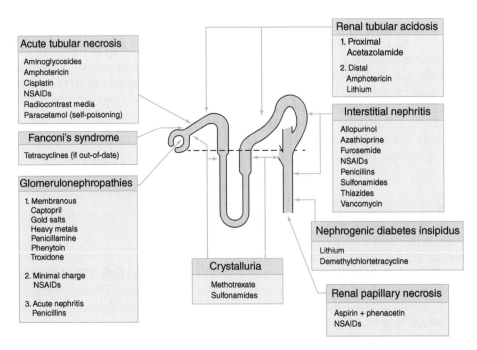

Figure 24.9   The adverse effects of certain drugs upon the kidney. *Source:* Aadapted from Grahame-Smith and Aronson (2002) John Wiley & Sons.

Management of AKI

AKI is preventable, therefore pre-renal or post-renal causes should be addressed in a timely fashion with early management being paramount, whilst intrinsic renal diseases require identification, diagnosis and treatment accordingly. The approach employed when assessing all critically ill patients is Airway, Breathing, Circulation, Disability and Exposure (ABCDE). Table 24.6 details some of the common clinical examination features of AKI and some of the evidence-based managementstrategies that may be used to treat this condition. Life-threatening emergencies should always be treated as they are identified.

Life-threatening emergencies

The most common life-threatening emergency associated with AKI is hyperkalaemia. Plasma levels greater than 7 mmol/L are associated with ventricular fibrillation and cardiac arrest. The Clinical Practice Guidelines should be followed for hyperkalaemia with treatment being dependent upon the severity of serum plasma levels and ECG changes as seen in Figure 24.10

Table 24.6   Clinical features and findings in AKI and how they may be interpreted.

Clinical features and findings		Interpretation
General appearance		This will give an immediate indication of the patient's airway status, level of consciousness and acuity of illness.
Airway and breathing	Pulmonary oedema • Bilateral crackles on auscultation • Chest x-ray – bilateral patchy opacification, pleural effusions	Fluid overload or cardiac failure
	Abnormal upper airway sounds	Uraemic encephalopathy and HRS can result in reduced level of consciousness, as evidenced by a decreased GCS. If the patients GCS is ≤8, this *may* lead to loss of normal airway reflexes.
	↑ respiratory rate	Compensatory mechanism due to metabolic acidosis
	↓ O$_2$ saturations	Pulmonary oedema, increased demand due to sepsis
	Breathlessness	Pulmonary oedema, fluid overload, metabolic acidosis
Cardiovascular	Hypertension	Blood pressure is often raised in renal disease
	Hypotension	Hypovolaemia, sepsis
	Tachycardia	Compensatory mechanism for hypovolaemia, sepsis
	Raised jugular venous pressure (JVP)	Fluid overload or cardiac failure
	Peripheral oedema	
	Prolonged capillary refill time (CRT)	Hypovolaemia or cardiac failure
	Rapid CRT	Vasodilatation due to sepsis
Disability	Altered mental status	Poor cerebral perfusion due to hypotension or uraemia
	Dizziness	Hypotension due to hypovolaemia
	Seizures	Uraemia
	Pain	Infection, inflammation, acute urinary obstruction
Exposure/ 'Everything else'	Old scars	Previous renal surgery or peritoneal dialysis
	Abdominal distension	Enlarged kidneys or bladder
	Enlarged prostate or palpable mass on PR examination	Acute urinary obstruction due to enlarged prostate or tumour
	Presence of blood on PR exam	GI bleeding leading to hypovolaemia
	Low urine output	Acute urinary obstruction, hypovolaemia, hypotension
	Urinary – frequency, urgency, hesitancy	Acute urinary obstruction, infection
	Dysuria	Infection or inflammation
	Haematuria	Tumour, rhabdomyolysis, glomerulonephritis, ATN, infection
	Muscle swelling	Rhabdomyolysis

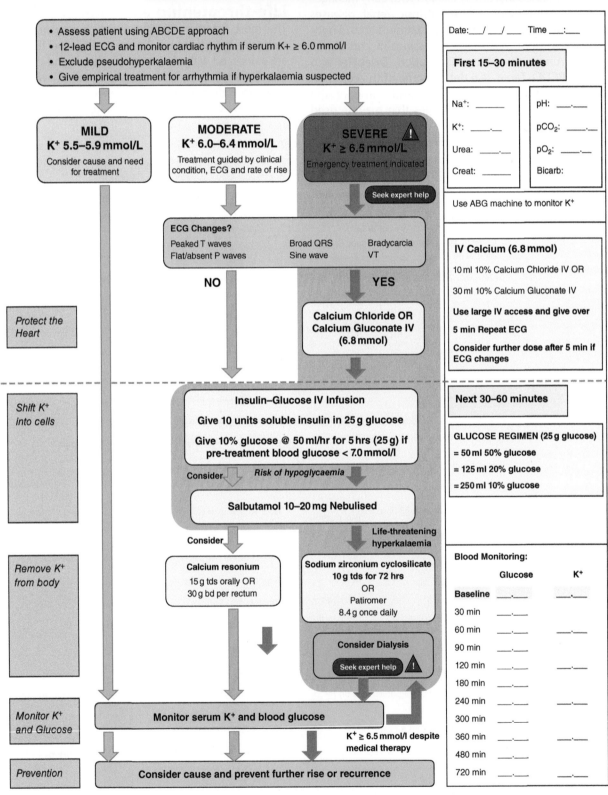

360

Figure 24.10 Treatment algorithm for hyperkalaemia. *Source:* Renal Association UK (2020) used with permission from UK Kidney Association.

(The Renal Association UK, 2020). Treatment of hyperkalaemia incorporates cardio protection (intravenous calcium chloride), shifting potassium into the cells (nebulised salbutamol, insulin dextrose) and removal of potassium from the body (potassium exchanging resins, diuretics, renal replacement therapy (RRT)).

Clinical features and examination

Pertinent information, from history taking and past medical history, may allow identification of risk factors for AKI. However, there are clinical features and findings on examination that may be present, indicating the onset or progression of an AKI, some of which are specific to disease processes. Figure 24.8 depicts clinical features and findings whilst Table 24.6 indicates how these may be interpreted in the context of AKI. It is important to have a systematic approach to assessment and the use of airway, breathing, circulation, disability and exposure (ABCDE) is recommended.

Management

In AKI significant uraemia and encephalopathy (HRS) may affect the patient's neurological status, compromising the airway. If the patient's Glasgow Coma Scale (GCS) is ≤8, it is likely that they will require intubation, ventilation and critical care admission.

Initial management of pulmonary oedema, secondary to fluid overload, requires the patient to be sat upright, application of oxygen to achieve targeted saturations and close monitoring. Diuretics may be utilised if renal function is preserved; however, it should be noted that many of these are nephrotoxic and may worsen AKI, as well as potentiate drug toxicity. Non-invasive CPAP or intubation and ventilation is indicated if respiratory failure worsens. Gas exchange and acid-base status can be monitored via placement of an arterial line. Metabolic acidosis, because of AKI, can cause the patient to increase their respiratory rate, augmenting carbon dioxide elimination, to correct the pH. Care must be taken with mechanical ventilator settings as once the patient is sedated, they will no longer can compensate for a metabolic acidosis, which may worsen, precipitating cardiac arrest.

Emergency management of hypotension requires immediate replacement of circulating volume with appropriate fluid resuscitation (blood products or crystalloid). Fluid management in HRS may be in the form of intravenous human albumin solution, due to the nature of the disease process. Intravenous sodium bicarbonate improves metabolic acidosis and causes urinary alkalinisation, reducing cast formation and flushing the renal tubules, if administered at a high rate, in the management of rhabdomyolysis.

Response to fluid resuscitation should be reassessed and consideration given to pre-existing cardiac disease and anuria, as repeated fluid challenges may be detrimental, resulting in fluid overload and pulmonary oedema. Inotropic support in the critical care setting may be necessary, enhancing renal perfusion once hypovolaemia has been

appropriately treated. As previously discussed, hypertension may be the initial clinical presentation of an acute renal disease requiring management with nitrates and opioids. Monitoring of electrolytes, such as potassium and magnesium, will ensure that cardiac arrhythmias are minimised.

Pupils, blood glucose and other causes of disordered consciousness (drugs) are included in disability assessment and those associated with AKI have been discussed previously. Exposure requires full examination of the body; potential sources of sepsis should be identified, and antibiotics commenced immediately. Drug charts should be interrogated for nephrotoxic drugs and stopped immediately.

One of the hallmarks of AKI is oliguria. It is essential that a urine output of <0.5 ml/kg/hr for more than 2 hours is recognised and reported to the medical team. This will allow early intervention, potentially preventing AKI. If diuretics are administered, urine output should be interpreted in caution as an increase may give false reassurance of improving renal function. The insertion of a urinary catheter will allow accurate assessment of urine volumes, but it is not without risk. Fluid balance is key to understanding the patient's overall volume status and this is achieved through accurate documentation of input and output. Insertion of a central line will add to assessment of the patient's intravascular volume in addition to providing intravenous access and inotropic support within critical care.

Renal USS and CT scan should be ordered urgently to investigate the cause of AKI if it is not apparent. Referral to the renal team may be appropriate as interventions such as nephrostomy or stenting could be required. Prompt renal replacement therapy (RRT) may be indicated and this is discussed in the subsequent part of this chapter.

361

Snapshot

Martha is a 76-year-old lady who has been admitted to hospital with severe diarrhoea and vomiting. She is currently in monitoring in the Emergency Department. Her symptoms started with nausea 3 days ago following a meal in a restaurant, but she has managed to continue to take her medications. Her past medical history includes hypertension, type II diabetes mellitus and COPD. A prescription she has brought in from home reveals that she takes lisinopril 20 mg once a day, amlodipine 5 mg once a day, metformin 500 mg twice a day and a salbutamol inhaler as required. She complains of feeling more unwell and a Registered Nurse (RN) finds the following on assessment:

Airway (A): patent, the patient is speaking in full sentences
Breathing (B): oxygen saturations of 94% on 4 L nasal cannulae (NEWS2 = 3), respiratory rate 24 (NEWS2 = 2)
Circulation (C): heart rate 110 (NEWS2 = 1), sinus rhythm, blood pressure 90/40 mmHg (NEWS2 = 3), cool peripherally with a peripheral capillary refill time of 4 seconds

Disability (D): patient is alert on the AVPU scale (NEWS2 = 0), pupils are size 3, equal and reactive to light, blood glucose is 7, temperature 36.7°C (NEWS2 = 0)

Exposure (E): there is nothing else to find on full body examination. One 20g cannula in the right antecubital fossa. There is no urinary catheter but Martha reports that she hasn't passed any urine for at least 24 hours

Total NEWS2: 9

Nursing actions:
- Medical team review requested
- Vascular accesses checked for patency
- Critical care outreach team contacted

Diagnosis
- Martha is significantly dehydrated and therefore hypovolaemic and hypotensive
- Intravenous fluids were prescribed by the medical team
- A urinary catheter was inserted with minimal output
- The antihypertensives on the drug chart were suspended
- Biochemistry demonstrated a urea of 14 and creatinine of 234
- An arterial blood gas was as follows: pH 7.26, pCO_2 2.8, pO_2 12, HCO_3 18 BXS -8
- The diagnosis of an AKI was made, and Martha was transferred to critical care for further management

362

Chronic kidney disease

Chronic kidney disease is defined as an abnormality in kidney function, demonstrated by glomerular filtration rate (GFR) of less than 60 mL/min per 1.73m², or markers of kidney damage, which has been present for more than three months, with associated health implications (KDIGO, 2013). Worldwide the estimated prevalence of CKD is 5–15%, with the main causes reported as diabetes, glomerular nephritis, pyelonephritis, polycystic kidney disease and hypertension (O'Callaghan, 2017; UK Renal Registry, 2020). The risk of developing CKD increases with age due to decline in renal function and increasing prevalence of diseases causing renal impairment (NICE 2015; O'Callaghan, 2017). There is an increased risk of myocardial infarction or stroke associated with CKD and premature death

is 5–10 times more likely, before progression to ESRD (Webster, 2017). Stratification of severity, as well as local and national guidance, informs healthcare professionals in the care and management of patients with CKD. Figure 24.11 depicts the stages of CKD and the risk of CKD. Those patients with stage 4 may require referral to renal specialists and in addition to specific interventions indicated in stage 3, whilst stage 5 CKD generally indicates the need for RRT (Davies, 2014).

The complications of CKD arise due to progressive loss of functioning nephrons leading to the accumulation of toxic metabolic products, inadequate production of erythropoietin and vitamin D. Clinical manifestations of CKD are depicted in Figure 24.12.

Management

The national guidance for the early identification and management of chronic kidney disease in adults in primary and secondary care makes recommendations regarding life style modification, dietary intervention, self-management, in addition to pharmacotherapy (NICE, 2015). Management of anaemia, blood pressure, mineral and bone disorders, volume status, electrolyte disturbance and metabolic acidosis are key to CKD.

Diabetic nephropathy

Diabetic renal disease remains the single most common cause of renal failure that requires treatment with renal replacement therapy (UK Renal Registry, 2020). Approximately 40% of Type I and Type II diabetic patients develop diabetic nephropathy, the incidence of which has only just recently plateaued and may be attributable to the development of clinical practice guidelines endorsing early diagnosis and prevention (Gross et al., 2005; Haneda et al., 2015). It is less common in Type II diabetic patients of European descent in comparison to African or Asian (O'Callaghan, 2017). Diabetic nephropathy may occur because of the long-term complications of diabetes mellitus, which cause damage to the structure and function of the kidney (Davies, 2014). When glycaemic control is poor, with protracted periods of hyperglycaemia, damage to vascular tissue occurs, significantly increasing the risk of death from cardiovascular disease (Davies, 2014; Gross et al., 2005; Nazar, 2014).

Snapshot

Paul is a 25-year-old who presented to hospital feeling generally unwell with malaise, nausea, shortness of breath and myalgia. When questioned further there had been a few months of general malaise. He has no past medical history and does not take any regular medications. The RN completes an assessment as follows:

Airway (A): patent, the patient is speaking in full sentences
Breathing (B): oxygen saturations of 84% on 4 L nasal cannulae (NEWS2 = 5), respiratory rate 24 (NEWS2 = 2)
Circulation (C): heart rate 114 (NEWS2 = 2), sinus rhythm, blood pressure 182/96 mmHg (NEWS2 = 0), warm peripherally with a peripheral capillary refill time of 2 seconds, there is evidence of bilateral lower limb oedema
Disability (D): patient is alert on the AVPU scale (NEWS2 = 0), pupils are size 3, equal and reactive to light, blood glucose is 8.2, temperature 37.1°C (NEWS2 = 0)

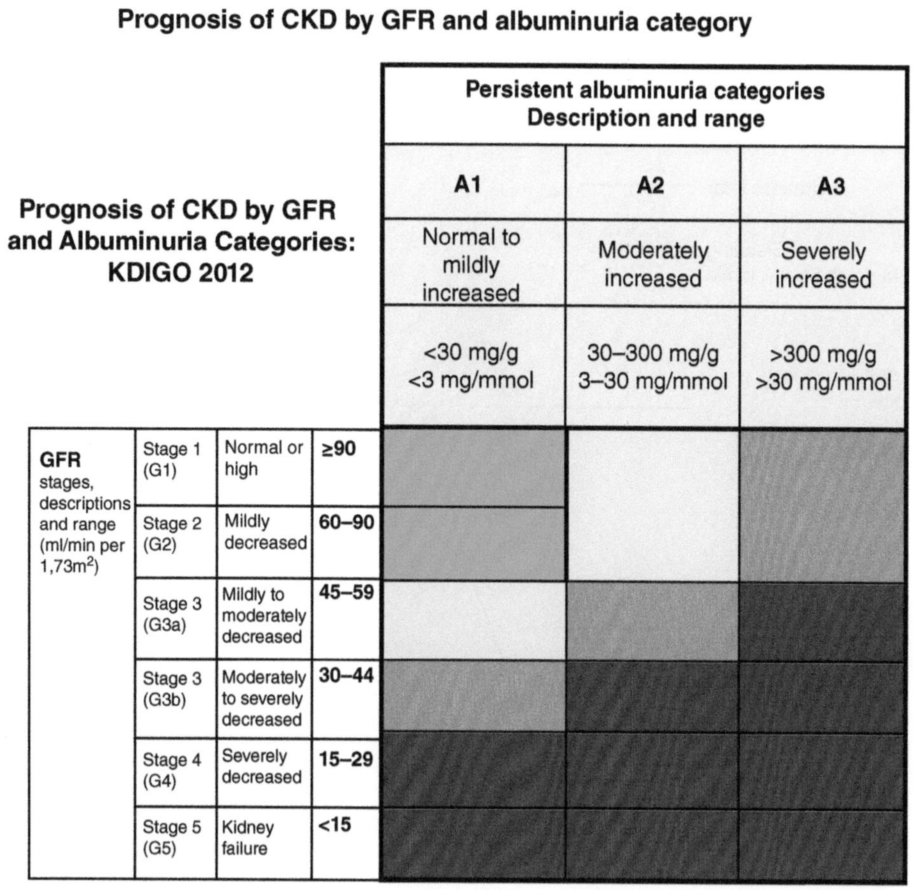

Prognosis of CKD by GFR and albuminuria category

Prognosis of CKD by GFR and Albuminuria Categories: KDIGO 2012			Persistent albuminuria categories Description and range		
			A1	**A2**	**A3**
			Normal to mildly increased	Moderately increased	Severely increased
			<30 mg/g <3 mg/mmol	30–300 mg/g 3–30 mg/mmol	>300 mg/g >30 mg/mmol
GFR stages, descriptions and range (ml/min per 1,73m²)	Stage 1 (G1)	Normal or high	≥90		
	Stage 2 (G2)	Mildly decreased	60–90		
	Stage 3 (G3a)	Mildly to moderately decreased	45–59		
	Stage 3 (G3b)	Moderately to severely decreased	30–44		
	Stage 4 (G4)	Severely decreased	15–29		
	Stage 5 (G5)	Kidney failure	<15		

Green: low risk (if no other markers of kidney disease, no CKD); Yellow: moderately increased risk; Orange: high risk; Red, very high risk.

Figure 24.11 KDIGO classification of CKD (2012). *Source:* Peate and Hill (2021) John Wiley & Sons.

Exposure (E): there is nothing else to find on full body examination. There is no urinary catheter.
Total NEWS2 = 8

Blood results:
- Urea 18.9
- Creatinine 185
- Potassium 7.2
- Phosphate 2.4
- Haemoglobin 52g/L

Arterial blood gas
pH 7.10 pCO_2 2.1 pO_2 7.6 HCO_3 11 BXS -18

Chest x-ray
Bilateral infiltrates

Nursing actions:
- Medical team review requested immediately.
- Patient transferred to a monitored bed due to the risk of arrhythmia.
- Critical care outreach team contacted.

Diagnosis:
- Paul has signs of acute fluid overload (pulmonary and peripheral oedema) due to newly diagnosed chronic renal failure
- His potassium level is dangerously high and requires treatment according to the hyperkalaemia management guideline
- Transfer to critical care is required for management of Paul's type I respiratory failure, fluid overload, hyperkalaemia and metabolic acidosis with mechanical ventilation and dialysis

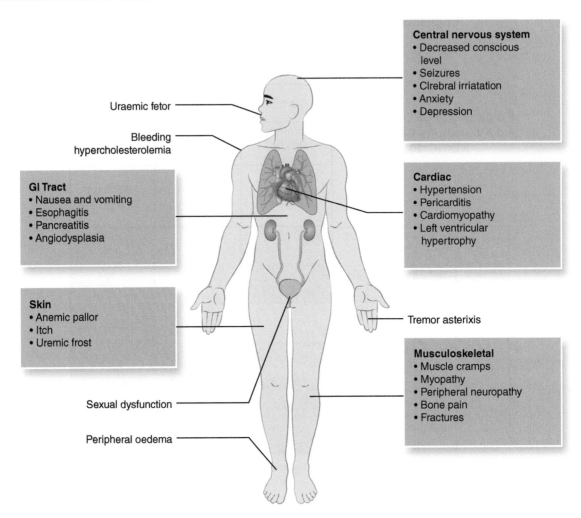

Central nervous system
- Decreased conscious level
- Seizures
- Clrebral irriatation
- Anxiety
- Depression

Uraemic fetor

Bleeding hypercholesterolemia

GI Tract
- Nausea and vomiting
- Esophagitis
- Pancreatitis
- Angiodysplasia

Cardiac
- Hypertension
- Pericarditis
- Cardiomyopathy
- Left ventricular hypertrophy

Skin
- Anemic pallor
- Itch
- Uremic frost

Tremor asterixis

Musculoskeletal
- Muscle cramps
- Myopathy
- Peripheral neuropathy
- Bone pain
- Fractures

Sexual dysfunction

Peripheral oedema

Figure 24.12 Clinical manifestations of CKD.

Continuous renal replacement therapy (CRRT)

As explored within the previous section of this chapter, the correction of potentially life-threatening consequences because of renal failure may require the institution of RRT. There are several modalities of RRT that can provided within ICU, these will largely be dependent on local practice. Figure 24.13 explores some of the indications for RRT within critical care and the principles behind some of the main modalities of RRT. In order to appreciate the underlying principles of RRT, one must understand the basis of osmosis, diffusion. This topic is explored in depth within O'Callaghan's (2017) text, but Table 24.7 outlines some of the fundamental principles surrounding the different modes of RRT. The dosing/intensity of RRT in the critically ill patient is controversial.

Dosing of CRRT

Dosing refers to the amount of eluent (ultrafiltrate) in ml/kg of body weight per hour (Davies et al., 2019). Several seminal studies have tested the efficacy of different RRT dosing strategies which ranged from 20ml/kg/hr to 70ml/kg/hr (Bellemo et al., 2009; Palevsky et al., 2008; Ronco et al., 2000; Tolwani et al., 2008; Van Wert et al., 2010). The typical dose of CRRT in the UK is 25–35 mL/kg/h; however, local practice may vary.

Anticoagulation

The aim of anticoagulation is to maintain patency of the extracorporeal circuit to ensure that optimal therapy can be delivered. There are various options for anticoagulation, with each having advantages and disadvantages. Table 24.8 explores some of the most common options, their mode of action and the potential complications that may rise because of their usage.

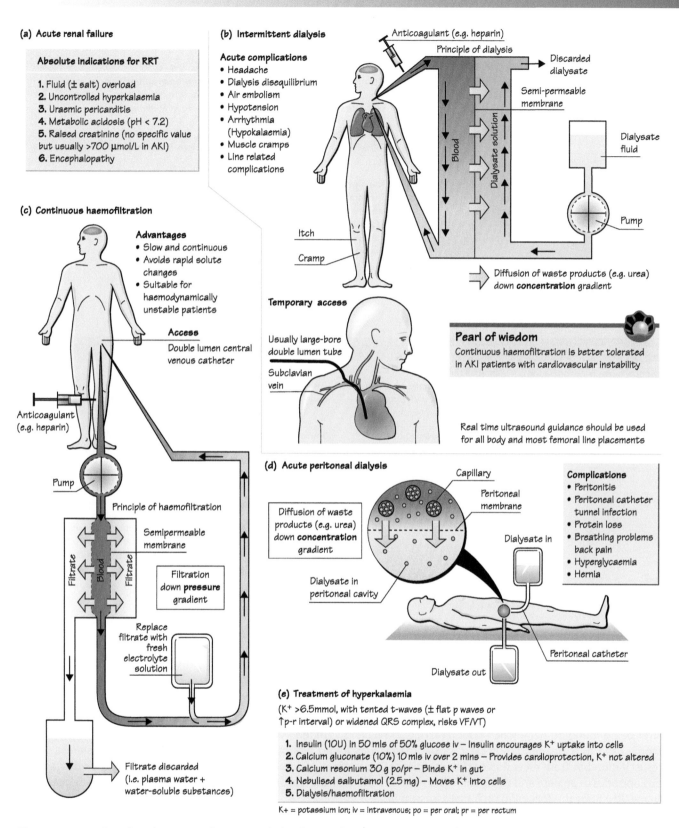

(a) Acute renal failure

Absolute indications for RRT

1. Fluid (± salt) overload
2. Uncontrolled hyperkalaemia
3. Uraemic pericarditis
4. Metabolic acidosis (pH < 7.2)
5. Raised creatinine (no specific value but usually >700 μmol/L in AKI)
6. Encephalopathy

(b) Intermittent dialysis

Acute complications
- Headache
- Dialysis disequilibrium
- Air embolism
- Hypotension
- Arrhythmia (Hypokalaemia)
- Muscle cramps
- Line related complications

Anticoagulant (e.g. heparin)

Principle of dialysis

Discarded dialysate

Semi-permeable membrane

Blood

Dialysate solution

Dialysate fluid

Pump

Itch

Cramp

Diffusion of waste products (e.g. urea) down **concentration** gradient

(c) Continuous haemofiltration

Advantages
- Slow and continuous
- Avoids rapid solute changes
- Suitable for haemodynamically unstable patients

Access
Double lumen central venous catheter

Anticoagulant (e.g. heparin)

Pump

Principle of haemofiltration

Semipermeable membrane

Filtrate

Blood

Filtrate

Filtration down **pressure** gradient

Replace filtrate with fresh electrolyte solution

Filtrate discarded (i.e. plasma water + water-soluble substances)

Temporary access

Usually large-bore double lumen tube

Subclavian vein

Pearl of wisdom

Continuous haemofiltration is better tolerated in AKI patients with cardiovascular instability

Real time ultrasound guidance should be used for all body and most femoral line placements

(d) Acute peritoneal dialysis

Capillary

Peritoneal membrane

Diffusion of waste products (e.g. urea) down **concentration** gradient

Dialysate in

Dialysate in peritoneal cavity

Dialysate out

Peritoneal catheter

Complications
- Peritonitis
- Peritoneal catheter tunnel infection
- Protein loss
- Breathing problems back pain
- Hyperglycaemia
- Hernia

(e) Treatment of hyperkalaemia

(K+ >6.5mmol, with tented t-waves (± flat p waves or ↑p-r interval) or widened QRS complex, risks VF/VT)

1. Insulin (10U) in 50 mls of 50% glucose iv – Insulin encourages K+ uptake into cells
2. Calcium gluconate (10%) 10 mls iv over 2 mins – Provides cardioprotection, K+ not altered
3. Calcium resonium 30 g po/pr – Binds K+ in gut
4. Nebulised salbutamol (2.5 mg) – Moves K+ into cells
5. Dialysis/haemofiltration

K+ = potassium ion; iv = intravenous; po = per oral; pr = per rectum

Figure 24.13 Renal replacement therapy and absolute indications. *Source:* Leach (2014) John Wiley & Sons.

365

Table 24.7   Fundamental principles of RRT in ICU. *Source:* Davies et al., 2019; Gemmell et al., 2017.

Modality	Underlying principles	Notes
Haemodialysis	• Ultrafiltration = fluid transport • Diffusion = solute transport	• The movement of **solutes** down a **concentration gradient**, from an area of higherconcentration to an area of lower concentration • Dialysate fluid is used to create a concentration gradient across the semi-permeablemembrane. • The waste dialysate is produced as effluent • Diffusion is more effective at removing low molecular weight molecules (<30 kDa) such as urea, creatinine, ions and ammonia.
Haemofiltration	1. Ultrafiltration =fluid transport 2. Convection = solute transport	• The movement of solutes with water flow = solvent drag. • The more fluid moved through the semi-permeable membrane, the more solutes areeventually removed. • Replacement fluid is used to create this phenomenon = convention. • Positive, negative and osmotic pressure is generated by non-permeable solutes through the filter
Haemodiafiltration	A combination of the above	

Table 24.8   Anticoagulation options for CRRT.

Anticoagulant	Mode of action	Advantages	Disadvantages/Cautions
Regional heparinanticogulation	• Inhibits thrombin • Potentiates naturally occurring inhibitors of activated Factor X (Xa) • See Chapter 11 for further details	• Cost-effective • Easily titratable • Easily reversed	• Haemorrhage • Heparin resistance • Heparin-induced thrombocytopenia (hit).
Regional citrate anticoagulation	• Binding andchelating free ionised calcium, which is a critical co-factor in both the intrinsic and extrinsic coagulation cascades	• Shown to preserve filter life longer than other agents	• Citrate toxicity resulting in worsening acidosis, liver failure and deranged coagulation • Haemorrhage • Requires intensive monitoring of pre and post filter calcium levels • Electrolyte disturbances; hypomagnesaemia, hypernatraemia, hypocalcaemia and hypercalcaemia • Cardiovascular collapse secondary to above
Regional or systemic prostacyclin/epoprostenol anticoagulation	• Potent inhibitor of platelet aggregation& potent vasodilator	• Easily titratable • Can be delivered regionally, or systemically	• Haemorrhage • Platelet consumption • Hypotensive episodes

Snapshot

Florence is a 48-year-old lady who works as a cleaner. She has been transferred to hospital to hospital by her partner after being found on her kitchen floor lethargic and having vomited. An empty bottle of 70% isopropyl alcohol (commonly used as a cleaner, disinfectant or degreaser) was found nearby. She has just been urgently transferred to a resuscitation bay from reception of the Emergency Department. Her documented past medical history includes previous episodes of anxiety and depression. Her records state that she does not take any regular medications. A Registered Nurse (RN) finds the following on initial assessment:

Airway (A): Snoring due to airway obstruction from tongue, relieved with a jaw thrust manoeuvre. Noted to have a 'fruity' odour to her breath.

Breathing (B): Shallow breathing pattern. Oxygen saturations of 71% on room air, rising to 81% when on 15 L via non re-breathe mask (NEWS2 = 5), respiratory rate 8 breaths per minute (NEWS2 = 3). On auscultation she has reduced air entry to the right lung base.Initial arterial blood gas results showed a severe mixed respiratory and metabolic acidosis.

Circulation (C): Heart rate 48 beats per minute (NEWS2 = 1), sinus bradycardia, blood pressure 82/40 mmHg (NEWS2 = 3), cool peripherally with a peripheral capillary refill time of 5 seconds.

Disability (D): Patient is responsive to pain on the AVPU scale (NEWS2 = 3), pupils are size 2, equal and reactive to light, but sluggish. Blood glucose is 9 mmol/L, temperature 35.2°C (NEWS2 = 1).

Exposure (E): There is nothing else to find on full body examination. A urine dipstick was positive for ketones and acetone

Total NEWS2: 16

Nursing actions:
- Registered nurse immediately informs senior nurse and medical team caring for the patient.
- Emergency assessment by critical care outreach nurse and critical care medic requested.

Diagnosis:
- Florence is critically ill and in a peri-arrest state.
- The history of her presentation and her examination findings suggest she likely ingested the 70% isopropyl alcohol (isopropanol), which can result in central nervous system, respiratory depression and circulatory failure.
- The presence of 'fruity' breath, along with her urinalysis results, suggest that this is indeed the case as isopropanol is metabolised to form acetone which can result in a classic fruit odours breath.
- Florence was intubated and ventilated, received intravenous fluids resuscitation and transferred to critical care urgently for further management with RRT.
- Isopropanol and acetone both have low molecular weights, low volumes of distribution, low protein binding, and hence are responsive to removal by extracorporeal/RRT techniques such as haemodialysis and hemodialfiltration.

Drug dosing and RRT

The pharmacokinetics of drugs in intensive care patients is complex and when RRT is added this becomes an additional challenge to ensure therapeutic dosing is maintained. Chapter 11 explores these factors in more detail and provides useful resources for promoting effective medicines management.

Kidney transplantation – critical care considerations

Kidney transplantation is the treatment option for patients with end-stage renal failure. In 2017 to 2018 3,272 renal transplants were performed within the UK (NHS Blood and Transplant, 2018). Approximately 30% of donors were living donors, with over 60% of donation following brain stem or cardiac death. Quality of life is significantly improved in comparison to dialysis, but organs are in short supply, with waiting list times of 2.5 to 3 years. It remains to be seen if the change in law, to an 'opt-out' system, in England in 2020, dramatically affects transplantation.

The most common complication following renal transplantation is rejection. Hyperacute rejection is rare and previously occurred due to mismatched tissue typing. Thrombotic occlusion of graft vasculature results in ischaemia and requires re-transplantation. Acute rejection is common and clinical manifestations include ongoing electrolyte imbalance, anuria, fluid retention and rising creatinine. Immunosuppressive therapy reduces rejection via inhibition of the immune response but is not without risk including infection and carcinoma. Other acute complications include post-operative problems following major surgery (bleeding, pain, infection), poor renal function (drug toxicity, ATN) and cytomegalovirus (CMV) infection. Graft versus host disease occurs when a immune response is mounted, resulting in fibrosis and necrosis of the skin, GI tract and liver. Incidence increases with age and HLA mismatch. Management includes corticosteroids and chemotherapy but if severe can lead to organ failure and death. Transplant patients within critical care require close monitoring for signs of rejection, infection, electrolyte disturbance, poor renal function and side effects of immunosuppressive therapy.

367

Orange Flag

The success of renal transplantation is not only governed by the surgical procedure, post-operative recovery and long-term medical management but also the psychological effects. Following transplantation there are profound changes to the social, psychological and relational aspects of both the patients and relatives lives.

Sleep hygiene is challenging within critical care and poor sleep quality leading to emotional fragility is recognised within this cohort of patients. Early detection of anxiety and depression, which are common following renal transplantation, is vital as psychological support may improve treatment compliance and adherence (De Pasquale et al., 2020).

Conclusion

As a student health care practitioner working with critically ill patients, you will undoubtedly be involved in the care of several patients with one or multiple types of renal disorder. These disorders can be very complex and have the potential to have detrimental effects on a patient's chance of survival to hospital discharge. The causes of renal disorders can be multifactorial and often are interlinked with other comorbidities such as cardiovascular disease and diabetes. The incidence of AKI continues to rise despite multiple public health campaigns and NHS initiatives. As such, it is crucial that the healthcare professionals involved in supporting this patient group to manage their acute and chronic disease process have a sound understanding of the physiology, pathophysiological, pharmacological and evidence base that underpins the promotion of safe and effective care.

Take home points

1. The renal system is both the intended and unintended target of multiple therapies within critical care practice; therefore, it is very important to have an understanding of the physiological principles pertaining to the renal system to aim to prevent associated complications.

2. AKI affects 26–67% of critically ill patients and is associated with poorer outcomes, such as CKD and end-stage renal disease (ESRD).

3. Chronic kidney disease is defined as an abnormality in kidney function, demonstrated by glomerular filtration rate (GFR) of less than 60 mL/min per $1.73m^2$.

4. Patients with underlying CKD who then go on to develop an AKI are at high risk of developing metabolic acidosis.

References

Adamczak, M., Masajtis-Zagajewska, A., Mazanowska, O. et al. (2018). Diagnosis and treatment of Metabolic acidosis in Patients with Chronic Kidney Disease – Position statement of the Working Group of the Polish Society of Nephrology. https://www.karger.com/Article/Pdf/490475 (accessed September 2019).

Basile, D.P., Anderson, M.D., and Sutton, T.A. (2012). Pathophysiology of acute kidney injury. *Compr Physiol* 2(2): 1303–1353.

Bello, A.K., Alrukhaimi, M., Ashuntantang, G.E. et al. (2017) Complications of chronic kidney disease: current state, knowledge gaps, and strategy for action. *Kidney International Supplement* 7(2): 122–129.

Bellomo, R., Cass, A., Cole L. et al. (2009). RENAL Replacement Therapy Study Investigators: Intensity of continuous renal-replacement therapy in critically ill patients. *N Engl J Med* 361(17): 1627–38.

Bellomo, R., Ronco, C., Kellum, J.A. et al. (2004). Acute renal failure – definition, outcome measures, animal models, fluid therapy and information technology needs: the Second International Consensus Conference of the Acute Dialysis Quality Initiative (ADQI) Group. https://ccforum.biomedcentral.com/articles/10.1186/cc2872 (accessed November 2020).

British National Formulary (2020a). Prescribing in renal impairment. https://bnf.nice.org.uk/guidance/prescribing-in-renal-impairment.html (accessed December 2020).

Chavez, L.O., Leon, M., Einav, S., and Varon, J. (2016). Beyond muscle destruction a systematic review of rhabdomyolysis for clinical practice. *Critical Care* 20 No 135.

Critical Care Networks-National Nurse Leads (CC3N) (2015). National Competency Framework for Registered Nurses in Adult Critical Care. Step 2 Competencies. https://www.cc3n.org.uk/uploads/9/8/4/2/98425184/02_new_step_2_final.pdf (accessed 15 October 2020).

Cumming, A. and Payne, S. (2009). The renal system. In: *Macleod's Clinical Examination*, 12e (ed. G. Douglas, F. Nicol, and C. Robertson), 217–234. China: Elsevier.

Davies, A. (2014). Acute kidney injury. In: *Renal Nursing*, 4e (ed. N. Thomas), 97–115. Hoboken, NJ: John Wiley & Sons.

Davies, T.W. Ostermann, M. & Gilbert-Kawai, E. (2019). Renal replacement therapy for acute kidney injury in intensive care. *British Journal of Hospital Medicine*. 80: 8.

De Pasquale, C., Pistorio, M.L., Veroux, M. (2020). Psychological and psychopathological aspects of kidney transplantation: a systematic review. https://www.ncbi.nlm.nih.gov/pmc/articles/PMC7066324/ (accessed December 2020).

Dutton, H. and Finch, J. (2018). *Acute and Critical Care Nursing at a Glance*. Hoboken, NJ: John Wiley & Sons.

Gemmell, L. Docking, R., and Black, E. (2017). Renal replacment therapy in critical care. *BJA Education* 17(3): 88–93.

Girling, B.J., Channon, S.W., Haines, R.W. et al. (2020). Acute kidney injury and adverse outcomes of critical illness: correlation or causation? *Clinical Kidney Journal* 13(2): 133–141. doi: 10.1093/ckj/sfz158.

Graeme-Smith, D.G. and Aronson, J.K. (2002). *Oxford Textbook of Clinical Pharmacology and Drug Therapy*, 3e. Oxford: Oxford University Press.

Gross, J.L., de Azevedo, M.J., Silverio, S.P. et al. (2005). Diabetic nephropathy: Diagnosis, prevention and treatment. *Diabetes Care* 28(1): 164–176.

Haneda, M., Utsunomiya, K., Koya, D. Babazono, T. et al. (2015). A new classification of diabetic nephropathy 2014: a report from Jint Committee on Diabetic Nephropathy. https://onlinelibrary.wiley.com/doi/full/10.1111/jdi.12319 (accessed November 2020).

Health Education England & The Faculty of Intensive Care Medicine (2020). e-Learning for Intensive Care Medicine. https://www.e-lfh.org.uk/programmes/intensive-care-medicine/ (accessed December 2020).

Hunter, J.D., Gregg, K., and Damani, Z. (2006). Rhabdomyolysis. *Continuing Education in Anaesthesia, Critical Care and Pain* 6(4): 141–143.

Kidney Care UK (2020). Facts and Stats. https://www.kidneycareuk.org/news-and-campaigns/facts-and-stats/ (accessed November 2020).

Kidney Disease Improving Global Outcomes (2012). KDIGO clinical practice guideline for acute kidney injury. *Kidney International Supplement* 2: 1–138.

Kidney Disease Improving Global Outcomes (2013). KDIGO clinical practice guideline for acute kidney injury. *Kidney International Supplement* 3: 1–150.

Kidney Research UK (2018). Annual Report and Financial Statements. https://kidneyresearchuk.org/about-us/annual-reports/ (accessed September 2019).

Lafayette, R. (2019). British Medical Journal Best Practice Acute Kidney Injury. https://bestpractice.bmj.com/topics/en-gb/83/pdf/83.pdf (accessed November 2020).

Leach, R. (2014). *Critical Care Medicine at a Glance*, 3e. West Sussex: John Wiley & Sons.

Makris, K. and Spanou, L. (2016). Acute kidney injury: definition, pathophysiology and clinical phenotypes. https://www.ncbi.nlm.nih.gov/pmc/articles/PMC5198510/ (accessed December 2020).

Mehta, R., Kellum, J., Shah, S. et al. (2007). Acute Kidney Injury Network: Report of an Initiative to Improve Outcomes in Acute Kidney Injury. https://ccforum.biomedcentral.com/articles/10.1186/cc5713 (accessed November 2020).

Morcos, R., Kucharik, M., Bansal, P. et al. (2019). Contrast-induced acute kidney injury: Review and practical update. *Clinical Care Medicine Insights: Cardiology* 13: 1–9.

Nair, M. (2018). The renal system and associated disorders. In: *Fundamentals of Applied Pathophysiology: An Essential Guide for Nursing and Healthcare Students*, 3e (ed I. Peate), 247–277. Wiley Blackwell.

National Confidential Enquiry into Patient Outcome and Death (NCEPOD) (2009). Adding insult to injury. A review of the care of patient who dies in hospital with a primary diagnosis of acute kidney injury (acute renal failure). https://www.ncepod.org.uk/2009report1/Downloads/AKI_report.pdf (accessed November 2020).

National Institute of Clinical Excellence (2013). Acute Kidney Injury: prevention, detection and management. Clinical Guideline 169. https://www.nice.org.uk/guidance/cg169 (accessed November 2020).

National Institute of Clinical Excellence (2015). Chronic Kidney Disease in adults: assessment and management. https://www.nice.org.uk/guidance/cg182 (accessed November 2020).

National Institute of Clinical Excellence (2017). Immunosuppressive therapy for kidney transplant in adults. Technology appraisal guidance TA481. https://www.nice.org.uk/guidance/ta481 (accessed December 2020).

National Institute of Clinical Excellence (2019). Chronic Kidney Disease. https://cks.nice.org.uk/chronic-kidney-disease#!topicSummary (accessed November 2020).

Nazar, C.M.J. (2014). Diabetic nephropathy: Principles of diagnosis and treatment of diabetic kidney disease. *Journal of Nephropharmacology* 3(1): 15–20.

Neal, M.J (2020). *Medical Pharmacology at a Glance*, 9e. Wiley-Blackwell.

NHS Blood and Transplant (2018). Annual Report on the kidney transplantation 2017/18. https://nhsbtdbe.blob.core.windows.net/umbraco-assets-corp/12256/nhsbt-kidney-transplantation-annual-report-2017-2018.pdf (accessed November 2020).

O'Callaghan, C. (2017). *The Renal System at a Glance*, 4e. Chichester: John Wiley & Sons.

Office for National Statistics (2018). Deaths that were caused by 'Acute Kidney Injury', by place of death and broad age group, England and Wales, registered 2001 to 2016. https://www.ons.gov.uk/peoplepopulationandcommunity/birthsdeathsandmarriages/deaths/adhocs/007984deathsthatwerecausedbyacutekidneyinjurybyplaceofdeathandbroadagegroupenglandandwalesregistered2001to2016 (accessed September 2019).

Palevsky, P.M., Zhang, J.H., Connor, T.Z. et al. (2008). VA/NIH Acute Renal Failure Trial Network: Intensity of renal support in critically ill patients with acute kidney injury. *N Engl J Med* 359(1): 7–20.

Peate, I. and Hill, B. (2021). *Fundamentals of Pharmacology: For Nursing & Healthcare Students*. Wiley-Blackwell.

Peate, I. and Nair, M. (2017). *Fundamentals of Anatomy and Physiology: For Nursing and Healthcare Students*. Wiley-Blackwell.

Prowle, J.R. (2018). Organ cross-talk in shock and critical illness. *ICU Management and Practice* 18(3): 175–178.

Resuscitation Council (2015). *Advanced Life Support Manual*. London: Resuscitation Council.

Ronco, C., Haapio, M., House, A.A. et al. (2008). Cardiorenal syndrome. *J Am Coll Cardiol* 52: 1527–1539.

Ronco, C., Bellomo, R., Homel, P. et al. (2000). Effects of different doses in continuous veno-venous haemofiltration on outcomes of acute renal failure: a prospective randomised trial. *Lancet* 356(9223): 26–30.

Shah, M.M. and Mandiga, P. (2020) Physiology, plasma osmolality and oncotic pressure. In: *StatPearls*. Treasure Island, FL: StatPearls Publishing. https://www.ncbi.nlm.nih.gov/books/NBK544365/ (accessed December 2020).

Simonetto, D.A., Gines, P., and Kamath, P.S. (2020). Hepatorenal syndrome: pathophysiology, diagnosis and management. *BMJ* 370.

Talley, N.J. and O'Connor, S. (2010). *Clinical Examination. A Systematic Guide to Physical Diagnosis*, 6e. Chatswood: Elsevier.

The Renal Association UK (2020). Clinical Practice Guidelines Treatment of Acute Hyperkalaemia in Adults. https://renal.org/sites/renal.org/files/RENAL%20ASSOCIATION%20HYPERKALAEMIA%20GUIDELINE%202020.pdf (accessed January 2020).

The UK Renal Registry (2020). UK Renal Registry 22nd Annual Report of the Renal Association. https://renal.org/sites/renal.org/files/publication/file-attachments/22nd_UKRR_ANNUAL_REPORT_FULL.pdf (accessed December 2020).

Tolwani, A.J., Campbell, R.C., Stofan, B.S. et al. (2008). Standard versus high-dose CVVHDF for ICU-related acute renal failure. *J Am Soc Nephrol* 19(6): 1233–1238.

Umanath, K. and Lewis, B. (2018). Update on Diabetic Nephropathy: Core Curriculum 2018. https://www.ajkd.org/article/S0272-6386(17)31102-2/fulltext (accessed December 2020).

Van Wert, R., Friedrich, J.O., Scales, D.C. et al. (2010). High-dose renal replacement therapy for acute kidney injury: systematic review and meta-analysis. *Crit Care Med.* 38(5): 1360–1369.

Vassalotti, J.A., Centor, R., Turner, B.J. et al. (2016). Practical approach to detection and management of chronic kidney disease for the primary care clinician. https://www.amjmed.com/article/S0002-9343(15)00855-4/pdf (accessed November 2020).

Wang, H.E., Munter, P., Chertow, G.M. et al. (2012). Acute kidney injury and mortality in hospitalized patients. *Am J Nephrol* 35: 349–355. https://www.karger.com/Article/Pdf/337487 (accessed November 2020).

Ward, J.P.T. and Linden, R.W.A (2017). *Physiology at a Glance*, 4e. Wiley Blackwell.

Webster, A.C., Nagler, E.V., Morton, R.L. et al. (2017). Chronic kidney disease. *Lancet* 389(10075): 1238–1252.

Yates, C.J., Fourlanos, S., Hjelmesaeth, J. et al. (2012). New-onset diabetes aster kidney transplantation – challenges and changes. *American Journal of Transplantation* 12: 820–828.

369

Chapter 25

Endocrine critical care

Geraldine Fitzgerald O'Connor and Emma Long

Aim

The aim of this chapter is to provide the reader with an evidence-based understanding of endocrine disorders for patients who are cared for in critical care settings.

Learning outcomes

After reading this chapter the reader will be able to:

- Understand the pathophysiology of the endocrine system.
- Show an ability to appreciate the complexities critical care patients undergo with the regulation of their endocrine system.
- Distinguish the key precipitating factors, history and clinical course for each disorder.
- Describe the treatment for the most common endocrine disorders in patients who are critically unwell.

Test your prior knowledge

- Name the glands of the endocrine system and discuss their functions.
- Name the three diabetic emergencies.
- Can you name the symptoms which are a good indicator of a thyroid crisis?
- Analyse the interventions for patients with DKA and HHS. Distinguish the primary differences.
- How can the danger of hypoglycaemia be prevented?

Fundamentals of Critical Care: A Textbook for Nursing and Healthcare Students, First Edition. Edited by Ian Peate and Barry Hill.
© 2023 John Wiley & Sons Ltd. Published 2023 by John Wiley & Sons Ltd.
Companion website: www.wiley.com/go/peate/criticalcare

Introduction

Chapter 25 explores the endocrine system and how this relates to patients who are critically unwell. Every cell in the human body is influenced by the endocrine system. The endocrine system acts to maintain equilibrium at the cellular level and is a vital link in homeostasis. When abnormalities occur, illness or death can result. Treatment usually requires managing a deviant hormone by either reducing or increasing its production or secretion from its associated endocrine gland. A thorough understanding of the endocrine system and how its functions is necessary for nurses and other healthcare professionals in accurately assessing and treating endocrine disorders.

The endocrine system usually produces classical signs and symptoms of dysfunction such as weight gain or loss, menstrual disturbance, excessive thirst, resistant hypertension, are a few examples and the stress of critical illness provokes a significant response by the endocrine system (Sole et al., 2017).

Endocrine disorders have effects on many of the body systems. At the same time, acute illness may lead to hypofunction, and occasionally hyperfunction of the endocrine system. This chapter will explore these disorders and the effect on the critically ill person.

Step 1 competencies: National Standards

1:5 Gastrointestinal System (Critical Care Networks – National Nurse Leads (CC3N) 2015)

You must be able to demonstrate through discussion essential knowledge of (and its application to your supervised practice): Causes of pancreatic dysfunction:

- Pancreatitis
- Diabetes Mellitus Type 1, and Diabetes Mellitus Type 2.

6Cs: Communication

Effective communication with a patient in ICU is paramount to adequately assess the patient's needs and care due to high levels of monitoring.

Thyroid and parathyroid glands

Thyroid gland

The thyroid gland is butterfly-shaped and has two lobes connected by the isthmus. It is located on the trachea, inferior to the larynx. The thyroid gland is the largest pure endocrine gland in the body (Marieb, 2015) and produces three active hormones: thyroxine (T4), triiodothyronine (T3) and calcitonin. Except for the adult brain, spleen, testes, uterus and the thyroid gland itself, thyroid hormones affect virtually every cell in the body (Marieb, 2015).

Calcitonin is responsible for lowering serum calcium level. This is achieved by reducing the rate of calcium release from bone and reducing the rate of formation of new osteoclasts. Calcitonin can correct high serum calcium levels quickly, and its secretion is enhanced when blood calcium levels are elevated above 2.6 millimoles per litre (mmol/L) (Adam et al., 2017).

The thyroid gland is one of the main regulators of metabolism. T3 and T4 typically act via nuclear receptors in target tissues and initiate a variety of metabolic pathways. High levels of T3 and T4 typically cause these processes to occur more frequently. Metabolic processes increased by thyroid hormones include:

- Basal metabolic rate
- Gluconeogenesis
- Glycogenolysis
- Protein synthesis
- Lipogenesis
- Thermogenesis

This is achieved in several ways, such as increasing the size and number of mitochondria within cells, increasing Na-K pump activity and increasing the presence of β-adrenergic receptors in tissues such as cardiac muscle (Clausen, 2003).

The main regulator of thyroid function is via a negative feedback mechanism. The anterior pituitary is stimulated to synthesise and secrete thyroid-stimulating hormone (TSH) by thyrotrophin-releasing hormone (TRH) produced by the hypothalamus. TSH stimulates the thyroid gland to synthesise and secrete the thyroid hormones T3 and T4. In turn, the secretion of T3 and T4 inhibits the release of further TSH (Adam et al., 2017).

Disorders of the thyroid gland

Hypothyroidism (myxoedema)

Myxoedema coma is the extreme manifestation of hypothyroidism, which, although rare, carries a mortality ranging from 30 to 60% (Bersten and Soni, 2014). It occurs when a patient with long-standing hypothyroidism suffers an additional significant stress. Infections and discontinuation of thyroid supplements are the major precipitating factors (Adam et al., 2017). The clinical presentation is often nonspecific making the diagnosis difficult. Three major features are (Waldmann et al., 2019):

- Altered mental status
- Hypothermia
- Clinical features of hypothyroidism

Immediate management (Wiersinga, 2018):

- ABC (Airway, Breathing, Circulation) – very low threshold for anaesthetic assistance owing to airway risk from coma or seizures
- Cautious correction of hypothermia by insulation, ensuring cardiac monitoring in place throughout
- Immediate thyroid replacement – large initial iv dose of 300–500 µg T4, if no response add T3

> # 6Cs: Courage
> Being courageous ensures everyone gets the quality of care they deserve.

Hyperthyroidism (thyrotoxicosis)

Hyperthyroidism is a medical condition caused by excessive levels of thyroid hormones. Graves' disease is the most common form of hyperthyroidism or it can be secondary to a pituitary tumour or excess administration of thyroxine. Over-secretion of thyroid hormones leads to increased cellular metabolism throughout the body, and symptoms may include (Baid et al., 2016):

- Weight loss
- Tachycardia
- Hyperactivity
- Fatigue
- Gastrointestinal hypermotility
- Muscle tremor
- Anxiety
- Exophthalmos

Patients will require admission to critical care when these symptoms are severe.

Treatment is aimed at reducing the effects of thyroxine on the cardiovascular system (anti-thyroid medication, β-blockers, steroids).

> # 6Cs: Competent
> Being competent allows us as nurses to have the knowledge required to make decisions to give the best possible care to our patients.

Thyroid crisis

Thyroid crisis is the life-threatening clinical extreme of hyperthyroidism. It is more common in women than in men, and with reported mortality ranging from 10% to 75% in hospitalised patients (Bersten and Soni, 2014). Characteristic features include hyperpyrexia, severe tachycardia, extreme restlessness, hypertension and dehydration (Waldmann

et al., 2019). The cause of a thyrotoxic storm is commonly Graves' disease precipitated by severe infection, surgery, trauma, or pregnancy. The management should involve supportive therapy, reduction of plasma thyroid concentration and blockade of peripheral effects of thyroxine (β-Adrenoceptor antagonists – propranolol, metoprolol, esmolol; iodine; corticosteroids; carbimazole) and treatment of precipitating factors (Holcomb, 2002).

> # Orange Flag
> Steroids have been shown to cause delirium in critically ill patients and therefore it is important to recognise, assess and support any noticeable signs of delirium.
> (Clegg and Young 2011)

Parathyroid glands

The parathyroid glands are in the posterior aspect of the thyroid gland. There are usually four, but the precise number varies. Parathyroid hormone (PTH), the protein hormone of these glands, is the single most important hormone controlling the calcium balance of the blood. It's release is triggered by falling blood calcium levels and inhibited by hypercalcaemia. PTH increases ionic calcium levels in blood by stimulating three target organs: the skeleton, the kidneys, and the intestine (Marieb, 2015). PTH and calcitonin have opposing effects; together, they maintain a plasma calcium level of 2.15–2.55 mmol/litre and an ionised calcium level (non-protein-bound) of 1.18–1.3 mmol/litre (Adam et al., 2017). Calcium plays an important role in many physiological pathways that include muscle contraction, the secretion of neurotransmitters and hormones, and coagulation (Firth et al., 2020).

Disorders of the parathyroid glands

Hypercalcaemia

The clinical presentation of hypercalcaemia varies from a mild, asymptomatic, biochemical abnormality to a life-threatening medical emergency. The causes vary from hereditary disorders causing primary hyperparathyroidism, malignancy, drugs, rhabdomyolysis, and sarcoidosis. Symptoms usually develop when serum calcium exceeds 3.50 mmol/litre (Firth et al., 2020). The signs and symptoms of hypercalcaemia are shown in Box 25.1.

Treatment of severe hypercalcaemia includes (Bersten and Soni, 2014):

- Volume expansion: 0.9% NaCl 200–300 ml/h to achieve urine output of >100 ml/h
- Enhance renal excretion: furosemide 40–100 mg 1–4 hourly

Box 25.1   Signs and symptoms of hypercalcaemia.

- Cardiac: short Q-T interval, prolonged P-R interval, AV block, AF
- Neurological: drowsiness, depression, confusion, coma
- GI: nausea and vomiting, abdominal pain, pancreatitis
- Renal: polyuria, renal stones, and renal failure
- Musculoskeletal: muscle weakness, general malaise, bone pain

- Calcitonin 4 IU/kg (increases excretion of calcium and inhibits bone reabsorption), works rapidly but may only remain effective for 24–48 hours.
- Bisphosphonates: (potent inhibitors of bone resorption): pamidronate (60–90 mg over 4 hours) or zoledronic acid (4 mg over 15 mins)
- Glucocorticoid therapy: hydrocortisone or dexamethasone
- Haemodialysis

Medications management: thyroxine/levothyroxine

Levothyroxine is a synthetically produced form of thyroxine, a hormone excreted by the thyroid gland. It is used primarily to treat hypothyroidism at a dose of 1.6 mcg/kg once daily and taken orally. The monitoring of thyroid-stimulating hormone (TSH) is required to establish appropriate dosing.

Side effects are generally caused by incorrect dosing and can result in abdominal pain, nausea, agitation, fever, muscle cramps and headaches

Hypocalcaemia

Hypocalcaemia is defined as a serum calcium level <2.0 mmol/litre. However, as plasma calcium levels may be inaccurate in the presence of hypoalbuminaemia, ionised Ca^{2+} or corrected serum Ca^{2+} should be used. The normal lower limit for ionised Ca^{2+} is 1.1 mmol/litre. In cases of hypoalbuminaemia a correction factor can be applied to serum calcium levels (Waldmann et al., 2019):

Corrected Ca^{2+} (mmol/L) = measured × (40 – albumin (g/L)) × 0.02

Causes:

- Septic shock
- Acute or chronic renal failure

- Citrate chelation (blood transfusion or regional citrate anticoagulation)
- Malignancy
- Hypomagnesaemia

Treatment of hypocalcaemia requires replacement of calcium either by oral supplementation or IV calcium depending on the level and speed of correction needed. Treatment for acute symptomatic hypocalcaemia is initially 10–20 mL, calcium gluconate injection 10% (providing approximately 2.25–4.5 mmol of calcium) should be administered with plasma-calcium and ECG monitoring, and either repeated as required or, if only temporary improvement, followed by a continuous intravenous infusion to prevent recurrence, alternatively (by continuous intravenous infusion), initially 50 mL/hour, adjusted according to response (Joint Formulary Committee, 2020).

Medicines management: steroids

Whilst steroid use in ICU is common practice side effects of use need to be recognised. Complications of steroid use in ICU are but not limited to

- Suppression of the adrenal axis
- Hyperglycaemia
- Myopathy
- Hypokalaemia
- Leucocytosis
- Delayed wound healing
- Immunosuppression
- Pancreatitis

Pituitary gland

The pituitary gland lies inferior to the hypothalamus, linked through the pituitary stalk. While anterior and posterior components of the gland are anatomically related, they are developmentally and functionally discrete (Webb et al., 2016). The functionality of the pituitary gland can be seen in Table 25.1.

Disorders of the pituitary gland

Syndrome of inappropriate antidiuretic hormone secretion

In Syndrome of Inappropriate Antidiuretic Hormone Secretion (SIADH) there can be either be an increase in secretion or increase in production of ADH. This increase

Table 25.1 Functionality of the pituitary gland. *Source:* Adam et al., 2017.

The anterior pituitary gland	The posterior pituitary gland
• Growth hormone (GH) affects, fat, protein, and carbohydrate metabolism • Thyroid-stimulating hormone (TSH) stimulates the thyroid gland to secrete thyroid hormones • Adrenocorticotrophic hormone (ACTH) controls the secretion of adrenocortical hormones • Gonadotrophic hormones involved in sexual functions	• Oxytocin stimulates contraction of the uterus and the muscles of the milk ducts in the breast • Antidiuretic hormone (ADH, vasopressin) stimulates reabsorption of water from the distal tubules of the kidney

in ADH occurs even though osmolality is normal and so it causes an increase in total body water and hyponatraemia. SIADH can be caused by a pituitary tumour, other malignant tumours, head trauma or drugs. Management of the condition is the same whatever the cause or type of SIADH. The underlying cause should be treated appropriately, and fluid restriction instituted to between 500 and 750 ml/24 h (Firth et al., 2020). In patients with severe symptomatic hyponatraemia (<120 mmol/L) hypotonic saline (3 or 1.8%) can be added to fluid restriction to restore serum sodium quickly. Excessive rapid correction (>0.5–1 mmol/L/hour) should be avoided to prevent the rare, but serious complication of central pontine myelinolysis (Webb et al., 2016) resulting in serious neurologic complications.

Medications management: vasopressin

Vasopressin is used to manage anti-diuretic hormone deficiency. Vasopressin is used to treat diabetes insipidus related to low levels of antidiuretic hormone. Vasopressin infusions are also used as second line therapy for septic shock patients not responding to fluid resuscitation or infusions of dopamine/noradrenaline. It is administered through an intravenous device, intramuscular injection, nasally or sublingually. Side effects are abdominal pain, diarrhoea, vomiting, chest pain, cardiac arrest, hypertension.

Learning event: reflection

Reflect on how much you understand about endocrine syndromes and how critical illness makes it difficult to identify the classic signs and symptoms of these syndromes.

Diabetes insipidus

Diabetes insipidus causes impaired renal conservation of water, resulting in polyuria (> 3 L in 24 hr). As long as the thirst centre remains intact and the person is able to respond to this thirst, fluid volume can be maintained. If the patient is unable to respond, severe dehydration results if fluid losses are not replaced (Sole et al., 2017).

Central diabetes insipidus results from a lack of ADH causing polyuria and polydipsia. The main causes being neurosurgery, head trauma, and hypoxic brain injury.

Nephrogenic diabetes insipidus is a primary renal tubular defect of water reabsorption in which there is a poor response to ADH. Main causes are drug-induced (lithium toxicity), hypokalaemia and renal disease (Adam et al., 2017).

The management of DI is led by:

• Prevention of dehydration
• Correction of sodium imbalance
• Prevention of further complications

It is essential to accurately record fluid intake and output to guide likely fluid requirements. The free water (FW) deficit may be calculated using the following formula (Baid et al., 2016):

$$FW\ deficit = 0.6 \times weight(kg) \times (current\ Na \div 14 - 1)$$

Management of DI should also focus on regular cardiovascular assessment to prevent cardiovascular compromise and other complications include seizures and encephalopathy.

In patients with excessive polyuria, administration of desmopressin (typically dosed at 1–2 µg BD) may be necessary to prevent significant volume contraction and hyperosmolality with severe hypernatraemia (Webb et al., 2016).

Patients with nephrogenic DI do not or only partially respond to desmopressin and treatment can include thiazide diuretics which may limit the polyuria via volume contraction and improved tubular water reabsorption.

6Cs: Compassion

Showing compassion for a patient during times of stress and distress is the fundamental building blocks for building a therapeutic relationship.

Pathophysiology

Pancreas

The pancreas has endocrine and exocrine functions. The exocrine assists in the digestion and absorption of nutrients. Clustered lobules and lobes (acini) of enzyme producing cells release secretions into the pancreatic duct. This occurs from vagal stimulation and release of hormone secretion and cholecystokinin control the rate of and number of pancreatic secretions daily. On average about 1000 ml of digestive enzymes are released (Adam et al., 2017). The endocrine function involves the islets of Langerhans which are a cluster of cells with the pancreas which perform the endocrine function of the pancreas. They contain:

- Alpha cells that produce glucagon, a hormone that stimulates glycogenolysis in the liver
- Beta cells that produce insulin to promote carbohydrate metabolism and
- Delta cells that produce somatostatin, the hormone that inhibits gastric secretion and somatotrophin release.

Glucagon and insulin have a profound effect upon metabolism. Insulin produced by the pancreatic beta cells (β), transports glucose into the cells, converts glucose into fats, promotes glucagon storage in the liver and muscle cells, inhibits fat metabolism and promotes tissue growth by protein deposition. Glucagon has the opposite effect to insulin. Its primary role is to increase blood sugar levels. This is done when the alpha cells detect low blood glucose levels.

Examination scenario: blood glucose monitoring

Blood glucose monitoring involves obtaining a drop of blood and using a testing strip designed for glucose monitoring that is read by a blood glucose monitor (please refer to local policy for calibration and training on the medical device you are using).

Diabetes mellitus

Hyperglycaemia occurs due to a deficiency, destruction (due to antibodies) or impaired effectiveness of insulin. There are two types:

- Type 1: insulin-dependent. This accounts for approximately 10% of diabetes and usually has its onset in childhood or adolescence. It is a result of and autoimmune destruction of beta cells in the pancreas.
- Type 2: non-insulin-dependent. Usually affecting people over 40 partially due to pancreatic decline and often seen in obese people due to fat causing insulin resistance

(Adam et al., 2017; Joint British Diabetes Societies Inpatient Care Group, 2012, 2013).

Medications management: short-acting insulin

Human insulin is the name that describes a synthetic insulin that is grown in laboratories. Short-acting insulin starts to act from 30 minutes after injecting to peak action occurring between 2 and 3 hours after injecting lasting up to 10 hours.

Secondary diabetes

Diabetes that results because of drug therapy, metabolic/endocrine disease, critical illness (including trauma and burns) and includes gestational diabetes. Insulin resistance is usually applied to this type of diabetes and may be due to problems of decreased secretion of insulin, the responsiveness of the cellular insulin receptors or modified pathways. With critical illness there is also an increased release of stress hormone (cortisol, catecholamines, glucagon and growth hormones) that antagonise the insulin's metabolic actions (Adam et al., 2017; Webb et al., 2016).

Snapshot

Noah, aged 55, had been admitted to ICU following developing sepsis at home from a urinary tract infection. He was sedated, ventilated, on inotropes and enterally fed and requiring insulin. He has now been extubated but remains on his enteral feed until he has been assessed by the Spech and Language Therapist.

His enteral feed had been stopped at 0800.

Airway (A): Airway is patent, patient is speaking.
Breathing (B): oxygen saturations 97% (NEWS2 = 0), on 2 litres nasal cannula (NEWS2 = 2), respiratory rate (RR) 26 breaths per minute (NEWS2 = 3).
Cardiovascular System (C): Blood Pressure (BP) is 95/65 (NEWS2 = 0), Heart Rate (HR) is 105 beats per minute (NEWS2 = 1), capillary refill time is (CRT) is 4 seconds, he is cool to touch.
Disability (D): Patient is alert (NEWS2 = 0), Body Temperature (T) is 37.5°C.
Exposure (E): Noah was sweating and shaking.
Total NEW2 Score: 6.

Nursing actions:

- A full head-to-toe assessment was performed including recording Noah's blood glucose level.
- A doctor was made aware of his raised NEW2 score

Diagnosis:
- His blood glucose level had dropped to 3.9 mmol/L
- His insulin infusion was stopped immediately and an infusion of 10% glucose 150mls and then his blood glucose was rechecked after 15 mins.

What other steps should be taken to care for Noah at this time?

Acute severe pancreatitis

Acute severe pancreatitis is caused by an obstruction to the Ampulla of Vater, which prevents acid chymne being neutralised and therefore stimulating continued release of pancreatic juices. Congestion then ruptures the ductules in the pancreases and release pancreatic juice directly onto the gland. It is through this process autodigestion occurs, causing oedema and resulting in insulin production being affected (Adam et al., 2017).

Hyperglycaemia in the critically ill

The critically ill patient is at risk of hyperglycaemia from many factors. Different stressors include their disease state, illness related hormonal response to stress and the environment itself. Risk factors include (Sole et al., 2017; Webb, 2016):

- Pre-existing diabetes mellitus
- Obesity
- Pancreatitis
- Cirrhosis
- Hypokalaemia
- Normal stress response release of cortisol, growth hormones, catecholamines, glucagon, glucocorticoids, cytokines (interleukin-1, interleukin-6 and tumour necrosis factor (TNF))
- Ageing
- Lack of muscle activity
- Insulin deficiency/ resistance
- Administration of exogenous catecholamines and glucocorticoids, dextrose solutions or nutritional support.
- Some drug therapies e.g., thiazides, beta-blockers, highly active antiretroviral therapy (HAART), phenytoin, tacrolimus, and cyclosporine.

Orange Flag

The interrelationship between hormonal abnormalities and psychological factors is complex and should be viewed in a multifactorial frame of reference (Sonino and Fava, 2004).

Although stress-induced hyperglycaemia is a normal physiologic response related to the flight-fight mode,

glucose elevation is associated with poor hospital outcomes with or without a formal diagnosis of diabetes (Webb et al., 2016). Effective control of a patient's blood sugar has been shown to improve outcomes (NICE-SUGAR Study Investigators, 2009). The landmark study by Van de Berghe et al. in 2001 demonstrated that tight glycaemic of hyperglycaemia in the critically ill surgical population reduced morbidity and mortality. Studies after this in a wider population showed that there was higher mortality and hypoglycaemia incidence when too tight control was applied.

6Cs: Commitment

Showing commitment demonstrates a willingness to improve the care and experience for all patients.

Diabetic emergencies

There are three types of diabetic emergencies:

- Diabetic ketoacidosis (DKA) characterised by hyperglycaemia, ketosis and acidosis and sometimes coma
- Hyperosmolar hyperglycaemic states (HHS) usually characterised by hyperglycaemia but with mild or no ketones
- Hypoglycaemic coma.

Red Flag

Some patients have hypoglycaemic unawareness and remain asymptomatic despite extremely low blood glucose levels. Elderly patients and those taking beta-blockers are at especially high risk.

Diabetic ketoacidosis

It occurs more frequently in patients with type 1 diabetes but is becoming more common in patients type 2 as well (Joint British Diabetes Societies Inpatient Care Group, 2013). Causes include infection, myocardial infarction or commonly non-compliance with medication. Coma is not always a feature, but conscious levels can vary according to the degree of increased serum plasma osmolality.

Diabetic ketoacidosis (DKA) is the most complex characterised by the presence of

- Hyperglycaemia: Insulin facilitates transfer of glucose into cells. Therefore, a lack of insulin results in an inability to utilise glucose derived from carbohydrate metabolism. Other 'stress' hormones (catecholamines, glucagon, cortisol, and growth hormone) are released in stress states; there is an antagonistic action insulin which further exacerbates hyperglycaemia.

- Acidosis: This is due to the accumulation of ketone β-hydroxybutyrate and acetoacetate and therefore the subsequent anion gap. The arterial pH is less than 7.3 and the anion gap often exceeds 20 mmol/L.
- Ketonemia the patient cannot utilise glucose derived from dietary carbohydrate because of insufficient insulin. Energy is increasingly provided from fat breakdown (lipolysis). These free fatty acids are converted into ketones in the body by the liver (acetone, acetoacetate and β-hydroxybutyrate) can cause profound metabolic acidosis.

Snapshot

Clinical presentation:
Zahara is a 22-year-old lady, normally fit and well, who was admitted to hospital via ED after being found by flat mates disoriented, smelling of alcohol and complaining of abdominal pain. She was admitted to ICU for monitoring with query pancreatitis or perforated appendix and is awaiting a CT scan.

Airway (A): Airway is patient and Zahara is speaking in sentences.

Breathing (B): Oxygen saturations on room air 96% (NEWS2=0) on room air (New2=0). Respiratory rate 32 and has Kussmaul respiration (NEWS2= 3).

Cardiovascular (C): Blood pressure (BP) is 92/60 (NEWS2=2), heart rate (HR) is 125 beats per minute (NEWS2= 2), capillary refill time (CRT) centrally is 4 seconds, and she is cool to touch. No urine passed since admission.

Disability (D): Zahara is responding to voice on the AVPU scale (NEWS2=3), body temperature is 37.1°C. Her blood glucose level is 17 mmol/L and ketones 4 mmol/L with point-of-care testing.

Exposure (E): Zahara is flushed and dry. Her mouth is dry and is asking for something to drink.

Total NEW2 Score: 10.

Nursing actions:
- Urgent medical review.
- Diagnostic test: laboratory test, Arterial blood gas (ABG) and urinalysis.
- Hourly observations.
- Insertion of urinary catheter.

Diagnosis:
- Zahara was diagnosed with diabetes ketoacidosis and started on a management plan to reduce her blood glucose levels and replace fluids lost. Her ABG showed acidosis with a pH of 7.25 and bicarbonate of 14.
- Further investigations and referral to the Diabetic team for type 1 diabetes.

Clinical Investigations: urinalysis

Urinalysis is a simple non-invasive test of urine using a reagent strip. It can be performed for screening, diagnosis, and management of conditions.

There are many different chemical reagent strips available from several manufacturers, but the following tests are commonly available on all variants:

- Blood
- Bilirubin and urobilinogen
- Nitrites
- Leucocytes
- Protein
- Ketones
- Glucose
- pH
- Specific gravity

It is important that professionals understand methods for collecting urine, limit the risk of contamination by using reagent strips correctly and accurately interpret results (Yates, 2016)

Management

The Joint British Diabetes Societies Inpatient Care Group (2013) recommends that care bundles are split into four times zones in the first 24-hour time period (hour 1: immediate management, 1–6 hours, 6–12 hours and 12–24 hours). The four areas for management to consider are:

1. Stabilisation: The patient's ability to maintain an airway, if conscious level as assessed by the Glasgow Coma Scale is low then intubation and mechanical ventilation are likely to be needed.
   - Self-ventilating patients will require oxygen to maintain normal saturations.
   - Frequent ABGS measurements to monitor O_2, CO_2 and pH levels.
2. Restoration of adequate circulation:
   - Significant fluid replacement is required as water deficits are likely to be high (estimated at 100 mL deficit/kg). It is recommended that a crystalloid replacement, with current guidelines suggesting a premixed potassium chloride in 0.9% saline, care should be taken to monitor for hypochloraemia (see Table 25.2). Rapid fluid replacement is recommended in adults only.
   - Target blood pressure is >90 mmHg. CVS monitoring and invasive fluid assessment (CVP) may be required.
   - Fluid balance should be closely monitored.
   - Patients with pre-existing CVS, renal impairment or other comorbidities will need extra vigilance during the assessment of fluid status.

Table 25.2 Saline and potassium replacement regime. *Source:* Joint British Diabetes Societies Inpatient Care Group, 2013.

Fluid	Volume
0.9% sodium chloride	1000 ml over the first hour
0.9% sodium chloride with potassium chloride	1000 ml over the next 2 hours
0.9% sodium chloride with potassium chloride	1000 ml over the next 2 hours
0.9% sodium chloride with potassium chloride	1000 ml over the next 4 hours
0.9% sodium chloride with potassium chloride	1000 ml over the next 4 hours
0.9% sodium chloride with potassium chloride	1000 ml over the next 6 hours
Reassessment of CVS status is mandatory at 12 hours as further fluid may be required.	

3. Glucose control:
   - A fixed-rate intravenous insulin infusion should be commenced, and this should be related to weight. The exception is in obese patients who should have a modified scale.
   - Current guidelines suggest a fixed-rate 0.1 international unit (iu) of insulin/kg/hour should be infused. Suggested rates in Table 25.3.
   - Regular blood glucose monitoring. If blood glucose concentration is >20 mmol/L or 'high' on point-of-care testing a sample should be sent to the laboratory.
   - Blood glucose concentration should drop by 3 mmol/hour. Urgent review if failure to obtain this level.
   - If blood glucose levels drop below 14 mmol/L in the first 6 hours, Intravenous glucose may be required.
   - Blood ketones should be assessed regularly and continued until ketoacidosis is corrected. If this is not possible, venous bicarbonate levels will need to be assessed.
   - Low-acting insulin can be administered subcutaneously if the patient already takes it as per local guidelines.

- The fixed-rate insulin infusion should be discontinued once the patient is stable. Normal medication administration should be recommenced following discussion with the medical team.

4. Electrolyte replacement
   - Administration of intravenous insulin will reduce serum potassium levels, therefore close observation is required.
   - The target range is 4–5 mmol/L.
   - Potassium should be replaced as per Table 25.4. If the levels are outside the normal reference range, medical review should be sought.
   - Monitor signs of cardiac arrhythmias linked to potassium abnormalities.
   - Regular assessment of other electrolytes is recommended and treated as per local guidelines.

Table 25.3 Suggested rates of insulin infusion. *Source:* Joint British Diabetes Societies Inpatient Care Group, 2013.

Patient weight (kg)	Insulin dose (iu/h)
60–69	6
70–79	7
80–89	8
90–99	9
100–109	10
110–119	11
120–129	12
130–139	13
140–149	14
>150	15 (refer to diabetic team)

Table 25.4 Potassium replacement. *Source:* Joint British Diabetes Societies Inpatient Care Group, 2013.

Potassium level in the first 24 hours (mmol/L)	Potassium replacement in mmol/L of solution
Over 5.5	Nil
3.5–5.5.	40
Below 3.5	Senior review as additional potassium needs to be given.

Clinical investigations: point-of-care testing

Point-of-Care (PoC) testing is a form of testing that can occur at or near the patient's bedside. The benefit of a bedside monitor is getting results back quickly compared to laboratory testing that will determine quick treatment escalation. Some examples of PoC testing are blood glucose, arterial blood gases (ABG's), blood ketones, urinalysis.

Hyperosmolar, hyperglycaemic states (HHS)

Hyperosmolar, hyperglycaemic states are common in patients with non-insulin-dependent diabetes mellitus. There is often a predisposing factor that triggers the condition. Some factors are age, infection, trauma (including burns), myocardial infarction, pancreatitis, hepatitis, renal failure, hypothermia, carbohydrate overload and some medications (Joint British Diabetes Societies Inpatient Care Group, 2013; Sole et al., 2017; Webb, 2016).

Hyperosmolar, hyperglycaemic states differ from diabetic ketoacidosis in the level of free fatty acids and counter-regulatory hormone is lower. This is due to sufficient insulin still being secreted to prevent lipolysis and hyperglycaemia. Therefore, ketosis may be mild or absent. The mortality rate is higher than diabetic ketoacidosis at around 15–25% (Joint British Diabetes Societies Inpatient Care Group 2013, Webb 2016). The condition tends to manifest over a period of days, resulting in severe dehydration and hyperosmolar state.

Management

The Joint British Diabetes Societies Inpatient Care Group (2013) recommends that care bundles are split into four times zones in the first 24-hour time period (hour 1: immediate management, 1–6 hours, 6–12 hours and 12–24 hours). The five areas for management to consider are:

1. Stabilisation: The patient's ability to maintain an airway, if conscious level as assessed by the Glasgow Coma Scale is low then intubation and mechanical ventilation are likely to be needed.

   - Self-ventilating patients will require oxygen to maintain normal saturations.
   - Frequent ABGS measurements to monitor O_2, CO_2 and pH levels.

2. Normalisation of serum osmolarity:

   - Patients will present with extreme fluid loss. It is estimated that the hyperglycaemic hyperosmolar state causes fluid depletion in the range of 100–220 mL/Kg.
   - Close monitoring of serum osmolarity should occur at least hourly. If point-of-care not available, then the following formula can be used and plotted on a graph (Joint British Diabetes Societies Inpatient Care Group, 2013):

$$\text{Serum osmolarity} = 2Na^+ + \text{glucose} + \text{urea}$$

   - Rapid changes may be harmful as it causes significant fluid shifts. Fluid replacement should be given cautiously.

3. Restoration of circulating volume:

   - Current recommendations are 0.9% sodium chloride as the principal IV fluid. If the patient osmolarity is not falling hypertonic solutions such as 0.45% (half-strength) sodium chloride may be used.
   - The aim of the treatment is to replace 50% of lost volume in the first 12 hours and the remainder in the next 12 hours.
   - Care should be given in vulnerable groups (e.g. cardiac and renal impairment) when given large volumes of fluid.

4. Normalisation of blood glucose levels:

   - Fluid replacement alone will reduce blood glucose levels as serum osmolarity decreases during the initial stages.
   - Insulin therapy should be commenced only after initial fluid resuscitation to avoid fluid shifts.
   - Insulin may be required earlier if there is a significant ketonemia.
   - Current guidelines from the Joint British Diabetes Societies Inpatient Care group (2013) suggest a fixed-rate 0.05 unit of insulin/kg/hour should be infused. Suggested rates in Table 25.5. The aim is to reduce blood glucose levels at a rate of 5 mmol/L/hr.

5. Restoration on electrolyte balance:

   - Sodium and potassium levels should be monitored.
   - Sodium levels may increase slightly during the initial fluid resuscitation. Further fluid may be required in the sodium levels continue to rise.
   - Sodium levels should not decrease too quickly and should not exceed 10 mmol in 24 hours.
   - Potassium shifts are less pronounced than in diabetic ketoacidosis. Potassium should be replaced as necessary.
   - Hypophosphateamia and hypomagnesaemia are common and should be replaced as per local policy.

Table 25.5 Suggested rates of insulin. *Source:* Joint British Diabetes Societies Inpatient Care Group 2013.

Patient weight (kg)	Insulin dose (units/h)
60–69	3
70–79	3.5
80–89	4
90–99	4.5
100–109	5
110–119	5.5
120–129	6
130–139	6.5
140–149	7
>150	7.5 (refer to diabetic team)

379

Table 25.6   Signs and symptoms.

- Headache
- Hunger
- Faintness
- Cool, moist skin
- Sweating
- Slurred speech
- Tachycardia/ bradycardia
- Irrational behaviour, agitation
- Coma

Hypoglycaemia

Patients who develop hypoglycaemia are usually known diabetics controlled either by insulin or oral hypoglycaemics. Occasionally liver failure or less commonly Addison's disease may precipitate hypoglycaemia. Signs and symptoms (see Table 25.6) result from low blood sugars that may be caused by insulin overdose.

Management of hypoglycaemia starts with prevention. Specific directions for hypoglycaemia avoidance and treatment should be written into hospital glucose management protocols for intensive care units especially for patients on intravenous insulin therapy (Bersten and Soni, 2014).

Management

- Stop any insulin.
- Increase blood glucose levels using the following administrations of glucagon (can take 15 minutes to work) or 10% (150–160 ml) or 20% (75–85 ml) glucose over 10–15 minutes.
- Reassess and close monitoring of blood glucose levels.
- Establish cause of episode.

Pathophysiology

Adrenals

Above each kidney there is a gland known as the adrenal. Each gland has an inner layer, the medulla, and an outer layer the cortex. The adrenal hormones help us cope with extreme (stressful) situations.

Adrenal cortex

The adrenal cortex has three cell layers. The zone glomerulosa is the outermost layer and produces mineralocorticoids, primarily aldosterone. The middle and largest layer produces glucocorticoids cortisol (hydrocortisone), cortisone and corticosterone. Some sex hormones (androgen and oestrogen) are produced. The outermost layer the reticularis produces mostly glucocorticoids and some sex hormones.

Mineralocorticoids

These regulate water and electrolyte haemostasis, the sodium and potassium concentrations in the extracellular fluid. The most important mineralocorticoid is aldosterone which makes up 95% of the mineralocorticoid activity (Tortora and Derrickson, 2017; Sole et al., 2017). The effect of aldosterone is to increase extracellular fluid sodium and chloride ions concentrations. Aldosterone acts on the distal loops and collecting ducts in the kidneys to increase their reabsorption of sodium from the forming urine and return into the bloodstream. Aldosterone's primary goal is maintaining sodium ion balance, the sodium reabsorption and the regulation of other ions (potassium, hydrogen, chloride, and bicarbonate). Based on the principle where sodium goes water follows, this event leads to changes in blood volume and blood pressure. Sodium ion regulation is crucial to the body's overall homeostasis. Aldosterone regulatory affects are brief therefore, electrolyte balance can be precisely controlled and modified continuously. Secretion is simulated by several factors, rising blood potassium levels, low blood levels of sodium and decreasing blood volume and pressure. The converse inhibits aldosterone secretion.

Mechanisms that regulate aldosterone secretion:

1. Renin-angiotensin pathway is the major regulator of aldosterone release, influencing both electrolyte-water balance of the blood and blood pressure. Specialised cells of the juxtaglomerular apparatus (within the kidney) become excited when blood pressure and volume declines or plasma osmolarity drops. The cells secrete renin into the blood and converts angiotensin (a plasma protein) into angiotensin I in the liver. As blood flows through lung capillaries, an enzyme called angiotensin-converting enzyme (ACE) converts angiotensin I into angiotensin II. Angiotensin II is a hormone that stimulates the adrenals to secrete aldosterone.
2. Fluctuating plasma concentrations of sodium and potassium directly influence the zona glomerulus cells. Increased potassium and decreased sodium are stimulatory and conversely is inhibitory.

Glucocorticoids

Glucocorticoids regulate the metabolism of fat, protein and carbohydrates and can enhance resistance to physical stress. There are three import glucocorticoids, cortisol (hydrocortisone), corticosterone and cortisone. Cortisol is responsible for about 95% of glucocorticoid activity. Glucocorticoids have the following effects:

1. Along with other hormones glucocorticoids promote normal metabolism. Their role is to make enough adenosine triphosphate (ATP) available. They increase the rate at which proteins are catabolised and amino acids are removed from cells, primarily muscle and transported to the liver. The amino acids are then synthesised into new proteins needed for metabolic reactions. If the body reserves of fat or glycogen are low the liver may convert

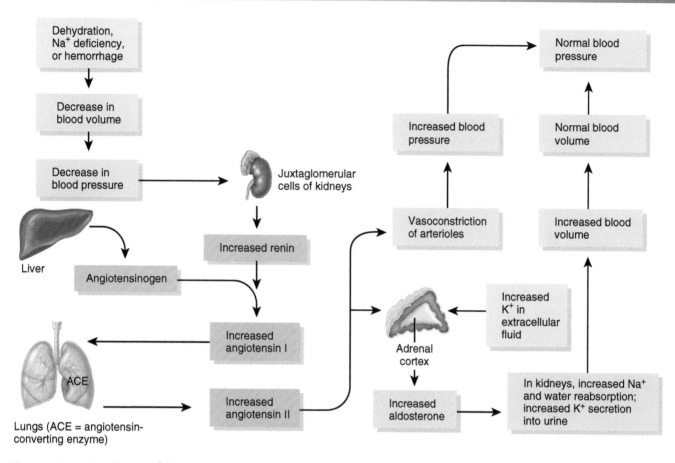

Figure 25.1   Regulation of the secretion of aldosterone by renin-angiotensin.

381

lactic acid or certain other amino acids into glucose (gluconeogeneisis).

2. Provide resistance to stress. Extra glucose is used by the tissues to produce adenosine triphosphate (ATP) for combating various stresses (fasting, fright, temperature extremes, high altitude, bleeding, infection, surgery, trauma and debilitating disease). They also make the blood vessels more sensitive to constriction. Thereby increasing blood pressure. This effect is an advantage if the stress happens to be blood loss, which tends to make blood pressure fall.

3. They have anti-inflammatory compounds that inhibit the cells and secretions participate in the inflammatory response. They reduce the number of mast cell production thus reducing histamine.

The control of glucocorticoid secretion is a negative feedback (Figure 25.2). Low blood levels, mainly cortisol, stimulate the hypothalamus to secrete corticotropin releasing hormone (CRH). Corticotropin releasing hormone and low levels of glucocorticoids both promote the release of adrenocorticotrophic hormone (ACTH) from the pituitary gland. Adrenocorticotrophic hormone is carried in the blood to the adrenal cortex where it stimulates glucocorticoid secretion.

Gonadocorticoids

The adrenal cortex secretes both male and female gonadocorticoids. Androgens, oestrogen and progesterone secretaries is relatively low compared to amounts secreted by the gonads.

Adrenal medulla

The adrenal medulla consists of hormone-producing cells called chromaffin cells that surround large blood vessels. These cells receive direct innervation from preganglionic neurons of the sympathetic division of the autonomic nervous system. They produce catecholamines and is considered a neuroendocrine structure due to the role catecholamines play in the autonomic nervous system.

Adrenaline (epinephrine) and noradrenaline (norepinephrine)

Events that activate the sympathetic nervous system, fear, hypoxia, hypotension, anger, cold, pain etc cause a release of adrenaline and nor-adrenaline. The joint action of the two hormones is to prepare the body for action ('fight or flight'). The immediate energy needs of the body must

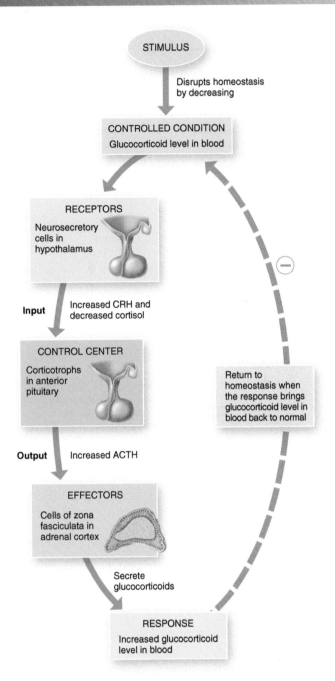

Figure 25.2 Adrenal glands.

be met, and blood flow and volume are increased to the essential organs (Tortora and Derrickson, 2017). Adrenaline constricts the blood vessels in the skin mucosa and dilates those in the skeletal muscle and the eyes. It relaxes the bronchioles and thereby increasing lung capacity, heart rate and cardiac output. Adrenaline also dilates the blood vessels of the brain, muscles and myocardium ensuring blood flow is maintained to these areas. Liver glycogen is mobilised and converted into glucose providing an immediate source of energy. Noradrenaline is the transmitting substance of the sympathetic nervous system and pre-ganglionic sympathetic fibres. It increases

blood pressure by constricting arterioles and veins (except in the essential areas where adrenaline counteracts this effect).

Disorders of the adrenal glands

Adrenal medulla

A tumour of the chromaffin cells of the adrenal medulla where adrenaline and noradrenaline are secreted is called a phaeochromocytoma. In 90% of patients the tumour originates in the medulla, with the remaining 10% occurring along the sympathetic chain (Adler et al., 2008). The tumours can metastasise and behave like a malignancy. The secretions on the catecholamines are intermittent and during acute attacks can result in the patient having headaches, tachycardia, hyperglycaemia, blurred vision, bowel disturbances and very severe hypertension (systolic blood pressure up to 300 mmHg).

Management

The treatment is surgical removal of the tumour. The blood pressure must be controlled well in advance, generally using alpha and beta-adrenergic blocking agents. Alpha blockage begins before beta otherwise severe hypertensive crisis can be precipitated. Two common pre-operative treatments are phentolamine or phenoxybenzamine, which have a short duration of action. Other drugs used are labetalol (alpha and beta effects) or propanol (beta effects). If severe hypertensive crisis occurs an intravenous infusion of sodium nitroprusside can be used to control blood pressure. Adrenoceptor blockage has usually withdrawn 12–36 hours post surgery. Therefore, post-operative care of the patient is paramount, with close monitoring of blood pressure and heart rate. Removal of catecholamine source during surgery can cause hypovolaemic collapse. If this occurs, large volume replacement is required to achieve homeostasis. Pre-operative preparation of these patients is paramount.

Adrenal cortex

Disorders causing adrenal insufficiency can be classified into three groups:

- Primary causes: autoimmune disease, congenital adrenal hyperplasia, adrenal adenoma, tuberculosis, AIDS, metastatic disease, sarcoidosis
- Secondary causes: impairment of the pituitary gland resulting in a deficiency of ACTH (cancer, head injury hypopituitarism).

- Tertiary causes: disease of the hypothalamus resulting in deficiency of corticotrophin releasing factor.

Addison's disease (Adrenal crisis).

Adrenal crisis is a life-threatening absence of cortisol (glucocorticoid) and aldosterone (mineralocorticoid) with severe signs and symptoms (Table 25.7). A deficiency of cortisol results in decreased production of glucose, decreased metabolism of protein and fat, decreased appetite, decreased intestinal motility and digestion, decreased vascular tone and diminished effects of catecholamines. If a patient who is deficient in cortisol is stressed, this deficiency can produce profound shock because of decreased vascular tone caused by reduced catecholamines. Deficiency of aldosterone results in decreased retention of sodium and water, circulating volume and increased potassium and hydrogen ion reabsorption, which forms the main sign of an Addisonian crisis.

Table 25.7 Signs and symptoms of reduced aldosterone and cortisol levels.

Effects of the lack of:	
Aldosterone	**Cortisol**
• polyuria • dehydration • thirst • hyponatraemia • hyperkalaemia • hypotension (postural) • cardiac arrhythmias	• muscle weakness • hypoglycaemia • gastrointestinal (nausea and vomiting, diarrhoea, abdominal pain) • emotional disturbances (depression, irritability) • susceptible to infection

Snapshot

Gary is a 61-year-old man was admitted to ICU after being intubated. He is thought to be in Addison's crisis after not taking his regular prednisolone for rheumatoid arthritis.

Airway (A): ETT.
Breathing (B): oxygen saturations 96% (NEWS2 = 0), on 40% oxygen (NEWS2 = 2), respiratory rate (RR) 12 breaths per minute (NEWS2 = 0).
Cardiovascular System (C): Blood Pressure (BP) is 90/65 (NEWS2 = 0), Heart Rate (HR) is 106 beats per minute (NEWS2 = 1), capillary refill time (CRT) is 4 seconds, he is cool to touch.
Disability (D) (neurological System), Patient is Unconscious (NEWS2 = 3), on the AVPU scale Body Temperature (T) is 38.0°C.
Exposure (E) no abnormal findings.
Total NEW2 Score: 6.

Nursing considerations on admission:
- A–E systems assessment.
- Oxygen and ventilatory support as directed by patient's condition and ABGs.
- Monitor vital signs for decreased cardiac output.
- 12-lead ECG.
- Monitor fluid balance.
- Regular monitoring of blood glucose levels.

What other investigations or treatment might Gary need?

Red Flag

Steroid use cannot be stopped abruptly; tapering the drug gives the adrenal glands time to return to their normal patterns of secretion.

The rate of withdrawal of the steroids depends on (NICE, 2020):

- The person's response to the withdrawal (if withdrawal symptoms are reported, resume a higher dose and continue the withdrawal at a slower rate).
- The disease being treated.
- The duration of treatment and dosage

Management

Immediate treatment is required as the patient will be in shock and will progress to circulatory collapse.

- Rehydration: with a colloid followed by 0.9% sodium chloride. It is not uncommon for 3–4 litres to be needed over the first few hours.
- Hypoglyceamia: corrected with infusions of hypertonic glucose and careful monitoring of blood sugar levels.
- Cortisol replaced without delay after baseline bloods are taken. Hydrocortisone 100–200 mg q.d.s or dexamethasone 4 mg q.d.s is given intravenously for immediate crisis. This is followed by an oral maintenance once the patient has stabilised.

Conclusion

The endocrine glands form a communication network throughout the body. The hormones from these glands control and regulate metabolic processes. Hormones are regulated via positive or negative feedback systems that control the release of hormones. It is important to assess and manage patients quickly when the glands do not function properly, as this can lead to morbidity and mortality. Nurses work within a multidisciplinary team to provide information and act quickly to prevent further deterioration and respond and evaluate treatment plans provided they are working within their competency range and scope of practice (ICS 2019, NMC 2018).

Take home points

1. Endocrine disorders can have serious consequences for all patients.
2. The clinical presentation of endocrine disorders can often be non-specific making the diagnosis difficult.
3. The thyroid gland is one of the main regulators of metabolism and produces three active hormones: T4, T3 and calcitonin.
4. The parathyroid glands produce PTH which is the single most important hormone controlling calcium balance in the blood; calcium plays a role in muscle contraction, coagulation and the secretion of neurotransmitters and hormones.
5. The hormones of the pituitary gland help regulate the functions of other endocrine glands.
6. The pancreas has two main functions: an exocrine function that helps in digestion and an endocrine function that regulates blood sugar.
7. Adrenal glands produce hormones that help regulate your metabolism, immune system, blood pressure, response to stress and other essential functions.

References

Adam, S., Osborne, S., and Welch, J. (2017). *Critical Care Nursing Science and Practice*, 3e. Oxford: Oxford University Press.

Adler, J.T., Meyer-Rochow, G.Y., Benn, D. et al. (2008). Phaeochromocytoma: Current appraoches and future directions. *The Oncologist* 13(7): 779–793.

Baid, H., Creed, F., and Hargreaves, J. (2016). *Oxford Handbook of Critical Care Nursing*, 2e. Oxford: Oxford University Press.

Bersten, A.D. and Soni, N. (2016). *Oh's Intensive Care Manual*, 7e. Butterworth Heinemann: Philadelphia.

Clausen, T. (2003). Na+-K+ Pump Regulation and Skeletal Muscle Contractility. *American Physiological Society* 83(4): 1269–1324.

Clegg, A. and Young, J.B. (2011). Which medications to avoid in people at risk of delirium: a systematic review. *Age and Ageing* 40(1): 23–29.

Firth, J., Conlon, C., and Cox, T. (2020). *Oxford Textbook of Medicine*, 6e. Oxford: Oxford University Press.

Holcombe, S.S. (2002). Thyroid diseases: A primer for the critical care nurse. *Dimensions of Critical Care Nursing* 21, 4 p127–133.

Intensive Care Society (2019). *Guidelines for Provision of Intensive Care Society*, 2e. https://www.ics.ac.uk/ICS/ICS/Pdfs/GPICS_2nd_Edition.aspx (accessed 1 December 2020).

Joint British Diabetes Societies Inpatient Care Group (2012). The management of the hyperosmolar hyperglycaemic states (HHS) in adults with diabetes. www.diabetes.nhs.uk (accessed 16 November 2020).

Joint British Diabetes Societies Inpatient Care Group (2013). The management of the diabetes in adults. www.diabetes.nhs.uk (accessed 16 November 2020).

Joint Formulary Committee (2020). British National Formulary. http://www.medicinescomplete.com (accessed 28 January 2021).

Marieb, E. (2017). *Essentials of Anatomy and Physiology*, 12e. Pearson Education Limited: Essex.

Mazzeo et al. (2019). Activation of pituitary axis according to underlying critical illness and its effect on outcome. *Journal of Critical Care* 54: 22–29.

NICE (2020). *Corticosteroids*. https://cks.nice.org.uk/topics/corticosteroids-oral/management/corticosteroids/ (accessed 1 March 2021).

NICE-SUGAR study Investigators (2009). Intensive versus conventional glucose control in critically ill patients. *New England Journal of Medicine* 260(13): 1283–1297.

NMC (2018). The Code. Professional Standards of Practice and Behaviour for Nurse, Midwives and Nursing Associates. https://www.nmc.org.uk/standards/code/ (accessed 1 December 2020).

Page, P. and Skinner, G. (2010). *Emergencies in Clinical Medicine*. Oxford: Oxford University Press.

Sole, M., Klien, D., and Moseley, M. (2017). *Introduction to Critical Care Nursing*, 7e. Elsevier: Missaouri.

Sonino, N. and Fava, G. (2004). Psychological aspects of endocrine disease. *Clinical Endocrinology* 49(1): 1–7.

Tortora, G.J. and Derrickson, B.H. (2014). *Tortora's Principles of Anatomy and Physiology*, 14e. Wiley: USA.

Van den Berghe, G. Wilmer, A. Hermans, G. (2001). Intensive insulin therapy in critically ill patients. New England Journal of medicine 345: 1359–1367.

Waldmann, C., Rhodes, A., Soni, N., and Handy, J. (2019). *Oxford Desk Reference: Critical Care*, 2e. Oxford: Oxford University Press.

Webb, A., Angus, D., Finfer, S. et al. (2016). *Oxford Textbook of Critical Care*. Oxford: Oxford University Press.

Yates, A. (2016). Urinalysis: how to interpret results. *Nursing Times* 2: 1–3.

Chapter 26

Haematological and immunological critical care

Barry Hill, Gerri Mortimore, and Pamela Arasen

Aim

The aim of this chapter is to provide the reader with an understanding of patients with complex haematological disorders that present in critical care for specialist medical and nursing interventions.

Learning outcomes

After reading this chapter the reader will be able to:

- Understand the pathophysiology of the haematological system and apply this in clinical practice.
- Understand and appreciate the complexities of care required for people who are critically unwell with a haematological disorder.
- Consider the clinical and therapeutic interventions required for patients presenting with acute and critical haematological and immune system issues.
- Understand human blood groups and indications for blood transfusion including the administration process and safety procedures.
- Be prepared to demonstrate the application of theory to practice when nursing people that have haematological related critical illness.

Test your prior knowledge

- What are the key cellular components of blood?
- What is anaemia?
- What are the causes of neutropenia?
- Which body system produces plasma proteins and clotting factors?
- What is sepsis and septic shock?

Fundamentals of Critical Care: A Textbook for Nursing and Healthcare Students, First Edition. Edited by Ian Peate and Barry Hill.
© 2023 John Wiley & Sons Ltd. Published 2023 by John Wiley & Sons Ltd.
Companion website: www.wiley.com/go/peate/criticalcare

Introduction

Haematological disorders such as thrombocytopenia including immune thrombocytopenia, coagulopathy, disseminated intravascular coagulation (DIC) and disorders affecting the immune system are frequently encountered by patients with critical care needs. The management of these haematological conditions are complex as their causes are generally multi-factorial, for example, induced by medications, disease, can be genetic or related to malignancies, and in the unstable person requiring critical care can be life-threatening. A systematic evaluation of a patient's history, clinical presentation, diagnostic and assessment laboratory findings is paramount to determine the cause of the haematological disorder and identify the subsequent critical care interventions and therapies. Although there is no set competency section in the National Competency framework for Registered Nurses in Critical Care regarding haematological and immunological care it is likely you will nurse patients with these.

Normal physiology

The haematological or haematopoietic system consists of blood, which makes up 8% of the human body weight, blood vessels and coordinates with blood-forming organs such as the bone marrow, spleen, liver, lymph nodes and thymus gland. The haematological system ensures adequate oxygen and nutrient delivery to the tissues, and is responsible for transport of hormones and antibodies, triggers the inflammatory and immune responses, removes waste and ensures homeostasis in the fluid-electrolyte and acid-based systems (Adam et al., 2017; Marieb, 2015).

Blood components

Blood can be divided into key components.

Plasma

Plasma is the liquid portion of blood. About 55% of human blood is plasma, and the remaining 45% are red blood cells, white blood cells and platelets that are suspended in the plasma. Plasma is 92% water and contains 7% vital proteins including albumin, gamma globulin and anti-haemophilic factor, and 1% mineral salts, sugars, fats, hormones, and vitamins. Plasma serves four essential functions: including the facilitation and maintenance of blood pressure and blood volume. It also supplies critical proteins for blood clotting and immunity. Plasma also carries electrolytes such as sodium and potassium to muscles. Finally, plasma supports pH balance in the body assisting cell function and homeostasis. Plasma contains the minor fractions including albumin, which is a protein produced in the liver and helps keep blood volume in a normal range. Clotting factors such as fibrinogen and von Willebrand factor, are another group of proteins also that flow in blood plasma. Immunoglobulins, also known as immune globulins, are antibodies which

can be separated from plasma to treat viruses and bacteria. White blood cells contain interferons, proteins to fight infection and interleukins, another group of proteins which help cells communicate with each other. Red blood cells contain haemoglobin, which are essential to carry oxygen and hemin, a salt which can block the release of substances such as porphyrins (Adam et al., 2017; Marieb, 2015).

Red blood cells

Every second, 2–3 million RBCs are produced in the bone marrow and released into the circulation. Also known as erythrocytes, RBCs are the most common type of cell found in the blood, with each cubic millimetre of blood containing 4–6 million cells. With a diameter of only 6 µm, RBCs are small enough to squeeze through the smallest blood vessels. They circulate around the body for up to 120 days, at which point the old or damaged RBCs are removed from the circulation by specialised cells (macrophages) in the spleen and liver. The mature RBC lacks a nucleus. This allows the cell more room to store haemoglobin, the oxygen-binding protein, enabling the RBC to transport more oxygen (Table 26.1). RBCs are also biconcave in shape; this shape increases their surface area for the diffusion of oxygen across their surfaces.

White blood cells

White blood cells, also called leukocytes or white corpuscles, are a cellular component of the blood that lacks haemoglobin, has a nucleus, is capable of motility, and defends the body against infection and disease by ingesting foreign materials and cellular debris, by destroying

Table 26.1   The red blood cells. *Source:* Peate, 2018 with permission of Elsevier.

Oxygen transportation	Oxygen is transported by haemoglobin (Hb) in the red blood cell (RBC). Each molecule of Hb carries with it up to four molecules of oxygen. This means that each RBC has a potential oxygen-carrying capacity of over 1 billion oxygen molecules. Oxygen transportation is dependent on the available Hb, therefore those patients who have active bleeding disorders, or those who are anaemic can potentially have altered oxygen delivery.
Haemopoiesis	The process in which blood cells are formed.
Destruction of erythrocytes	The lifespan of an erythrocyte is around 120 days, after this they break down (this is called haemolysis). The body retains the iron that has been released from the broken down cells and the bone marrow then uses this to create new cells.
Blood groups	There are four blood groups, known as A, B, AB and O. Blood group O is normally referred to as 'universal'. When providing care to those patients who need a blood transfusion, it is essential that the nurse understands the A, B, AB and O system.

infectious agents and cancer cells, or by producing antibodies. Among the white blood cells are:

- **Monocytes:** They have a longer lifespan than many white blood cells and help to break down bacteria.
- **Lymphocytes:** They create antibodies to fight against bacteria, viruses, and other potentially harmful invaders.
- **Neutrophils:** They kill and digest bacteria and fungi. They are the most numerous types of white blood cell and are the first line of defence during infection
- **Basophils:** These small cells secrete chemicals such as histamine, a marker of allergic disease, that help control the body's immune response.
- **Eosinophils:** They attack and kill parasites and cancer cells and help with allergic responses.

Platelets

Platelets or thrombocytes are small, colourless cell fragments in the blood that form clots and stop or prevent bleeding. Platelets are made in bone marrow which contains stem cells that develop into red blood cells, white blood cells, and platelets. Platelets control bleeding and are essential to surviving surgeries such as organ transplant, as well as fighting cancer, chronic diseases, and traumatic injuries. Donor platelets are given to patients who do not have enough of their own, a condition known as thrombocytopenia, or when a person's platelets are not working appropriately. Raising the patient's blood platelet count reduces the risk of dangerous or even fatal bleeding.

Haematopoiesis

Haematopoiesis is the process which occurs in the bone marrow and through which the haematological system makes new blood cellular components which are all derived from haematopoietic stem cells. These pluripotent stem cells produce different types of bloods cells called myeloid and lymphoid. Myeloid cells include neutrophils, basophils, eosinophils, erythrocytes, macrophages, and platelets. Lymphoid cells are T cells and B cells. The components of blood are shown in Figure 26.1.

Haemoglobin is the iron-containing oxygen transport protein and 1 molecule of haemoglobin binds with 4 molecules of oxygen or 1.34 mL of oxygen, forming oxyhaemoglobin. Oxygen-carrying capacity in blood depends on how much haemoglobin it contains and the more haemoglobin molecules in RBC, the more oxygen they will be able to transport. Clinically, normal blood contains 12–18 g haemoglobin per 100 mL blood. Normal haemoglobin counts are 13–18 grams per decilitre (g/dL) in men and 12–15 g/dL in women (Marieb, 2015).

Oxygen readily dissociates from haemoglobin in the tissues through diffusion as the concentration of oxygen in the cells is lower than in blood. Haemoglobin also carries 20% of carbon dioxide which binds to the haem protein and forms carbaminohaemoglobin. The efficient transport of O_2, CO_2 and H^+ in the blood depend on the enzyme carbon anhydrase, RBC specific membrane, cytoplasmic proteins, and the distinctive intracellular RBC environment. In addition, RBC have high 2,3-diphosphoglyceric acid (2,3-DPG), an organic phosphate which maintains the redox state stability. An increase in 2,3-DPG, seen in anoxia, will cause the oxyhaemoglobin dissociation curve to shift to the right and more oxygen to be released at a given oxygen tension. Decreases in 2,3-DPG concentration, seen in states such as septic shock and hypophosphatemia, cause a leftward shift.

Disorders of erythrocytes

Blood disorders affect the RBCs (Figure 26.2). They include polycythaemia which can be primary, when there is an excessive production of red cell count or Hb> 180g/L, and secondary where red cell count proliferates due to chronic hypoxaemia in conditions such as chronic obstructive pulmonary disease or following increased erythropoietin production in response to high altitudes (Adam et al., 2017).

The second type of disorders is related to the membrane of the RBC. Hereditary spherocytosis is caused by changes in genes relating to membrane proteins that allow for red blood cells to mutate into a sphere shape, instead of a biconcave disk shape. Finally, anaemia is a low level of haemoglobin or haematocrit and a lowered ability of the blood to carry oxygen. Causes of anaemia include decrease in RBC number which result from haemorrhage such as gastrointestinal bleeding or the lysis of RBC in bacterial infection; decreased production of red blood cells in iron deficiency, also known as sideropaenia, is caused by lack of iron in diet and symptoms include increased tiredness, shortness of breath, low exercise tolerance.

B12 vitamin deficiency

B12 vitamin deficiency can cause megaloblastic anaemia. Deficiency in B12 prevents erythrocytes from maturing and to become macrocytic (large) and nucleated. These large erythrocytes are destroyed prematurely, leading to anaemia. The most common cause of B12 deficiency is an autoimmune condition called pernicious anaemia. This type of anaemia is due to a lack of intrinsic factor (IF), a protein which is produced by glands in the gastric mucosa. IF must bind with B12 to enable the absorption of this vitamin in the terminal ileum of the small intestine. Hence, pernicious anaemia is a form of malabsorption. It is rare that dietary deficiency causes B12 deficiency, but it can occur in people who consume excessive amounts of alcohol, are anorexic or in the elderly population.

Signs of B12 deficiency are glossitis; smooth, sore red tongue and koilonychia in which fingernails initially flatten out and then become concave or spoon-shaped. It can take several years to deplete B12 stores hence why observing patients' fingernails flattening out, can alert the clinician a long time before they become 'spoon-shaped'

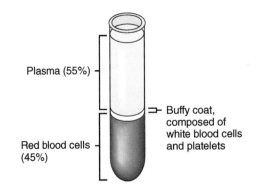

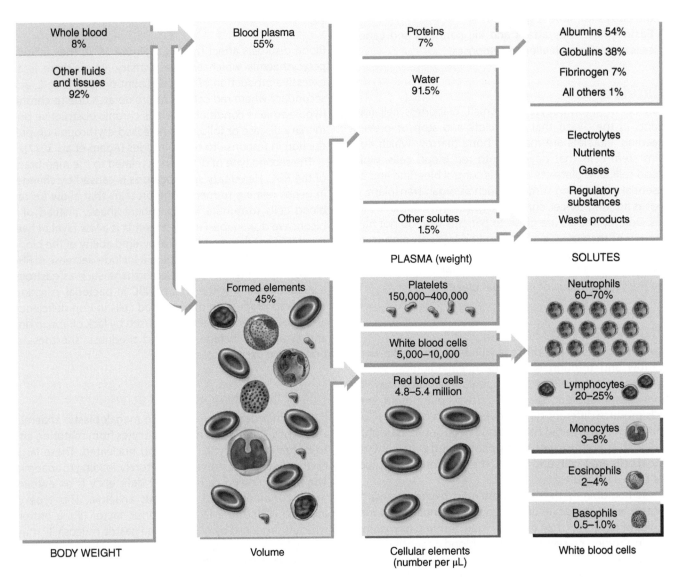

Figure 26.1   Components of blood. *Source:* Peate (2021) with permission of John Wiley & Sons.

i.e. koilonchyia. Symptoms of vitamin B12 deficiency can be seen in Figure 26.3.

Sickle cell anaemia

Sickle cell anaemia is a genetic disorder, where abnormal haemoglobin in RBCs occurs due oxygen content of blood being lower than normal and results in the haemoglobin become sharp and sickle-shaped, instead of the doughnut shape. The deformed, crescent shape and stiff erythrocytes collapse easily and would dam up in small blood vessels, causing an interference with oxygen delivery. In the event of a crisis, people with sickle cell anaemia (mostly of African descent), would experience extreme respiratory distress and excruciating pain, requiring pharmacological interventions including primary analgesic treatments such as

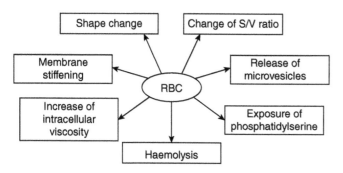

Figure 26.2   Change in RBCs.

non-steroidal anti-inflammatory drugs (NSAIDs) strong opioids, corticosteroids and low molecular heparin dose. During an acute painful sickle cell episode, evidence from studies indicate that patients perceived a lack of monitoring of their pain and their vital signs. Inherited blood disorders such as thalassaemia can also cause decreased haemoglobin production. there are two main types of thalassaemia, alpha thalassaemia and beta thalassaemia.

Genetic haemochromatosis

Although anaemias are well recognised within the medical and nursing fraternity, a condition that is very rarely considered is iron overload. One of the main causes of iron overload is genetic haemochromatosis. The most common is Type 1 genetic haemochromatosis (there are five types of haemochromatosis) which is an autosomal recessive condition, meaning that you must inherit a variant gene from both sets of parents to inherit the condition. If you inherit only one copy, you are termed a carrier.

It is surprising that although this is the most common genetic condition affecting Caucasians of Northern European descent, it is underdiagnosed in this UK. Early symptoms of lethargy, fatigue, abdominal pains, cognitive difficulties such as brain fog and abdominal pains are generic and as such, diagnosis is often missed, delayed, or misdiagnosed. If left untreated, the high levels of circulating iron are deposited in all organs of the body including joints and the skin, giving it a bronzed appearance. However, as the liver is the main storage place for iron, liver disease generally precedes disease in other organs.

Diagnosis is made on blood tests. It is recommended that a ferritin level (abnormal is >300 ug in males and >200 ug in females) is checked alongside a transferrin saturation (abnormal is >50% in males and 45% in females). If the ferritin levels are elevate, bearing in mind females can still have normal ferritin levels, then a haemochromatosis gene (HFE) gene test should be requested.

Treatment consists or regular venesections, usually weekly depending on the initial ferritin level until ferritin

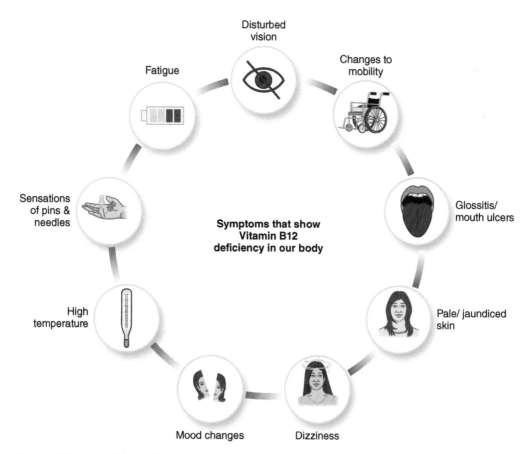

Figure 26.3   Signs of Vitamin B12 deficiency.

and transferrin saturation levels are brought down to below 50 ug if the patient tolerates. Once de-ironed then maintenance therapy is initiated, usually at 3 monthly intervals for the rest of the patient's life.

Haemostasis

Haemostasis is the process to prevent and halt blood loss from a damaged blood vessel and is the first stage of wound healing. After an injury such as a skin tear or the rupture of a blood vessel, primary haemostasis occurs as vascular spasms and accumulation of platelets such as fibrinogen causes a platelet plug at the site temporarily slow or stop blood loss.

Secondary haemostasis occurs when platelets and tissue factor trigger the clotting cascade, leading to the formation of fibrin threads. Fibrin traps red blood cells and forms a blood clot. But the antithrombotic control mechanisms activate the release of plasmin which causes fibrinolysis and clot degradation allowing the blood vessels to become patent and free from clots (Adam et al., 2017; Marieb, 2015). The components of haemostasis can be seen in Figure 26.4 and the three pathways that make up the classical blood coagulation pathway are shown in Figure 26.5.

The three major types of blood cancer are:

- Leukaemia – cancer that starts in the bone marrow. It produces abnormal white blood cells that cannot fight infection. Preventing the bone marrow from producing healthy red blood cells and platelets. Two types of leukaemia usually affect adults. They are acute myelogenous leukaemia (AML) and chronic lymphocytic leukaemia (CLL).
- Lymphoma – cancer that starts in a type of white blood cell called lymphocytes; lymphocytes help the body fight infection. Over time, these cancerous cells build up inside the lymph nodes and damage the immune system. There are two types of lymphoma called Hodgkin lymphoma and non-Hodgkin lymphoma.
- Multiple myeloma – cancer that begins in the plasma cells. It prevents the body from fighting infection, weakens bones and can damage kidneys.

There are also a variety of blood disorders that are not cancerous but can contribute to a person becoming critically unwell (Table 26.2). These include:

- Haemophilia – an inherited condition that prevents blood from clotting properly.

Lymphoma

Another common haematological condition is lymphoma. The term lymphoma covers a variety of malignant blood cancer conditions, usually of B-cell origin. These are characterised as lymphomas because of the production of lymphoid cells, starting in the lymph nodes or lymph tissues within the lymphatic system. Lymphomas belong to two

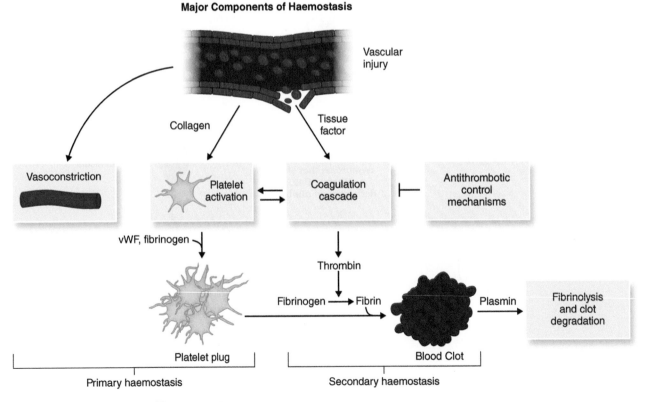

Major Components of Haemostasis

Vascular injury

Collagen

Tissue factor

Vasoconstriction

Platelet activation

Coagulation cascade

Antithrombotic control mechanisms

vWF, fibrinogen

Thrombin

Fibrinogen → Fibrin

Plasmin

Fibrinolysis and clot degradation

Platelet plug

Blood Clot

Primary haemostasis

Secondary haemostasis

Figure 26.4   Components of haemostasis.

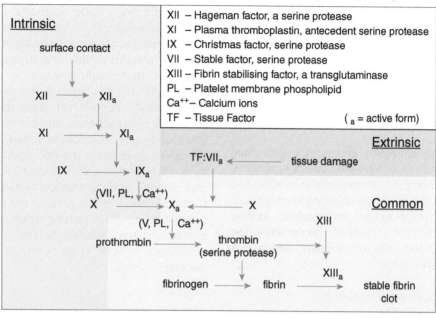

The three pathways that makeup the classical blood coagulation pathway

XII – Hageman factor, a serine protease
XI – Plasma thromboplastin, antecedent serine protease
IX – Christmas factor, serine protease
VII – Stable factor, serine protease
XIII – Fibrin stabilising factor, a transglutaminase
PL – Platelet membrane phospholipid
Ca++– Calcium ions
TF – Tissue Factor ($_a$ = active form)

Figure 26.5 Blood coagulation pathways.

Table 26.2 Haematological disorders.

Anaemia	Bleeding disorders	Malignant immunoproliferative diseases	Vasculitis
Iron-deficiency anaemia	Disseminated intravascular coagulation (DIC)	Lymphoma	Autoimmune haemolytic anaemia
Vitamin deficiency anaemia	Thrombocytosis	Leukaemia	Lupus antiphospholipid antibody syndrome
Anaemia of chronic disease	Thrombocytopenia	Myeloma	Vasculitis
Aplastic anaemia	Idiopathic thrombocytopenic purpura (ITP)	Malignant immunoproliferative diseases	
Anaemias associated with bone marrow disease	Haemophilia		
Autoimmune haemolytic anaemias (AIHA)			

groups: Hodgkin lymphoma (HL) and non-Hodgkin lymphoma (NHL).

Hodgkin lymphoma

Lymphoma means cancer of the lymphatic system. The lymphatic system is a system of thin tubes and lymph nodes that run throughout the body. Lymph nodes are bean shaped glands. The thin tubes are called lymph vessels or lymphatic vessels. Tissue fluid called lymph circulates around the body in these vessels and flows through the lymph nodes. The lymphatic system is an important part of the immune system. It plays a role in fighting bacteria and other infections, and it tries to destroy old or abnormal cells, such as cancer cells.

Hodgkin lymphoma was named after the doctor who first recognised it. It used to be called Hodgkin disease. Hodgkin lymphoma has a particular appearance under the microscope and contains cells called Reed–Sternberg cells. Non-Hodgkin lymphoma (NHL) looks different under the microscope and does not contain Reed–Sternberg cells. It is important that health care professionals can tell the differ-

ence between Hodgkin lymphoma and NHL. They are two different diseases and the treatment for them is not the same.

Risk factors for Hodgkin lymphoma

The risk factors include older age, genetics and lifestyle, with lifestyle accounting for approximate 45% of cases. Epstein–Barr virus (human widespread herpes virus) is the highest-ranking lifestyle risk factor for HL. As a risk factor, it is weighted at 45% (in the UK population), whilst other conditions such as human immunodeficiency virus (HIV), immunological problems, being overweight and having weight-related conditions, as well as smoking, all increase the risk of developing HL.

Signs and symptoms

Ninety percent of HL patients will identify a palpable nonpainful lump within their lymph nodes (see Fig. 30.6). The clinical term for this is 'painless lymphadenopathy'. According to Cancer Research UK (2018b), the first symptom of HL is usually a swelling in the neck, axilla or inguinal canal. The swellings are usually painless, but some people may find that they ache. Other symptoms may include any of the following:

- Drenching and/or frequent sweats, especially at night
- Unexplained pyrexia
- Weight loss
- Tiredness
- A cough or breathlessness
- A persistent itch all over the body.

The most common symptoms are pyrexia, drenching night sweats and weight loss. These are called 'B symptoms'. Other symptoms, such as pain, tenderness and swelling, will depend on where in the body the enlarged lymph nodes are. Some people with HL may have abnormal cells in their bone marrow when they are diagnosed. This can lower the number of healthy blood cells in the blood, which may cause the following symptoms:

- Breathlessness (dyspnoea) and tiredness
- An increased risk of infection
- Excessive bleeding, such as nosebleeds (epistaxis), very heavy menstrual periods (menometrorrhagia), or tiny spots of blood under the skin (multiple petechiae). Very rarely, some people with HL may have pain in the affected lymph node when drinking alcohol. Many of these symptoms are common to many other conditions and most people with these symptoms will not have HL.

Non-Hodgkin lymphoma

In NHL, white blood cells (lymphocytes) divide abnormally. Normal white blood cells have resting time, but people with lymphoma will not have this. This means that white cells divide continuously, so too many are produced. also, they do not naturally die off as white blood cells normally do.

These cells start to divide before they are fully mature. So, they cannot fight infection as normal white blood cells do. The abnormal white blood cells start to collect in the lymph nodes, or in other places such as the bone marrow or spleen. They can then grow into tumours and begin to cause problems in the lymphatic system, or in the organ in which they are growing. For example, if a lymphoma starts in the thyroid gland, it can affect the normal production of thyroid hormones and cause airway obstruction. Lymphoma is most noticed in the lymph nodes in the neck. It is quite common to find it in the liver or spleen. But it can also be found in other body organs, such as the stomach, small bowel, bones, brain, testicles or skin. Although very uncommon, it can also affect the eye.

There are many different types of NHL. These types can be classified in several different ways. One way is by the type of cell affected. NHL affects certain white blood cells called lymphocytes. Two types of lymphocytes can be affected – B cells and T cells. So, people can have a B-cell lymphoma or a T cell lymphoma. Most people with NHL have B-cell lymphomas. T cell lymphomas are more common in teenagers and young adults.

Risk factors for Non-Hodgkin lymphoma

The risk factors include older age, genetics and lifestyle (Cancer Research UK, 2018c). As this blood cancer is so rare, with so many subtypes and variables, most contemporary evidence remains limited. It is suggested that a variety of infections, particularly *Helicobacter pylori*, are linked to NHL. Within the UK, lifestyle risk factors include certain occupational exposure, such as constant exposure to diesel fumes, ionising radiations, and being a farmer or machinist (Karunanayake et al., 2008), and medicines (such as chemotherapy) may increase the risk. Additionally, some studies have suggested that certain drugs used to treat rheumatoid arthritis, such as methotrexate and tumour necrosis factor inhibitors, might increase the risk of NHL (American Cancer Society, 2017). Ionising radiation, HIV, immunological problems, being overweight and having weight-related conditions, as well as smoking, all increase the risk of developing NHL.

Signs and symptoms of NHL

According to MacMillian Cancer Support (2017), the most common patient presentation is from painless swelling in the lymph nodes in one area of the body, usually in the neck, axilla or inguinal canal. Some people have other symptoms relating to where the lymphoma is in their body. This could lead to the following symptoms:

- A cough, difficulty swallowing (dysphagia) or breathlessness (dyspnoea) (if the lymphoma is in the chest area)
- Indigestion (dyspepsia), abdominal pain or weight loss (if the lymphoma is in the stomach or bowel). If NHL spreads to the bone marrow, it can reduce the number of blood cells. This can cause:
  - Tiredness (too few RBCs)
  - Difficulty fighting infections (too few WBCs)
  - Bruising or bleeding (too few platelets).

NHL can also cause general symptoms, including:

- Heavy, drenching sweats at night
- Pyrexia that comes and goes without any obvious cause
- Unexplained weight loss
- Tiredness
- Itching of the skin (pruritus) that does not go away.

Diagnosis of NHL

The most current NICE guideline for diagnosis and management of NHL is NG52 (NICE, 2017). NG52 covers diagnosis and management of NHL in people aged 16 years and over. It aims to improve care for people with NHL by promoting the best tests for diagnosis and staging and the most effective treatments for six of the subtypes: follicular lymphoma, mucosa-associated lymphoid tissue (MALT) lymphoma, mantle lymphoma, diffuse B-cell lymphoma, Burkitt lymphoma and peripheral T cell lymphoma. A variety of diagnoses require different management; for specific advice, please refer to NG52 (NICE, 2017).

Care and treatment of people with NHL

According to Cancer Research UK (2018c), it is typical within the UK to have a '2 weeks' wait' standard for a diagnosis of blood cancers, with the highest proportion of cases diagnosed early. Referral is most frequently made by the General Practitioner. Patients in the UK report very good or excellent experiences of their episodes of care, with all patients having a Clinical Nurse Specialist. NICE guideline NG52 (NICE, 2017) recommends tests and treatments, suggesting biopsy, radiotherapy, immunochemotherapy and BMT/ stem cell transplantation.

Disseminated intravascular coagulation

Disseminated intravascular coagulation (DIC) is a syndrome characterised by the systemic activation of the coagulation system in the body which consist firstly of the clotting mechanism, responsible in preventing excessive blood loss and secondly of the fibrinolytic mechanism which ensures the blood vessels remain patent and free of clots. Disseminated intravascular coagulation (DIC) is characterised by systemic activation of blood coagulation, which results in generation and deposition of fibrin, leading to microvascular thrombi in various organs and contributing to multiple organ dysfunction syndrome (MODS). The common causes of DIC include sepsis and severe infection – the most common cause (organ failure type of DIC); trauma (neurological trauma); organ destruction (eg pancreatitis); malignancy – solid tumours or leukaemia (bleeding type of DIC); severe transfusion reactions; obstetric complications – amniotic fluid embolism, abruptio placentae; haemolysis, elevated liver enzymes, low platelets (HELLP) syndrome; eclampsia – (bleeding type or major bleeding type of DIC); retained dead fetus syndrome; vascular abnormalities – large vascular aneurysms (bleeding type of DIC); severe hepatic failure; severe toxic reactions – snake bite, transfusion reactions, and transplant rejection; heat stroke; and hyperthermia. This process can be seen in Figure 26.6.

Pathophysiology of DIC

DIC is an inappropriate, accelerated systemic activation of clotting cascade leading to formation of fibrin within the circulation. Clotting cascades activated (usually by the extrinsic pathway) – damage to endothelium (burns, trauma, head injury), cytokine release and bacterial endotoxin cause release of tissue factor. Tissue Factor and Factor VIIa released leading to *explosive* production of thrombin. The human body's natural anti-thrombin agents (e.g., proteins C and S, anti-thrombin) are overwhelmed by persistent thrombin formation and their own subsequent reduced synthesis. Platelets aggregate (systemically) and clotting factors are rapidly consumed. Haemorrhaging will then

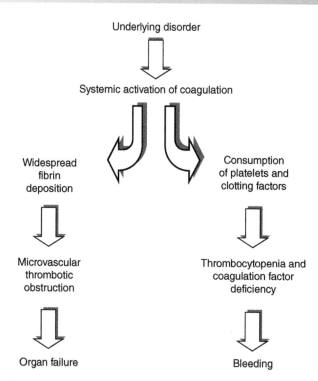

Figure 26.6   The process of DIC. *Source:* Levi et al. (2009) with permission of John Wiley & Sons.

begin. Excessive clotting leads to microvascular thrombosis and macrovascular occlusion. The body then activates the fibrinolytic pathway. Fibrin is degraded by plasmin and fibrinogen degradation products are released into the blood. The latter impair the subsequent production of fibrin which causes further bleeding.

A pro-thrombotic state develops when there is an increase in thrombin and plasminogen activator inhibitor Type 1. There is a decrease in anti-thrombin tissue factor pathway inhibitor and activated protein C. These substances normally regulate coagulation and haemostasis, and both are rapidly consumed in sepsis. Continuing pro-thrombotic state leads to platelet sludging, microthrombi formation, microvascular permeability, hypoperfusion and disseminated intravascular coagulation syndrome (Adam et al., 2017).

Signs and symptoms of DIC

The main clinical presentation is bleeding, but in approximately 5–10% of the population it is manifested with microthrombotic lesions, such as gangrenous limbs. In most patients nursed in hospital, excessive bleeding may be seen after venepuncture, or around cannula sites, sutures, wound drains, and wounds. Because of the high probability of bleeding, the nurse must be cautious of nonvisible bleeding. Generalised bleeding in the gastrointestinal tract, mouth, throat, lung and urinary tract and vaginal bleeding may become severe.

Additional signs and symptoms include:

* Infections
* Malignancy
* Vascular abnormalities

393

- Hypersensitivity reactions
- Obstetric complications.

Less frequently, thrombi may cause acute kidney injury and ischaemia, and can sometimes cause gangrene within affected organs.

Diagnosis of DIC

The diagnosis of DIC is not made from a single laboratory value. It will be made based on the collection of a variety of data, beginning with a characteristic patient history and physical examination, investigations for prolonged clotting times, deranged fibrinogen levels (fibrin degradation and D-dimer) and a declining platelet count. The International Society for Thrombosis and Haemostasis DIC scoring system provides objective measurement of DIC. Where DIC is present, the scoring system correlates with key clinical observations and outcomes. It is important to repeat the tests to monitor the dynamically changing scenario, based on laboratory results and clinical observations (British Society of Haematology, 2009).

Pathogenesis is believed to be a key event underlying DIC and comes from the increased activity of tissue factor. Damaged tissue will inevitably be released into the circulating volume from damaged cells or tumours, or because of increased cell release secondary to normal inflammatory processes (such as proinflammatory cytokine release by monocytes and endothelial cells). It is usual that blood is taken and sent to pathology for clotting focused testing when:

- Patients present as being more pale regardless of sin tone, and complaining of fatigue
- Patients present with abnormal bleeding, such as prolonged bleeding or with an inability to stop bleeding
- When organ function is impaired, in multi-organ failure
- When liver failure is suspected.

In cases such as these, it would be pertinent to explore partial thromboplastin time (PTT) and activated PPT. PTT is a test that measures the overall speed at which blood clots, by means of two consecutive series of biochemical reactions known as the intrinsic and common coagulation pathways.

Care and treatment of DIC

The British Society of Haematology (2009) give the following guidelines for the diagnosis and management of DIC. Transfusion of platelets or plasma (components) in patients with DIC should not primarily be based on laboratory results and should in general be reserved for patients who present with bleeding. In patients with DIC and bleeding or at high risk of bleeding (e.g. post-operative patients or patients due to undergo an invasive procedure) and a low platelet count, transfusion of platelets should be considered. Nurses and nursing associates must ensure that patients are monitored appropriately and that they use national early warning scores (NEWS) to recognise

deterioration and escalate concerns as they arise. Patients who are actively bleeding and have an inability to clot are at greater risk of hypoxia and bleeding, as well as anxiety and fear about their condition. Nurses must observe for any obvious bleeding, including lower gastrointestinal tract (such as melena) and upper gastrointestinal tract (such as haematemesis) and observe the patient for non-obvious bleeding (such as colour changes, temperature, abdominal distention and new bruising) as this might indicate bleeding within the body. It is important to recognise that there are clinical conditions that appear very similar to DIC include sever liver failure, heparin-induced thrombocytopenia and idiopathic purpura fulminans.

Thrombocytopenia

Thrombocytopenia intensifies the risk of bleeding and related complications and consequently patients require platelet transfusions which is the cornerstone in treatment (Russell et al.,2017). However, a growing body of evidence show that prophylactic transfusion of platelets should be avoided in thrombocytopenic non-intensive care patients (ICU) patients. In addition, studies indicate that many patients with a malignant haematological condition who received blood products such as cryoprecipitate could have complications such as infectious and non-infectious serious hazards of transfusion (Russell et al., 2017).

Neutropenia and sepsis

Neutropenia

Neutropenia can be associated with life-threatening infection. It is most significant when the total neutrophil count is $< 0.5 \times 10^9$/L. Causes of neutropenia include:

- Infections – particularly viral (including HIV), also malaria, typhoid, TB. Acute changes are often noted within 1 to 2 days of infection and may persist for several weeks.
- Drugs – neutropenia with antipsychotic medication has been a significant problem in recent years.
- Autoimmune diseases – SLE, rheumatoid arthritis, anaphylaxis.
- Nutritional – B12 deficiency, folate deficiency, alcohol dependency, anorexia nervosa.
- Splenomegaly.
- Bone marrow pathology e.g., leukaemia, myelodysplasia, aplastic anaemia.

Critically unwell neutropaenic patients are at substantial risk of infections, especially unusual or atypical infections, including fungal or viral infections. Patients are often on prophylactic anti-fungal, antiviral or anti-pneumocystis (pneumocystis jerovicii) medications, and these should be continued while on ICU unless the dose or drug requires adjustment to treat, rather than prevent, active infection.

All neutropaenic patients should be reverse-barrier nursed wherever possible; in addition, it is worth noting that they are also at particular risk from individuals infected with varicella. Iatrogenic infections such as ventilator-acquired pneumonia, catheter-related bloodstream infection (CRBSI) and urinary catheter infections are common in neutropaenia; in the early stages of a critical illness, it may be desirable to avoid invasive procedures such as bladder catheterisation, tracheal intubation, or central venous access where possible.

Neutropaenic patients who develop symptoms of infection (e.g. pyrexia or rigors) should be suspected of having an infection even where there is no evidence of a specific source. They are less likely to develop suppurative symptoms and may not develop classical chest X-ray appearances of pneumonia. A full septic screen of urine, blood, and sputum should be performed, and this is likely to need repeating, sometimes daily.

Sepsis

Sepsis is a complex clinical syndrome, of physiological, pathological and biochemical abnormalities related to infection and in spite of latest advances, still remains a cause of public health concern. The incidence of sepsis is still growing at an alarming rate worldwide reflecting the ageing populations with comorbidities, affects largely the patients with cancer, HIV with immunosuppression and causes 48,000 deaths each year in the UK only (UK Sepsis Trust, 2020). With a previous excessive focus on inflammation, misleading its diagnosis and delaying its treatment, the leading experts in sepsis had to redefine it in the third international consensus (2016), 'as a life-threatening organ dysfunction caused by a dysregulated host response to infection'. Sepsis can occur by any pathogenic microbe and the leading sources are pneumonia, urinary tract infection and infection of the skin (Brent, 2017).

Pathophysiology of sepsis

The complex pathophysiology of sepsis encompasses cellular changes such as cytology, morphology, and the activation of the pro and anti-inflammatory pathways. In response to the invading organisms, the immune system attempts to locally avoid pathogen spread, eliminate the organisms and to repair tissue damage. The pattern recognition receptors recognise the organisms as pathogen associated molecular patterns and trigger an inflammatory cascade. Chemical mediators known as cytokines are released from the white blood, and act through cell surface receptors and are crucial to the innate immune system as they fight off infections, but they can become dysregulated and pathological in inflammation and sepsis, leading to a cytokine storm, immune cell hyperactivation and could cause a life-threatening systemic inflammatory syndrome. These mediators can cause vasodilation and increased capillary permeability, manifested by severe hypotension in the clinical presentation of the septic patient. The symptoms of sepsis are not only related to infection and the immune response that it triggers but also the large alterations in immunosuppression. As the vascular endothelium

is activated by the invading organisms and is likely to be damaged, the coagulation cascade is activated but as intravascular coagulation, fibrinolysis and rapid consumption of the clotting factors occurs, the septic patient is also at risk of coagulation disorders such as disseminated intravascular coagulation and multi-organ dysfunction.

Risk factors of sepsis

Certain age groups are at a higher risk of developing sepsis. These are the very young, under the age of one year, and people aged 75 years and above. Other risk factors are the frail, diabetic, immunocompromised which includes those taking immunosuppressant drugs for medical reasons, people taking long-term steroids, intravenous drug users and anyone who has had a breach in skin integrity. This includes post-operative patients, or people who have experienced burns, accidental cuts, and blisters. Other groups who are at significant risk from sepsis are those with intravenous or arterial lines, parenteral feeding, or indwelling catheters (NICE, 2016).

Further consideration should be given to pregnant females especially to those who have miscarried, underwent Caesarean section or forceps delivery, or termination of pregnancy (NICE, 2016).

Signs and symptoms of sepsis

Septic shock is a subset of sepsis, characterised by a need for vasopressors to maintain a mean arterial pressure of 65 mmHg and a serum lactate of > 2 mmols/L in the absence of hypovolaemia. In septic shock, the excessive systemic vasodilation, a limited vascular response to circulating catecholamines due to inflammatory mediators and the production of reactive oxygen species such as nitric oxide, produced by the vascular endothelium would all lead to a reduced systemic vascular resistance. Moreover, the capillary leak is systemic causing a reduction in circulating volume. The net effect of these pathological conditions is hypotension. To compensate for the low blood pressure, the heart works harder to attempt to compensate, and this is known as compensatory tachycardia. In the early stage of sepsis, the patient may have warm peripheries, a normal capillary refill time, subtle changes in behaviour but as sepsis progresses, the patient will show clinical signs such as cold and clammy skin, an altered mental status, delayed capillary refill time, reduced urine output and a raised lactate (Nagalingam, 2018). Lactic acidosis will occur due to decreased oxygen transfer across the alveoli, following proteins and fluids leaking into the tissues of the lungs. The reduced surface area for gas exchange and the consequent ventilation and perfusion mismatch causes hypoxaemia. The body attempts to compensate for poor delivery of oxygen to the tissues and anaerobic metabolism with a raised respiratory rate, which is a crucial indicator of deterioration. An awareness of the physiological processes and the signs and symptoms will assist in diagnosis, avoid delay in treatment of sepsis and reduce mortality (Table 26.3).

395

Table 26.3   Examples of different types of shock.

Types of Shock		
Type	**Reason**	**Possible causes**
Hypovolaemic shock	Loss of blood, plasma, or dehydration	Haemorrhage Burns Dehydration Pancreatitis Peritonitis
Septic shock also known as endotoxic shock	Severe infection causes vasodilation	Gram-negative bacteria Multiple infections
Anaphylactic	Sudden release of histamine and other chemicals causing systemic vasodilation with a sudden drop in blood pressure	Medications, Food such as nuts, shellfish and others.
Cardiogenic shock	Diminished ability of the heart to pump blood around the body	Myocardial infarction especially affecting the left ventricle Heart failure Pulmonary embolus Cardiac tamponade Chest injuries
Neurogenic shock		Traumatic brain injury Spinal cord injury

The Royal College of Physicians (2017) introduced the tract and trigger system the National Early Warning Score (NEWS) 2, including changes in altered mental status to the patient's observations to determine sepsis. The quick Sequential (Sepsis-related) Organ Failure Assessment (qSOFA), must be used as a bedside clinical score, to score adult patients who have an infection, who have subsequent high risk of organ dysfunction with score of 2 points or more, which is associated with an in-hospital mortality greater than 10%. The qSOFA definition and diagnostic criteria include the following three criteria: a respiratory rate > 22 breaths per minute, hypotension with systole < 100 mmHg and an altered mental status. This clinical tool, initially developed for the out-of-hospital setting, the emergency department and ward settings was later revised for the critical care setting.

Management of sepsis and septic shock

According to NICE (2016), if sepsis is suspected, blood tests which include blood gas analysis and blood cultures should be taken. Fluid and antimicrobials should be prescribed and administered within the first hour of admission. All patients suspected to have a diagnosis of sepsis should be immediately seen by a senior clinician for escalation of further aggressive resuscitation and may require admission to high dependency unit (HDU) or ICU. Admission to critical care units occurs when septic shock is unresponsive to fluid

therapy and vasopressor support is required to bolster blood pressure (Martin, 2019). Noradrenaline is recommended if, despite intravenous fluid input, mean arterial pressure fails to improve (Nee, 2006).

Surviving Sepsis Campaign Guidelines 2021

When nursing a patient with suspected sepsis it is imperative to complete a rapid assessment and implement the use the sepsis 6 care bundle which includes giving (1) oxygen, (2) fluids, (3) antimicrobials and taking (4) cultures, (5) bloods and an arterial blood gas and (6) urine output. Rapid assessment includes history and clinical examination, tests for both infectious and non-infectious causes of acute illness, and immediate treatment of acute conditions that can mimic sepsis. Whenever possible, this should be completed within 3 hours of presentation so that a decision can be made as to the likelihood of an infectious cause of the patient's presentation and timely antimicrobial therapy provided if the likelihood is thought to be high. The timing of administration of antimicrobial must be within the first hour whether sepsis is definite or possible (SSC, 2021).

Vasoactive agent management should include norepinephrine as a first-line vasopressor, with a target Mean Arterial Pressure (MAP) of 65 mmHg. It is suggested that consideration should be placed on insertion of an arterial line to measure blood pressure measurement via invasive monitoring. If central access is not available, then safe peripheral vasopressors can be used. If MAP is remains less than 65 mmHg then vasopressin should be considered to supplement the existing norepinephrine. If cardiac dysfunction with persistent hypoperfusion is present despite adequate volume status and blood pressure, it is imperative to consider adding dobutamine or changing to epinephrine (SSC, 2021).

The aim of fluid resuscitation is to replace lost intravascular volume. Administering intravenous fluid, increases oncotic pressure, which assists to move fluid from the interstitial spaces back into the circulation (Epstein and Waseem, 2021; Mandal, 2016; Martin, 2019; Tigabu et al., 2018). This reduces the inflammation cascade. The increased intravascular volume in turn increases the stroke volume and cardiac output which helps to improve tissue and organ perfusion minimising or reversing any organ dysfunction and physiological abnormalities (Martin, 2019).

Vasculitis

Vasculitis is a rare condition that causes inflammation of the blood vessels, causing them to narrow. There are many forms of vasculitis (Table 26.4).

Because of the multiple complications that can occur with vasculitis, e.g., sight loss, hearing loss, organ damage and death, diagnosis is key and apprising patients of treatment-related information is a high priority. According to Boyer and Mortimore, (2020) nurses are well placed to deliver this information which in turn, can reduce the negative effects of treatment regimens and compliance.

Table 26.4   Some types of vasculitis (*Source*: https://www.nhs.uk/conditions/vasculitis/).

Name	Signs and symptoms	Treatment
Eosinophilic granulomatosis with polyangiitis (Churg–Strauss syndrome) Also known as ANCA-associated vasculitis Affects adults aged 30–45	· Asthma · Allergic rhinitis · Temperature of 38°C or above · Muscle and joint pain · Tiredness · loss of appetite and weight loss · Affects the nerves, causing weakness, pins and needles or numbness · Damages the kidneys or heart muscle	Corticosteroids
Giant cell arteritis (temporal arteritis) arteries in the head and neck especially the temples are often affected. Occurs in adults over 50 years of age. It also commonly occurs alongside polymyalgia rheumatica.	· Aching and discomfort around the temples · Jaw muscle pain while eating · Headaches · Double vision or vision loss · Can cause blindness and/or stroke	Corticosteroids
Polymyalgia rheumatica (is closely associated with giant cell arteritis and people are often diagnosed simultaneously)	· Pain and stiffness in the shoulders, neck and hips, which is often worse after waking up · A high temperature · Extreme tiredness · Loss of appetite and weight loss · Depression	Corticosteroids usually prescribed in lower doses than for giant cell arteritis.
Granulomatosis with polyangiitis (Wegener's granulomatosis) Also known as ANCA-associated vasculitis Mainly affects blood vessels in the nose, sinuses, ears, lungs and kidneys. It mainly affects middle-aged or elderly people.	· A high temperature · Night sweats · Sinusitis · Nose bleeds · Shortness of breath and haemoptysis · Kidney injury · Can cause organ failure	Corticosteroids
Henoch–Schönlein purpura Affects children	· Purpura – appear like small bruises or reddish-purple spots · Joint pain · Abdominal pain · Diarrhoea · Vomiting · Haematuria · Blood in faeces It is not usually serious	Usually improves without treatment
Takayasu arteritis Mainly affects young women. Rare occurrence in the UK	· Extreme tiredness · A high temperature · Weight loss · muscle and joint pain · Dizziness · Shortness of breath · Painful, numb or cold limbs	
Buerger's (also known as Thromboangiitis obliterans) is a disease of the small and medium arteries and veins that restricts blood flow to the hands and feet. Thrombi can develop inside the blood vessels. It is not clear whether this is a true vasculitis. Affects almost exclusively smokers, mainly in young men aged 20–40 years, although more recently has been diagnosed in patients over the age of 50, mainly women.	· Numbness and tingling to fingers and toes · Skin ulcers and gangrene in the fingers and toes which may require amputation.	Immediate smoking cessation Anti-inflammatory and immunosuppressant treatments have not shown to be effective in Buerger's Disease.

397

Blood transfusions in adults

A blood transfusion is a clinical procedure involving the transfer of whole blood, or one of its components, from a donor to a recipient. It can be life-saving for patients.

Careful donor selection, processing, storage and distribution of blood components by healthcare staff is required to ensure safe and effective blood transfusion practice. However, the British Society for Haematology (BSH) (2017) has identified that errors still occur in the requesting, collection and administration of blood components, which can lead to significant risks for patients. These risks and adverse events are monitored by the Serious Hazards of Transfusion (SHOT), which is the UK's independent, professionally led haemovigilance scheme. In 2019, 84.1% (2857/3397) of all reports (including near miss and right blood right patient reports), were due to errors (Narayan and Poles, 2020).

Although it is often a medical responsibility to prescribe blood components, the completion of pre-transfusion sampling, bedside checks, and monitoring of the patient during transfusion is most often the responsibility of the nurse (Vasiliki, 2011). The National Institute for Health and Care Excellence (NICE) (2015) has produced guidelines for the assessment and management of blood transfusions. It includes information on patient safety during the blood transfusion process to further reduce errors, as well as providing alternatives to blood transfusion.

The UK national haemovigilance surveillance programme, SHOT, repeatedly identifies that patient are harmed, and some die, because of being given the incorrect type of blood.

The Chief Medical Officer and Chief Nursing Office recognised in a CAS alert (Department of Health, 2017) that in 2014 a patient died because of an ABO-incompatible transfusion in a high-profile case. The nurse collected, then administered a unit intended for another patient with a similar name. This would have been prevented if the final bedside check had been undertaken correctly. There were seven ABO-incompatible transfusions reported to SHOT in 2015, and three in 2016. All of these were preventable. In addition to the risk of non-biocompatible transfusion, patients may have other specific, and sometimes critical, transfusion requirements such as irradiated blood, CMV-negative serology blood and extended phenotype blood. Two critical points occur in preparation for transfusion; the first is to correctly identify the patient and label the sample when taking blood for a pre-transfusion blood sample, and the second is to check the details on the unit of blood and the patient's identity at the point of transfusion. Evidence from SHOT shows that the bedside check performed at the point of transfusion is not always undertaken correctly and that this puts patients at risk of serious complications or death.

Blood sample collections

Blood sample collection procedures are a critical step in ensuring the safety of transfusion. Blood sampling from patients, whether in hospital or in the community, is a regular and important part of health care. Nevertheless, as with all interventions, it is not without risk.

Correctly linking the blood sample to the patient from whom it was taken is fundamental, thus confirmation of the patient's identity and labelling the blood sample at the bedside is essential. If the sample in the tube does not belong to the patient whose name is on the tube, and this is not detected, then many different consequences may follow. Wrong blood in tube (WBIT) errors, where the blood in the tube is not that of the patient identified on the label, may lead to catastrophic outcomes, such as death from ABO-incompatible red cell transfusion (Bolton-Maggs et al., 2015).

Blood groups

In the early 1900s it became apparent that some patients were dying after blood transfusions and scientists discovered that there was incompatibility between some blood groups. There are more than 300 blood groups, but only a minority cause clinically significant transfusion reactions (Joint UK Blood Transfusion and Tissue Transplantation Services Professional Advisory Committee (JPAC), 2014a).

The two most important blood groups in clinical practice are ABO and RhD. The ABO system includes four main blood groups: A, B, AB and O. All of these groups are named because of the antigens on the surface of the red blood cells (RBCs). Antibodies can be formed against the antigens which the recipient lacks and can be naturally occurring or stimulated through pregnancy, transfusion or transplantation. Blood groups and compatibility of RBCs are shown in Table 26.5.

RBCs sometimes have the RhD antigen. If this is present, then the blood group is RhD-positive. If there is no RhD antigen present, the blood group is RhD-negative.

A patient's Rh status is particularly important in patients with childbearing potential. If a pregnant woman is RhD-negative and the fetus is RhD-positive this can stimulate the formation of antibodies in the woman that may cross

Table 26.5 Blood groups and compatibility in relation to red blood cells only. *Source:* adapted from American Society of Hematology, 2021.

	Type A	Type B	Type AB	Type O
Antigen (no red blood cells)	Antigen A	Antigen B	Antigen A + B	Neither A nor B
Antibody (in plasma)	Anti-B antibody	Anti-A antibody	Neither antibody	Both antibodies
Blood recipients and donors	Cannot have B or AB blood. Can have A or O blood	Cannot have A or AB blood. Can have B or O blood	Can have any type of blood. Is the universal recipient	Can only have O blood. Is the universal donor

the placenta and destroy the RBCs in the fetus. This is called sensitisation. This process does not normally affect the first pregnancy but, if a subsequent pregnancy with a RhD-positive fetus occurs, the woman's body will produce antibodies immediately, which can cross the placenta and cause haemolytic disease of the fetus and newborn (HDFN). Today, pregnant women are offered anti-D immunoglobulin injections during pregnancy to help remove the RhD fetal blood cells before they cause sensitisation. If a woman has already developed anti-D antibodies in a previous pregnancy (she is already sensitised) the immunoglobulin injections are contraindicated and more monitoring of the pregnancy will occur and the baby will require treatment after delivery. Administration when anti-D antibodies are present exposes the patient unnecessarily to a blood product (NHS website, 2021; Norfolk, 2013).

Compatibility

A donor's blood group must be compatible with the recipient's blood group. If it is not, an acute or delayed haemolytic transfusion reaction may occur. For example, if someone with blood group A (antigen A on the RBCs) is given blood group B RBCs the anti-B antibodies in the plasma will attack the group B cells. Therefore, group A RBCs must never be given to someone who has group B blood. Blood group AB has both antigen A and antigen B on its RBCs and no antibodies in the plasma. Those with type AB blood can receive blood from any of the blood groups (see Table 26.5). RBCs of blood group O do not have any A or B antigen on their surface, therefore the recipient's body will not react against group O RBCs and therefore group O RBCs can be given to a patient of any blood group. However, the presence of RhD has to be taken into consideration, with blood group O negative (no Rh factor) referred to as the 'universal donor' and this is most often given to patients in an emergency when the patient's blood group is not known. Type O negative RBCs have no antigens, it will not trigger an immune response, even if the recipient has a different blood type. Blood group AB positive is referred to as the 'universal recipient'. It is important to note here that in almost all cases patients are transfused with the same blood group as their own so there is less risk of incompatibility.

Indications for blood transfusions

The Blood Safety and Quality Regulations (BSQR) (legislation.gov.uk, 2005) define blood components as a therapeutic constituent of blood (such as RBCs, platelets, fresh frozen plasma (FFP), cryoprecipitate or granulocytes),. There are also licensed medicinal products derived from whole blood or plasma such as solvent detergent (SD) plasma, albumin and anti-D immunoglobulin (JPAC, 2014b). Whole blood is rarely used for transfusion now and patients are given a blood component only where there is a deficiency, which prevents unnecessary use of blood components (Lister et al., 2020).

Red blood cells

RBCs, also called erythrocytes, are the most abundant cell type in the blood. The primary function of RBCs is to transport oxygen to body cells and deliver carbon dioxide to the lungs. RBCs are transfused to patients to restore oxygen-carrying capacity in patients with anaemia or blood loss where alternative treatments are ineffective or inappropriate (JPAC, 2014a). Although local policies will vary, evidence suggests that most patients can tolerate anaemia with a haemoglobin of 70 g/litre in the absence of active bleeding (Lister et al., 2020). Most people can cope with losing a moderate amount of blood without needing a blood transfusion, as this loss can be replaced with other fluids to improve circulating volume. However, if larger amounts of blood are lost, a blood transfusion may be the best way of replacing blood rapidly. A blood transfusion may be needed to treat severe bleeding during or after an operation, childbirth or after a serious accident, for example. A major haemorrhage can be defined as (NICE, 2015):

- The loss of more than 1 blood volume within 24 hours (around 70 mL/kg, or more than 5 litres in a 70 kg adult)
- The loss of 50% of total blood volume in under 3 hours
- Bleeding in excess of 150 mL/minute in adults.

As a practical clinical definition, major haemorrhage is bleeding that leads to:

- A systolic blood pressure of less than 90 mmHg or
- A heart rate of more than 110 beats per minute in adults.

Additionally, blood component transfusions may be given to those patients who are deemed at risk of severe bleeding, such as patients with bleeding disorders (eg disseminated intravascular coagulation and platelet dysfunction).

Haemoglobin within RBCs transports oxygen around the body, therefore if there are fewer RBCs, there is less oxygen transportation, and consequently an increased chance of organ failure and even death.

Sometimes the bone marrow, which produces blood cells, cannot make enough RBCs. This may be due to disease or a failure of the bone marrow to work properly. It may be temporary or a longer-term problem. Some treatments, such as chemotherapy, can also affect the bone marrow in this way. In some cases, the anaemia can be treated with medicines; in other cases, a blood transfusion may be the best treatment (NHS Blood and Transplant, 2018).

Platelets

Platelet transfusions are offered to patients with thrombocytopenia who have clinically significant bleeding. In thrombocytopenia patients have low platelet production or increased destruction, therefore a transfusion can be beneficial to prevent or treat bleeding (Lister et al., 2020).

Fresh frozen plasma (FFP)

Plasma is obtained from whole blood donations or component donation by apheresis and is frozen soon after collection to protect its blood-clotting factors. It may be transfused to patients with significant bleeding but without major haemorrhage if they have abnormal coagulation test results and alternative therapies (eg prothrombin complex concentrate) are not available.

Cryoprecipitate

Cryoprecipitate is made from donated FFP, which is then thawed, centrifuged and the precipitate collected. It is used for patients with or without major haemorrhage who have clinically significant bleeding and low fibrinogen levels below 1.5 g/litre (2 g/litre in obstetric bleeding). Additionally, dried fibrinogen is now available for prescription as described in the British National Formulary (BNF). This can be administered by intravenous injection (IV), or by intravenous infusion (Joint Formulary Committee, 2021). It should be noted that the licence for fibrinogen concentrate is very restrictive.

Granulocytes

Transfusion of granulocytes is uncommon (these include neutrophils, which are phagocytic white blood cells) but may be indicated in patients with life-threatening soft tissue or organ infections with bacteria or fungi and low neutrophil counts, usually in the setting of severe, prolonged neutropenia after cytotoxic chemotherapy (JPAC, 2014a).

Procedural safety

All hospitals must have a transfusion policy with clear guidelines on blood transfusion practice. Regular training and competency assessment of all staff involved in the blood transfusion process is vital for transfusion safety (NICE, 2015).

Pre-procedure and sampling

The decision to transfuse must be based on a clinical assessment and consideration given to alternative treatments and issues such as religious belief, where patients may refuse a blood transfusion. Once a decision is made that the patient requires a transfusion, consent will be gained from the patient if possible and recorded in the patient's notes (Safety of Blood, Tissues and Organs (SaBTO), 2020). A request is made by the prescribing doctor or registered practitioner and sent to the transfusion laboratory. This will include a blood sample from the patient for their ABO, Rh status, antibody screening and cross match (Vasiliki, 2011) to ensure compatible blood is ordered for the patient. The patient's identity with surname, forename, date of birth and unique identity number retrieved from the patient computer system should be included on the patient's wristband. More widespread use of electronic management systems using barcodes on ID bands and blood components and hand-held scanners linked to the laboratory system will continue to enhance blood transfusion practice (JPAC, 2014a). Collection of the sample and labelling of the sample tubes must be performed as one uninterrupted process involving one competent staff member.

Blood components are stored under temperature-controlled conditions to prevent damage to the product. RBCs are stored in a designated blood component refrigerator under controlled temperatures in a laboratory and contain anti-coagulant to prevent clotting of the infused blood. These must never be stored in ward or drug fridges at any time. Once the blood component is ready in the transfusion laboratory, nurses will ensure the patient is prepared with intravenous access and that the blood component is prescribed correctly before requesting delivery of the blood. The blood should be collected by a staff member who is trained and competent in this process as errors in removal from storage and transportation have been identified as a source of error (Lister et al., 2020). A request slip or transfusion prescription is used to check against the blood collected before signing the blood out to the clinical area. Today, computerised checking systems use bar codes and can scan staff IDs to reduce handwritten documentation and improve safety. Only one unit of blood should be collected at any one time unless it is an emergency requiring rapid transfusion and all blood components should be administered as soon as possible.

Pre-transfusion observations should be carried out on the patient, including blood pressure, temperature, heart rate and respirations no more than 60 minutes before the transfusion (Hurrell, 2014). Equipment should be prepared in advance and cannula access gained.

Administration of the blood product

The identity check between the patient and the blood component to be transfused is usually considered the last opportunity to identify errors made earlier in the process, as well as being the final point at which errors can occur. It is predominantly the responsibility of the nurse to ensure that the right patient receives the right blood. This must be performed at the bedside (Lister et al., 2020). The key principles of safe bedside administration are outlined in Box 26.1. If there are interruptions during the checking

Box 26.1 Bedside check.

The use of a formal bedside checklist has been mandated since the 2017 CAS alert **(Department of Health, 2017)**

Positive patient identification

- Confirm patient's full name and date of birth
- Ensure information matches the patient's identity wristband
- Ensure patient's hospital ID number is on the form returned to the lab when the transfusion is started

Patient details on component pack

- Check the details match with the patient's identity wristband and prescription

Correct prescription

- Check that the right component has been prescribed correct component
- Check it is the correct component
- Check that the component is compatible with the recipient's ABO blood group
- Check expiry date
- Ensure that the donation number and blood group matches the laboratory report label
- Check pack for signs of leakage and inspect for any defects

Any specific requirements

- Does the patient need any irradiated blood or specially selected units?
- Does the patient require a diuretic prescription in the case of fluid overload, heart (pump) failure?

Source: Based on Bellamy, 2018

---

process it must start again and if there are any discrepancies the blood transfusion should not go ahead and discrepancies must be reported to the laboratory (JPAC, 2014a). All relevant documentation should be signed by the person administering the blood and the component donation number, date, time of starting and stopping the transfusion, dose/volume of component transfused, and name of the administering practitioner should be recorded. Blood components must be given using a designated giving set and an infusion device can be used to control the rate of infusion (Lister et al., 2020). Once the transfusion has started, observations including blood pressure, heart rate, respiratory rate and temperature should be recorded on a transfusion record or an electronic patient record within 15 minutes. Most serious reactions such as ABO incompatibility will occur during this time (JPAC, 2014a). It is also important to observe and monitor the patient throughout the transfusion. Any concerns by the nurse or expressed by the patient would indicate the need to

perform additional observations. In the event of a reaction, the transfusion should be stopped immediately, resuscitation measures begun if required and contact made with both medical staff and the transfusion lab. Possible reactions are listed in Box 26.2. Nursing considerations are listed in Box 26.3 (JPAC, 2014c).

Post-procedural care

At the end of each unit transfused, the time and volume infused must be recorded. Transfusion should be completed within 4 hours of leaving controlled temperature storage (JPAC, 2014d). It is important that the patient's heart rate, blood pressure, respiratory rate and temperature are recorded no more than 60 minutes after the end of the transfusion (Lister et al., 2020). Inpatients should be observed for late reactions, which can occur up to 24 hours after a transfusion. Day-care patients should be advised to report symptoms developing after discharge. If there is any suspicion of a reaction during the hospital stay, the blood component pack and all records must be sent back to the transfusion lab. Where there are no issues, all documentation must be filed in the patient record. For patients requiring ongoing transfusions, the blood giving set should be changed every 12 hours (Robinson et al., 2018). Once the transfusion is complete all equipment, including the component pack, should be discarded as clinical waste.

Traceability

The UK Blood Safety and Quality Regulations 2005 (as amended) defines 'traceability' as 'the ability to trace each individual unit of blood or blood component from the donor to its final destination (whether this is a recipient, a manufacturer of medicinal products or disposal) and from its final destination back to the donor' (legislation.gov.uk, 2005; JPAC, 2014a). The regulations place an obligation on both blood establishments (regulation 8) and hospital blood banks (regulation 9) 'to ensure full traceability of blood and blood components'.

The expectation is that traceability information will therefore be available for all blood and blood components and retained in a retrievable form for 30 years. However, it is acknowledged that, occasionally, the final fate of a specific blood component cannot be confirmed. In such cases, steps should be taken by the blood establishment or hospital blood bank to monitor and investigate each traceability failure.

In clinical practice, it is usually hospital policy that the blood product paper label or sticker is detached following transfusion. If using paper notes the sticker will be placed in the clinical notes. If using electronic notes, this code will be scanned in or typed into the clinical notes system. The blood product label will also be kept in a designated box and sent to the pathology laboratory for recording and storage purposes.

Box 26.2   Common signs and symptoms of acute transfusion reactions.

Urticaria/itching

Urticaria (hives) and/or itching can be the presenting sign of a mild allergic reaction but can also be associated with the onset of a life-threatening anaphylactic reaction. The transfusion should be stopped, and the patient should be carefully monitored for progression of symptoms.

Fever/chills

Fever and/or chills are most commonly associated with a febrile, non-haemolytic reaction. However, they can also be the first sign of a more serious acute haemolytic reaction, transfusion-related acute lung injury (TRALI), or septic transfusion reaction. If the patient's temperature rises by 1°C or higher than the temperature at the start of transfusion, the transfusion should be stopped. Acute haemolytic reaction or bacterial contamination should be suspected if there is a greater rise in temperature, or more serious symptoms (such as rigors).

TRALI

Transfusion-related acute lung injury (TRALI) is defined as new acute lung injury (ALI) that occurs during or within 6 hours of transfusion, not explained by another ALI risk factor. Transfusion of part of one unit of any blood product can cause TRALI. The mechanism may include factors in unit(s) of blood, such as antibody and biologic response modifiers. In addition, yet to be described factors in a patient's illness may predispose them to the condition. The clinical presentation of TRALI is related to pulmonary permeability oedema, thought to occur secondary to the release of various leucocyte interleukins, and may include fever, hypotension, tachycardia and rarely a transient drop in the peripheral neutrophil count (Murphy et al., 2020).

Respiratory distress/dyspnoea

Dyspnoea, or shortness of breath, is a concerning sign that can often be seen with more severe reactions, including anaphylaxis, TRALI, and transfusion-associated circulatory overload (TACO). It can also be seen by itself without accompanying symptoms.

Hypotension

Hypotension can be seen with an acute haemolytic reaction, septic transfusion reactions, anaphylaxis, and TRALI.

Hypothermia

Hypothermia can be seen with large volume transfusions of refrigerated components. The only intervention needed is warming the patient and/or blood component.

Source: Modified from Suddock and Crookston, 2019.

Box 26.3   Nursing considerations.

No drugs or other intravenous fluid must be added to or administered via the same cannula during the transfusion of any blood component.

Flushing through the remainder of the blood in the line with 0.9% sodium chloride is unnecessary and is not recommended because it may result in particles being flushed through the filter.

If another IV infusion is to take place after the blood transfusion, a new IV fluid administration set must be used to reduce the risk of incompatible fluids or drugs causing haemolysis of any residual red cells that may be left in the administration set.

If multiple units of red blood cells are being transfused, the administration set should be changed at least every 12 hours to prevent bacterial growth. Additionally, in cases of massive haemorrhage, where different components are to be given in rapid succession, it is common clinical practice to use a new set for each component.

Source: JPAC, 2014c.

Patient information

NICE (2015) recommends that clinical staff provide verbal and written information to patients who may have or who have had a transfusion, and their family members or carers (as appropriate). This should include the reason for the transfusion, the risks and benefits, the transfusion process, any alternatives and that they would not be eligible to donate blood in future.

Alternatives to blood transfusions

It is important to acknowledge that blood transfusions are only administered if there are no other alternatives and clinical assessment indicates the need for a blood transfusion. Tranexamic acid may be given to patients who are undergoing surgery where potential blood loss is >500 ml (NHSBT, 2021). According to NICE (2015), erythropoietin can be given if the patient has anaemia and meets the criteria for blood transfusion, but declines it because of religious beliefs or other reasons, or the appropriate blood type is not available because of the patient's red cell antibodies. Additionally, intravenous or oral iron can be offered before and after surgery to patients with iron-deficiency anaemia (NICE, 2015).

Summary of SaBTO recommendations on consent

According to the guidelines from the expert advisory committee on the Safety of Blood, Tissues and Organs (SaBTO) (2020) on patient consent for blood transfusion, it is recommended that:

> Informed and valid consent for transfusion is completed for all patients who will likely, or definitely, receive a transfusion. These recommendations apply to transfusion of whole blood, red blood cells, platelets, fresh frozen plasma (FFP), cryoprecipitate and granulocytes, as well as those who are exposed to blood or blood components. These recommendations also apply to where transfusion might occur during a procedure where the patient is incapacitated, for example, where blood is routinely requested prior to surgery or where a 'group and save' or 'cross-match' sample is taken pre-procedure. Such shared decision-making discussions should be documented in the patient's clinical record.

Patients who have been given a blood transfusion and were not able to give informed and valid consent prior to the transfusion are informed of the transfusion prior to discharge and provided with relevant paper or electronic information.

All patients who have received a transfusion have details of the transfusion (type(s) of component), together with any adverse events associated with the transfusion, included in their hospital discharge summary to ensure both the patient and their family doctor are aware. The patient should also be informed that they are no longer eligible to donate blood (except for individuals who have received convalescent plasma from donating convalescent plasma to treat individuals with SARS-CoV-2 infection/COVID-19).

The UK Blood Services provide a standardised source of information for patients who may receive a blood transfusion in the UK.

Training in consent for transfusion is included in all relevant undergraduate healthcare practitioners' training, followed by continuous, regular knowledge updates (minimum 3-yearly) for all healthcare practitioners involved in the consent for transfusion process.

There is a centralised UK-wide information resource for healthcare practitioners to facilitate consent for transfusion discussions, indicating the key issues to be discussed when obtaining informed and valid consent for a blood transfusion, and providing up-to-date information on the risks of transfusion. This resource should be provided by the UK Blood Services. The feasibility of developing and maintaining this resource should be completed by the UK Blood Services within 6 months of the publication of these recommendations.

All UK healthcare organisations who provide blood transfusions employ mechanisms (such as audit) to monitor the implementation and compliance with these SaBTO recommendations, with subsequent improvement plans developed and implemented if indicated.

The transfusion of blood components is common in clinical practice but is a complex process that requires nurses and other health staff to be vigilant in all aspects of transfusion practice to ensure patient safety is maintained throughout. Clinical guidelines and appropriate education and training are essential to standardise blood transfusion practice and reduce avoidable errors, which are most often attributed to human error (Booth and Allard, 2017). There is now clinical evidence to support the process of 'patient blood management', which is an evidence-based multidisciplinary approach aimed at optimising the individual and holistic needs of patients and reducing avoidable use of blood components when alternatives may be suitable (Gallagher et al., 2015). Most blood transfusion reactions occur because of human error. Some reactions can be severe, but many are benign. Anaphylactic reactions to a blood transfusion are very rare but often result in a fatality (American Society of Anesthesiologists, 2014). Transfusion in the UK is generally safe and SHOT data for the 5 years to 2019 show the risk of death from transfusion as 0.87 per 100 000 components issued (Narayan and Poles, 2020). Patients on any ward can receive a blood transfusion and so all nurses must know the potential complications and how to manage them.

403

Snapshot 1

David is 59-year-old gentleman is two days post surgery following an open appendicectomy for a ruptured appendix. Repeated problems with urinary retention post-operatively have led to insertion of a urinary catheter.

His past medical history includes hypertension for which he normally takes Ramipril 2.5 mg and Amlodipine 5 mg. He is currently on a surgical ward and complains of feeling unwell; cold and shivery. He is reviewed by the critical care outreach team due to deteriorating status.

AIRWAY Look, Listen, Feel	Assess patency
	• Listen for signs of decreased air entry or for course crackles which might denote consolidation. Stridor, snoring, wheezing, gurgling denoting airway obstruction. Airway sounds clear • Note ability to cough and clear airway secretions. If coughing sputum check, colour, consistency, and volume • ACTIONS appropriately: Sit patient up and send sputum culture for Microscopy Culture and Sensitivity
BREATHING Look Listen Feel	Observes patient skin colour for changes regardless of skin tone Centrally – lips and oral mucosa for cyanosis (Nil central cyanosis) • Peripherally-fingers for cyanosis/clubbing (Nil clubbing noted) • Coughing thick, green sputum • Mouth and lips very dry
Measure	Observes position Sat up, mouth breathing • Use of accessory muscles (yes, looks distressed) • Trachea midline yes – no deviation noted which could be indicative of lung collapse or large tumour or pleural effusion • No pneumothorax • Looks and feel for bilateral chest expansion shallow respirations • Uses a stethoscope to auscultate the lungs using a ladder pattern to assess air entry and breath sounds: Adventitious sounds: Right basal late inspiratory crackles – fluid in the alveoli/pneumonia
	Feel limbs noting warmth and perfusion. • Note's temperature change along all limbs (may complete this under circulation) (cool fingers and toes, feels clammy) • Check colour of skin if mottled, pale, flushed, face pale, legs, look mottled
	• Note oxygen percentage and delivery method AIR • Assesses oxygen saturations identifying acceptable ranges for patient 91% (target range 94–98%)
	Observes patient's breathing for one full minute, noting rate, 25 breaths per minute: • Rhythm, regular • Depth, shallow
	ACTIONS appropriately e.g. • Oxygen as required for target 94% (5 L face mask or equivalent) Respiratory rate down to 21 • Sits patient up.

CIRCULATION Look Listen Feel	• Temp 39.1°C • Assesses capillary refill in finger (applies pressure for 5 seconds with finger above heart level) (Cap refill < 2 secs)
Measure	Feel limbs noting warmth and perfusion.
	• Notes temperature change along all limbs (may complete this under breathing) cool at peripheries,
	• Palpates radial pulse for 60 seconds noting rate, (HR 110) • Rhythm regular and bounding
	Palpates with thumb for 5 seconds for signs of pitting oedema (none)
	• Records blood pressure (100/70 mmHg) • MAP > 70 mmHg • Pulse pressure 30 mmHg – narrow – fluid depleted
	• Assesses urine output at > 0.5 mL/kg/hour urinary catheter, output 30 mL last 2 hours weight 80 kg) Urinalysis SG raised
	• Assesses fluid balance: Feeling nauseated so not drinking, no fluid chart present, skin turgor poor, mouth dry. • Actions check IV access, • 45° passive leg raise • Considers sepsis/ dehydration/ AKI
DISABILITY	• Uses ACVPU to correctly assess level of wakefulness (A) Orientated and able to respond appropriately to questions • Checks Blood glucose level (Normal) • ACTIONS appropriately
EXPOSURE	• Inspects wounds/drains, skin for rashes/erythema. • Checks catheter site • Checks wound site • Both calves same size, no warmth or tenderness • Venflon in situ, looks clean. Visual Infusion Phlebitis (VIP) score of 0
Investigations	Sputum for culture was sent off, CXR: Right basal consolidation, Hospital-Acquired Pneumonia (HAP) – ? Chest Sepsis ECG: sinus tachycardia with ventricular ectopic rate 100 Hb, 138g/L (13.8 g/dL), Urea 17.6 mmol/L, Creatinine (122 µmol/L) (NR 64–104 µmol/L) Electrolytes K+ 3.3 mmol/L Na+ 145 mmmoL/litre C-reactive protein (CRP) 55 mg/L WCC 12 × 10^9 Sample arterial blood gas analysis pH 7.32, PaO$_2$ 9.0kPa PaCO$_2$ 4.0 kPa, HCO$_3^-$ 19 Base Excess (BE) −4 (on oxygen), Lactate 2.5 mmol/L Wells Score/D Dimers/Clotting considered (Pulmonary Embolism) As NEWS2 >5, consider sepsis and tools such as qSOFA. Sepsis 6 – blood culture, urine culture, lactate

Management:

Observations and monitoring in accordance with NEWS2 (Royal College of Physicians, 2017).

ECG – Sinus tachycardia with ventricular ectopic rate 100

Correct electrolytes, potassium, magnesium to allow the potassium-pump and cardiac cells functions to be restored.

Sepsis 6 – fluids 30 mL/kg. Encourage patient to drink more orally. Strict fluid balance.

Multidisciplinary approach: Microbiologist involvement for advice on treatment. Send cultures.

Antibiotics within 1 hour. If blood pressure does not improve – consider vasopressors – noradrenaline is the first inotrope.

Consider nebulisers – saline to manage secretions. Humidified oxygen and chest physiotherapy.

Keep patient informed. Health promotion. Encourage deep breathing exercises.

Snapshot 2

Theresa is a 67-year-old retired woman, who has a ten-month history of overwhelming tiredness, arthralgia and feeling low of mood. Over the last month arthralgia pains have worsened and has lost 3 kg in weight.

Over the last 2 days Theresa feels that she is short of breath and a purpuric rash has developed over her lower and upper extremities. Headache and abdominal pains have developed This has led to admission to hospital for further tests and investigations.

Past medical history: Commenced on citalopram 20 mg once daily, 3 months ago, for low mood.

Drug history: No known allergies, no recent prescription for medicines other than citalopram but takes paracetamol and ibuprofen for joint pains

No relevant family history

Social history: Divorced, no children, retired art teacher.

Smokes 10–15 cigarettes/day and has done since the age of 15

Glass of wine most evenings

Pets: dog called Syd.

On examination: Looks unwell, pale and non-blanching purpuric rash noted on arms, legs and abdomen.

Airway (A): Airway is patent, patient is speaking.

Breathing (B): Oxygen saturations 92% (NEWS2 = 2), on 3/L oxygen, respiratory rate (RR) 26 breaths per minute (NEWS2 = 3). Chest examination reveals fine crackles mid to lower zones

Cardiovascular system (C): Blood Pressure (BP) is 114/75 (NEWS2 = 0), Heart Rate (HR) is 85 beats per minute (NEWS2 = 0), capillary refill time (CRT) is 2 seconds, she is warm to touch.

Disability (D) (neurological system), Patient is alert (NEWS2 = 0), on the AVPU scale (see Chapter 14), Body temperature (T) 36.7C

Exposure (E) Urinalysis reveals 2+ blood, 3+ protein. No finger clubbing but leuchonychia noted.

Total NEW2 Score: 5.

Nursing actions: contacts doctor to discuss rash.

Differential diagnosis considered: Thrombocytopenia. Vasculitis affecting lungs and kidneys. Undiagnosed COPD A full examination, assessment and diagnostic tests including blood tests: FBC, LFTs, CRP, ESR, auto antibody screen, immunoglobulins.

Kidney biopsy: glomerular nephritis

CXR reveals ground glass appearance

Final diagnosis: ANCA-associated granulomatous vasculitis (formerly known as Wegener's vasculitis).

6Cs: Compassion

Without prompt medical intervention and treatment, ANCA-associated granulomatous vasculitis can be fatal. This is due to the inflammation of blood vessels leading to organ damage and failure. In this case study, the patient required a kidney biopsy to assess the extent of kidney damage. Mortality is highest in the first year of diagnosis of vasculitis. Nurses are best placed to offer care and compassion for patients diagnosed with this rare disorder. The symptoms can be distressing and cause great anxiety. Patient education, especially regarding treatment is paramount. Informing patients of potential relapse signs and symptoms can be life-saving. Although rare, nurses should have a knowledge of vasculitis to offer empathy, emotional support and understanding to both the patient and their loved ones.

Medication management

Treatment is with a tapering course of corticosteroids, and long-term immunosuppression therapy. Unfortunately, treatment does not cure the condition but can lead to remission. Patients must be informed of the risks of immunosuppression and to avoid being near people with infections and to take care in the sun, as the incidence of skin cancer can increase. Depending on the type of immunosuppression prescribed, patients will require regular surveillance screening to monitor FBC and kidney function. Nurses also need to be mindful that protein and blood in the urine is indicative of relapse and frequent urinalysis is also required.

Steroids can induce diabetes and cataracts. Patients should be monitored for this occurring. In addition, once steroids are commenced, vitamin D and calcium should be prescribed to prevent steroid induced osteoporosis.

Snapshot 3

35-year-old man admitted to surgical ward with pancreatitis secondary to gallstones. Within 12 hours of admission patient's condition deteriorated.

Airway (A): Airway is patent.
Breathing (B): Oxygen saturations 92% on air (NEWS2 = 2), respiratory rate (RR) 27 breaths per minute (NEWS2 = 3).
Cardiovascular System (C): Blood pressure (BP) is 86/55 (NEWS2 = 3), Heart rate (HR) is 126 beats per minute (NEWS2 = 2), capillary refill time (CRT) is 4 seconds, he is cool to touch.
Disability (D) (neurological System), Patient is drowsy but responds to verbal stimuli (NEWS2 = 1), on the AVPU scale (see Chapter 14), Body temperature (T) is 38.8°C (NEWS2 =1).

After medical review he was transferred to ICU, where he was and commenced on inotropes to maintain blood pressure and later ventilated. Over the next 24hours blood test were taken (see clinical investigation)

Clinical Investigation

Routine bloods, i.e. FBC; noted a falling platelet count with increasing INR/prothrombin time.
D-dimer: Arterial line and IV sites were oozing blood. bruising noted on left flank and around umbilicus.
D-dimer raised.
The ISTH DIC scoring system was utilised and scored 5.

Test	0 points	1 point	2 points	3 points
INR or PT prolongation	INR ≤ 1.3<3 seconds	INR 1.3–173–6 seconds	INR >1.7>6 seconds	
Fibrinogen	>100 mg/dL	<100 mg/dL		
D-dimer	<400 ng/dL		400-4,000 ng/ml	>4,000 ng/ml
Platelets	>100,000/uL	50,000-100,000/uL	<50,000 uL	

1. Interpretation of total score:
2. ≥5 points: Positive for DIC
3. < 5 points: Negative, but patients could still have 'non-overt DIC' which could evolve into frank DIC. If there is ongoing concern for DIC, coagulation labs may be repeated in 12–24 hours.

Diagnosis: DIC secondary to organ destruction caused by severe pancreatitis.

No one blood test can diagnose DIC but rather a combination of patient's history such as acute pancreatitis (organ destruction) and combined blood test results; decreasing platelets, raised D-dimer, increased clotting time and generalised overt bleeding from areas such as intravenous and arterial cannula sites.

6Cs: Courage

DIC is a life-threatening condition where clotting factors and platelets are consumed which results in fibrin deposition in the microcirculation leading to clot formation. Haemorrhagic events are due to reduced clotting factors. This can scare both the patient and their family members. Use courage to support people regarding this serious complication, as it is associated with a poor prognosis and a high mortality rate and can be traumatising. Careful consideration should be given on how to break the news to family. Nurses are best placed to an emotionally support families during difficult times such as this.

Learning event: reflection

In pancreatitis, the auto destruction of the pancreas causes pancreatic enzymes to spill out to surrounding areas of tissue and fat, destroying it. If blood vessels are damaged or destroyed it can lead to haemorrhage which can manifest as bruising round the umbilicus known as Cullen's sign and bruising along left flank, known as Grey Turner's sign. The damaged pancreatic tissue can become necrotic and infected. IV antibiotics would be prescribed, and the necrotic tissue could be surgically removed if appropriate. In some instances, the necrosis can cause systemic inflammatory response syndrome (SIRS) to occur.

Medications management

It is essential to treat the underlying condition leading to DIC.

Supportive treatment consists of replacing clotting factors such as platelets, fresh frozen plasma and cryo-precipitate in patients who are bleeding. It is often helpful to discuss the case with the lab scientists to determine amount of blood products required.

Conclusion

This chapter has provided an evidence-based discussion regarding people who encounter a haematological disorder and require critical care intervention. The treatment and potential complications and special needs of haematology patients within critical care environment have been discussed. Knowledge gained in this chapter will assist ICU nurses to care for any critically unwell patient with a haematological disorder who is transferred to and cared for in their intensive care unit. Greater understanding of all these aspects of care will ensure that the patients with a haematological malignancy in ICU and their family receive the most appropriate care.

Take home points

1. People with haematological disorders who are critically unwell will require complex multi-organ support in a critical care unit that provides level 2 and 3 care.
2. Critically unwell people with haematological disorders will present with abnormal vital signs due to altered pathophysiology.
3. Haemoglobin is the iron-containing oxygen transport protein and 1 molecule of haemoglobin binds with 4 molecules of oxygen or 1.34 mL of oxygen, forming oxyhaemoglobin. Consequently, patients that do not create enough RBCs such as those with bone marrow cancers will present breathless and pale.
4. There are three blood coagulation pathways: intrinsic, extrinsic and common.
5. Neutropenic patients should always be reverse-barrier nursed.
6. Sepsis is common in critically unwell haematological patients and can lead to septic shock. Understanding the sepsis 6 and the altered pathophysiology of shock is fundamental for critical care nurses.
7. Blood component transfusion will be a routine practice for critically unwell patients with haematological disorders.
8. Blood component transfusion is a complex procedure and blood groups, and components, must be understood by critical care nurses undertaking these procedures.
9. People who are critically unwell with hepatological disorders require nurses to practise the 6Cs at all times.
10. People with haematological disorders have long-term conditions and their stay in critical care is associated with an exacerbation of their illness to manage multi-organ failure. Family and friends can help nurses provide holistic care.

References

Adam, S., Osborne, S., and Welch, J. (2017). *Critical Care Nursing: Science and Practice*, 3e. Oxford: Oxford University Press.

American Cancer Society (2017). Non-Hodgkin's lymphoma risk factors. https://www.cancer.org/cancer/non-hodgkinlymphoma/causes-risks-prevention/riskfactors.html.

American Society of Anesthesiologists. Top blood transfusion-related complication more common than previously reported. 16 December 2014. Science Daily. https://tinyurl.com/ym6yszcu (accessed 19 April 2021).

American Society of Hematology. Blood safety and matching. https://tinyurl.com/zmwk2vxa (accessed 19 April 2021).

Arwyn-Jones, J. and Brent, A.J. (2019). Sepsis. *Surgery* 37(1).

Bellamy M. (2018). Foreword. In: *Serious Hazards of Transfusion (SHOT) Steering Group. Annual SHOT Report 2017*. https://tinyurl.com/hfx8p4wc (accessed 19 April 2021).

Bolton-Maggs, P.H.B., Wood, E.M., and Wiersum-Osselton, J.C. (2015) Wrong blood in tube – potential for serious outcomes: can it be prevented? *Br J Haematol*. 168(1): 3–13.

Booth, C. and Allard, S. (2017). Blood transfusion. *Medicine (Baltimore)* 45(4): 244–250.

Boyer, H., Mortimore, G. (2020). Anti-neutrophil cytoplasmic antibodies-associated vasculitis: a guide and case study. *British Journal of Nursing* 29(22): 1333–1340.

Brent, A. (2017). Sepsis. *Medicine* 45(10): 649–653. doi: 10.1016/j.mpmed.2017.07.010.

British Society for Haematology (2017). Administration of blood products. https://tinyurl.com/k7rdumnb (accessed 19 April 2021).

British Society of Haematology (2009). Diagnosis and management of disseminated intravascular coagulation (1). http://www.b-s-h.org.uk/guidelines/guidelines/diagnosis-and-management-of-disseminated-intravascular-coagulation-1/.

British Society of Haematology (2017). Guidelines. http://www.b-s-h.org.uk/guidelines/guidelines/ (accessed March 2022).

Cancer Research UK (2018a). Hodgkin lymphoma symptoms. https://www.cancerresearchuk.org/about-cancer/hodgkin-lymphoma/symptoms (accessed March 2022).

Cancer Research UK (2018b). Hodgkin lymphoma: incidence statistics. https://www.cancerresearchuk.org/health-professional/cancer-statistics/statistics-by-cancer-type/hodgkin-lymphoma/ (accessed March 2022).

Cancer Research UK (2018c). Non-Hodgkin lymphoma statistics. http://www.cancerresearchuk.org/health-professional/cancer-statistics/statistics-by-cancer-type/non-hodgkin-lymphoma (accessed March 2022).

Department of Health (DH) (2010). Equality and diversity: Equality Act 2010. https://www.gov.uk/government/organisations/department-of-health/about/equality-and-diversity (accessed March 2022).

Department of Health (2017). Safe transfusion practice: Use a bedside checklist. CAS alert. CEM/CMO/2017/005. https://tinyurl.com/5c4ckuh5 (accessed 5 July 2021).

Epstein, E.M., Waseem, M. (2021). *Crystalloid Fluids*. https://www.ncbi.nlm.nih.gov/books/NBK537326/ (accessed 8 August 2021).

European Society for Medical Oncology (2014). Clinical practice guidelines: Hodgkin's lymphoma: ESMO clinical practice guidelines for diagnosis, treatment and follow-up. *Ann. Oncol.* 25(3): 70–75.

Gallagher, T., Darby, S., Vodanovich, M. et al. (2015). Patient blood management nurse vs transfusion nurse: is it time to merge? *Br J Nurs* 24(9): 492–495.

Gyawali, B., Ramakrishna, K., and Dhamoon, A.S. (2019). Sepsis: The evolution in definition, pathophysiology, and management. *Sage Open Medicine* 7(1).

Hurrell, K. (2014). Safe administration of blood components. *Nurs Times* 110(38): 16–19.

Joint Formulary Committee (2021). Fibrinogen, dried. British National Formulary (online). London: BMJ Group and Pharmaceutical Press. https://tinyurl.com/c3rz2hb7 (accessed 19 April 2021).

Joint United Kingdom Blood Transfusion and Tissue Transplantation Services Professional Advisory Committee (2014a). Traceability update 2014. https://tinyurl.com/7pzdsc (accessed 19 April 2021).

Joint United Kingdom (UK) Blood Transfusion and Tissue Transplantation Services Professional Advisory Committee (2014b). Providing safe blood – blood products. Transfusion handbook. https://tinyurl.com/ysvna9yw (accessed 5 July 2021).

Joint United Kingdom (UK) Blood Transfusion and Tissue Transplantation Services Professional Advisory Committee (2014c). Technical aspects of transfusion. Technical aspects of transfusion. Transfusion handbook. https://tinyurl.com/arpup2z (accessed 19 April 2021).

Joint United Kingdom (UK) Blood Transfusion and Tissue Transplantation Services Professional Advisory Committee (2014d). Safe transfusion – right blood, right patient, right time and right place. Transfusion handbook. https://tinyurl.com/6xb6tm2a (accessed 19 April 2021).

Karunanayake, C., McDuffie, H.H., Dosman, J.A. et al. (2008). Occupational exposure and non-Hodgkin's lymphoma: Canadian case-control study. Environmental Health. https://ehjournal.biomedcentral.com/articles/10.1186/1476069X-7-44#Bib1.

Legislation.gov.uk. (2005). *Blood Safety and Quality Regulations*. SI 2005/50. https://tinyurl.com/3ankvncj (accessed 19 April 2021).

Levy, M.M., Toh, C.H., Thachil, J., and Watson, H.G. (2009). Guidelines for the diagnosis and management of disseminated intravascular coagulation. *British Journal of Haematology* 145(1): 24–33.

Levy, M.M., Evans, L.E., and Rhodes, A. (2018). The surviving sepsis campaign bundle: 2018 update. *Critical Care Medicine* 46(6). doi: 10.1097/ccm.0000000000003119.

Lister, S., Holland, J., Grafton, H. (eds) (2020). *The Royal Marsden Manual of Clinical Nursing Procedures*, 10e. Professional edn. Chichester: John Wiley.

MacMillian Cancer Support (2017). Signs and symptoms of non-Hodgkin's lymphoma (NHL). https://www.macmillan.org.uk/information-and-support/lymphoma/lymphoma-non-hodgkin/understanding-cancer/signs-and-symptoms.html (accessed March 2022).

Mandal, M. (2016). Ideal resuscitation fluid in hypovolemia: The quest is on and miles to go! *International Journal of Critical Illness and Injury Science* 6(2): 54–55.

Marieb, E.N. (2015). *Essentials of Human Anatomy and Physiology*, 11e. Harlow: Pearson.

Martin G.S. (2019). Optimal fluid management in sepsis. *Qatar Medical Journal* 2019(2): 40. doi: 10.5339/qmj.2019.qccc.40.

Murphy, C.E., Kenny, C.M., Brown KF. (2020). TACO and TRALI: visualising transfusion lung injury on plain film. *BMJ Case Rep* 13(4): e230426.

Nagalingam, K. (2018). Understanding sepsis. *British Journal of Nursing* 27(20). doi: 10.12968/bjon.2018.27.20.1168.

Narayan, S. and Poles, D. (2020). Headline data: deaths, major morbidity and ABO-incompatible transfusions. In: *Serious Hazards of Transfusion (SHOT) Steering Group. Annual SHOT Report 2019*. https://tinyurl.com/hux25dkx (accessed 19 April 2021).

National Institute for Health and Care Excellence (NICE) (2016). Sepsis: recognition, diagnosis and early management. NICE guideline [NG51] Published: 13 July 2016 Last updated: 13 September 2017. https://www.nice.org.uk/guidance/ng51/chapter/Recommendations#identifying-people-with-suspected-sepsis (accessed 12 July 2021).

National Institute for Health and Care Excellence (2015). Blood transfusion. NICE guideline NG24. https://www.nice.org.uk/guidance/ng24 (accessed 19 April 2021).

National Institute for Health and Care Excellence (2017). Non-Hodgkin's lymphoma: diagnosis and management. https://www.nice.org.uk/guidance/ng52/chapter/Recommendations (accessed March 2022).

Nee, P., A. (2006). Critical care in the emernecy department: Severe sepsis and septic shock. *Emergency Medical Journal* 23: 713–717.

NHS Blood and Transplant (2018). Blood types. https://tinyurl.com/3rbdfpew (accessed 19 April 2021).

NHS Blood and Transplant (2021). Patient blood management checklist 1. In: *PBM Toolkit*. https://hospital.blood.co.uk/pbm-toolkit/ (accessed 6 July 2020).

NHS Direct (2017). Sepsis. https://111.wales.nhs.uk/encyclopaedia/s/article/sepsis (accessed March 2022).

NHS England (2017) Sepsis guidance implementation advice for adults. https://www.england.nhs.uk/wp-content/uploads/2017/09/sepsis-guidance-implementation-advice-for-adults.pdf (accessed March 2022).

NHS England (2018). Clinical commissioning policy: Bendamustine with rituximab for first-line treatment of advanced indolent non-Hodgkin's lymphoma (all ages). https://www.england.nhs.uk/wp-content/uploads/2018/07/1605-bendamustine-with-rituximab-for-nhl.pdf (accessed March 2022).

NHS UK (2017). Thalassaemia. https://www.nhs.uk/conditions/thalassaemia/ (accessed March 2022).

NHS (2021). Overview. Rhesus disease. https://tinyurl.com/bc3jm7rb (accessed 19 April 2021).

Norfolk, D. (ed) (2013). *The Handbook of Transfusion Medicine*, 5e. Norwich: TSO. http://www.transfusionguidelines.org.uk/transfusion-handbook (accessed 19 April 2021).

Peate, I. (2018). *Learning to Care: The Nursing Associate*. London: Elsevier.

Robinson, S., Harris, A., Atkinson S. et al. (2018). The administration of blood components: a British Society for Haematology guideline. *Transfusion Med* 28(1): 3–21.

Safety of Blood, Tissues and Organs (advisory committee). Guidelines from the expert advisory committee on the Safety of Blood, Tissues and Organs (SaBTO) on patient consent for blood transfusion. 17 December 2020. https://tinyurl.com/2yzn36ue (accessed 5 July 2020).

Suddock, J.T. and Crookston, K.P. (2019). Transfusion reactions. Treasure Island (FL): StatPearls Publishing. https://www.ncbi.nlm.nih.gov/books/NBK482202/ (accessed 19 April 2021).

Surviving Sepsis Campaign Guidelines. (2021). https://www.sccm.org/Clinical-Resources/Guidelines/Guidelines/Surviving-Sepsis-Guidelines-2021 (accessed 1 March 2022).

Tigabu, B.M., Davari, M., Kebriaeezadeh, A., and Mojtahedzadeh, M. (2018). Fluid volume, fluid balance and patient outcome in severe sepsis and septic shock: A systematic review. *Journal of Critical Care* 48: 153–159.

Vasiliki, K. (2011). Enhancing transfusion safety: nurse's role. *Int J Caring Sci* 4(3): 114–119.

Webb, A. Angus, D., Finfer, S. et al. (2016). The haematological system. In: *Oxford Textbook of Critical Care*, 2e (ed. A. Webb, D. Angus, S. Finfer et al.), 1261–1312. Oxford: Oxford University Press.

Chapter 27

Musculoskeletal considerations in critical care

Clare L. Wade and Helen Sanger

Aim

This aim of this chapter is to provide an evidenced-based understanding of both primary and secondary musculoskeletal complications experienced by patients in critical care.

Learning outcomes

After reading this chapter the reader will be able to:

* Understand the varying nature, mechanism, presentation, and management of traumatic injury.
* Describe how to carry out a comprehensive assessment of musculoskeletal injury or impairment.
* Recognise the complex nature of intensive care unit-acquired weakness (ICUAW), its management, and persistent functional impact.
* Describe the physiological assessment necessary to determine appropriateness for early mobilisation, understanding precautions and relative contraindications.

Test your prior knowledge

* How is major trauma defined and how is severity of injury determined?
* What is damage-control surgery and why is it commonly used in the management of major trauma?
* Why is physical and functional impairment after critical illness often associated with poor quality of life?
* Can you describe some of the pathophysiological processes that lead to ICUAW?
* What are some of the key physiogical considerations when determining safety and appropriateness to mobilise?

Fundamentals of Critical Care: A Textbook for Nursing and Healthcare Students, First Edition. Edited by Ian Peate and Barry Hill.
© 2023 John Wiley & Sons Ltd. Published 2023 by John Wiley & Sons Ltd.
Companion website: www.wiley.com/go/peate/criticalcare

Introduction

Chapter 27 explores musculoskeletal considerations for patients in critical care. Musculoskeletal impairment can either be primary in nature, and the reason for admission (i.e., in the event of traumatic injury), or a secondary effect of critical illness and its management. All healthcare practitioners in critical care should have an understanding of musculoskeletal anatomy and physiology, and be able to assess for and recognise impairment. Musculoskeletal impairment can prolong rehabilitation and recovery, and potentially lead to longer-term functional disability. This chapter will explore the mechanisms and management of traumatic injury, the pathophysiology and assessment of ICUAW, and provide an evidence-based overview of assessment for early mobilisation.

Trauma

Major trauma is defined as an injury or combination of injuries that is life-threatening and has the potential to cause long-term disability (National Institute for Health and Care Excellence (NICE), 2016). The majority of people suffering major trauma will require critical care for advanced monitoring and management, the primary principles of which are to restore homeostasis, continue resuscitation and monitor closely for potential complications (Tisherman and Stein, 2018). Severity of traumatic injury is graded using the Abbreviated Injury Scale (AIS); a severity scoring system which uses an ordinal scale to classify each injury in every body region according to relative importance (Table 27.1).

The majority of patients suffering major trauma will be cared for in a specialist trauma critical are unit within a Major Trauma Centre (MTC), patients with less severe injuries may be managed in a non-specialist critical care unit.

6Cs: Courage

Courage is essential when discussing life-changing trauma with patients. Honesty is key.

Table 27.1   The Abbreviated Injury Scale. *Source:* Based on AACM, 2020.

1	Minor
2	Moderate
3	Serious
4	Severe
5	Critical
6	Maximum (Currently untreatable)

Mechanism of injury

Major trauma is the largest cause of mortality in adults under 45 years. In these cases, the overwhelming mechanism of injury is high impact, such as in the case of road traffic collisions. Although major trauma was previously associated with the younger population, Kehoe et al. (2015) recently demonstrated that the majority of patients suffering major trauma in the UK are over the age of 50. Adults aged 60 years and over account for more than 50% of severely injured patients admitted to critical care. Currently, the most predominant mechanism of injury resulting in major trauma in the UK is a low-energy fall (TARN, 2017). Regardless of the type or severity of injury, older patients suffer more complications and have higher mortality risk than their younger counterparts (Gillies, 1999; TARN, 2017). Trauma in the over-75 age group is often referred to as 'Silver Trauma'.

Musculoskeletal injury

Musculoskeletal injuries are the most common reason for surgery in severely injured patients following trauma, with more than 70% of patients requiring at least one orthopaedic operative procedure (Balogh et al., 2012). Injury to limbs may result in nerve injuries, vascular injuries or muscle damage. Fractures are often defined by the amount of damage to the soft tissue around the bone. When a fracture is associated with an open wound, it is termed an 'open' or 'compound' fracture. An open fracture is associated with significant soft tissue damage, wound contamination and a high risk of infection and further complications. With a closed fracture, there is no penetration of protrusion of the bone through the skin. It is important to recognise that a closed fracture may be still be complex in nature, with associated damage to the surrounding soft and connective tissue. Musculoskeletal injury is commonly associated reduced functional outcome and reduced quality of life and persistent pain (Gabbe et al., 2012).

A crush injury to skeletal muscle can cause the direct release of intracellular muscle components, such as myoglobin, creatine kinase, lactate dehydrogenase and electrolytes in the bloodstream (Torres et al., 2015). This destruction of skeletal muscle tissue and release of enzymatic content is known as rhabdomyolysis. It can lead to systemic complications, most notable acute kidney injury (AKI) (Chavez et al., 2016). Refer to Chapter 24 for further discussion about the renal complications associated with rhabdomyolysis.

Pelvic injury

High-impact injury often results in complex pelvic trauma, which has one of the highest associated mortality rates of skeletal injury (Coccolini et al., 2017). The pelvis is rich in blood supply, so traumatic injury can lead to haemorrhage, caused by damage to internal organs and blood vessels. In severe pelvic injury, the application of a non-invasive external pelvic compression, in the form of a pelvic binder or a circumferential sheet, is required to temporarily stabilise the pelvis and reduce bleeding (Weaver and Heng, 2015; Coccolini et al., 2017). This should not be removed without the documented consent of the appropriate specialist team. External fixation may be used to stabilise the pelvis in the presence of haemodynamic instability.

The severity of the pelvic injury and the respective operative or non-operative management will often dictate the approach to mobilisation. In some cases, a period of bed rest may be required. In others, weight-bearing and mobilisation within pain limitations may be advocated (Van Aswegen, 2016).

Chest trauma

Chest trauma is highly associated with mortality and morbidity. Injuries to the chest wall can result in complications including pneumonia, haemothorax, pulmonary contusion and chronic pain. The main objective of chest trauma care in critical care is to reduce pain and promote pulmonary hygiene, limit secondary respiratory complications and monitor closely for signs of deterioration.

Recent studies have focused on the implementation of multidisciplinary integrated bundles or pathways of care in order to prevent complications, and recognise and treat deteriorations quickly (Curtis, 2016; Kelley, 2019). Pathways include early and optimal analgesia, often employing the use of regional anaesthetic techniques; respiratory adjuncts such as CPAP, NIV or HFNC; early recognition of deterioration using screening for patients at risk and/or target inspiratory capacity measurements; and complication prevention including surgical fixation, early mobilisation and intensive physiotherapy (Battle et al., 2013).

6Cs: Compassion

If people remember not what you say to them, but how you made them feel, then compassion is essential for all healthcare professionals.

Management of traumatic injury

The management of a patient who has suffered major trauma will differ depending on the mechanism of injury, injuries sustained, and the teams involved in the operative/non-operative management. The concept of damage-control orthopaedics uses little operative intervention until the patient is physiologically stable enough to undergo definitive fixation (Balogh et al., 2012; Van Aswegen, 2016).

Red Flag: Spinal injury/instability

It is unsafe to mobilise a patient with spinal injury prior to confirmation of stability, or surgical fixation. Depending on the mechanism of injury and individual's symptoms, it may be necessary to carry out full in-line spine immobilisation (NICE, 2016).

External fixation

External fixation is commonly used in the management of traumatic limb injuries or pelvic injuries to provide rapid, stable fixation when a patient is not physiologically stable enough to tolerate a more invasive surgical procedure (Pacheco and Saleh, 2004; Balogh et al., 2012). This can be particularly common in the presence of polytrauma, or in the case of severe intra-articular or open fractures. Metal pins or wires are placed into the bone and are then attached to an external frame of bar outside of the skin, allowing for the segments of the fracture to be held in a desirable position (e.g. Figure 27.1). The sites where the pins or wires enter the skin are called pin sites. Pin sites should be cleaned regularly, and closely monitored for signs of infection (Timms and Pugh, 2012; Walker, 2018).

Surgical fixation

Once a patient is physiologically stable, definitive care may involve surgical fixation of fractures and/or soft tissue injuries. This will often consist of open reduction and internal fixation (ORIF), to realign the bone and insert hardware, like plates, screws, or an intra-medullar (IM) rod to hold the realigned bone together. Post-operative complications may include infection, pain, and limb compartment syndrome.

Conservative management

In some cases, fractures may be managed conservatively (or 'non-operatively'). This can often be the case in non-displaced upper limb fractures such as clavicle or humeral fractures), foot or ankle fractures, or stable pelvic fractures. In these cases, it is important for all members of the multidisciplinary team have a clear understanding of the management plan as set out by the responsible orthopaedic team. This may include a period of joint or limb immobilisation in a cast, splint or sling; physiotherapy and progressive rehabilitation; or mobilisation and provision of walking aid to facilitate preferred load-bearing status. Table 27.2 provides an overview of the load-bearing equivalent of common weight-bearing terms. It is important to recognise that any form of reduced weight-bearing can increase energy expenditure during ambulation when compared to the non-injured, healthy population (Hoyt et al., 2015). This should be taken into consideration when considering appropriateness to mobilise.

413

(a)   (b)

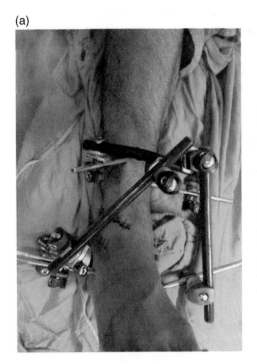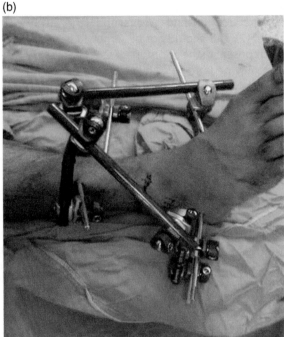

Figure 27.1   Post-operative photographs of the ankle after stabilisation via multiplanar external fixator. *Source:* Sayit et al. (2017) with permission of John Wiley & Sons.

Table 27.2   Load-bearing equivalent of common weight-bearing terms. *Source:* Based on Thompson et al., 2018.

FWB	Full weight-bearing	100% of body weight as pain allows
PWB	Partial weight-bearing	30–50% of body weight
TTWB	Toe-touch weight-bearing	20% of body weight
NWB	Non-weight-bearing	No weight

6Cs: Competence

Assess your own competence against the competencies in this chapter. If you are unsure, discuss them with your mentor.

Trauma competencies

T6a – Musculoskeletal Injuries and Compartment Syndrome (National Major Trauma Nursing Group (NMTNG), 2017)
   Undertake in a safe and professional manner:

- Care and management of the patient with skin and/or skeletal traction
- Care and management of the patient with external fixation including pin site care and documentation
- Care, management and removal of a pelvic binder (application and skin care)
- Care and management of the patient with plaster of Paris
- Care and management of the patient with splints

Snapshot: Polytrauma

Alice is a 45-year-old woman, admitted to hospital 2 days ago, following an RTC. She has fractures to her left acetabulum, patella, shaft of tibia and sternum. She also sustained abdominal bruising under her seatbelt, and splenic laceration. The orthopaedic trauma surgeons performed an ORIF of her acetabulum and stabilised the tibial shaft fracture with intramedullary (IM) nail. Her sternal and patella fractures, and splenic laceration are being managed conservatively.

Airway (A): Patent.
Breathing (B): SpO$_2$ 95% (NEWS2 = 1), on 40% FiO$_2$, with 40 L/min flow, via HFNC (NEWS2 = 2), respiratory rate (RR) 29 breaths per minute (NEWS2 = 3).
Cardiovascular System (C): Blood Pressure (BP) is 115/85 (NEWS2 = 0), Heart Rate (HR) is 102 beats per minute (NEWS2 = 1), warm peripheries.
Disability (D) Patient is Alert (NEWS2 = 0). Temperature is 37.6°C.

Exposure (E) Sitting up in bed, pain at rest is documented as 6/10.

Total NEWS2 score: 8.

Actions

- Clarify location and type of pain with Alice.
- Check prescribed analgesia, offer PRN analgesia if able.
- Check orthopaedic post-operative instructions for pelvic ORIF and tibial IM nail.
- Check management instructions for splenic laceration – has bed rest been recommended?
- Perform neurovascular observations, with particular focus on left foot.

Diagnosis:

- Alice's main source of pain is around her pelvis, and the site of her acetabular ORIF.
- She has PRN opiate analgesia prescribed, and her pain at rest reduces to 2/10 on a numerical pain rating scale, 20 minutes after liquid morphine (oramorph).
- The orthopaedic post-operative instructions for the tibial nail are to 'weight bear as tolerated', but for the pelvic ORIF to 'toe-touch weight bear on left'.
- The general surgeons have not requested any limitation in mobility in their non-operative management of Alice's splenic injury.

Snapshot: silver trauma

Mohammed is a 78-year-old retired GP. He tripped whilst out walking, and was admitted to hospital via A+E. His medical history includes hypertension. His CT scan showed undisplaced fractures to his 6th, 7th, 8th and 9th ribs on the left side. After initial admission to the trauma ward, the nursing staff on this ward requested an urgent medical review due to his NEWS2 score of 9. He has been transferred to the HDU for observation, pain management, and respiratory support as required.

Airway (A): Own.

Breathing (B): Self-ventilating on 4 L/min O_2 nasal cannula (NEWS2 =2). SpO$_2$ 93% (NEWS2 = 2), RR35 (NEWS2 = 3), able to talk in short sentences only.

Cardiovascular System (C): Unsupported. HR 110 (NEWS2 = 2), BP 150/85.

Disability (D) neurological status: Alert and orientated. Temperature 37.

Exposure (E) everything else: Sitting slumped in bed, reports 9/10 pain on inspiration.

NEWS2: 9.

Actions required:

- Urgent review by the medical team and/or pain team. Assessment for possible regional anaesthesia.
- Escalation of respiratory support to achieve target SpO$_2$ of 94–98%
- Complete any blunt chest trauma assessments used in your hospital. Some hospitals measure inspiratory capacity.
- Monitor vital signs closely. Tachycardia, tachypnoea and low oxygen saturations may further deteriorate whilst pain remains severe.
- Discuss Mohammed's care with him – does he understand why he has been admitted to HDU, what the current plan of treatment is, and why? Remember to use language and detail appropriate to his level of understanding.
- Report and document findings.

Intensive care unit-acquired weakness

Muscle weakness remains one of most commonly reported complications of critical illness. Acquired muscle weakness can lead to delayed recovery, increased post-critical care dependency and disability, increased morbidity and decreased quality of life for critical illness survivors (Hermans and Van den Berghe, 2015; Herridge et al., 2011). Although there are primary neuromuscular disorders that can trigger profound muscle weakness, leading to the need for critical care intervention (see Table 27.3 for examples), the overwhelming majority of muscle weakness suffered by those in critical care develops as a secondary disorder while they are being treated for their critical illness (Vanhorebeek et al., 2020). Studies have shown an average of 45% (range 25–70%) of critically unwell patients can develop muscle weakness of a result of their critical illness (Puthucheary et al., 2013).

The pathophysiology by which this muscle weakness occurs is still not fully understood, but there are processes that are known to contribute. Severe muscle atrophy and

415

Table 27.3 Differential conditions that can be the cause of weakness in critical care patients.

Rhabdomyolysis
ICUAW
Guillain–Barré
Myasthenia gravis
Spinal cord injury

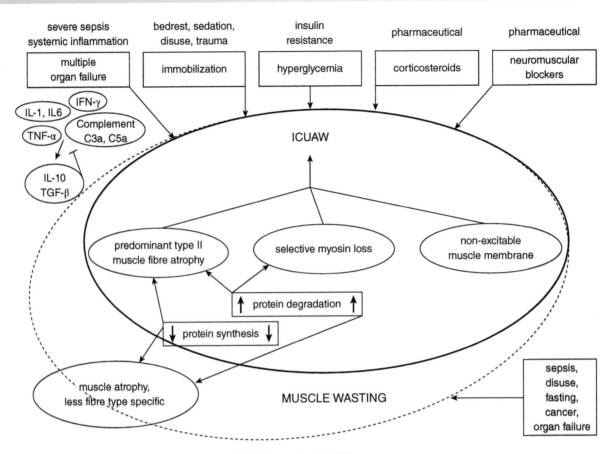

Figure 27.2   Pathophysiological processes and risk factors in ICUAW.

weakness can occur due to critical illness myopathy (CIM), critical illness polyneuropathy (CIP) or a combination of both, known as critical illness neuromyopathy (CINM) (Hermans and Van den Berghe, 2015). Differentiating between neurogenic dysfunction (dysfunction originating from the disturbance of the nervous system) and myogenic dysfunction (dysfunction originating from the disturbance of the skeletal muscle) often involves complex or invasive electrodiagnostic or histological testing. For this reason, generalised muscle weakness that occurs in critical illness is often referred to under the umbrella term Intensive Care Unit-Acquired Weakness, or ICUAW.

Pathophysiology

Most ICUAW is myogenic in origin (CIM) and occurs due to dysfunction in muscle protein homeostasis, skeletal muscle inflammation and mitochondrial dysfunction. Critical illness polyneuropathy (CIP) occurs less frequently but is associated with slower functional recovery than myopathy. CIP is caused by injury to the neuron and axonal degeneration, believed to be caused by dysfunctional microcirculation. In addition to specific polyneuropathies and myopathies that occur within the process of critical illness, other variables such as drug effects, metabolic affects and disuse atrophy due to reduced physical activity can also contribute to ICUAW (Kress and Hall, 2014) (Figure 27.2).

Medications management: neuromuscular blocking agents (NMBAs)

Also called paralysing agents. The most common paralysing agents used in critical care are non-depolarising NMBAs. These act as competitive acetylcholine antagonists at the neuromuscular junction, examples include rocuronium, atracurium, and vecuronium. Accepted best clinical practice is to achieve deep sedation prior to and during neuromuscular blockade.

Muscle protein homeostasis

Critical illness is a complex metabolic state, characterised mostly by hypermetabolism due to a profound physiological stress. Physiological stress results in an increased release of catabolic hormones and a reduction in anabolic hormones. This net catabolic state leads to an increased rate of muscle protein (Puthucheary et al., 2013) breakdown, and a depletion of protein reserves within the skeletal muscle, leading to rapid loss of muscle mass early on within the period of critical illness (van Gassel et al., 2020). The rate of muscle breakdown is known to correlate with the severity of critical illness and multi-organ dysfunction (Puthucheary et al., 2013)

Skeletal muscle inflammation and structural disorganisation

Higher levels of circulating inflammatory markers are associated with marked decrease in muscle strength and mass (Tuttle et al., 2020). Muscle biopsies from critically unwell patients have demonstrated inflammation, cellular infiltrates and necrosis on day 7 of critical illness (Puthucheary et al., 2013).

Bioenergetic disturbance

Mitochondrial dysfunction in skeletal muscle is a recognised complication of sepsis and multi-organ failure (Arulkumaran et al., 2016). Altered mitochondrial function is likely to compromise ATP production, and thus the ability to generate energy required for muscle contraction and force generation. Immobilisation also results in decreased mitochondrial efficiency (Bear et al., 2017).

Disuse atrophy

Although not the primary cause of ICUAW, disuse atrophy due to immobilisation, can exacerbate the skeletal muscle degradation that occurs due to the complex pathophysiological processes outline above. The musculoskeletal effects of 'bed rest' and physical inactivity, outside of the context of critical illness are well recognised. Immobilisation and disuse results in an overall reduction in muscle mass, a reduction in muscle fibre size and a reduction in type II muscle fibres compared with type I muscle fibres (Parry and Puthucheary, 2015). This results in a reduced force-generating capacity and overall reduction in muscle strength.

Axonal degeneration

The mechanisms of axonal degeneration leading to CIP is not completely understood. It is suggested that disruption to microcirculation, and microvascular changes in the endoneurium caused by sepsis, lead to axonal degeneration and neuronal injury in critical illness polyneuropathy. This can be exacerbated by hyperglycaemia (Hermans and Van den Berghe, 2015; Kress and Hall, 2014).

Clinical presentation

ICUAW typically presents as generalised, symmetrical weakness, which affects the limbs and respiratory muscles. Facial and ocular muscles are often spared. Proximal limb muscles are usually more affected than distal limb muscles which can often impact on joint stability in joints such as the shoulders and hips. Anti-gravity muscles, such as the quadriceps muscles, gluteal muscles and erector spinae muscles, are often most affected, leading to functional dysfunction in sitting, standing and walking.

Tendon reflexes are generally reduced, although these are not often assessed at the bedside. Patients with CIP may present with altered or impaired sensation, although this is often difficult to assess in the critically unwell patient.

Prolonged weaning from mechanical ventilation is often a complication of ICUAW, due to atrophy of the diaphragm and respiratory muscles. Peak cough flow (PCF) and the

Table 27.4   Clinical investigations: MRC scale.

MRC grade	Muscle state
0	No contraction
1	Flicker of contraction
2	Active movement with gravity eliminated
3	Active movement against gravity
4	Active movement against gravity and resistance
5	Normal power

ability to clear secretions effectively can be compromised due to reduced strength in the abdominal muscles.

Diagnosis and assessment of ICUAW

ICUAW is diagnosed with the use of the Medical Research Council (MRC), whereby a sum score of less than 48 is indicative of ICUAW.

Examination scenario: the MRC sum score

The MRC sum score (MRC-SS) is made up of 12 measurements of strength, 6 on each side of the body (3 in the upper limb, and 3 in the lower limb).

The MRC grading scale is used assess each movement listed below, and the 12 scores are added together. The MRC-SS has a minimum score of 0, and maximum of 60.

1. Shoulder abduction
2. Forearm flexion
3. Wrist extension
4. Hip flexion
5. Knee extension
6. Ankle dorsiflexion

Procedure: Assess each movement on both the left and right sides, grading them out of 5 using the MRC scale (Table 27.4). Add the 12 measurements together to give the MRC-SS.

Learning event: reflection

Reflect on the differences between the pathophysiology and management of primary injury to the musculoskeletal system (trauma), versus injury to the musculoskeletal system secondary to critical illness (ICUAW).

417

Assessment of musculoskeletal impairment or injury

Assessment of musculoskeletal injury or impairment will need to be specific to the patient and how they are presenting. This is likely to include joint range of motion, muscle power and pain. In the presence of traumatic injury, neurovascular observations are also recommended.

Joint range of motion

Joint range of motion (ROM) refers to the distance and direction a joint can move. The movement that is available at any joint is determined by the articulating surfaces of the joint, the type of joint and the movement allowed for by the regional muscles, ligaments and the joint capsule. Active movement at the joint is created by muscle contraction, whilst ligaments and joint capsules exist to limit excessive movement at a joint. Each joint has an available ROM, expressed in degrees, and moves through specific planes of movement (Muscolino, 2016).

Separate assessment of passive ROM and active ROM should take place. Passive ROM assessment determines the available range that the joint can be taken through passively, by an applied external force, such as a therapist. Passive ROM of a joint can be limited by swelling, surrounding capsular and ligamentous structures, shortened muscles or connective tissue. Active ROM is determined by the contraction of the agonist muscle creating a force on the bones

of a joint. Active ROM is often limited by muscle weakness, muscle imbalance and pain.

Muscle power

In critical care, manual muscle testing usually follows the Medical Research Council (MRC) system as in Figure 27.3.

Pain

Musculoskeletal injury is commonly accompanied by pain, both at rest and particularly with movement. Assessment and management of pain is particularly important when passively moving or engaging a patient in active mobilisation. Pain intensity can be assessed using a number of simple tools. The Numerical Rating Scale (NRS) is commonly used with alert patients in the critical care unit. Patients are asked to identify a number which best fits their pain intensity, usually on a scale of 0 and 10 (Haefeli and Elfering, 2006).

In patients who are unable to self-report their pain, due to reduced consciousness, sedation and intubation, the Critical Care Pain Observation Tool (CPOT) can be used to assess pain (Severgnini et al., 2016).

Clinical investigations: numerical rating scale

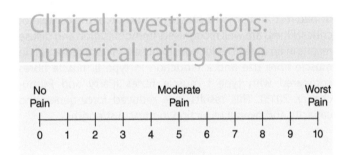

418

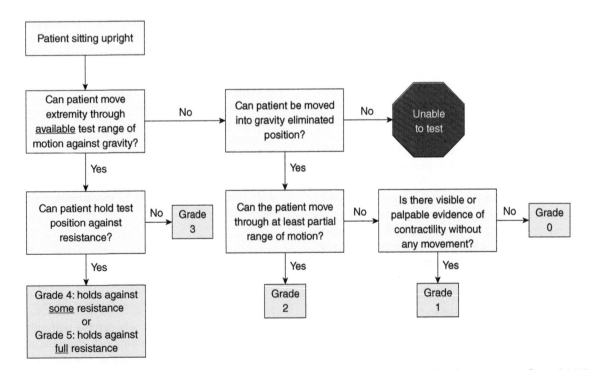

Figure 27.3 Manual muscle testing algorithm. *Source:* Ciesla et al. (2011) reproduced with permission from OASIS group, John Hopkins University.

Medications management: analgesia

Effective pain management is essential for all critical care patients, but particularly important to consider prior to mobilisation. Opioid agonists, such as morphine or fentanyl, are commonly used analgesics on critical care. Morphine can be prescribed orally, intravenously (IV), intramuscularly (IM), subcutaneously, rectally, intrathecally or rectally. Fentanyl can only be given IV.

Neurovascular assessment

It is crucial that neurovascular assessment is undertaken for patients admitted to the critical care unit following musculoskeletal trauma, orthopaedic surgery (both internal and external fixation) or crush injury (Johnston-Walker and Hardcastle, 2011). Neurovascular assessment is performed to evaluate the sensory and motor function of a limb and the peripheral circulate to allow for the early identification of neurovascular compromise or impairment (Schreiber, 2016). Healthcare professionals managing trauma patients should be competent in carrying out a neurovascular assessment and in recognising impairment or early signs of acute compartment syndrome. The Royal College of Nursing (2022) emphasise that of the neurovascular observations, pain is deemed the most important indicator of compartment syndrome, particularly pain experienced on passive stretch of the muscle group affected, or that is out of proportion to the injury.

Examination scenario: neurovascular observations

Neurovascular observation of limb extremities is essential, particularly in the case of long bone injury, or in the presence of any risk factors for compartment syndrome. When completing a neurovascular examination, it can be helpful to think of the '6 Ps':

1. Pain
2. Poikilothermia (cool Peripheries)
3. Paraesthesia
4. Paralysis
5. Pulselessness
6. Pallor

When completing neurovascular observations, remember that compromise could be caused by one or more pathophysiological mechanisms. These include acute compartment syndrome, cellulitis, deep vein thrombosis, neuropraxia, or peripheral arterial injuries (Donaldson et al., 2014). Use the findings of the neurovascular examination as part of a holistic assessment to narrow down a differential diagnosis.

Management of musculoskeletal injury and impairment

Joint positioning and passive movements

Positioning of the critical care patient should aim to reduce risk of joint damage and contracture. Joint contracture is a limitation in the passive range of motion, secondary to shortening of the connective tissues and muscle. It commonly occurs when a muscle is immobilised in a shortened position (Farmer and James, 2001). Periods of prolonged immobility often associated with severe critical illness predispose patients to joint contractures, which can persist after the critical illness has resolved, and have functional implications (Clavet et al., 2008). Joint position should aim to maintain the natural alignment of the limbs wherever possible, using pillows, splints or specialist equipment as indicated (Christie, 2008; Griffiths and Gallimore, 2005). Care should particularly be shown in the handling and positioning of shoulders, especially within the context of ICUAW. Gustafson et al. (2018) demonstrated high prevalence of shoulder impairment and subsequent upper limb dysfunction 3–6 months post-ICU discharge. They recognise that the rapid loss of muscle mass in ICUAW is likely to place the glenohumeral joint at risk of increased instability. Handling and positioning of the shoulder should be performed in a way which does not place the joint at risk of repetitive subluxation.

It is recommended that passive joint movements, through full available range of motion, are carried out daily to assess for joint contractures or changes in muscle tone in the unconscious patient (Sommers et al., 2015). It may be judicious to avoid full shoulder flexion or abduction past 100–120° with a patient in supine, due to restricted scapular movement.

419

Orange Flag: Psychological distress

Acute distress is common among critical care patients. The environment, sleep deprivation, discomfort, isolation from friends and family, inability to participate in work or leisure activities, and worry about their own health can all contribute.

This distress may present differently in different individuals, perhaps as low mood, or anxiety. Its presence can make it difficult for an individual to engage in physical rehabilitation.

6Cs: Commitment

Healthcare professionals must be committed to their own continuing professional development. Ensure you are up to date with your knowledge and understanding.

Early mobilisation

Early mobilisation is a key component of an evidence-based approach to optimise ICU patients' recovery and outcomes.

Physiological assessment for mobilisation

When considering how appropriate it is to commence a mobilisation intervention with a patient, it is important to first understand the physiological effects of activity and movement. This will allow you to make an informed decision as to the physiological stability of a patient and the safety of the intervention.

Red Flag: Bleeding

Patients with known uncontrolled active bleeding should not be mobilised. Those with suspicion of active bleeding or increased bleeding risk may not be appropriate to mobilise, particularly if the risk of an adverse event such as a fall or line displacement is considered non-negligible.

Medications management: anticoagulation

Anticoagulant drugs commonly used in critical care include low molecular weight heparins (e.g., heparin, enoxaparin, tinzaparin); factor Xa inhibitors (e.g., rivaroxaban, fondaparinux, apixaban); or direct thrombin inhibitors (e.g., dabigatran).

Airway

The presence of an endotracheal tube does not, itself, contraindicate mobilisation. In fact, multiple research studies have attested to the safety and feasibility of early mobilisation of the intubated and ventilated patient (Clarissa et al., 2019). Despite this it is still not routine practice in UK critical care units to mobilise patients on mechanical ventilation delivered via endotracheal tubes. This is less to do with the presence of the ETT per se, but because these patients are often less physiologically stable, and therefore unable to safely engage in physical activity.

When engaging any patient with an artificial airway in out-of-bed mobilisation, it is important that somebody has delegated responsibility for maintaining the safety of the airway. Length of ETT should be clearly noted prior to and after mobilisation to assess for any inadvertent displacement.

Breathing

Any active physical movement will increase cellular respiration within skeletal muscle, leading to an increase in partial pressure of carbon dioxide (pCO_2) in the blood. This increase in pCO_2 will cause the respiratory control centres in the hypothalamus to send signals to the respiratory muscles to increase the force of contraction, resulting in increased tidal volume and overall minute ventilation. Once the increase in tidal volume alone is not sufficient to meet the increased need to expire CO_2, the rate of breathing will also increase. It is key to note that many patients with ICUAW have respiratory muscle weakness and may have a reduced ability to generate sufficient muscle contraction to increase tidal volume adequately, leading to premature increase in respiratory rate. For this reason, if a patient already has an increased respiratory rate or work of breathing at rest, it may not be appropriate to engage in a mobilisation intervention which will increase their respiratory effort further.

An increase in cellular respiration within skeletal muscle will also increase oxygen (O_2) demand. If a patient is requiring a high concentration of supplemental oxygen at rest, i.e., in the presence of a pathology which causes a physiological shunt, they may not be able to supply a significant increased demand of oxygen at skeletal muscle tissue. In some instances, the cause of the physiological shunt (i.e. atelectasis or secretion retention) may respond favourably to mobilisation and positioning (Pathmanathan et al., 2015). In such cases, clear clinical reasoning, appropriate monitoring and ensuring adequate availability of supplementary oxygen in crucial. Liaison and joint assessment with other MDT specialists may be indicated.

Circulation

The cardiovascular response most commonly associated with increased physical activity is an increase in cardiac output to supply the increased demand of oxygen-rich blood at working skeletal muscle tissue. This manifests as an increase in both stroke volume and an increase in heart rate. Therefore, if a patient has a high resting heart rate it may be advisable to monitor the cardiovascular response to physical activity closely.

420

Red Flag: Cardiovascular instability

This may present as extreme brady or tachycardia, such as HR <50 or HR >150; hypo or hypertension, most commonly assessed via a target range for either mean arterial pressure (MAP), or systolic pressure; some rhythm abnormalities, such as new or uncontrolled fast atrial fibrillation.

Any active mobilisation will place an increased demand on the cardiovascular system, at least temporarily, so instability at rest is likely to contraindicate active mobilisation.

A period of immobility is often associated with a reduction in normal orthostatic responses. This often manifests as orthostatic hypotension on changes of postural set on commencement of mobilisation. Assessment of mean arterial pressure (MAP), the amount of vasoactive support that is required to maintain adequate MAP and any associated symptoms is key prior to mobilisation intervention.

Medicines management: treating hypotension

Medical management of blood pressure is complex, and optimal therapy depends on the pathological cause of hypo or hypertension.

Hypotension is commonly treated with one or more drugs that have a vasopressor or inotropic effect. These include pure vasopressors, such as phenylephrine and vasopressin; and inotropic vasopressors ('inopressors'), such as noradrenaline and adrenaline.

Blood pressure increases during physical activity and exercise to provide oxygenated blood to skeletal muscle. In the event of a hypertensive crisis, or when patients are requiring intravenous antihypertensive therapy, the risks associated with exercise are likely to outweigh the benefits (Hodgson et al., 2014).

Disability

Mobilisation and exercise should be avoided with the very agitated, combative or difficult to rouse patient. Ideally, sedation should be interrupted prior to engaging a patient in mobilisation or activity. As discussed previously, assessment of pain, muscle power, joint range and consideration of any limitation to movement or weight-bearing should be considered.

Orange Flag: Delirium

Acute delirium is common in critical care. Delirium is frequently characterised by a disturbance in attention and awareness, disorientation, reduction in cognitive ability, and sometimes altered consciousness. These symptoms provide an obvious challenge for safe active mobilisation. However, delirium does not contraindicate mobilisation, and in fact mobilisation may help to reduce delirium.

Exposure/Environment

It is important to be aware of wounds and skin breakages to limit any potential further damage to vulnerable areas. Open surgical wounds (such as an open abdomen) may limit the ability to engage in mobilisation and should be discussed with the responsible surgeon.

There are few attachments that would limit engagement in early mobilisation intervention if physiological assessment deems it safe to proceed. It is, however, key to ensure that attachments are adequately secured and not put under undue tension. Risk assessment of attachments, including drains, intravenous therapies and monitoring devices; environment, including footwear and obstacles; and moving and handling, including competence and number or personnel should all be considered.

As there are no current internationally accepted physiological parameters that determine the safety of mobilisation in critical care, healthcare professionals should adhere to any locally published guidance which reflects the practices within their units. It is important to have regular discussions as a multidisciplinary team to determine safety and readiness for mobility and physical rehabilitation interventions. Hodgson et al. (2014b) developed a Red-Amber-Green (RAG) rating system based on clinical expert consensus which healthcare professionals may find useful to aid in clinical decision making (see Figure 27.4). These parameters are expert consensus-based guidance and should be used as such. They are not exhaustive, and do not replace the need for a comprehensive clinical assessment by one or more suitably qualified members of the ICU MDT prior to each mobilisation episode.

6Cs: Communication

Effective communication is a lynchpin of any MDT, for all pathways of care.

Measuring mobility and function

Measuring physical function in the critical care unit is important to monitor the efficacy of rehabilitation interventions, document patients' progress and recovery and to identify patients at risk of poor physical outcomes (Parry et al., 2017). One simple and appropriate outcome measure is the ICU Mobility Scale, shown in Figure 27.5.

Is it safe to mobilise? RAG rating

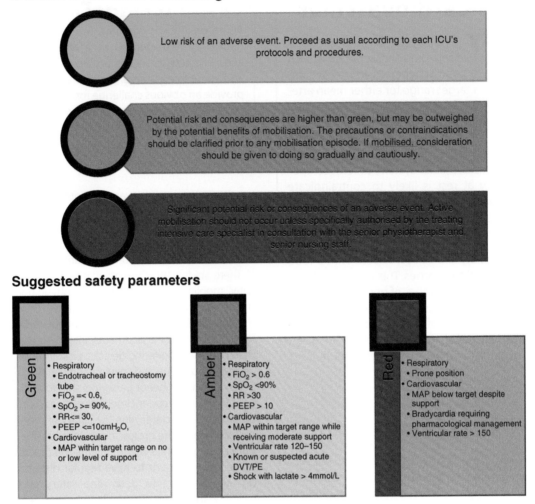

Low risk of an adverse event. Proceed as usual according to each ICU's protocols and procedures.

Potential risk and consequences are higher than green, but may be outweighed by the potential benefits of mobilisation. The precautions or contraindications should be clarified prior to any mobilisation episode. If mobilised, consideration should be given to doing so gradually and cautiously.

Significant potential risk or consequences of an adverse event. Active mobilisation should not occur unless specifically authorised by the treating intensive care specialist in consultation with the senior physiotherapist and senior nursing staff.

Suggested safety parameters

Green
- Respiratory
  - Endotracheal or tracheostomy tube
  - FiO_2 =< 0.6,
  - SpO_2 >= 90%,
  - RR<= 30,
  - PEEP <=10cmH$_2$O,
- Cardiovascular
  - MAP within target range on no or low level of support

Amber
- Respiratory
  - FiO_2 > 0.6
  - SpO_2 <90%
  - RR >30
  - PEEP > 10
- Cardiovascular
  - MAP within target range while receiving moderate support
  - Ventricular rate 120–150
  - Known or suspected acute DVT/PE
  - Shock with lactate > 4mmol/L

Red
- Respiratory
  - Prone position
- Cardiovascular
  - MAP below target despite support
  - Bradycardia requiring pharmacological management
  - Ventricular rate > 150

Figure 27.4   Critical care. Expert consensus and recommendations on safety criteria for active mobilisation of mechanically ventilated critically ill adults. *Source:* Adapted from Hodgson et al. (2014).

Level 1 Patient and Enhanced Care Areas Competencies

7.2.1 – Physiological changes to acute illness – Promoting independence through function:

Demonstrate through discussion:

- The physiological impact of reduced physical function/immobility on the body's systems.
- Awareness of how acute and chronic medical conditions impact on a patient's physical function ability.
- Clinical presentation of patients who are recovering from an acute illness and may be deconditioned/suffering with muscle wasting and/or fatigue.
- Awareness of when patients are too medically unstable to engage in functional activities.

Demonstrate through practice:

- Accurate social history taking to establish previous levels of function.
- A comprehensive risk assessment including
  - Moving and handling.
  - Falls.
- Encouragement of independent function by:
  - Ensuring a safe environment.
  - Limiting constraints such as catheters, drips etc.
  - Management of pain.
- Education of patients and relatives of the benefits of maintaining independent function.
- An ability to follow instruction provided by other MDT specialists outlining safe moving and handling, equipment requirements and strategies to achieve 24-hour approach to rehabilitation.
- Referrals to relevant multidisciplinary team members if strategies to promote independent function are unsuccessful or patient is not at baseline level.

ICU Mobility Scale

	Classification	Definition
0	Nothing (lying in bed)	Passively rolled or passively exercised by staff, but not actively moving.
1	Sitting in bed, exercises in bed	Any activity in bed, including rolling, bridging, active exercises, cycle ergometry and active assisted exercises; not moving out of bed or over the edge of the bed.
2	Passively moved to chair (no standing)	Hoist, passive lift or slide transfer to the chair, with no standing or sitting on the edge of the bed.
3	Sitting over edge of bed	May be assisted by staff, but involves actively sitting over the side of the bed with some trunk control
4	Standing	Weight bearing through the feet in the standing position, with or without assistance. This may include use of a standing lifter device or tilt table.
5	Transferring bed to chair	Able to step or shuffle through standing to the chair. This involves actively transferring weight from one leg to another to move to the chair. If the patient has been stood with the assistance of a medical device, they must step to the chair (not included if the patient is wheeled in a standing lifter device).
6	Marching on spot (at bedside)	Able to walk on the spot by lifting alternate feet (must be able to step at least 4 times, twice on each foot), with or without assistance.
7	Walking with assistance of 2 or more people	Walking away from the bed/chair by at least 5 metres (5 yards) assisted by 2 or more people.
8	Walking with assistance of 1 person	Walking away from the bed/chair by at least 5 metres (5 yards) assisted by 1 person.
9	Walking independently with a gait aid	Walking away from the bed/chair by at least 5 metres (5 yards) with a gait aid, but no assistance from another person. In a wheelchair bound person, this activity level includes wheeling the chair independently 5 metres (5 yards) away from the bed/chair.
10	Walking independently without a gait aid	Walking away from the bed/chair by at least 5 metres (5 yards) without a gait aid or assistance from another person.

Figure 27.5   The ICU Mobility Scale. *Source:* Hodgson et al. (2014a) used with permission from Elsevier.

Snapshot: ICUAW

James is a 58-year-old man who was admitted to critical care with pneumonia 2 weeks ago. He was intubated and ventilated for 8 days and extubated onto HFNC 6 days ago. Prior to this hospital admission James was still working (as an administrator at the local council offices), and walked and cycled regularly. He is an ex-smoker, with a 20-pack-year history, who quit 10 years ago. When his sedation stopped 6 days ago, the MDT ward round noted that he has ICUAW. Yesterday James was able to step-transfer from his bed to a chair with the assistance of a nurse, a physiotherapist, and a zimmer frame. He reports that he was 'knackered' after this.

How would you assess James' musculoskeletal function?

1. Calculate James' MRC-SS.
2. What else would you assess or document in relation to James' physical function?
3. Are you able to utilise clinical guidelines or quality standards to suggest a plan for James' rehabilitation? Who else might be involved in this plan?

6Cs: Care

Remember that **self-care** is also important, to ensure that you can provide the best care to patients. Consider how you manage your own physical, psychological, and spiritual wellbeing during your training, and career.

Conclusion

Musculoskeletal injury in critical care can be complex in its management. Comprehensive assessment, and liaison with relevant speciality teams and multidisciplinary colleagues are essential. Long-term disability and reduction in physical function is common after a period of critical illness.

Take home points

1. Musculoskeletal complications following critical illness are common, particularly for patients who have a protracted critical stay.
2. Major traumatic injury and ICUAW are just two examples of musculoskeletal and/or neuromuscular causes of weakness and impaired function in critical care.
3. The key to safe early mobilisation for patients recovering from critical illness is thorough physiological, clinical and environmental assessment.
4. Multidisciplinary communication is important for coordinating early and ongoing physical rehabilitation intervention.

References

Arulkumaran, N., Deutschman, C., Pinsky, M. et al. (2016). Mitochondrial function in sepsis. *Shock (Augusta, Ga.)* 45(3): 271–281. doi: 10.1097/SHK.0000000000000463.

Association for the Advancement of Automotive Medicine [AACM] (2020). *Abbreviated Injury Scale (AIS), Association for the Advancement of Automotive Medicine.* https://www.aaam.org/abbreviated-injury-scale-ais/ (accessed 20 December 2020).

Balogh, Z.J., Reumann, M., Gruen, R. et al. (2012). Advances and future directions for management of trauma patients with musculoskeletal injuries. *Lancet (London, England)* 380(9847): 1109–1119. doi: 10.1016/S0140-6736(12)60991-X.

Battle, C., Hutchings, H., and Evans, P.A. (2013). Blunt chest wall trauma: A review. *Trauma* 15(2):156–175. doi:10.1177/1460408613488480.

Bear, D., Parry, S., and Puthucheary, Z. (2017). Can the critically ill patient generate sufficient energy to facilitate exercise in the ICU? *Current Opinion in Clinical Nutrition and Metabolic Care* 21: 1. doi: 10.1097/MCO.0000000000000446.

Chavez, L.O., Leon, M., Einav, S., and Varon, J. (2016). Beyond muscle destruction: a systematic review of rhabdomyolysis for clinical practice. *Critical Care (London, England)* 20(1): 135. doi: 10.1186/s13054-016-1314-5.

Christie, R.J. (2008). Therapeutic positioning of the multiply-injured trauma patient in ICU. *British Journal of Nursing* 17(10): 638–642. doi: 10.12968/bjon.2008.17.10.29477.

Ciesla, N., Dinglas, N., Fan, E. et al. (2011). Manual muscle testing: A method of measuring extremity muscle strength applied to critically ill patients. *Journal of Visualized Experiments: JoVE*, (50). doi: 10.3791/2632.

Clarissa, C., Salisbury, L., Rodgers, S., and Kean, S. (2019). Early mobilisation in mechanically ventilated patients: a systematic integrative review of definitions and activities. *Journal of Intensive Care* 7. doi: 10.1186/s40560-018-0355-z.

Clavet, H., Hébert, P., Fergusson, D. et al. (2008). Joint contracture following prolonged stay in the intensive care unit. *CMAJ: Canadian Medical Association Journal* 178(6): 691–697. doi: 10.1503/cmaj.071056.

Coccolini, F., Stahel, P., Montori, G. et al. (2017). Pelvic trauma: WSES classification and guidelines. *World Journal of Emergency Surgery; London* 12. doi: 10.1186/s13017-017-0117-6.

Donaldson, J., Haddad, B., and Khan, W.S. (2014). The pathophysiology, diagnosis and current management of acute compartment syndrome. *The Open Orthopaedics Journal* 8: 185–193. doi: 10.2174/1874325001408010185.

Farmer, S.E. and James, M. (2001). Contractures in orthopaedic and neurological conditions: a review of causes and treatment. *Disability and Rehabilitation* 23(13): 549–558. doi: 10.1080/09638280010029930.

Gabbe, B.J., Simpson, P., Sutherland, A. et al. (2012). Improved functional outcomes for major trauma patients in a regionalized, inclusive trauma system. *Annals of Surgery* 255(6): 1009–1015. doi: 10.1097/SLA.0b013e31824c4b91.

van Gassel, R.J.J., Baggerman, M.R., and van de Poll, M.C.G. (2020). Metabolic aspects of muscle wasting during critical illness. *Current Opinion in Clinical Nutrition and Metabolic Care* 23(2): 96–101. doi: 10.1097/MCO.0000000000000628.

Gillies, D. (1999). Elderly trauma: They are different. *Australian Critical Care* 12(1): 24–30. doi: 10.1016/S1036-7314(99)70509-6.

Griffiths, T. and Gallimore, D. (2005). Positioning critically ill patients in hospital. *Nursing Standard (Royal College of Nursing (Great Britain)* 1987(19):56–64; quiz 66. doi:10.7748/ns2005.06.19.42.56.c3902.

Gustafson, O.D., Rowland, M., Watkinson, P. et al. (2018). Shoulder impairment following critical illness: A prospective cohort study. *Critical Care Medicine* 46(11): 1769–1774. doi: 10.1097/CCM.0000000000003347.

Haefeli, M. and Elfering, A. (2006). Pain assessment. *European Spine Journal* 15(Suppl 1): S17–S24. doi: 10.1007/s00586-005-1044-x.

Hermans, G. and Van den Berghe, G. (2015). Clinical review: intensive care unit acquired weakness. *Critical Care (London, England)* 19: 274. doi: 10.1186/s13054-015-0993-7.

Herridge, M.S., Tansey, C., Matté, A. et al. (2011). Functional disability 5 years after acute respiratory distress syndrome. *New England Journal of Medicine* 364(14): 1293–1304. doi: 10.1056/NEJMoa1011802.

Hodgson, C., Needham, D., Haines, K. et al. (2014a). Feasibility and inter-rater reliability of the ICU Mobility Scale. *Heart & Lung: The Journal of Cardiopulmonary and Acute Care* 43(1): 19–24. doi: 10.1016/j.hrtlng.2013.11.003.

Hodgson, C.L., Stiller, K., Needham, D. et al. (2014b). Expert consensus and recommendations on safety criteria for active mobilization of mechanically ventilated critically ill adults. *Critical Care* 18(6): 658. doi: 10.1186/s13054-014-0658-y.

Hoyt, B.W., Pavey, G., Pasquina, P., and Potter, B. (2015). Rehabilitation of lower extremity trauma: A review of principles and military perspective on future directions. *Current Trauma Reports* 1(1): 50–60. doi: 10.1007/s40719-014-0004-5.

Johnston-Walker, E. and Hardcastle, J. (2011). Neurovascular assessment in the critically ill patient. *Nursing in Critical Care* 16(4): 170–177. doi: 10.1111/j.1478-5153.2011.00431.x.

Kehoe, A., Smith, J., Edwards, A. et al. (2015). The changing face of major trauma in the UK. *Emergency Medicine Journal: EMJ* 32(12): 911. doi: 10.1136/emermed-2015-205265.

Kelley, K.M., Burgess, J., Weireter, L. et al. (2019). Early use of a chest trauma protocol in elderly patients with rib fractures improves pulmonary outcomes. *The American Journal of Surgery* 85(3): 288–229.

Kress, J.P. and Hall, J.B. (2014). ICU-acquired weakness and recovery from critical illness. *The New England Journal of Medicine* 370(17): 1626–1635. doi: 10.1056/NEJMra1209390.

Muscolino, J.E. (2016). *Kinesiology: The Skeletal System and Muscle Function*, 3e. Elsevier.

National Institute for Health and Care Excellence [NICE] (2016). *Major trauma: assessment and initial management (NICE Guideline 39)*, 23. https://www.nice.org.uk/guidance/ng39/resources/major-trauma-assessment-and-initial-management-pdf-1837400761285.

National Major Trauma Nursing Group (NMTNG) (2017). National Competency Framework for Adult Critical Care Nurses: Trauma. https://www.cc3n.org.uk/uploads/9/8/4/2/98425184/step_1_trauma_competencies.pdf (accessed March 2022).

Pacheco, R.J. and Saleh, M. (2004). The role of external fixation in trauma. *Trauma* 6(2): 143–160. doi: 10.1191/1460408604ta308oa.

Parry, S.M. and Puthucheary, Z.A. (2015). The impact of extended bed rest on the musculoskeletal system in the critical care environment. *Extreme Physiology & Medicine*. 4. doi: 10.1186/s13728-015-0036-7.

Parry, S.M., Huang, M., and Needham D.M. (2017). Evaluating physical functioning in critical care: considerations for clinical practice and research. *Critical Care* 21(1). doi: 10.1186/s13054-017-1827-6.

Pathmanathan, N., Beaumont, N., and Gratrix, A. (2015). Respiratory physiotherapy in the critical care unit. *Continuing Education in Anaesthesia Critical Care & Pain* 15(1): 20–25. doi: 10.1093/bjaceaccp/mku005.

Puthucheary, Z., Rawal, J., McPhail, M. et al. (2013). Acute skeletal muscle wasting in critical illness. *JAMA* 310(15): 1591–1600. doi: 10.1001/jama.2013.278481.

Royal College of Nursing (2022). Peripheral neurovascular observations for acute limb compartment syndrome: RCN consensus guidance. https://www.rcn.org.uk/professional-development/publications/peripheral-neurovascular-observations-for-alcs-uk-pub-009-905 (accessed 16 March 2022).

Schefold, J.C., Bierbrauer, J., and Weber-Carstens, S. (2010). Intensive care unit – acquired weakness (ICUAW) and muscle wasting in critically ill patients with severe sepsis and septic shock. *Journal of Cachexia, Sarcopenia and Muscle* 1(2): 147–157. doi: 10.1007/s13539-010-0010-6.

Schreiber, M.L. (2016). Neurovascular assessment: An essential nursing focus. *Medsurg Nursing; Pitman* 25(1): 55–57.

Severgnini, P., Pelosi, P., Contino, E. et al. (2016). Accuracy of Critical Care Pain Observation Tool and Behavioral Pain Scale to assess pain in critically ill conscious and unconscious patients: prospective, observational study. *Journal of Intensive Care* 4(1): 68. doi: 10.1186/s40560-016-0192-x.

Sommers, J., Engelbert, R., Dettling-Ihnenfeldt, D. et al. (2015). Physiotherapy in the intensive care unit: an evidence-based, expert driven, practical statement and rehabilitation recommendations. *Clinical Rehabilitation* 29(11): 1051–1063. doi: 10.1177/0269215514567156.

TARN (2017). *Major Trauma in Older People*. Manchester: TARN.

Thompson, S.G., Phillip, R.D., and Roberts, A. (2018). How do orthopaedic surgeons and rehabilitation professionals interpret and assess 'toe touch' weight bearing and 'partial' weight bearing status in the rehabilitation setting? *BMJ Open Sport & Exercise Medicine* 4(1): e000326. doi: 10.1136/bmjsem-2017-000326.

Timms, A. and Pugh, H. (2012). Pin site care: guidance and key recommendations – ProQuest. *Nursing Standard* 27(1): 50–56.

Tisherman, S.A. and Stein, D.M. (2018). ICU management of trauma patients. *Critical Care Medicine* 46(12): 1991–1997. doi: 10.1097/CCM.0000000000003407.

Torres, P.A., Helmstetter, J., Kaya, A. et al. (2015). Rhabdomyolysis: pathogenesis, diagnosis, and treatment. *The Ochsner Journal* 15(1): 58–69.

Tuttle, C.S.L., Thang, L.A.N., and Maier, A.B. (2020). Markers of inflammation and their association with muscle strength and mass: A systematic review and meta-analysis. *Ageing Research Reviews* 64. doi: 10.1016/j.arr.2020.101185.

Van Aswegen, H. (2016). Cardiorespiratory management of special populations – trauma. In: *Cardiorespiratory Physiotherapy: Adults and Paediatrics*, 5e (ed. E. Main and L. Denehy), 700–709. Edinburgh: Elsevier.

Vanhorebeek, I., Latronico, N., and Van den Berghe, G. (2020). ICU-acquired weakness. *Intensive Care Medicine* 46(4): 637–653. doi: 10.1007/s00134-020-05944-4.

Walker, J. (2018). Assessing and managing pin sites in patients with external fixation, *Nursing Times* 114(1): 18–21.

Weaver, M.J. and Heng, M. (2015). Orthopedic approach to the early management of pelvic injuries. *Current Trauma Reports* 1(1): 16–25. doi: 10.1007/s40719-014-0005-4.

Chapter 28

Burn care within a critical care setting

Nicole Lee

Aim

The aim of Chapter 28 is to provide the reader with an understanding of the needs of a burn-injured patient requiring critical care. The focus is on the immediate 72 hours post-burn until a definitive burn bed is identified and the patient prepared for transfer.

Learning outcomes

After reading this chapter the reader will be able to:

- Understand the pathophysiological changes that occur following a burn injury, including systemic effects.
- Understand the initial burn assessment including burn size, depth of injury and fluid requirements.
- Discuss appropriate care of critically ill burn-injured patients.
- Understand the holistic needs of burn-injured patients, including infection control and multiprofessional collaboration to improve outcomes.
- Understand the psychological impact on patients and those important to them.

Test your prior knowledge

- Can you name an injury tool for a *burn size* assessment?
- What *burn depths* are included in the *burn size* calculations?
- What formula is often used to calculate the fluid resuscitation requirements in the first 24 hours following burn injury?
- What clinical care is required to improve burns injured patients' outcomes?
- When is it important to ensure limb perfusion assessment?

Fundamentals of Critical Care: A Textbook for Nursing and Healthcare Students, First Edition. Edited by Ian Peate and Barry Hill.
© 2023 John Wiley & Sons Ltd. Published 2023 by John Wiley & Sons Ltd.
Companion website: www.wiley.com/go/peate/criticalcare

Introduction

It is essential for critical care nurses to be able to demonstrate knowledge of first aid and the initial emergency management of a burn-injured patient within the critical care setting. The initial care of any burn-injured patient must follow basic first aid principles set out by the Resuscitation Council (UK). This follows an ABCDE approach after ensuring that it is safe for first responders to carry out burn first aid (Resuscitation Council, 2015). Understanding the mechanism of the burn event is vital because dangers may not be obvious, especially following electrical and chemical burns, and first responders must not become casualties themselves while providing first aid.

The overall aim of first aid following a thermal injury is to stop the burning process by removing the heat source, followed by a period of cooling before covering the wound. Cooling of a burn requires cool running water to be applied to the wound for 20 minutes as soon as possible after the injury. This can be effective up to 3 hours post injury (British Burns Association, 2018). This method is the Gold Standard treatment with strong evidence that it reduces the depth and progression of injury and improves outcomes for patients of all ages. Over-zealous cooling can lead to hypothermia, which increases morbidity and mortality (Hostler et al., 2013). Remember to cool the burn but warm the patient.

Burn-injured patients often require active warming to maintain normothermia, which can be achieved by:

- Use of a warm environment
- Covering the burn wound once first aid is completed – cling film is an ideal primary dressing
- Warm coverings to the patient with blankets or warming devices
- Warm fluids

Non-adherent clothing must be removed, especially if wet, as well as all jewellery that may cause constrictive complications as oedema develops (EMSB, 2020).

6Cs: Care

Burn-injured patients will require long stays within hospital needing large amounts of care from the full MDT.

Special burns first aid considerations include:

- Prolonged water irrigation for chemical injuries
- The use of commercial rinsing solutions for chemical injuries *if* available
- The use of specific treatments for hydrofluoric acid injuries
- High index of suspicion in electrical injuries for latent or obscure complications anywhere between entry and exit

wounds along the path taken by the current including unanticipated muscle necrosis, compartment syndrome, fractures, and cardiac dysrhythmias; an early electrocardiogram (ECG) is necessary.

Initial primary and secondary surveys should take place with an understanding of the importance of not being distracted by the burn injury to ensure that other, potentially life-threatening, injuries are not overlooked. Photographs must be taken to prevent unnecessary distress to the patient by repeatedly disturbing the wounds. After being fully assessed, stabilised and photographed, the patient must be referred to the local burn service. In the UK, burn services are organised into a hierarchical system within networks to prioritise the needs of each patient. Once referred, the specialist burn care team will identify an appropriate service for the patient and provide advice on how to care for the patient.

The mnemonic SKIN can be used to assess the initial care considerations of a burn-injured patient.

> S – Sensory
> K – Knowledge of fluid management
> I – Infection
> N – Normothermia

Comprehensive assessment of burn injuries requires an understanding of the burn event itself including what was happening at the time and how the burn occurred, how long the burning process occurred, and what first aid was provided. This will help to anticipate patterns and possible progression of different types of injury, such as scalds, flame burns or contact injuries. Burn wound assessment determines the burn size and depth of injury to address the needs of each patient.

6Cs: Commitment

The MDT need to work collaboratively and require commitment to time, effort and resources to support the recovery of critically ill patients with burn injury.

Classification of burn wound depths

There are several burn injury classifications based on depth. These are described below (see also Table 28.1).

Erythema

This involves inflammation of the outermost layer of the skin only. The skin remains intact with a capillary refill time (CRT) <2 seconds. Erythema is not considered 'burn-injured tissue' and does not count towards the burn size calculation (Figure 28.1).

Table 28.1   Classification of burn depth. Source: adapted from NICE, 2020.

Depth of the burn	The skin layers that are affected	Examination of the person's skin
Superficial epidermis; (such as, exposure to the sun; sunburn)	Epidermis affected, dermis remains intact	Red and painful skin, no blistering. Capillary refill, skin blanches very quickly but then refills
Superficial dermal, partial thickness	Epidermis and the upper layers of the dermis are involved	The person's skin is red or pale pink and it is painful. There is blistering. Capillary refill, skin blanches however it regains it colour slowly
Deep dermal, partial thickness	The epidermis, the upper and the deeper layers of the dermis become involved, underlying subcutaneous tissues however, are not involved	The skin is dry, blotchy or mottled, it is red and usually it is painful as a result of the superficial nerves that have been exposed. Capillary refill does not blanch.
Full thickness	Here the burn will have extended through to all skin layers, to the subcutaneous tissues. If severe, this extends to the muscle and the bone	The person's skin appears white, brown or black (if charred), there are no blisters present. The skin can be dry, leathery or waxy, it is painless. Capillary refill does not blanch.

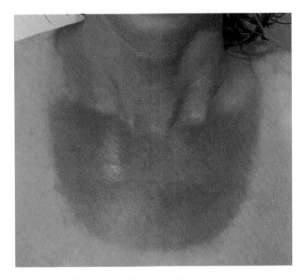

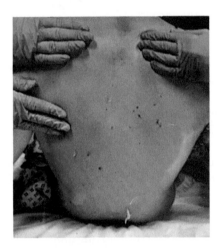

Figure 28.2   Superficial dermal injury (Wollinger, 2022).

Figure 28.1   Erythema (Lee, 2020).

Superficial dermal (or superficial partial thickness)

This involves damage to the epidermis and uppermost dermis leading to separation of the two layers. Fluid accumulates underneath intact epidermis to form blisters (Figure 28.2). Blister fluid is pro-inflammatory and will cause a burn to deepen the longer it is in contact with the wound bed. Blister management is controversial but larger blisters will rupture leading to an open wound prone to infection and pain. Ideally, they should be de-roofed in a controlled clinical environment. Intact blisters also prevent evaluation of the wound bed leading to inaccurate depth of injury assessment and planning. The wound bed is hyperaemic with a CRT <2 seconds.

The management of blisters requires careful planning, including:

- Empathy and explanation to the patient
- Pain relief before the procedure that is appropriate to the size of the injury
- Prompt application of dressings
- Medical photography
- Liaison with burns services for advice

Deep dermal (or deep partial thickness)

This involves damage to the deeper dermis. Damaged blood vessels in the upper dermis are coagulated or ruptured and appear as fixed staining. The burn may or may not be painful depending on how many nerve endings remain to be stimulated. The wound bed has a slower CRT of 3–4 seconds but can still heal with good wound care and optimal dressings. Intact hair follicles are a positive sign because the epithelial cells lining them promote wound healing (Figure 28.3).

Full thickness

This involves damage to all layers of the skin. There is little or no CRT. The surface feels firm and cool to touch, often with a pale waxy appearance. However, the colour can vary depending on the mechanism of injury and the history helps with diagnosis. Apart from the smallest burns, the treatment is surgical removal of the dead tissue (Figure 28.4).

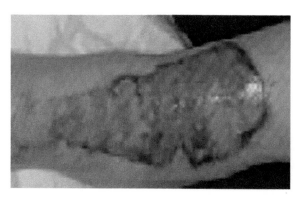

Figure 28.3   Deep dermal injury (London and South East Burn Network, 2015).

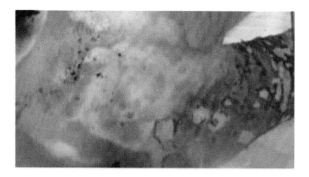

Figure 28.4   Full thickness injury (Wollinger, 2022).

Learning event

Most burn wounds are 'mixed depth' because the heat source is not distributed over the skin evenly during any injury. The burn depth is usually worse at the site of injury and lessens as the heat dissipates further away from it. Some areas may be deeper where the contact time is longer, for example, where clothing has not been removed in a timely manner or where first aid has been suboptimal. However, the normal skin thickness and perfusion can also influence burn depth and progression.

Pathological considerations

Jackson in 1947 proposed three zones of damage within the burn wound (Hettiaratchy et al., 2005):

1. **Zone of coagulation:** Irreversible damage caused by the direct effect of heat coagulating tissues and denaturing proteins.

2. **Zone of stasis:** Reduced tissue perfusion that is salvageable if blood flow is restored promptly. This zone can be further compromised by additional insults such as infection, hypotension, and oedema, and may spread into the zone of hyperaemia.

3. **Zone of hypernatraemia:** This area has the least damage and represents an appropriate inflammatory response to the burn.

If perfusion of burn-injured tissue is maintained, the zone of stasis can recover limiting the injury to the zone of coagulation only. However, if care is suboptimal, ongoing ischaemia causes irreversible damage and deepening of the burn. This is known as *burn wound progression*. In practice, this commonly occurs due to cardiovascular instability and the need for inotropes, chronic respiratory failure, renal failure and the need for renal replacement therapy, infection, hypothermia, nutritional depletion, and constrictive dressings.

There is a sudden, and initially uncompensated, release of cytokines and inflammatory mediators following a burn injury. As the burn size increases, the inflammatory storm is much harder to control, and a profound systemic response is observed. Critical care nurses must be aware of the respiratory, cardiovascular, metabolic and immunological derangement that occurs in larger burns (see Figure 28.5, Burns Response). These effects are seen for burns >10% TBSA in children and >15 % TBSA in adults (Herndon, 2012).

Respiratory problems include bronchoconstriction and potential inhalational injuries involving direct damage to the lung tissues or systemic effects from the inhaled toxic products of combustion. *Cardiovascular* problems include vasodilation that reduces systemic vascular resistance causing hypotension, increased capillary permeability leading to protein loss from the capillaries causing increased hydrostatic pressure and fluid shifts into the interstitial space, and reduced cardiac contractility. *Metabolic* problems include increased basal metabolic rate (up to three times normal) leading to increased nutritional needs in order to meet basic requirements and additional needs for healing. This results in increased heart rate and core temperature due to resetting of the hypothalamus. Early enteral feeding maintains gastrointestinal integrity and prevents bacterial translocation. *Immunological* problems are related to prolonged immunosuppression.

Learning event

One of the most important things that I have noticed in burn care is the value of a full MDT to plan the holistic care of these complex patients.

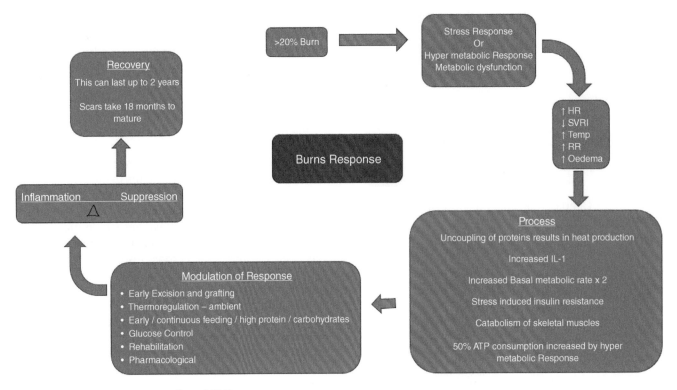

Figure 28.5 Burns response (Lee, 2021).

Burn size estimation

Burn size estimation is achieved by using a recognised tool to calculate the percentage of Total Body Surface Area (TBSA) burned (Figures 28.6, 28.7, 28.8 and 28.10). It is important to remember that differences exist between adults and children, which is recognised in the Lund and Browder chart (see Figure 28.6).

It is important to identify a circumferential burn. As the swelling increases, a torniquet effect can arise in the limbs, causing impaired peripheral perfusion, or constriction to the chest, causing inadequate ventilation. A surgical escharotomy may be needed to release the constriction and restore normal perfusion or ventilation.

Learning event

Having worked in a large burns ITU for 12 years, the question I am most often asked is, 'If the patient suffers a large burn injury, is it better to let nature take its course and allow them to die with dignity?' Answer: No. I have seen patients with 96% TBSA burns survive while those with smaller burns have died. At the scene, it is almost impossible to identify survivors as you don't have all the information available, and we know that individuals respond to injuries and treatment differently. There are always exceptions to any rule! Burn specialists use frailty scores and other scoring systems to support their decision-making processes but also have the resources and experience to provide holistic care to the patient and their relatives. Therefore, I believe it is important to deliver good pre-hospital care and initial stabilisation with prompt transfer so that burns specialists with the necessary knowledge and skills can make the definitive decisions that improve survival and outcomes.

Infection control

Critical Care Nurses must be able to demonstrate knowledge and understanding of Infection Control measures in burn-injured patients. All wounds must be swabbed on admission for routine surveillance. Antibiotic stewardship is essential because burned patients remain in critical care environments for many weeks and multidrug resistant infections will emerge. Wound surveillance identifies colonising organisms and their sensitivities so that targeted antimicrobials can be used if systemic signs of infection develop. Meticulous wound care and infection control principles must be considered at every stage of burn care. Side rooms with negative pressure are often better for patients with large burn wounds to be nursed to protect them and others from the bacterial load of their wounds.

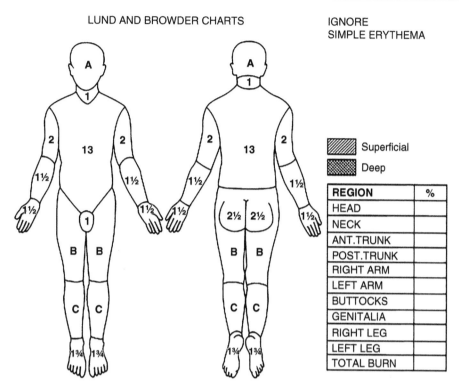

LUND AND BROWDER CHARTS

IGNORE
SIMPLE ERYTHEMA

RELATIVE PERCENTAGE OF BODY SURFACE AREA
AFFECTED BY GROWTH

AREA	AGE 0	1	5	10	15	ADULT
A = ½ OF HEAD	9½	8½	6½	5½	4½	3½
B = ½ OF ONE THIGH	2¾	3¼	4	4½	4½	4¾
C = ½ OF ONE LEG	2½	2½	2¾	3	3¼	3½

Figure 28.6   Lund and Browder. *Source:* Herndon (2012) with permission of Elsevier.

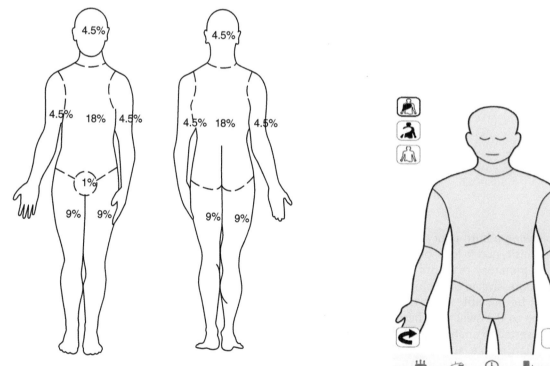

Figure 28.7   Wallace Rule of Nines. *Source:* Herndon
(2012) with permission of Elsevier.

Figure 28.8   Mersey burns app (Mersey Burns app, 2020).

Case study

A 30-year-old male caught fire while welding under a car in his garage, sustaining a 60%TBSA burn. His estimated weight on admission is 80 kg.

1. Calculate this patient's fluid requirements in the first 24 hours.
2. What is the hourly volume in the first 8 hours.
3. What is the hourly rate in the next 16 hours.

6Cs: Compassion

Critical care staff must show compassion to patients, relatives and friends during the patient's admission as this is a very traumatic and emotional episode of care for someone that they love.

Learning event

The second question that I am most frequently asked relates to intravenous fluid resuscitation therapy, 'Does the patient require this much fluid, and does it make a difference?' Answer. Yes. Individualised fluid resuscitation therapy, guided by end-organ perfusion such as urine output or invasive cardiovascular monitoring, really does compensate for burn shock, prevents progression of the burns, reduces the need for surgery, and improves the outcomes for patients. But, over-resuscitation and 'fluid creep' results in significant complications – remain vigilant!

An ABCDE approach to burn care

Airway

Airway oedema following a burn injury can be intrinsic (airway injury) or extrinsic, due to local burns of the neck or the systemic inflammatory response. Intubation is required if there is progressive airway compromise. Once inserted, it may not be possible to change the tube for up to a week due to the swelling. The largest tube possible should be inserted to enable bronchoscopy and regular passing of large size suction catheters for chest physiotherapy and airway toileting. The tube must remain uncut to ensure it protrudes sufficiently as facial swelling develops, which can be dramatic and is often underestimated.

Nursing care

- Regular evaluation of tube ties and release/re-tie as swelling develops
- Nurse in a head up position to reduce swelling
- Regular mouth care as this will be a dirty airway
- Regular face care every 4–6 hours
- Ensure sedation levels are at a safe level to secure the airway

Learning event

Severe swelling can occur in even relatively minor burns of the face, head and neck, and I have seen cut endotracheal tubes migrate into the mouth – please keep tubes uncut until the risk of swelling has passed.

Medication management

Critical care nurses must be able to provide burn-injured patients with appropriate interventions for their inevitable pain and administer them safely. Sedation and adequate pain relief must be carefully titrated to the patients' needs. In general, follow local protocols for analgesia and sedation but always consider discussing individual needs with the local burn service.

Pain relief includes morphine, fentanyl, and alfentanil. Pre-procedure boluses will need to be prescribed as PRN additional pain relief in order to meet the care needs of the patient, such as rolling and repacking. Almost every procedure will be painful and an appropriate plan must be in place to deliver the best holistic care possible. Anticipatory pain can be difficult to manage.

Learning event

It is common practice in burn care to give an additional pre-procedure bolus before most interventions. However, you must allow enough time for the medication to take effect before starting. Be sure you understand the pharmacology of medications you use as some can take up to 20 minutes to take effect.

Breathing

As well as standard breathing assessments based on a look, listen, and feel approach and appropriate observations, critical care nurses dealing with burn-injured patients must explore the mechanism of injury to appreciate additional risks associated with an enclosed space, such as smoke inhalation injury, metabolic poisoning from inhaled toxic products of combustion, or associated trauma caused by blast or explosions.

Signs of inhalation injury

- Burns to face, lips, tongue, mouth, (oro)pharynx
- Soot in sputum, nose or mouth
- Dyspnoea
- Stridor
- Singed nasal hair
- Change of voice
- Decreased consciousness
- Clinical hypoxaemia (saturations <94% on room air)
- Increased COHb levels

Clinical investigation

Measurement of carboxyhaemoglobin (COHb) level can diagnose possible smoke inhalation injury. Normal levels are <3% for non-smokers or <12% for smokers but can also be high in new-born babies. Levels can be measured on most blood gas analysis machines. Treatment for carboxyhaemoglobinaemia is 100% oxygen to flush out the COHb that is attached to red blood cells. Remember, high COHb levels confuse oxygen saturation probes, which will show 100% saturation despite some of the haemoglobin being unusable for oxygen transport. The true PaO_2 must be checked on a blood gas.

The diagnosis of an inhalation injury is supported by chest X-ray and bronchoscopy findings. Bronchial lavage is useful to remove adherent soot and contaminant particles that may encourage ventilator-associated pneumonias. Inhalational protocols vary slightly across the country so contact your local burns service for advice. Treatment includes high flow oxygen with intubation if needed, the use of an inhalation nebuliser regime, enhanced chest physiotherapy, and regular sputum sampling.

Nursing Care

- Nurse the patient sat upright and from side to side to help with postural drainage of soot filled mucus
- Good mouth care to clear the oral cavity
- Assistance to optimise chest physiotherapy
- Timely nebulisation regimes

6Cs: Courage

Courage is needed by the MDT when caring for burn-injured patients ensuring they feel safe and supported during their recovery.

Clinical Investigation

Cyanide poisoning is another possibility for patients with burns from fires in enclosed spaces. Clinical features include

- Reduced GCS
- Hypotension <110 mmHg or hypertension >180 mmHg
- Early lactic acidosis

If suspected, hydroxocobalamin (Cyanokit) 5g is recommended to be given early.

Cardiovascular

Initial cardiovascular assessment will often show increased heart rate, decreased blood pressure from vasodilation, low temperature, reduced CRT, and reduced urine output. It is important that critical care nurses can demonstrate the ability to care appropriately for a patient receiving large volume fluid resuscitation. Guides for fluid management include the use of cardiac output studies and assessment of end-organ perfusion. High urine outputs indicate over-resuscitation and must be avoided. Low urine output is more common and require additional fluid challenges on top of the fluid resuscitation calculation. Remember, fluid resuscitation calculations are a guide and must be tailored to the individual needs of the patient.

Nursing Care

- Meticulous fluid resuscitation monitoring
- Aggressive temperature management (see image 28.8)
- Regular limb assessment to check perfusion

6Cs: Competence

Competence with burns assessment and management strategies is proven to improve patient outcome.

Case Study

The core temperature is noted to be 35°C.

1. What measures are you going to put in place to increase the patient's temperature?
2. How often will you reassess it?

Disability (neurological assessment)

It is vital to check both eyes early for injury as this may be the only time for the next week that they will be visible due to systemic swelling and periorbital oedema. The use of fluorescein sodium 2% eye drops identifies damaged areas as green when using the blue light on an ophthalmoscope. If possible, an ophthalmology assessment is recommended. Blood glucose levels must be monitored and a sliding scale started if necessary to keep blood sugars <10 mg/dL.

Exposure (and everything else)

Now is the time to reassess the mechanism of injury and look for missed injuries or other issues. The patient may have an underling health condition that led to the injury, or it may have been an acute episode resulting in trauma from an explosion. It is imperative that the critical care nurse completed the following:

- Assess burn size
- Routine microbiology swabs
- Baseline medical photographs
- Clean the area with a betadine wash under appropriate pain relief then dress with a non-adherent first layer and thick absorbent second layer to soak up fluid loss from wound bed. Dressings quickly become sodden and will need to be changed regularly, perhaps 6 hourly, during the first 24–48 hours.
- Insert nasogastric tube and start early enteral feeding to meet calorie needs
- Consider additional clinical investigations such as creatine kinase in electrical injuries (creatine kinase levels should be less than 198 U/L)
- Chemical injuries may require regular wound bed pH monitoring
- Check tetanus vaccine is up to date (EMSB, 2020)
- Check intra-abdominal pressures regularly in large volume resuscitaitons or high risk injury mechanisms

Psychological support

It is important that critical care nurses can demonstrate an appreciation of the diverse biopsychosocial issues that affect patients with burn injuries, including interventions that may be useful in the short and long term. The nature of burn injuries often leaves a devastating impact on patients, families, and witnesses to the injury, as well as nurses and healthcare professional not used to managing them. Local burn services have trained psychotherapists who can offer advice and support if needed. However, in the early stages, psychological support tends to be quite practical, with links and access to help within local community.

Case Study

During a house fire, George continued to try to put a fire out when he realised he had no contents insurance. He sustained a 45% TBSA flame burn with smoke inhalation. His wife is now left with no home, two children that saw the incident, and a husband in critical care. George is a self-employed plumber and is the only earner for the family, which have no savings or critical illness cover.

George will require a protected airway, rapid sequence induction (RSI), sedation and mechanical ventilation – which will delay psychological support for him until awake. However, the needs of the wife and children in the first 72 hours will be much greater and signposting for support such as temporary accommodation, access to emergency funds, or maybe supported time to visit her husband will be rewarding. Remember to speak to your local burn service for advice as there are charities and support systems in place that can help these patients and their relatives.

6Cs: Communication

Effective communication is imperative in critical care. The MDT must utilise effective and appropriate communication techniques in every contact with the patient, their family and those important to them.

Nursing care

Supporting a relative to see a loved one in ITU is common and requires preparatory work so that they understand the roles of the equipment and what to expect from the patient. Burns injuries are often highly distressing and their loved one will look very different due to marked swelling and bulky dressings. The impact on relatives must be considered at all times. Relatives with often imagine what it must be like for their loved one and become overwhelmed. If not dealt with compassionately, it will add to their emotional trauma and ability to help with rehabilitation later. Dressings placed over the affected areas can help (Figure 28.9).

Burns Patient Warming Management Strategies

Temperature <35 degrees is showed to increase mortality in burn injured patients

Aggressive warming is required to increase core temperature and aid skin perfusion

- Warm room temperature
- Warm fluid management
- Covering of the burn wound with dressing
- Use of a warming blanket device
- Wrapping of the head of the patient
- Warm feeds or NG water

Additional measures if remains < 35 degrees

- Warm bladder what outs
- Removal of any wet cold outer layers of dressing from wound exudate
- Warm betadine added to me soft gauge and placed on the wounds
- Renal replacement therapy with heater on set covered with warming blanket

Nicole Lee, 2020

Figure 28.9 Burns patients warming management strategies (Lee, 2020).

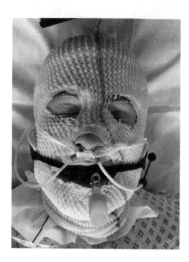

Figure 28.10 Facial dressing concealing a facial burn injury (Lee, 2020).

Learning event: reflection

Think about the SKIN mnemonic:

S – Sensory – give pain relief
K – Knowledge of fluid management – Parkland formula
I – Infection – swab and dressings
N – Normothermia – Active warming required

Be sure to make early referrals to your local burn services for advice and support.

Examination scenario

Smriti is a 75 kg 56-year-old female. She was cooking at home when her sari caught fire from the gas hob. Her husband heard her scream and made her stop, drop and roll to put out the flames sustaining hand burns himself. The emergency services advised her to shower with cool water as first aid for 20 minutes.

A – Ambulance arrived. She had a hoarse voice and burns to her face and neck. She was intubated uneventfully at the scene.

B – COHb level of 30% recorded. She is on mechanical ventilation set to BIPAP using a pressure control of 20, PEEP +8, FiO$_2$ of 1.0, and a set respiratory rate of 18 breaths per minute.

C – Heart rate is 90 bpm with a manual BP currently 80/40 and a CRT of 5 seconds

D – Sedated on fentanyl and propofol with a RASS of -4

E – Burns (Figure 28.11)

Are you able to:

1. Work out %TBSA burned
2. Work out fluid resuscitation using the Parkland formula
3. Plan the first 24 hours of care using ABCDE approach

435

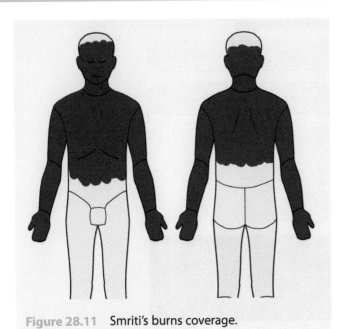

Figure 28.11 Smriti's burns coverage.

Carboxyhaemoglobin (COHb) level reference ranges

Adults: <2.3% (0.023); <3% saturation of total haemoglobin

- Smokers: 2.1–4.2% (0.021–0.042); other sources suggest: 2–5%
- Heavy smokers (>2 packs/day): 8–9% (0.08–0.09); other sources suggest: 5–10%

Haemolytic anaemia: Up to 4%
New-born babies: ≥ 10–12%
Critical values: >20%

Acknowledgement

I am grateful for support with comments and review from Mr Niall Martin, Consultant Burns Surgeon at St Andrews Burns Centre Chelmsford.

Examination scenario

Bob is a 75-year-old male with a past medical history (PMH) of hypertension high hypercholesterolemia and dementia. Bob got himself in hot bath unattended in early hours of the morning found by wife at 7.00am wondering around the house in distress with no clothes on and scald injury.

A – Clear
B – Bilateral air entry RR 20, oxygen Saturations 98% on room air
C – Heart rate 110bpm, BP 110/60, urine output – <25 mls last hour
D – Alert and responding to staff but confused and upset. Core temperature 36°C
E – burns (Figure 28.12)

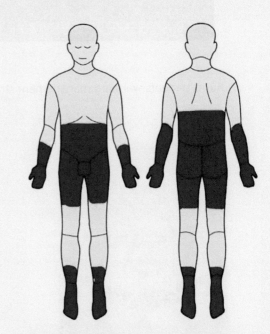

Figure 28.12 Bobs Burn Injury coverage.

1. Work out Bob's TBSA
2. Work out his Parkland formula
3. Discuss the ABCDE approach and apply it to Bobs scenario

References

British Burns Association, 2018. First Aid clinical practice Guidelines. www.britishburnsassociation.org (accessed March 2022).
British Burns Association (2020). *Emergency Management of Severe Burns*. Australia and New Zealand Burn Association.

CC3N, 2019. Specialist Burns Competencies for Use in Non Specialist Units. https://www.cc3n.org.uk/uploads/9/8/4/2/98425184/burns_comps_single_pages.pdf (accessed March 2022).
CYANOKIT Training Presentation | Cyanokit. https://cyanokit.com/getmedia/d3c6ad54-19cd-437e-9dec-e33375f65d2e/CYANOKIT-Training-Presentation_Nov2021 (accessed March 2022).

Herndon, D.N. (2012). *Total Burn Care*, 4e. London: Saunders Elsevier.

Hettiaratchy, S., Papini, R., and Dziewulski, P. (2005). *ABC of Burns*. Blackwell Publishing/BMJ Books.

Hostler et al., 2013. Admission temperature and survival in patients admitted to burn centres. *Journal of Burn Care Research* 34(5): 498–506.

London and South East Burn Network, 2015. LSEBN Burn Depth Assessment. https://www.lsebn.nhs.uk (accessed March 2022).

NICE (2020). Burns and scalds. https://cks.nice.org.uk/topics/burns-scalds/diagnosis/assessment/ (accessed 10 April 2021).

Resuscitation Council, 2015. The ABCDE Approach. https://www.resus.org.uk/library/2015-resuscitation-guidelines/abcde-approach (accessed March 2022).

Chapter 29

Maternal critical care

Wendy Pollock

Aim

The aim of this chapter is to introduce nursing and healthcare students to the fundamental knowledge and underpinning evidence base required to care for critically ill pregnant and postpartum women.

Learning outcomes

After reading this chapter the reader will be able to:

- Describe key physiological adaptations of pregnancy pertinent to critical care nursing practice.
- Discuss recognition of clinical deterioration in the pregnant woman and how it may differ to the non-pregnant patient.
- Understand the common conditions that lead to critical care admission during pregnancy and postpartum.
- Discuss strategies to encourage maternal-infant bonding when mother and baby are separated by maternal critical illness.
- Recall the adaptations to basic life support needed for maternal resuscitation in the second half of pregnancy.

Test your prior knowledge

- State two physiological adaptations that occur in the cardiovascular system and two adaptations in the respiratory system.
- Identify four red flag signs and symptoms in a pregnant woman.
- What are the normal vital signs in pregnancy?
- Why is anti-D immunoglobulin given to some women?
- Explain why a left-lateral tilt or manual uterine displacement is needed during cardiopulmonary resuscitation (CPR) in the second half of pregnancy ($\geq$ 20 weeks' gestation)?

Fundamentals of Critical Care: A Textbook for Nursing and Healthcare Students, First Edition. Edited by Ian Peate and Barry Hill.
© 2023 John Wiley & Sons Ltd. Published 2023 by John Wiley & Sons Ltd.
Companion website: www.wiley.com/go/peate/criticalcare

Introduction

Giving birth is a healthy, normal life event for most women. However, for some women, pregnancy and childbirth can be associated with a life-threatening event that may require admission to critical care. The aim of this chapter is to provide an initial overview of the knowledge and skills needed to care for critically ill pregnant and postpartum women. In particular, the adapted physiology of pregnancy, common conditions in pregnancy and postpartum that lead to admission to a critical care unit, and details on the nursing and medical management.

Many women who experience a pregnancy complication, or who have underlying medical conditions, have complex care needs during pregnancy and postpartum. Most of these women stay in the care of maternity services and receive care in areas such as birth suite or a maternity high dependency unit (HDU). Depending on the capability of the maternity service, women requiring level 2 critical care can usually be cared for by specialist midwives. There are 'enhanced maternity care' competencies to guide the knowledge and skill development of midwives caring for women who need level 2 critical care (Royal College of Anaesthetists (RCoA), 2018). For women that need level 3 care intervention provided in intensive care units (ICU's), there are specialist maternal competencies for critical care nurses available (Critical Care Networks-National Nurse Leads (CC3N), 2019). The intent of these competency frameworks is to close the service gap, as historically, midwives and critical care nurses were ill-prepared to care for critically ill pregnant and postpartum women. Consequently, women sometimes received sub-optimal care, such as delay in the recognition of severity of illness, and this, along with other systemic issues, contributed to adverse outcomes including maternal death (Knight et al., 2019). Thus, the focus of 'enhanced maternity care' works on the basis that 'the starting point when considering care of the critically ill obstetric patient is that the quality of that care should be of the same standard as for the nonpregnant patient' (Jardine et al., 2019, p. vii). Crucially, the provision of maternal critical care must consider:

- Adapted physiology of pregnancy
- Pregnancy conditions and complications
- The presence of the fetus

Epidemiology

Globally, by far the most common conditions that require pregnant and postpartum women to be admitted to critical care are obstetric haemorrhage and preeclampsia, with maternal sepsis a distant third (Pollock et al., 2010). Most women are admitted in the early postpartum period, often on the day that they have given birth. However, women admitted to critical care units when pregnant are more likely to have a non-obstetric condition that requires specialist care, such as pneumonia.

The rate of maternal admission to level 3 critical care in the UK is 2.24/1000 births; however, this does not include any woman whose pregnancy ended before 24 weeks' gestation (Jardine et al., 2019). Maternal admissions make up 1.3% of the UK ICU population (Simpson et al., 2020). In the UK, risk factors for maternal admission to ICU are women of advanced maternal age ($\geq$ 35 years), black ethnicity, Body Mass Index (BMI) over 35 and parity of 3 or more (Jardine et al., 2019). About 18% of maternal admissions in the UK are pregnant.

The median ICU length of stay for a maternal admission in the UK is 29 hours, though women admitted with a non-obstetric diagnosis, such as pneumonia, have a longer stay than those admitted with an obstetric diagnosis, for example postpartum haemorrhage (Simpson et al., 2020). Importantly, maternal admission to ICU during the postpartum period usually involves separation of the mother from her baby. Some women have no memory of the birth event and do not see their baby for several days. This separation has the potential to negatively impact on maternal-infant bonding.

6Cs: Commitment

Demonstrate commitment to both mother and partner in supporting them in early parenthood to create a connection with their new baby as soon as possible.

Adapted physiology

All body systems are affected by pregnancy and the changes begin at the time of conception. Various hormones associated with pregnancy induce widespread changes, for example to the cardiovascular and respiratory systems, and these changes are highly relevant for critical care nursing practice. A brief overview of key physiological changes in pregnancy is provided below. Please explore a specialist text for more detail. Suggestions include van de Velde et al., (2013), and Einav et al., (2020).

Cardiovascular system

There is widespread vasodilation early following conception, and water and sodium retention, both occurring under the influence of various hormones associated with pregnancy, such as progesterone. This results in a slight reduction of blood pressure during the second trimester, with a mild progressive increase during the third trimester (Green et al., 2020). During pregnancy, circulating volume increases by 45% (De Haas et al., 2017). Heart rate increases progressively during pregnancy by 8–10 beats per minute with a slight levelling off towards the end of pregnancy (Green et al., 2020). Due partially to the increase in heart rate, but mainly due to an increase in stroke volume, cardiac output increases during pregnancy 30–50% (Robson et al., 1989). Maternal position can affect cardiac output and BP. The weight of the uterus compressing on major vessels in the supine position impede venous return and reduces cardiac output, and placental flow (Humphries et al., 2019). Consequently, pregnant women in the second half of pregnancy should not be nursed flat on their back. Instead, a left-lateral tilt should be maintained using a wedge, or a side-lying or sitting up position. Likewise, if a woman in the second half of pregnancy requires cardiac compressions (i.e., CPR), a left-lateral tilt or manual displacement of the uterus is required to facilitate effective CPR (Chu et al., 2020). Further, if CPR is ongoing past four minutes, perimortem Caesarean section is recommended to improve the survival of the mother (Knight et al., 2020).

Although there is an increase in the production of red blood cells (RBCs), due to the large increase in plasma volume, the increase is not enough to maintain the concentration of haemoglobin. Consequently, anaemia in pregnancy is defined as a haemoglobin concentration <110 g/l in first trimester and <105 g/l in second and third trimesters (Pavord et al., 2020). There is a slight reduction in platelet levels though the non-pregnant normal levels are usually maintained ($\geq 150,000 \times 10^{-3}$). Many clotting factors are increased in pregnancy; most notably, fibrinogen levels double by the end of pregnancy in preparation for the birth event and potential haemorrhage (Katz and Beilin, 2015). The combination of venous stasis and increased clotting factors increases the likelihood of thrombosis in pregnancy. The first month post-partum is also associated with an increased likelihood of thrombosis. Strategies to prevent deep vein thrombosis should be considered in all critically ill pregnant and postpartum women (Royal College of Obstetricians and Gynaecologists (RCOG), 2015).

Respiratory system

The mother provides oxygen to the fetus and removes the by-products of fetal metabolism, including carbon dioxide. Oxygen and carbon dioxide diffuse across the placenta based on the partial pressure differences. Thus, the mother's oxygen level is always higher than the fetal level and the mother's carbon dioxide level is always lower than the fetal level. An increase in maternal progesterone is thought to affect the respiratory centre in the brain stem, altering the sensitivity to carbon dioxide. The effect is to increase the maternal stimulus to breathe, reducing the normal $PaCO_2$, facilitating the removal of carbon dioxide from the fetus across the placental membrane. The increase in ventilation is achieved by a 36–50% increase in tidal volume (Patil et al., 2020) with the respiratory rate unchanged during pregnancy (Green et al., 2020). The kidneys increase excretion of bicarbonate to maintain a normal pH, resulting in a compensated respiratory alkalosis.

A pregnant woman is considered to have a 'high-risk' airway, with failed intubation occurring eight times more often in the pregnant woman than non-pregnant women (Quinn et al., 2013). Furthermore, with a reduction in the functional residual capacity (FRC), the pregnant woman is vulnerable during any period of apnoea (e.g., prior to intubation; sleep apnoea) and may experience rapid desaturation. Pre-oxygenation, a clinician who is experienced in complex airway management and access to a difficult airway protocol is recommended should a pregnant woman require tracheal intubation.

Renal system

The kidneys receive an increase of blood flow due to an increase in cardiac output (CO) and increased circulating volume causing an increase in the glomerular filtration rate (GFR). During pregnancy, large volumes of ultrafiltrate results in lower serum urea and creatinine levels. However, there are no validated values indicating renal injury in pregnancy, so a 1.5–1.9 times baseline, or >0.3 mg/dl (>26.5 μmol/l) increase in serum creatinine is recommended to signal acute kidney injury (Hall et al., 2019). The impact of the increase of glomerular filtration on urine output is unknown. Some glycosuria and proteinuria (< 300 mg/24 hrs) are normal in pregnancy, as the active transport mechanisms used to reabsorb glucose and protein back into the maternal circulation are overwhelmed. Women who have urinary catheters are vulnerable to urinary tract infection due to glycosuria. There is no relationship between glycosuria and serum glucose levels in pregnancy.

Liver and gastro-intestinal system

Under the influence of pregnancy hormones, all smooth muscle throughout the gastro-intestinal tract relaxes during pregnancy. This slows peristalsis in the gut, reduces cardiac sphincter tone and results in sluggish bile motility. Consequently, these changes increase the likelihood of constipation, gastric reflux (heartburn), cholelithiasis and cholecystitis during pregnancy (Al-Shboul et al., 2019).

The liver increases production of albumin but due to the large increase in plasma volume during pregnancy, the overall result is a reduction in measured serum albumin (30–40 g/L) contributing to the development of dependent oedema. This is common in pregnancy, in part due to the reduced colloid osmotic pressure. Additionally, there are changes to hepatic enzymes responsible for drug metabolism altering the pharmacokinetics of some medication (Feghali et al., 2015).

Immune system

The immune system is very complex and not all the changes that occur in pregnancy are well understood. It is likely that the immune system has fluctuating pro-inflammatory and anti-inflammatory patterns depending on the stage of pregnancy (Mor et al., 2017). Pregnant women are more vulnerable to some infections, such as varicella (chicken pox) and malaria.

440

Table 29.1   Physiological changes of pregnancy pertinent to critical care nursing.

System	Change in pregnancy
Cardiovascular	
Blood volume	↑ 40–50%
BP	small ↓ (mid-trimester)
systolic	small ↓ (mid-trimester)
diastolic	↑ 8–10 bpm
HR	↑ 30–50%
Cardiac output	
Respiratory	
Tidal Volume	↑ 36–50%
Minute Volume	↑ 40–50%
Respiratory rate	unchanged 12–20bpm
PaO_2 ↑	12.3–14.3 kPa
$PaCO_2$ ↓	3.3–4.4 kPa
pH	7.40–7.45
HCO_3 ↓	18–22 mmol/L
Renal	
Serum urea ↓	≤ 4.5 mmol/L
Serum creatinine ↓	< 78 µmol/L

Table 29.2   Normal vital signs in pregnancy.

Vital sign	Normal range in pregnancy
Temperature	36.0–37.2°C
BP	
systolic	95–139 mmHg
diastolic	55–89 mmHg
HR	60–105 beats per minute
RR	12–20 breaths per minute
SpO2	95–100%

6Cs: Competence

Recognising your own practice limitations is imperative. Adhere to your professional code of conduct and maintain proficiency. Ask for help if you are required to work outside your scope of your practice.

The placenta

The placenta is formed and functioning about 10–12 weeks following fertilisation and is the maternal-fetal interface (Bailey, 2020). The placenta has seven key functions to sustain the pregnancy and fetus: respiration (gaseous exchange), nutrition, storage, excretion, protection, transport and endocrine.

Recognising clinical deterioration

There is no national Maternal Early Warning Score (MEWS) in use in England, Wales or Northern Ireland, though one is in development. However, Scotland introduced their national MEWS chart in 2018 (Healthcare Improvement Scotland, 2018). Most obstetric units in the UK have a local MEWS in use, though they vary from trust to trust (Smith et al., 2017). MEWS charts should be used for all pregnant and postpartum women in hospital, regardless of the type of ward in which they are being cared e.g., emergency department, medical ward, postnatal ward (Knight et al., 2020). Sometimes MEWS charts are called MEOWS (Modified Early Obstetric Warning Score).

Early recognition of clinical deterioration in pregnant and postpartum women can be challenging due to the physiological adaptations of pregnancy. For example, with the additional circulating volume and increased cardiac output, women can lose a substantial amount of blood (>1500 mL) before showing any change in vital signs. Subtle changes and listening to the woman about how she feels is important for early identification of deterioration.

Examination scenario: estimate gestation

As a rough estimate, if the top of the fundus is at the level of the woman's umbilicus, the gestation is about 20 weeks. This is highly clinically relevant information as any woman who is in the second half of pregnancy (i.e., ≥ 20 weeks' gestation) needs to have the weight of the uterus shifted off her major vessels by either a left-lateral tilt or other positioning, if the woman is being nursed in bed. Importantly, this also needs to be done as part of CPR if the woman needs cardiac compressions.

Assessment of fetal wellbeing

If a pregnant woman is admitted to a critical care unit, consideration must be given to the assessment of fetal wellbeing in conjunction with a management plan. Fetal viability is about 22–24 weeks' gestation, though babies born this premature carry a significant risk of death or disability (Wilkinson et al., 2018; Smith et al., 2019). Any decision to deliver the baby early should be made collaboratively, with the mother and her partner as able, and be based on what is in the best interest of the woman (this is a situation when what is best for the woman is also best for the baby). There are risks and benefits for both the woman and the fetus in relation to birth around the time of maternal critical illness.

441

Medication management: antenatal corticosteroid

Betamethasone and dexamethasone are corticosteroids. In pregnancy, either may be used to enhance lung maturity of the fetus, resulting in an increase in surfactant production of the fetal lungs, reducing the incidence of respiratory distress syndrome and mortality in the preterm neonate. Betamethasone and dexamethasone are equally effective, and both are administered intramuscularly to women in the 24–48 hours prior to expected or likely pre-term birth (Crowther et al., 2019). All women expected to give birth prior to 34 weeks' gestation should be offered a course of antenatal corticosteroids, for example, two doses of betamethasone 12 mg given intramuscularly 24 hours apart or four doses of dexamethasone 6 mg given intramuscularly 12 hours apart (NICE, 2015-updated 2019). Further, antenatal corticosteroids should be considered for some women up to 36 weeks' gestation e.g., women at risk of preterm birth with preterm premature ruptured membranes.

If the gestation is at a stage where delivery may be considered based on the fetal wellbeing, it is reasonable to routinely monitor fetal wellbeing and to have a delivery plan in place. However, the usual methods used to monitor fetal wellbeing are not easily transferred to the critical care environment. For instance, a cardiotocograph (CTG) is commonly used to assess fetal wellbeing, but if the woman is receiving sedation/opioid agents e.g. midazolam, fentanyl, the fetus may also be sedated and this impairs the interpretation of the CTG. Likewise, a sedated fetus impacts the use of fetal movement and breathing patterns to assess fetal wellbeing for the same reason. Specialist obstetric input should be sought to assess fetal wellbeing.

Nursing considerations and recommendations for practice

Specialist knowledge and skills are required to care for critically ill pregnant and postpartum women.

Maternal Specialist Competencies (CC3N, 2019)

M1 Anatomy and physiology

- State the normal vital signs for pregnancy
- Locate the MEOWS chart and chart maternal observations

M2 Obstetric common conditions and relate to pathophysiology

- List some common obstetric conditions that lead to maternal critical care admission
- Discuss one common obstetric condition and outline the pathophysiology

M3 Obstetric national guidelines and resources

- Locate the national available resources for maternal critical care
- Discuss the local Trust guideline for maternal resuscitation

M4 Management of obstetric haemorrhage

- Describe the maternal assessment related to obstetric haemorrhage

M5 Management of reduced fetal movement (RFM)

- Discuss the methods used to assess fetal wellbeing in a critically ill pregnant woman

M6 Management of spontaneous rupture of membranes (SROM)

- Define SROM and discuss the relevance of this happening

M7 Management of hypertensive disorders of pregnancy

- Define preeclampsia, eclampsia and HELLP syndrome
- Discuss the use of magnesium sulphate in the prevention of eclampsia

M8 Sepsis

- List the common sources of sepsis in a pregnant and recently pregnant woman

M9 Maternal collapse and amniotic fluid embolism

- Outline the required variations to basic life support for a woman in the second half of pregnancy

M10 Timely escalation

- Outline the obstetric team referral process used when a pregnant woman is admitted to ICU

M11 Lactation

- Explain how lactation could be promoted and established in the ICU environment

M12 Wound and vaginal (PV) management

- Describe normal PV loss in the first week following birth

M13 Psychological care and family inclusion

- Discuss the importance of the maternal-infant bond and the potential effect of separation following birth

MEOWS Modified Early Obstetric Warning Score; HELLP Haemolysis, Elevated Liver enzymes and Low Platelets.

Snapshot: Antenatal pneumonia

Jane is 38 years old and is 30 weeks pregnant with her third child. Her previous pregnancies were uncomplicated, and she is a stay-at-home mum with her 2- and 5-year-old children. Jane has no relevant medical history apart from being obese, her BMI is 32. Over the past two days, Jane has started to feel unwell with a fever, general aches and chills, and a hacking cough. She presented to the hospital with vital signs showing BP 105/65; HR 115; RR 26; T 38.2°C; SaO$_2$ 94% on room air. Additionally, it was noted that Jane had not noticed any changes to fetal movements, that her abdomen was soft with no pain or evidence of contractions and there was no abnormal vaginal discharge.

Nursing actions:
- RN contacts the obstetric medicine team to come and review Jane; support the midwife to apply a cardiotocograph (CTG) to assess fetal wellbeing.
- Ensure that Jane is sitting up and in a comfortable position, apply oxygen as prescribed, provide reassurance.
- Conduct a full head-to-toe assessment and act on any immediate concerns; complete all documentation.
- Prepare for collection of blood cultures, indicated blood tests and IV cannulation.
- Obtain a sputum specimen.
- Prepare to transfer Jane for a chest X-ray.

Diagnosis:
- Jane had influenza A which was complicated by a community-acquired pneumonia (CAP).
- Jane's condition deteriorated and she was transferred to ICU for non-invasive ventilation (NIV) and critical care.
- Jane's blood cultures were negative following microscopy, culture and sensitivity (MC&S), but her sputum specimen grew staphylococcus aureus which was sensitive to clindamycin.

- Jane improved over the next three days with intravenous (IV) clindamycin and critical care organ support interventions.
- The fetus remained well with reassuring CTG and normal movements felt by Jane.
- Jane was transferred to the general ward and as she continued to improve, was discharged home after two days on oral antibiotics.

Red Flag: maternal sepsis

Maternal sepsis is a life-threatening condition defined as organ dysfunction resulting from infection during pregnancy, childbirth, post-abortion, or postpartum period (WHO, 2017). Maternal sepsis continues to be a cause of potentially preventable maternal death in the UK. The physiological adaptations in pregnancy may obscure signs and symptoms of infection and sepsis making detection of sepsis more challenging. The most common types of infection are endometritis, chorioamnionitis, urine tract infection and pneumonia. Early recognition and prompt treatment of sepsis is needed to reduce adverse outcomes for women and their babies. However, there is no universally recommended early warning tool in use. The Sepsis 6 are equally important in the effective management of maternal sepsis as they are in the non-pregnant population.

6Cs: Communication

Ensure to communicate with all members of the multidisciplinary team.

Clinical investigation: diagnostic imaging

Diagnostic imaging should be undertaken in pregnancy based on the clinical indication, just the same as in the non-pregnant patient (Lowe, 2019). This includes radiological procedures and nuclear medicine scans, such as, x-ray, CT scan and V/Q scan. The UK and Ireland Confidential Enquiries into Maternal Deaths and Morbidity often determine either a delay or absence of adequate investigation into the maternal condition contributed to maternal death (Knight et al., 2019). They emphasise the need to make a diagnosis and not simply exclude a diagnosis and recommend that diagnostic imaging should be undertaken as clinically indicated. The advice of a medical physicist can be taken to minimise exposure to the fetus from diagnostic imaging, such as, chest x-ray with perfusion scanning (Q) only, instead of a full V/Q scan. Appropriate shielding of the fetus should be utilised when able e.g., lead sheet across the abdomen prior to chest X-ray.

Red Flag: Cardiac disease in pregnancy

Cardiovascular diseases have been the leading cause of maternal death in the UK for over 20 years (Knight et al., 2019) and cardiac disease is consistently the largest single cause of indirect maternal death (Knight et al., 2020). The vast majority of women who die from cardiac disease in the UK (about 80%) are not known to have a pre-existing cardiac problem. Many of the physiological changes in pregnancy obscure the interpretation of signs and symptoms of developing heart failure in the pregnant woman e.g., breathlessness, oedema. Breathlessness at rest, or when lying down (i.e., unable to sleep flat with one pillow as usual) are red flags and warrant further examination. Likewise, chest pain should be fully investigated, using the same suite of diagnostic investigations as used in the non-pregnant population. Troponin levels can be interpreted the same as in non-pregnancy; however, there are gestation-specific B-type natriuretic peptide (BNP) levels.

6Cs: Care

Be kind and thoughtful in your care of a critically ill pregnant or postpartum woman (& partner), so that their experience of critical illness is as positive as it can be.

Snapshot: Antepartum haemorrhage

Georgia is a 26-year-old woman having her second child., Georgia presented to hospital at 35 weeks' gestation with severe, persistent abdominal pain. She felt and looked unwell. Her vital signs showed a BP 90/55; HR 125; RR 24; T 36.5°C; SaO$_2$ 99%. Georgia last felt her baby move that morning, but not since the abdominal pain started. Her abdomen was tense and firm on palpation. Georgia was diagnosed with placental abruption and went to theatre for an emergency Caesarean section. The baby was born in poor condition with Apgar scores of 3 at 1 minute and 6 at 5 minutes. The baby was transferred to the Neonatal Intensive Care Unit (NICU) for ongoing care. Georgia was estimated to have lost 2.4 L and the haemorrhage was controlled after delivery of the placenta. Georgia was transferred to the High Dependency Unit for ongoing care.

Nursing actions:
- Introduce self to Georgia and orient her to her surroundings and events.
- Conduct a head-to-toe assessment, including assessment of the fundus and lochia – whilst the haemorrhage was controlled before Georgia was transferred to HDU, it is possible for the uterus muscle to relax again and for bleeding to restart. Making sure that the fundus stays firm and contracted, and observing for the volume of lochia loss per vagina (PV) is part of her postpartum care.
- Check all IV lines and orders, medication chart, postoperative orders, and blood test results.
- Invite Georgia's partner into HDU to sit with Georgia.
- Check the blood group of Georgia – if she has a Rh-negative blood group she will need anti-D immunoglobulin. The dose is guided by a Kleihauer test.
- Check on the condition of the baby and communicate findings as appropriate.
- Ask Georgia about how she plans to feed her infant.
- If Georgia condition remains stable, discuss with the multidisciplinary team (MDT) whether Georgia may be taken to NICU to visit her baby.

Clinical investigation: Kleihauer test

If a woman who has a RhD-negative blood group carries a RhD-positive fetus, there is a risk that the woman will be exposed to fetal RhD-positive red blood cells, for example at the time of miscarriage, trauma, or birth. The woman may develop antibodies that act against RhD-positive blood cells which can become a major problem, especially in a subsequent pregnancy with a RhD-positive fetus, as the maternal antibodies cross the placenta, cause haemolisation of the fetal red blood cells and can result in severe anaemia in the fetus. To prevent this process called RhD sensitisation from occurring, RhD-negative women are given anti-D immunoglobulin. The anti-D immunoglobulin nullifies any RhD-positive cells that may have entered the mother's blood, and this stops the mother from generating the antibodies.

Rh-D negative women are routinely offered prophylactic anti-D immunoglobulin during pregnancy at 28–32 weeks' gestation, and again within 72 hours of birth. However, the routine dose may not be enough in some circumstances as an excessive amount of fetal blood may have entered the maternal circulation. When this might be the case, a maternal blood test is taken, called the Kleihauer test, which determines the size of the feto-maternal haemorrhage and identifies the dose of anti-D immunoglobulin required to 'mop up' all the fetal red blood cells. The recommended dose needs to be administered within 72 hours of the sensitising event to prevent maternal antibodies from being formed. Examples of sensitising events that commonly require a Kleihauer test to be ordered are abdominal trauma, fetal death in utero and antenatal haemorrhage.

Red Flag: Preeclampsia

Preeclampsia is a common disorder of pregnancy affecting 5–8% of the childbearing population. The condition results from a dysfunctional placenta which releases various mediators causing endothelial damage and widespread vasospasm. Hypertension developing in the second half of pregnancy is usually a feature of the condition and can lead to cerebral haemorrhage if not controlled (NICE, 2019). Other signs and symptoms of organ damage, e.g., acute kidney injury, pulmonary oedema, liver impairment, signal severe disease. Eclampsia, generalised tonic-clonic seizures, may occur, with magnesium sulphate the drug of choice to both prevent and treat eclampsia. Haemolysis, Elevated Liver enzymes and Low Platelets (HELLP) syndrome occurs in a distinct sub-group of women with these signs and similarly, they signal severe preeclampsia. Babies of women with preeclampsia are more likely to be small for their gestational age, and more likely to be born preterm or stillborn.

Severe headache, right upper quadrant pain (indicating liver involvement), visual disturbances (e.g., blurred vision) and over-responsive reflexes (e.g., patellar reflex) should be reported to the obstetric team.

Medication management: magnesium sulphate

Magnesium in a common electrolyte in the body, however, there are two unique uses of medication containing magnesium in pregnancy.

To prevent and treat eclampsia

Women with the pregnancy complication preeclampsia may develop tonic-clonic seizures called eclampsia. Magnesium sulphate has proven superior to regular anticonvulsant medication, such as, phenytoin, to prevent and treat eclamptic seizures. When administered to women, either by intravenous infusion or by intramuscular injection, magnesium sulphate halves the chance of a woman with preeclampsia developing eclampsia. Consequently, magnesium sulphate is the first-line drug of choice to prevent and treat eclampsia. The usual dosage is:

- A loading dose of 4 g should be given intravenously over 5 to 15 minutes, followed by an infusion of 1 g/hour maintained for 24 hours. If the woman has had an eclamptic fit, the infusion should be continued for 24 hours after the last fit.
- Recurrent fits should be treated with a further dose of 2–4 g given intravenously over 5 to 15 minutes (NICE, 2019).

Care is needed to monitor for signs of hypermagnesaemia (high serum magnesium level) including the assessment of deep tendon reflexes and observing for adequate urinary output as magnesium is excreted by the kidney.

To prevent the development of cerebral palsy in the baby

When a woman is expected to give birth to a pre-term baby, consideration should be given to the administration of magnesium to the pregnant woman in the 24 hours prior to the expected birth. This indication, so-called neuroprotection, has been shown to halve the chance of a pre-term baby developing cerebral palsy. All women expected to give birth prior to 30 weeks' gestation should be offered magnesium for neuroprotection, and consideration should be given to women expected to give birth between 30–34 weeks' gestation.

The recommended dosage for neuroprotection of the newborn is:

- Give a 4 g intravenous bolus of magnesium sulphate over 15 minutes, followed by an intravenous infusion of 1 g per hour until the birth or for 24 hours (whichever is sooner) (NICE, 2019).

Care needs to be taken to monitor for signs of hypermagnesaemia.

Snapshot: Postpartum haemorrhage

Salma is a 32-year-old woman who had her first baby this morning. She had no medical history. She developed preeclampsia at 36 weeks' gestation and underwent induction of labour. Initially her labour and birth went well. However, immediately following the spontaneous vaginal birth, the midwife noticed significant bleeding from the vagina and assessed the fundus to be boggy (uterus relaxed) and not contracted adequately. The first-line management for postpartum haemorrhage (PPH) was not effective. Salma was transferred to theatre where the haemorrhage was eventually controlled using uterine balloon tamponade, under a general anaesthetic. Her total blood loss was 2.7 L and she received 6 units of red blood cells (RBCs), 4 units of cryoprecipitate and 1g of tranexamic acid intravenously. Her observations on arrival to the critical care area were T 36.1, HR 105, BP 110/65, RR 18, SpO$_2$ 98% and she was sleepy, but responded to voice by opening her eyes. The fundus was firm, central and at the umbilicus, and a PV pad is in situ. She has two large-bore peripheral IVs in situ: one has a 1 L flask of Hartmann's with 40 units of syntocinon running at a 6 hourly rate; the other has the remainder of the last unit of RBCs, due to finish in about 30 minutes. Her urinary catheter is on hourly measurements and the uterine balloon is not draining any blood.

Nursing actions:
- Introduce self to Salma and orientate her to her environment.
- Conduct a head-to-toe assessment and identify any immediate red flags.
- Review blood test results and identify what and when new tests need to be drawn and sent off.
- Look at the medication chart and administer as required.
- Ensure Salma has good pain management and thromboprophylaxis strategies in place.
- Read the surgical report, look at the anaesthetic chart and birth suite partogram.
- Ask the whereabouts of the partner and ensure they are contactable and invited to be with Salma.
- Ask the whereabouts and clinical condition of the baby – communicate with the partner about telling the woman about the baby; see whether it is feasible for the baby to visit.
- Ask Salma and her partner what Salma's how she intends to feed her infant.
- Discuss the plan of care with the multidisciplinary team and develop a nursing plan for the rest of the shift.
- Document all observations and nursing actions.

6Cs: Compassion

Remember to communicate with Salma's partner and be welcoming to their presence in the critical care environment.

Examination scenario: Assess the fundus post-birth

As the most common reason a woman will need admission to ICU is following a postpartum haemorrhage, assessment of the fundus post-birth is a necessary skill to acquire. On the day of birth, the fundus is usually at the level of the umbilicus, and it should be central and feel very firm on palpation (feel as hard as a cricket ball when palpating via the abdomen). Normally, the uterus undergoes involution – where the uterus gets smaller and re-positions back to the pre-pregnant position in the pelvis – over a period of 7–10 days (Figure 29.1). Each day the uterus gets smaller and deeper to feel, with the fundus usually measured in relation to the position to the umbilicus (e.g., one finger-breadth above the umbilicus), the tone of the fundus (contracted/firm or boggy) and the centrality (central or to the left or right). The most common cause of postpartum haemorrhage is uterine atony – when the uterus is not contracted firmly allowing blood to flow from the placental site.

If the woman has undergone a hysterectomy as part of the postpartum haemorrhage management, there is no fundus to assess. In this situation, assessment of the abdominal wound is necessary (the same as for any surgical wound), as is assessment of any vaginal loss. Again, with the uterus removed, there will be no lochia to assess so any vaginal loss will be coming from a surgical wound.

Medications management: Oxytocin

The medication oxytocin is a synthetic manufactured version of the naturally occurring hormone oxytocin. It acts on the oxytocin receptors in uterine muscle (myometrium) to induce uterine contraction. It is used to induce and/or augment labour and may be part of the active management of the third stage of labour (delivery of the placenta) to prevent postpartum haemorrhage.

Oxytocin is commonly administered by continuous intravenous infusion to induce/augment labour and following Caesarean section to prevent postpartum haemorrhage. It is usually administered by intramuscular injection after the vaginal birth of the baby to prevent postpartum haemorrhage.

Women have different sensitivity to oxytocin so there is a range of dosage to induce/augment labour that is titrated according to the uterine response. Too much oxytocin will cause uterine hyperstimulation (too strong uterine contractions that come too quickly, not allowing the uterine muscle much resting time in between) and this is associated with uterine rupture, amniotic fluid embolism and fetal distress.

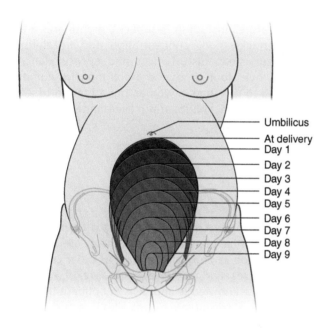

Umbilicus
At delivery
Day 1
Day 2
Day 3
Day 4
Day 5
Day 6
Day 7
Day 8
Day 9

Figure 29.1   Involution of the uterus.

Medications management: ergometrine maleate

Ergometrine is a manufactured ergot alkaloid (naturally produced by a fungus) that induces contraction of the uterus. Although the precise mechanism of action is not fully understood, it is thought to act as an alpha-receptor agonist, inducing uterine muscle contraction. Thus, the action is quite different to oxytocin and is unrelated to any de-sensitivity the oxytocin receptors may have developed through induction of labour. Ergometrine is often used to treat postpartum haemorrhage, especially if oxytocin is ineffective. However, ergometrine can cause widespread vasoconstriction and its use is contraindicated in some women, such as, those with cardiac disease, hypertension in pregnancy e.g., preeclampsia. Ergometrine is usually administered as an intramuscular injection, and nausea and vomiting are common side effects.

Supporting breastfeeding

Maternal critical illness is not a reason in itself to stop the woman from breastfeeding, if that is her choice of infant feeding. However, there are several things to consider including maternal consent, medications and resources to support her choice.

Consent should be obtained from the woman, or if she is not well enough, from her partner in conjunction with prior maternal preference. Many medications used in ICU have incomplete data on the safety for breastfeeding. However, breastmilk is of vital importance to the baby, and especially the preterm baby. Two helpful resources to check the safety of the breastmilk for the infant are the pharmacist and the neonatologist. Sometimes there is a short-term need to discard expressed breastmilk, e.g., if the woman has received imaging using an ionising agent. In this situation, the expressed breastmilk can be discarded for 48 hours, whilst not interfering with the establishment of lactation and the provision of breastmilk in the long term.

If the mother's choice is to breastfeed, she should be supported to establish lactation and to provide breastmilk for her baby. A combination of hand expressing and machine pumping may be used to establish lactation, which is usually conducted 3–4 hourly. See a midwifery text such as *Myles Textbook for Midwives* for detailed information on how to express and store breastmilk (Marshall and Raynor, 2020). Liaise with the midwifery team and/or the lactation consultant in the special care nurseries for assistance with establishing lactation in the critically ill woman.

If the mother chooses not to breastfeed, the best management of the breasts is to leave them alone and observe for any signs and symptoms of mastitis. In most women who experience critical illness, without the stimulation of the baby suckling or breast expression, limited milk is generated, and engorgement is not usually an issue. It is unlikely that the woman will require medication to suppress lactation.

Supporting the maternal-infant bond

Where possible, the mother and baby should be kept together. If the baby is well but not able to stay with the mother in ICU, baby visits should be facilitated. If the baby is not able to visit the mother, then strategies to enhance the maternal-infant connection should be used. Such strategies include talking about the baby, showing the mother photos of the baby, using video calls, asking the nursery/midwifery staff or partner to create a baby diary for the mother. Also, a piece of fabric laid against the mother's skin can be placed with the infant (and vice versa) to help with the connection using smell.

Orange Flag: mother-baby separation

Mothers that have no recollection of the birth event and who do not meet their baby for several days may have trouble feeling that the baby they are given is theirs. It is important to create a connection as early as you can and encourage interaction with the baby whenever possible.

Psycho-social considerations

Understandably, most women and their partners expect an uncomplicated and safe birth of their baby. Given most maternal admissions to a critical care area are unplanned (i.e., unexpected), there is the potential for the experience of critical illness to have an adverse effect on women, their partners and on their family and infant relationships. Caring communication including orientation of the woman to the events, the nurse introducing themselves and explaining where the woman is, and what happened to result in her admission to ICU, is important. If there has been a perinatal loss, involvement of a social worker, pastoral carer or bereavement counsellor may provide support to the woman and family.

Orange Flag: post-traumatic stress disorder

Post-traumatic stress disorder (PTSD) occurs in some people who have experienced a potentially life-threatening event, such as, critical illness. PTSD is known to occur in patients admitted to ICU and is more common in patients with a previous mental health problem and in patients with a negative ICU experience (Lee et al., 2020). PTSD is characterised by notable impairment in social functioning including a feeling of detachment and emotional numbing, and other features including flashbacks, nightmares and panic attacks, poor concentration and irritability, mood and sleep disturbances and hypervigilance. PTSD is over four times more common in women admitted to ICU than in women not admitted to ICU associated with childbearing (Hernández-Martinez et al., 2019).

Conclusion

Whilst caring for a critically ill pregnant or postpartum woman is a relatively rare event, the woman deserves equity of access to the same quality of care as other critically ill patients. Nurses and midwives can develop 'enhanced maternity care' knowledge and skills to optimise the provision of maternal critical care to critically ill women. Interdisciplinary communication, consultation and collaboration are vital for coordinated care and to achieve the best outcomes. Effort should be made to keep mother and baby together whenever possible, and to support the woman to breastfeed if she chooses to. The needs of the woman's partner should also be considered as part of the care of the woman. Psychological care for both the woman and her partner should be part of routine care, including the option for a post-ICU debrief and consultation.

Take home points

1. Increasing numbers of women experience a need for critical care during or soon after pregnancy.
2. Physiological adaptations occur across all body systems in pregnancy, beginning at conception and returning to the pre-pregnant state over a period of weeks after the pregnancy ends.
3. Most critical illness occurs in women who were previously well and as a result of an obstetric complication – with ICU admission usually occurring as an emergency and not a planned, elective admission.
4. Interdisciplinary communication, consultation and collaboration are vital for optimal care.
5. There are specialist maternity competencies that nurses can acquire to develop the necessary knowledge and skills to care for critically ill pregnant and postpartum women.
6. Be kind when providing care to a critically ill woman and her partner.

7. Nurture a mother-baby bond, i.e., enable the baby to visit the mother in ICU. Furthermore, even if the mother and baby have been separated to facilitate the provision of critical care, use photos, video calls and a diary, for example, to create a connection between mother and baby.

8. Support the mother's choice in infant feeding, including the establishment of lactation and breastfeeding/breast milk expression.

9. Ensure effective handover when the mother is transferred to a step-down or maternity ward.

10. Once the woman is fully recovered, offer the woman and her partner the opportunity to discuss her critical illness and management.

References

Al-Shboul, O.A., Al-Rshoud, H.J., Al-Dwairi, A.N. et al. (2019). Changes in gastric smooth muscle cell contraction during pregnancy: effect of estrogen. *Journal of Pregnancy* Article ID 4302309. doi: 10.1155/2019/4302309.

Bailey J. (2020). The placenta. In: *Myles Textbook for Midwives*, 17e. (ed. J. Marshall and M. Raynor), 133–143. Edinburgh: Churchill Livingstone Elsevier.

CC3N (Critical Care Networks-National Nurse Leads) (2019). National Competency Framework for Registered Nurses in Adult Critical Care Maternal Specialist Competencies. https://www.cc3n.org.uk/uploads/9/8/4/2/98425184/maternal_comps_final.pdf (accessed 5 December 2020).

Chu, J., Johnston, T.A., Geoghegan, J., on behalf of the Royal College of Obstetricians and Gynaecologists (2020). Maternal collapse in pregnancy and the puerperium. *BJOG* 127:e14–e52.

Crowther, C.A., Ashwood, P., Andersen, C.C. et al. (2019). Maternal intramuscular dexamethasone versus betamethasone before preterm birth (ASTEROID): a multicentre, double-blind, randomised controlled trial. *The Lancet Child & Adolescent Health*. 3(11): 769–780.

Davey M-A, Flood, M., Pollock, W. (2020). Risk factors for severe postpartum haemorrhage: a population-based retrospective cohort study. *Aust & NZ J Obstet Gynaecol*. 60: 522–532.

De Haas, S., Ghossein-Doha, C., Van Kuijk, S.M. et al. (2017). Physiological adaptation of maternal plasma volume during pregnancy: a systematic review and meta-analysis. *Ultrasound in Obstetrics & Gynecology*. 49: 177–187.

Einav, S., Weiniger, C.F., Landau R. (eds) (2020). *Principles and Practice of Maternal Critical Care*. Cham: Springer Nature.

Feghali, M., Venkataramanan, R., and Caritis S. (2015). Pharmacokinetics of drugs in pregnancy. *Seminars in Perinatology* 39(7): 512–519.

Green, L.J., Mackillop, L.H., Salvi, D. et al. (2020). Gestation-specific vital sign reference ranges in pregnancy. *Obstetrics & Gynecology* 135: 653–664.

Hall, D.R. and Conti-Ramsden, F. (2019). Acute kidney injury in pregnancy including renal disease diagnosed in pregnancy. *Best Practice & Research Clinical Obstetrics & Gynaecology* 57:47–59.

Healthcare Improvement Scotland. The Scottish Maternity Early Warning System (MEWS) 2018. Available from: https://ihub.scot/improvement-programmes/scottish-patient-safety-programme-spsp/maternity-and-children-quality-improvement-collaborative-mcqic/maternity-care/national-mews/ (accessed 30 January 2021).

Hernández-Martínez, A., Rodríguez-Almagro, J., Molina-Alarcón, M. et al. (2019). Postpartum post-traumatic stress disorder: Associated perinatal factors and quality of life. *Journal of Affective Disorders* 249: 143–150.

Humphries, A., Mirjalili, S.A., Tarr, G. et al. (2019). The effect of supine positioning on maternal hemodynamics during late pregnancy. *Journal of Maternal – Fetal & Neonatal Medicine* 32: 3923–3930.

Jardine J. (2019). *NMPA Project Team. Maternity Admissions to Intensive Care in England, Wales and Scotland in 2015/16: A Report from the National Maternity and Perinatal Audit*. London: RCOG.

Katz, D. and Beilin Y. (2015). Disorders of coagulation in pregnancy. *BJA: British Journal of Anaesthesia* 115(suppl_2): ii75–ii88.

Knight, M., Bunch, K., Tuffnell, D. et al. (eds) on behalf of MBRRACE-UK (2019). *Saving Lives, Improving Mothers' Care: Lessons Learned to Inform Maternity Care from the UK and Ireland Confidential Enquiries into Maternal Deaths and Morbidity 2015–17*. Oxford: National Perinatal Epidemiology Unit, University of Oxford. https://www.npeu.ox.ac.uk/mbrrace-uk/reports (accessed 6 December 2020).

Knight, M., Bunch, K., Tuffnell, D. et al. (eds) on behalf of MBRRACE-UK (2020). *Saving Lives, Improving Mothers' Care – Lessons Learned to Inform Maternity Care from the UK and Ireland Confidential Enquiries into Maternal Deaths and Morbidity 2016–18*. Oxford: National Perinatal Epidemiology Unit, University of Oxford. https://www.npeu.ox.ac.uk/mbrrace-uk/reports (accessed 16 January 2021).

Lee, M., Kang, J., and Jeong Y.J. (2020). Risk factors for post-intensive care syndrome: A systematic review and meta-analysis. *Australian Critical Care* 33(3): 287–94.

Lowe S. (2019). Diagnostic imaging in pregnancy: Making informed decisions. *Obstetric Medicine* 12(3): 116–122.

Marshall, J. and Raynor, M. (eds). *Myles Textbook for Midwives*, 17e. Edinburgh: Churchill Livingstone Elsevier.

Mor, G. (2017). The unique immunologic and microbial aspects of pregnancy. *Placenta* 57: 226.

NICE (2019). Hypertension in pregnancy: diagnosis and management. https://www.nice.org.uk/guidance/ng133 (accessed 5 December 2020).

NICE (2015; updated 2019). Preterm labour and birth. https://www.nice.org.uk/guidance/ng25 (accessed 5 December 2020).

Patil, H., Kataria, A., Teli, A. et al. (2020) Analysis of pulmonary function and serum progesterone level during pregnancy: A cross-sectional study. *Journal of South Asian Federation of Obstetrics and Gynaecology*. 12: 216.

Pavord, S., Daru, J., Prasannan, N. et al. (2020). UK guidelines on the management of iron deficiency in pregnancy. *Br J Haematol* 188: 819–830.

Pollock, W., Rose, L., Dennis, C.-L. (2010). Pregnant and postpartum admissions to the intensive care unit: a systematic review. *Intensive Care Medicine*. 36(9): 1465–1474.

Quinn, A., Milne, D., Columb, M. et al. (2013). Failed tracheal intubation in obstetric anaesthesia: 2 yr national case-control study in the UK. *British Journal of Anaesthesia* 110: 74–80.

Robson, S.C., Hunter, S., Boys, R.J., and Dunlop W. (1989). Serial study of factors influencing changes in cardiac output during human pregnancy. *American Journal of Physiology-Heart and Circulatory Physiology*. 256(4): H1060–H1065.

Royal College of Anaesthetists (RCoA). Care of the critically ill woman in childbirth; enhanced maternal care 2018. RCoA, London. https://www.rcoa.ac.uk/sites/default/files/documents/2020-06/EMC-Guidelines2018.pdf (accessed 6 December 2020).

Royal College of Obstetricians and Gynaecologists (RCOG) (2015). Reducing the risk of venous thromboembolism during pregnancy and the puerperium. Green Top Guideline 37a. London: RCOG. https://www.rcog.org.uk/globalassets/documents/guidelines/gtg-37a.pdf (accessed 5 February 2020).

Simpson, N.B., Shankar-Hari, M., Rowan, K.M. et al. (2020). Maternal risk modeling in critical care – development of a multivariable risk prediction model for death and prolonged intensive care. *Critical Care Medicine* 48(5): 663–672.

Smith, G.B., Isaacs, R., Andrews, L. et al. (2017). Vital signs and other observations used to detect deterioration in pregnant women: an analysis of vital sign charts in consultant-led UK maternity units. *International Journal of Obstetric Anesthesia.* 30: 44–51.

Smith, L.K., Draper, E.S., Manktelow, B.N. et al. (2019). *MBRRACE-UK Supplementary Report on Survival up to One Year of Age of Babies Born Before 27 Weeks Gestational Age for Births in Great Britain from January to December 2016.* Leicester: The Infant Mortality and Morbidity Studies, Department of Health Sciences, University of Leicester.

Van de Velde, M., Scholefield, H., and Plante L.A. (eds). (2013). *Maternal Critical Care: A Multidisciplinary Approach.* Cambridge: Cambridge University Press.

WHO Statement on Maternal Sepsis (2017). https://www.who.int/reproductivehealth/publications/maternal_perinatal_health/maternalsepsis-statement/en/ (accessed 5 December 2020).

Wilkinson, D., Verhagen, E., and Johansson S. (2018). Thresholds for resuscitation of extremely preterm infants in the UK, Sweden, and Netherlands. *Pediatrics* 142(Suppl 1): S574–S584.

Chapter 30

Critical care transfers

Kirstin Geer, Mark Cannan, and Stuart Cox

Aim

The aim of this chapter is to provide the reader with an evidence-based understanding of inter-hospital and intra-hospital transfer of the critically ill adult patient.

Learning outcomes

After reading this chapter the reader will be able to:

- Be introduced to different types of transfer.
- Understand the risks associated with transferring a critically ill adult.
- Understand the transfer process.
- Appreciate the roles and responsibilities of professionals within the transfer team.
- Apply the ABCDE approach to the transfer process.

Test your prior knowledge

- What types of transfers are there?
- Name the risks associated with the transfer of critically ill adults.
- What is the standard process of transfer?
- What is the role of the nurse/ODP throughout transfer?
- Identify how ABCDE is applied to a critically ill adult patient during transfers.
- CCN Critical Care Competencies

Fundamentals of Critical Care: A Textbook for Nursing and Healthcare Students, First Edition. Edited by Ian Peate and Barry Hill.
© 2023 John Wiley & Sons Ltd. Published 2023 by John Wiley & Sons Ltd.
Companion website: www.wiley.com/go/peate/criticalcare

This chapter will enhance your ability to understand the underpinning principles of the CCN Step Two competencies regarding critical care transfer (Box 30.1).

6Cs: Competence

Competence ensures that all those involved in critical care transfers must have the ability not only to understand an individual's health and social needs, but have the expertise through training, clinical and technical knowledge to undertake critical care transfers. The competence and treatment throughout the critical care transfer should be based on research and evidence.

Inter-hospital and intra-hospital patient transfers

The intra- and inter-hospital patient transfer is an important aspect of patient care which is often undertaken to improve upon the existing management of the patient. It may involve transfer of patients within the same facility for any diagnostic or therapeutic procedures or transfer to another facility with more advanced care services. The main aim in all such transfers is maintaining the continuity of medical care. As the transfer of critically ill patients may induce various physiological alterations (which may adversely affect the prognosis of the patient), it should be initiated systematically and according to the evidence-based guidelines (Kulshrestha and Singh, 2016).

Inter-hospital transfer is the process of moving a patient from one hospital to another either by road or air. This could be for an upgrade of care to a tertiary centre, or due to staffing or bed pressures within the referring hospital or could be a repatriation after specialist treatment. As such, critical care staff must be able to transfer patients not just from intensive care, but from other departments such as Accident & Emergency or Coronary Care Departments. The aim of the inter-hospital transfer is for the continuation of high-quality care throughout the transfer process so that the patient reaches the destination hospital in an efficient and safe manner (Droogh et al., 2015).

An intra-hospital transfer, on the other hand, occurs within the existing hospital in which the patient resides and is the more frequent type of transfer. For example, patients may be required to attend the radiology department for therapeutic or diagnostic purposes or be moved between wards or departments when escalating or de-escalating care within the hospital. The same considerations, preparation and risk assessment should be completed in the same manner for intra-hospital transfer as it is with inter-hospital transfers (Bourn et al., 2018).

Although there is no data to highlight the number of intra-hospital transfers annually, guidelines produced by the Intensive Care Society (2019) quote an 'under-reported' UK figure of 10,750 inter-hospital critical care transfers annually. This is said to be increasing in real terms year on year. It was noted that there was a general even spread through Monday to Friday while fewer transfers occurred during the weekend days. However, more (56%) were occurring during the hours of 18:00 and 07:59. A breakdown of the above figures showed 35.5% of inter-hospital transfers originated from general critical care units, 27.8% were from the emergency department, 25% were from 'other areas', 11% from specialist critical care areas and 13% were repatriations (1.8% of which were from abroad (ICS, 2019)).

6Cs: Care

Care is at the core of the NHS. The care we deliver on a critical care transfer must ensure the individual person receives the same level of care as they would receive on a critical care unit. This can be achieved by an assessment before transfer of the team composition and a multimodal training package

Transfer of the critically ill adult

Transfers are becoming more common due to centralisation of specialist centres and increasing demand on critical care beds putting pressure on critical care networks (Droogh at al., 2015). However, transfer of the critically ill adult is not without risk. Adverse events are widely reported in transfer between 12.5% (Droogh et al., 2012) to 62% (Flabouris et at., 2006). Main risks of transfer include problems with the patient or equipment, non-technical issues including communication, crew resource and organisational issues (Flabouris et al., 2006).

6Cs: Communication

Communication is central to successful caring relationships, to effective team working and is integral to a critical care transfer. Communication on a critical care transfer involves multiple parties including the patient, their family, referring and receiving unit and the ambulance service, whilst on transfer communication and updates should be provided to the receiving unit and a comprehensive ABCDE and medication handover provided on arrival.

The aim of transfer is to maintain high-quality care and ensure the safety of the patient and the transfer crew. Currently in the UK there is not a standardised transfer service nationwide. Scotland and Wales have a dedicated transfer service but there is currently no coordinated transfer service

Box 30.1   Intra- and inter-hospital transfer. *Source:* CC3N, 2015.

- Policies/procedure/guidelines related to the transport of the critically ill patient:
  - ICS guidelines
  - Regional standards
  - Risk assessment
  - Local policy
  - Bed management systems
  - Transfer audit documentation
- Role of team members when arranging and carrying out an intra- and inter-hospital transfer
- Complete a comprehensive risk assessment in collaboration with the MDT to ensure the patient is fit or suitable for transfer
- Identify the potential risks associated with transferring critically ill patients
- Indications for transfer from critical care including the:
  - Nature: repatriation, specialist treatment, investigation, continuing care
  - Sequence of expected event
  - Urgency and time-critical transfers
  - Reasons for reviewing individuals' priorities, needs and the time frame with which this should be undertaken
- Transfer process including the different considerations for clinical and non-clinical transfer decisions:
  - Communication with relatives and on-going updating of the situation as required
  - Ethical issues
  - Legal requirements
  - Local escalation policies
  - Bed management system
  - Referral to receiving hospital (including critical care and specialty consultants)
  - Responsibility of care during transfer
  - Indemnity insurance
  - Competency and skills of transferring personnel
  - Risk assessment of patient's physiological requirements and maintenance of homeostasis during transit
  - Contingency planning/back-up considerations
  - Drug administration during transfer
  - Type of transport required, time-critical issues, bariatric patients
  - Communication with receiving hospital prior to transfer
  - Documentation and audit
- Differing types of transport available and make recommendations for which is the most appropriate
- Process for organising the appropriate transport:
  - Ambulance service
  - Vehicle specification (including on board resources and equipment)
  - Ambulance equipment
  - Types of transfer trolley available
  - Storage of transport equipment in transit
  - Time-critical transfer issues
- Process for preparing to undertake an intra/inter-hospital transfer of a critically ill patient:
  - Gathering of extra battery packs, alternative equipment in case of malfunction
  - Clinical notes/radiology reports/recent blood profiles/investigations
  - Assessment of patient's physiological requirements during transfer
  - Accuracy of portable monitoring and equipment
  - Re assess safety/risk factors prior to transfer
- Process and sequence of communication required for providing oral reports/discussions:
  - Information and informed consent in the conscious patient
  - Discussion with family members
  - Verbal referral and handover of patients condition to receiving unit/service
  - Handover of condition and physiological requirements to the transfer team/personnel

- Sharing information with the team in relation to safety,
- risk assessments and contingency planning
- Contact receiving unit/service on departure
- Formal handover to receiving unit/service on arrival
- Documentation that needs to be completed in an accurate, concise and systematic manner during an inter-hospital transfer, with appropriate duplications:
  - Transfer form
  - Physiological observation chart
  - Nursing evaluation
  - Reporting of clinical incidents
  - Audit tool
- Prepare the patient for transfer by assisting the wider MDT in the physiological optimisation/stabilisation
  - Assess potentially competing needs of the patient for pre-transfer optimisation and specialist care
  - Assess clinical condition of patient before leaving the critical care unit
- Maintain the safety of the patient during transfer:
  - Assessment of the extra physiological stresses experienced by the patient during inter-hospital transfer
  - Anticipation of potential problems and planning to reduce the likelihood of their occurrence
  - Maintenance of situational awareness and readiness to respond to threatening situations if and as they occur
- Demonstrate awareness of situational factors that could impact on the quality and safety of a critical care transfer
- Identify areas in your own transfer practice that could be improved
- Reflect on your own transfer experience

in England (Grier et al., 2020). Critical Care transfer guidelines have been published by NICE (2018) and the Intensive Care Society (2019). However, adherence to guidance is not widely recorded. Regional critical care networks deliver transfer training for critical care staff and audit transfers within the region. Individual organisations should utilise local policy that is based on national guidance.

Preparation is key to maximise safety and avoid the risks identified above. Patient selection is an important aspect of this and each transfer should be justified based upon clinical need. Transfers that are not for an upgrade of care (such as bed pressures or staff shortages) should select the most stable patient who requires the least organ support.

Failure of equipment is the most common adverse event during transfers (Parmentier-Decrucq et al., 2013).

Equipment issues can be avoided by using standardised kit that staff are familiar with their use and ensuring robust processes are in place to check and maintain transfer equipment (Intensive Care Society, 2019). Specifically designed critical care transfer trollies should be utilised (Figure 30.1). Transfer bags with critical care equipment should be taken on transfer (Figure 30.2). Staff undertaking transfers must be familiar with and competent to use the transfer equipment. Some transfers may require the use of a bariatric transfer trolley and an ambulance suitable to transport it. This must be flagged up to the ambulance service at the earliest opportunity to ensure an appropriate vehicle is dispatched. It is important that transferring staff are familiar with and be able to connect the transfer trolley to the oxygen and electrical supply of the ambulance.

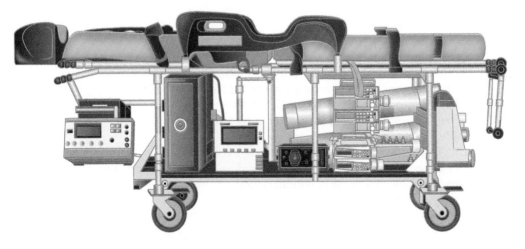

Figure 30.1 Example of CC transfer trolley.

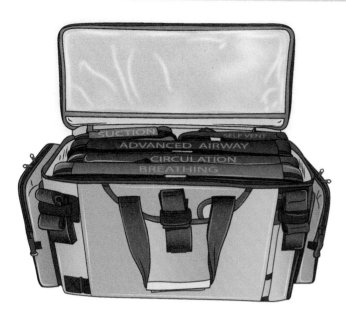

Figure 30.2 A consensus to determine the ideal critical care transfer bag.

The transducer must be connected to the ambulance. This should be confirmed by ensuring the transfer ventilator, drug infusion pumps and monitors are charging prior to departure.

Red Flag: Monitoring

Ensure that inotropes are used in clinical areas or critical care transfers where patients' haemodynamic status can be monitored adequately. Continuous monitoring of mean arterial blood pressure (MAP), cardiac output (CO) and central venous pressure (CVP) allows haemodynamic changes to be detected and addressed rapidly.

Transfers can be complex and involve multi healthcare professionals. Risks related to communication are commonly reported and account for 9% of all adverse events on critical care transfers (Flabouris et al., 2006). Key communications relating to transfer are between the sending and receiving centres, inter-departments of the sending hospital such as radiology and transfusion laboratory, between the transfer team, and with the patient and patients' relatives. Transfers between centres can be particularly daunting for relatives, to alleviate some of these worries, it is important to provide them with contact numbers, visiting times and directions of the receiving hospital if that information is known

Communication can be improved by ensuring accurate and up-to-date records of all stages of the transfer are maintained. Medical records in paper form may need to be copied and travelled with the patient. Any electronic records including images should be made available to the receiving unit prior to transfer. The transfer form, which includes the checklist,s must be completed and patient observations recorded en route.

Handover is a crucial point in ensuring quality of the transfer. A structured verbal handover (such as SBAR) should be utilised and commence either before or after the patient is safely moved from the trolley and monitors, ventilation and infusions are established and it is vitally important that both teams are focused, handover is not complete until the receiving team are satisfied with the handover and all queries have been clarified. After the transfer is completed a regional audit form must be submitted (either paper or electronic – region-specific).

6Cs: Courage

Courage enables us to do the right thing for the people we care for, to speak up when we have concerns. It means we have the personal strength and vision to innovate and to embrace new ways of working. Critical care transfers are a high-risk and challenging aspect of critical care. Staff must be supported before, during and after the transfer process with a debrief after every critical care transfer with the ability to speak up at any stage. This must be a standard approach even if it is an intra or inter-hospital transfer.

The transfer of critically ill adult patients is not at present standardised throughout the UK. There are some guidelines that have been published. However, they do cause some degree of inconsistency (National Institute of Health and Clinical Excellence (NICE), 2018). Currently there are large numbers of critically ill patients who require transfer between critical care units which poses significant risks. It is also more than likely that these numbers will increase over the coming years with data that shows transfers are poorly performed. Therefore, we need to look at all different ways this could be implemented and gather the evidence to make a strong enough recommendation to improve the transfer of these patients. There are also many transfers of critically ill patients for therapeutic or diagnostic purposes within the same hospital. This also needs to be looked at for staff to have some degree of instruction in order to achieve the best possible outcome for these patients.

Due to the complexity and potential risks of transfers, all staff who perform transfers are required to undertake formal critical care transfer training (ICS, 2019). This is usually provided by regional Critical Care Networks. The learning this chapter provides supports the National Competency Framework for Registered Nurses in Adult Critical Care Step Two Competencies (Critical Care Networks-National Nurse Leads, 2015).

Critical care bed and repatriation

In 2000, the Department of Health's (DoH) publication titled *Comprehensive Critical Care* made planning for inter-hospital transfer of the critically ill patient mandatory at local, regional, and national level, with transport services organised and coordinated to deliver safe, efficient and timely inter-hospital transfer, of all critically ill or injured patients (DoH, 2000). To facilitate this, managed clinical networks were established with responsibility for the coordination and development of transfer services, within defined geographical areas. Changes to commissioning arrangements following the Health and Social Care Act 2012, led to a review of these clinical networks. The NHS Commissioning Board (NHS CB) concluded that clinical networks had been responsible for significant and sustained improvements in quality of patient care and outcomes.

A framework for the continued provision of clinical networks as Operational Delivery Networks (ODNs) was published, with a focus on the coordination of patient pathways between providers over a wide area to ensure access to specialist resources and expertise. Twenty critical care ODNs were established in England, Wales and Northern Ireland, with responsibility for the oversight of effective referral pathways and safe and effective transfer processes.

There is no recent published data that provides an accurate estimate of the scale of critical care transfers in England per annum, but historical data estimated 10,000 in Great Britain in 1988 and over 11,000 in 1994. Increasing centralisation of specialist services in the National Health Service (NHS) and the establishment of major trauma networks in the United Kingdom (UK) are likely to have accelerated demand for both emergency transfers to access specialist resources and subsequent repatriation to the referring hospital for ongoing care. Pandemics such as the ongoing SARS-CoV-2 outbreak will also see exponential increases in non-clinical critical care transfers, both regionally and nationally, when units come under strain and demand exceeds supply.

In England, the responsibility for implementing these standards is devolved to regional Critical Care Networks. The ICS guidelines recommend that critical care networks should consider whether the development and use of dedicated transport teams is appropriate to best meet the transport needs of their patient population.

There are several instances when such management may be followed by further (secondary) transfer to another acute hospital:

- Clinical transfer: when the facilities needed for definitive treatment are not available at the initial hospital.
- Capacity transfer: when the initial hospital has inadequate equipment, bed capacity, staffing or monitoring to provide the necessary care.
- Repatriation: highly specialised hospitals may need to transfer patients to ensure they can treat the next patient who needs their specialist facilities. Patients

may also be moved back to hospitals nearer to their home and family. In these cases, patients will have had their specialist treatment and are almost always stable. The transfer may involve a step-down in the level of their care.

Orange Flag

Effective and open communication is key to establishing effective relationships with critically unwell patients, their family, and friends. Critical care transfer is a worrying event that is usually happening because of deterioration i.e. a head CT, or diagnostics processes for further treatment, or possibly to a referral centre for specialist treatment. Transfer has its own risks so critical care nurses must ensure they consider and alleviate the psychological impact this will have on people that don't understand what's happening.

Commonly used transfer terms are established in Table 30.1.

Table 30.1 Commonly used transfer terms.

Adult	Patient more than 18 yr of age
Critically ill	Patient requiring a level of care greater than that normally available on a standard ward (ICS level of care 1–3)
Primary transfer	Movement of patients from scene of injury or illness, to the nearest receiving hospital
Extended primary transfer	Movement of a patient from the scene of injury or illness to a specialist centre or trauma centre, bypassing the nearest hospital to reach a centre more appropriate to the needs of the patient
Secondary transfer	Movement of a patient from any hospital facility (emergency department/ward/critical care facility/operating theatre) to another centre
'Clinical' transfer	Patient transfer for speciality treatment or investigation not provided at referring hospital
'Capacity' transfer	Patient transfer for specialist treatment or investigation normally provided at referring hospital, but which is not currently available. The use of the term 'non-clinical transfer' should be avoided. Transfers for capacity reasons may still be clinically necessary and are sometimes critical
Repatriation	Patient transferred back to referring hospital or a hospital nearer the patient's home address
Inter-hospital transfer	Transfer of a patient between hospitals
Intra-hospital transfer	Transfer of a patient between areas/departments within the same hospital site

The risks of critical care transfer

Concerns regarding the safety of these transfers have been expressed for many years and variability in service provision exists despite the publication of national recommendations. The key elements of safe transfer involve decisions to transfer, communication, pre-transfer stabilisation and preparation, choosing the appropriate mode of transfer, i.e., land transport or air transport, personnel accompanying the patient, equipment and monitoring required during the transfer, and finally, the documentation and handover of the patient at the receiving facility. These key elements should be followed in each transfer to prevent any adverse events which may severely affect the patient prognosis.

Medical staff report a difficulty or complication during two thirds of intra-hospital transfers. Incident reporting has shown that one third of inter-hospital complications result in adverse outcomes including major physiological derangement (15%), patient/relative dissatisfaction (7%), prolonged hospital stays (4%), psychological injury (3%), and death (2%). The authors believed these events are under-reported and the true incidence of complications to be higher. Clinicians do not routinely undertake any other work with such a high rates of potential patient harm. Reassuringly, outcomes can be improved, and adverse incidents reduced with careful patient selection, transfer planning and equipment preparation, and, reassuringly, most (52–91%) of these incidents are preventable.

A hospital critical care department has a large team with experts and equipment on hand to help interventions, but clearly these are not available in transit. Transfers involve small teams working in isolation, and these teams are often unfamiliar with each other and the patient. Common management issues with communication and liaison between the ICU and sites of destination or origin have been identified as risks to patient safety.

A clear structure of governance is essential for safe practice and stressed by the Association of Anaesthetists Great Britain and Northern Ireland (AAGBI), Royal College of Anaesthetists (RCoA) and Intensive Care Society (ICS). The RCoA outlines that each Trust and Critical Care Network should have a designated consultant who is responsible for transfers, guideline production, training, documentation, data capture and audit, encouraging best practice and standardisation of protocols, equipment and documentation.

6Cs: Commitment

A commitment to our patients is a cornerstone of what we do with the ability to always improve the care and experience of our patients on critical care transfers. This commitment should be to adhere to all of the 6s and specifically in critical care transfers it should be to gain competency before undertaking a critical care transfer and to continuously refresh and upskill competency through training and reflection.

Transfer places burdens on both the preparing and remaining staff. Transfer must not jeopardise other patients or work within the hospital. Admission and transfer delays are independently associated with ICU morbidity and mortality and must be kept to a minimum.

Accompanying staff must be safely and promptly returned to their base after transfer, although it should be noted that the transferring platform may not always be able to fulfil this task. Late finishes need to be acknowledged with rest times observed. A dedicated transfer service has many advantages and is the preferred method of transferring patients requiring specialist treatment or who require prolonged transport.

The transfer process can be broken down as shown in Table 30.2.

Roles and responsibilities for critical care transfers are shown in Table 30.3.

Table 30.2   The transfer process.

1	Identify need to transfer a patient
2	Agreement between referring and accepting senior clinicians
3	Handover from critical care staff to transfer team
4	Transfer between care facilities
5	Handover from transfer team to accepting team
6	Return transfer team and equipment to base

Table 30.3   Roles and responsibilities for critical care transfers.

Referring Critical Care Consultant
- To give comprehensive verbal handover to the receiving critical care consultant
- Ensure accompanying doctor is familiar with the patient's condition and history and suitably trained
- Ensure written documentation is completed
- Maintain full responsibility for the patient until handover has been complete at the receiving hospital.

Referring Specialist Consultant
- To give comprehensive verbal handover to the receiving specialist consultant
- Ensure written documentation is complete

Nurse Lead on Transferring Unit
- To find an appropriate bed to transfer to
- To organise transfer
- Ensure accompanying nurse is familiar with the patient's condition and history and is suitably trained
- Ensure all written documentation is complete
- Telephone the receiving unit when the patient is leaving

457

(Continued)

Table 30.3 (Continued)

Transferring Team (Doctor and Nurse)
• Maintain continuation of medical and nursing treatments and cares throughout the transfer
• Ensure all equipment required for transfer is available and in full working order
• Complete transfer documentation throughout the transfer
• Give a full and comprehensive handover to the receiving team
• Take appropriate part of transfer form and place in the patient's notes at the transferring hospital
• Complete the online audit at the destination hospital once the patient is handed over
Ambulance Crew
• To provide a safe, appropriate transfer of patient and staff from the transferring to receiving hospital
• Ensure requested equipment/gases are available within the vehicle
• Ensure that ambulance is fully stocked with functional, standard equipment
• Return the trolley and transferring team to the referring hospital
Receiving Critical Care Medical Staff
• Accept referral and verbal handover from referring critical care consultant
• Accept full responsibility for the patient following handover from the transferring doctor
• Sign transfer form including any appropriate comments
Receiving Specialist Consultant
• Accept referral and verbal handover from referring specialist consultant
• Visit and assess the patient as soon as possible following the transfer
Receiving Nurse
• Accept full nursing responsibility for the patient following handover from the transferring nurse

Table 30.4 MINT mnemonic entails considerations for personnel, equipment, and transportation methods/modes. *Source:* Malpass et al., 2012.

M	Medical	• Doctor • Advanced practitioner • Grade required (consultant/registrar/advanced practitioner/trainee advanced practitioner)
I	Instrumentation	• Transfer bag – Preferably set out in ABCDE approach • Alternative oxygen delivery means (bag-valve mask or a Mapleson circuit) • Oxygen cylinders (calculate requirements) • Advanced airway (endotracheal tube/tracheostomy/surgical airway kit) • Suction • Invasive and noninvasive ventilator • Monitors (ECG, NiBP, arterial, CVP, capnography, SpO2, BG, temperature) • Defibrillator (with externally pacing) • Syringe drivers with a spare device • Additional device batteries • Drugs (both maintenance and emergency) • Fluids (crystalloids including hypertonic saline or mannitol; colloids including blood products)
N	Nursing	• Nurse (ITU, ED, CCOR, CCU)? • Operating department practitioner (ODP)? • Paramedic?
T	Transportation	• Certified bed/trolley for transfer • Patient transport service • Blue light double crewed ambulance (paramedic +/− emergency care assistant or a technician) • Air ambulance (including land ambulance transfer at base and destination)? • Expected journey time?

Preparation for transfer

Preparation for transfer can be and is a dauntingly demanding experience, even for those more experienced medical professionals. By using mnemonics such as seen in Table 30.4 (time permitting), health professionals can be sure that the transfer is well thought through, minimising the risk of error, however, in some situations, a 'scoop and run' approach may be necessary for time-critical transfers. This applies for both intra and inter-hospital transfers.

ABCDE process during critical care transfer

Airway

A secure airway is paramount for a safe transfer. A patient who is maintaining their own airway must be assessed to ensure there is no risk of deterioration from a neurological or physical perspective.

If there is any doubt about the safety of the airway, it should be secured and protected for transfer. Intubated patients must be sedated, have muscle relaxants administered and be established on the transfer ventilator.

Endo-tracheal tube (ETT) position must be confirmed by $EtCO_2$, chest auscultation and CXR. The tube must be secured and the length of the tube at the lips or incisors recorded.

Patients with tracheostomy must also have the above checks, as well as ensuring tracheal dilators, spare tracheostomy tubes the same size, and the size below are immediately available.

In transit, intubation/reintubation is suboptimal in the extreme and should be avoided by anticipating potential decline and taking all precautions in securing tracheal tubes (avoiding tube ties with neurological transfers). However, equipment to intubate and staff with advanced airway skills must be present on the transfer (Intensive Care Society, 2019). Before transfer, tracheal tube placement should be checked, radiologically confirmed (with images transferred to the receiving hospital) and recorded.

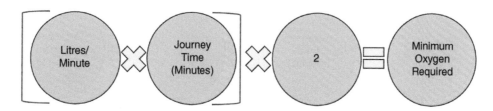

Figure 30.3 Oxygen calculations for the spontaneously breathing patient.

Red Flag: Cushing's Triad

When on a critical transfer with a patient with a traumatic brain injury (TBI) it is important to be aware of worsening deterioration. Cushing's triad refers to a set of signs that are indicative of increased intracranial pressure (ICP), or increased pressure in the brain. Cushing's triad consists of bradycardia (also known as a low heart rate), irregular respirations, and a widened pulse pressure.

Breathing

Care should be taken to ensure that ventilation is optimal, whether spontaneous or mechanical. Patients must be established on adequate ventilation prior to transfer, an arterial blood gas will confirm this. Spontaneously breathing patients must be stable, with no increase in work of breathing or oxygen requirements.

Ventilated patients should be stable on the transfer ventilator prior to transfer. Mode of ventilation including ventilation settings, oxygen requirements, tidal volume, respiratory rate, end-tidal CO_2 ($EtCO_2$) and sats must be recorded. 'Peg' saturation probes can be temperamental so consider either ear or single-use adhesive probes.

Red Flag: Hypoxia

Hypoxaemia is reduced arterial oxygen tension (below 8 kPa). Hypoxia is an inadequate oxygen supply to the tissues. Hypoxaemia can result from a ventilation/perfusion (V/Q) mismatch, anatomical (intrapulmonary, intracardiac) shunt, diffusion limitation, and/or hypoventilation. In clinical practice, a combinati:n of these factors is usually responsible. On critical care transfer it is imperative that oxygen tubing and oxygen cylinders are checked and safe to use and that spares are available.

Any pneumothoraces must be identified, decompressed and drained prior to transfer. The chest drain must remain in situ for the duration of the transfer. They should not be clamped and kept below the level of the patient to prevent re-accumulation of pneumothoraces.

Table 30.5 Oxygen cylinder capacities.

Cylinder size	Cylinder capacity (when full)
D	340
E	680
F	1360

Oxygen requirements should be calculated prior to transfer. It is prudent to anticipate that the patient's oxygen requirements may rise during transfer due to the supine position required for transfer, atelectasis caused by the upward pressure on the abdominal contents and diaphragm and acceleration forces affecting pulmonary blood flow. Therefore, the recommended minimum amount of oxygen taken on transfer should be calculated as twice the expected journey time (or if it is less than 1 hour, then you should take a minimum of 1 hour). See Table 30.5 and Figures 30.3 to 30.5 for cylinder capacities and oxygen calculations for both the spontaneously breathing and ventilated patient.

A critical care transfer bag with a bag-valve mask and Mapleson C circuit should be carried at all times in case of oxygen and/or ventilator failure.

Oxygen calculations – spontaneously breathing patient on face mask or nasal cannula oxygen

Example: A patient is requiring 40% (10 L/min) O_2 via venturi face mask. Journey time is 1 hour. Therefore: (10 L/min × 60 minutes) × 2 = 1200 Litres of oxygen is required (1 × F size cylinder or 2 × E size cylinders).

Oxygen calculations – ventilated patient

First, work out the minute ventilation (and add on the ventilator driving gas which is ventilator-specific), e.g: 600 mL × 15 bpm = 9000 mL + 1000 mL. Therefore, the minute ventilation will be 10 litres per minute (Oxylog 2000 ventilators

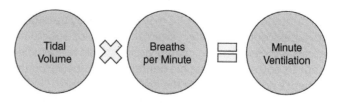

Figure 30.4 Minute volume calculation.

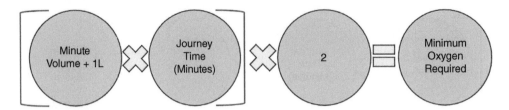

Figure 30.5 Oxygen calculation for the ventilated patient.

use approximately 1000 mL/min driving gas). Now that the MV is known, this needs to be calculated to double the journey time.

Example: For a 1-hour journey, this would calculate as: (10 L × 60 min) × 2 = 1200 litres of oxygen will be required (1 × F size cylinder or 2 × E size cylinders).

Circulation

Patients should be resuscitated and stabilised prior to transfer (but may be required en route in the case of time-critical inter-hospital transfers). A thorough assessment that includes heart rate, blood pressure, quality of the pulses, peripheral perfusion, and capillary refill should be completed prior to transfer.

Red Flag: Bradycardia

Bradycardia in mechanically ventilated, critically ill patients may be an incidental finding or it may represent serious pathology. In mechanically ventilated patients, bradycardia is associated with a relatively limited differential diagnosis. After determining whether a patient's bradycardia is a sinus bradycardia or whether it is due to a brady-dysrhythmia, clinicians should quickly consider and treat the cause, these may be medication effects, conduction system disease, myocardial damage and metabolic or endocrinologic abnormalities.

Acceleration in the ambulance can cause blood to be forced towards the patient's feet, which decreases venous return and reduces cardiac output and blood pressure. Any patients with cardiovascular instability should have a fluid challenge administered and be reassessed following this. Remember – full patients travel better.

Secure adequate intravenous access must be obtained prior to transfer. At a minimum this should include two wide bore peripheral access but may require central venous access (note that femoral CVC may kink and may be difficult to access during transfer; internal jugular or subclavian access is preferable). The point of access should be identified prior to, and easily accessible during transfer, ideally on the patient's right side (due to the ambulance layout).

Non-invasive blood pressure monitoring is unreliable during road travel. Invasive blood pressure monitoring is required, arterial lines and transducers must be well secured and appropriately positioned. Non-invasive blood pressure cuff should be in place pretransfer in case of arterial blood pressure failure.

Inotropes and or vasopressors may be required during transfer.

Medication management: noradrenaline

Because noradrenaline acts primarily via α1 receptors, it is usually used as a vasopressor (increasing systemic vascular resistance to maintain mean arterial blood pressure) rather than an inotrope. It is often used with other inotropes, such as dobutamine, to maintain adequate perfusion. Noradrenaline (norepinephrine) should only be administered as an intravenous infusion via a central venous catheter to minimise the risk of extravasation and subsequent tissue necrosis. Noradrenaline (norepinephrine) should be infused at a controlled rate using an infusion pump.

Medication management: adrenaline

Adrenaline has activity at all adrenergic receptors (predominantly acting as a β agonist in low doses and an α agonist at higher doses); other more specific inotropes are often preferred over adrenaline. Adrenaline is used mainly during resuscitation after cardiac arrest (in this case it is given as a bolus). It is not recommended for use in cardiogenic shock because of metabolic side effects, including hyperlactataemia and hyperglycaemia.

Medication management: isoprenaline

Isoprenaline is predominantly a β1 agonist and therefore increases cardiac contractility and heart rate. It also acts at β2 receptors causing vasodilation and decreases afterload. Because of this vasodilation, and to ensure adequate MAP is achieved, it may be necessary to administer dobutamine in combination with a vasopressor (eg, noradrenaline). The main side effects of Isoprenaline are increased heart rate, arrhythmias and raised myocardial oxygen demand which can cause myocardial ischaemia. Isoprenaline has a similar profile to dobutamine but tends to cause more tachycardia. It is sometimes used for bradycardic patients requiring inotropic support.

Inotropes should be attached to and running on a dedicated CVC lumen, they must be clearly labelled, easy to titrate, and be attached to a fully charged pump that is easily accessible. Drug giving sets must be positioned appropriately to ensure they are not pulling or under pressure. Pumps must be stowed safely underneath the transfer trolley. Transfer trolleys usually have space or 3 or an absolute maximum of 4 infusion pumps. Drugs that are a priority for level 3 transfers are sedation, analgesia and inotropes or vasopressors. Drugs such as neuromuscular blockade agents can be given as a bolus, while drugs which are not immediately required such as actrapid or TPN should be detached. Drug calculations must be calculated prior to transfer to ensure there is sufficient supply for the transfer, including any unforeseen circumstances (such as a broken lift, route diversion, or breakdown). Drugs must be calculated to last double the journey time, or a minimum of one hour. Drugs that are being infused at high rates can be concentrated to double or quadruple the concentration. If undertaking international transfers, it is important to be aware of restrictions related to taking controlled drugs across international borders. Any non-essential infusions such as electrolytes, insulin and feed should be discontinued for transfer.

Medication management: catecholamines

The most used inotropes are the catecholamines; these can be endogenous (eg, adrenaline, noradrenaline) or synthetic (e.g. dobutamine, isoprenaline). These medicines act on the sympathetic nervous system. Most commonly their cardiac effects are attributed to stimulation of alpha- and beta-adrenergic receptors (specifically $\alpha 1$, $\beta 1$, and $\beta 2$). However, this is a simplification: there are several subtypes of $\alpha 1$ receptors as well as $\alpha 2$, $\beta 3$ and various dopaminergic receptors that are involved.

Ideally blood products should be administered prior to transfer but appropriate blood products should be transported with the patient. If they are not used, they should be returned to the referring hospital's laboratory; a pre-transfusion sample may be useful for the receiving lab.

Specialist equipment including balloon pump, intracerebral pressure monitoring, pacing equipment, etc. should be discussed on a patient-by-patient basis.

Disability

Awake patients should be assessed to ensure there is no or minimal risk of neurological deterioration. Pain should be well controlled and analgesia available to be administered while en route if required. If opiates are being utilised, naloxone should also be available.

Ventilated patients must have adequate sedation (Propofol) as a continuous infusion and an opioid (e.g. morphine, fentanyl, alfentanil, or remifentanil depending on local practice and personal experience) for analgesia and should be titrated to response. Periods of increased stimuli during transfer should be preempted. Use of neuromuscular blockade agents is often advantageous during transfer to prevent coughing, line or tube misplacement and raised intracranial pressure.

Blood glucose should be checked prior to transfer and during specific circumstances. Ideally patients should not require administration of glucose or insulin during transfer, but if that is the case, a mode of checking blood glucose should be available intra-transfer.

Seizures should be controlled prior to transfer, and a strategy for treatment of raised intracranial pressure (hypertonic saline or mannitol) agreed upon in conjunction with the receiving specialist centre.

It may be simpler to administer routine medications/feed, either before or after transfer, if appropriate, to limit the number of lines and infusions.

Exposure

The patient should be exposed prior to transfer to ensure no injuries or clinical signs have been missed. The trauma patient should have their cervical spine, pelvic and long bone fractures immobilised as appropriate. All drains and lines should be securely fixed in place. There is an increased risk of hypothermia during transfer, so ensure that uncovering of the patient is limited and heat loss considered (e.g. vacuum mattresses, blankets, bubble wrap, active warming have all been used). Continuous temperature monitoring is recommended. For a full A–E assessment, including likely considerations at each phase, please see Table 30.6.

Consideration also needs to be taken regarding the transfer team using the mnemonic PERSONAL which encompasses considerations such as communications devices and contact numbers, money, clothing/personal protective equipment (PPE), planned route, staff food and mode of return transport. This can is demonstrated in Table 30.7.

An important aspect of transfer is liaising with the ambulance service to ensure the effective coordination of the transfer and the time frame appropriate to the type of transfer is requested. Local ambulance services have protocols for category of transfer and response. This should be confirmed by the referring hospital (Figures 30.6 and 30.7).

Table 30.6 A–E approach and considerations pre-transfer. *Source:* Malpass et al., 2012.

A	Airway(with C spine)	• Is the patient self-ventilating or invasively ventilated?
		• Is the endotracheal/tracheostomy secure and patent?
		  • Migration (what level is the endotracheal at the lips)?
		  • Cuff inflation pressure (is there a leak)?
		• Does the patient require immobilisation, with a vacuum mattress, scoop stretcher, or long spine board equivalent, cervical collar and/or head blocks and tape?

B	Breathing(with ventilation)	• Breathing assessment including auscultation and a chest X-ray • Chest drains below the level of the heart and secured? They are not pulling and ensuring they are swinging, draining or bubbling? • What is the ventilation mode (BiPAP, SIMV, PS, CPAP) is the patient including settings (RR, Tidal/Minute volume, FiO_2)? • Ventilator tubing secured? • Is there CO_2 capnography? • Has there been a blood gas within the last 15 minutes before departure whilst on the transport ventilator? • Does the blood gas show adequate oxygenation/ventilation? (If not, can this be optimised?) • What are the calculated oxygen requirements?

C	Circulation(with haemorrhage control)	• Cardiovascular assessment including inotropic support (which inotrope, strength, rate and mcg/kg/min)
		• What are the calculated infusion requirements?
		• Are there any haemorrhage concerns?
		  • Does any coagulopathy need to be reversed?
		  • Does the patient require blood products for transfer?
		• All monitoring leads (ECG, Invasive/Non-Invasive BP, SpO_2) are running centrally along the patient and will not cause skin damage?
		  • Are they on and all working?
		• All IV, CVC and arterial lines secure and are accessible from the patient's right-hand side
		  • at least two IVs accessible?
		• Have all non-essential infusions been detached?
		• Are there IV bolus fluids attached?
		• Urinary catheter is running centrally down the patient?

D	Disability(with neurological control)	• Neurological assessment including pupils, Blood glucose and noting any seizure activity? • Is the patient 15–30 degrees head up? • ETT ties appropriate if suspected raised intracranial pressure • Has secondary neurological injury prevention been considered? • Is the patient adequately sedated? • Are muscle relaxants required? • Are anticonvulsants required?
E	Exposure(with temperature regulation)	• Are there any patient temperature concerns? • Does the patient require active or passive warming or cooling? • Have all attempts of minimising pressure damage been considered? • Have all wounds been dressed? • Is the patient secured to the stretcher and stretcher secured to the ambulance?

Table 30.7 PERSONAL mnemonic.

P	Phone	• Is it a personal mobile? • Is it charged, and do you need a charging cable?
E	Enquiry number and name	• Do you have the receiving unit's phone number and the name of the receiving consultant? • Do you have your consultants phone number in case of emergency and requiring advice/help en route?
R	Revenue	• Has the transfer team got money in case of an emergency or a return taxi is required?
S	Safe clothing	• Has everyone got high visibility clothing? • Are there sufficient gloves, aprons, eye protection for personal protection? COVID PPE? • Warm clothing?
O	Organised route	• What is the route? • Is there a backup route in case of obstruction? • Do you have the correct hospital site?
N	Nutrition	• Is there food and water for the transfer team (if a prolonged transfer)?
A	A-Z map	• Is there one? • If using GPS, do you have the correct postcode?
L	Lift Home	• Is the ambulance bringing the team home? • Proposed method of returning to base location? • What if the ambulance gets re-diverted on the way back?

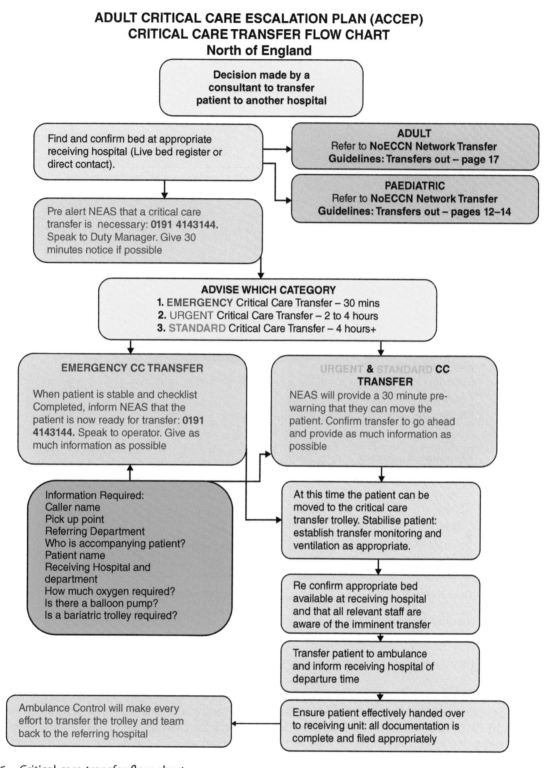

ADULT CRITICAL CARE ESCALATION PLAN (ACCEP)
CRITICAL CARE TRANSFER FLOW CHART
North of England

Decision made by a consultant to transfer patient to another hospital

Find and confirm bed at appropriate receiving hospital (Live bed register or direct contact).

ADULT
Refer to NoECCN Network Transfer Guidelines: Transfers out – page 17

PAEDIATRIC
Refer to NoECCN Network Transfer Guidelines: Transfers out – pages 12–14

Pre alert NEAS that a critical care transfer is necessary: **0191 4143144.** Speak to Duty Manager. Give 30 minutes notice if possible

ADVISE WHICH CATEGORY
1. EMERGENCY Critical Care Transfer – 30 mins
2. URGENT Critical Care Transfer – 2 to 4 hours
3. STANDARD Critical Care Transfer – 4 hours+

EMERGENCY CC TRANSFER
When patient is stable and checklist Completed, inform NEAS that the patient is now ready for transfer: **0191 4143144.** Speak to operator. Give as much information as possible

URGENT & STANDARD CC TRANSFER
NEAS will provide a 30 minute pre-warning that they can move the patient. Confirm transfer to go ahead and provide as much information as possible

Information Required:
Caller name
Pick up point
Referring Department
Who is accompanying patient?
Patient name
Receiving Hospital and department
How much oxygen required?
Is there a balloon pump?
Is a bariatric trolley required?

At this time the patient can be moved to the critical care transfer trolley. Stabilise patient: establish transfer monitoring and ventilation as appropriate.

Re confirm appropriate bed available at receiving hospital and that all relevant staff are aware of the imminent transfer

Transfer patient to ambulance and inform receiving hospital of departure time

Ambulance Control will make every effort to transfer the trolley and team back to the referring hospital

Ensure patient effectively handed over to receiving unit: all documentation is complete and filed appropriately

Figure 30.6 Critical care transfer flow chart.

463

TRANSFER CHECKLIST HANDOVER

Airway ETT Intubation grade Indication for intubation **Breathing** FiO2 Ventilator settings CXR ABG **Circulation** Access Fluids / output CV support / inotropes **Disability / drugs** GCS and pupils Glucose / temperature Antibiotics Insulin / infusions **Exposure / equipment** Infusions labelled Log roll Drains Other	Date of admission: Date of transfer: Patient details Affix sticker **Patient** PMH Medication Allergies **Problem** PC / HPC Diagnosis Examination / key findings Investigation results Critical incidents **Plan** Surgical LMWH / UFH Antibiotics Drains Feeding Family aware Outstanding issues Targets MAP UO PaO$_2$ PaCO$_2$

Consultant critical care _____   Parent speciality consultant _____

Figure 30.7 Transfer checklist handover.

Snapshot 1

Patient T is a 45-year-old female who has been in intensive care for 6 days due to community-acquired pneumonia. She had a tracheostomy performed on Day 4 of her stay. She has not required sedation or inotropes since then. She is ventilated on CPAP ASB, PEEP 10, PS 10 on 35% oxygen. She has been delirious but is calm and following commands. The rehabilitation practitioner has suggested a trip outside into the fresh air to aid her recovery.

Suitability for transfer

Patient T is ventilated via a tracheostomy. However, she is on single organ support and her oxygen requirement is low. As per ICS Guidelines (2021) she is deemed high risk and should therefore be accompanied by a nurse and an advanced practitioner or doctor. Although she is classified as high risk, she is clinically stable and the benefit of the transfer to the outdoors to her recovery justifies this risk

Risk assessment

A transfer to the outdoors raises considerations that other transfers may not. A risk assessment of the environment to ensure its suitability and how this may change in different weather conditions should be undertaken (e.g. will the surface become slippery when wet). The patient may need extra equipment such as blankets, sun cream or a sun hat. Emergency equipment must be readily available and the ability to contact the intensive care unit in case of

Checklist
A transfer checklist should be completed as per any inter-hospital transfer, see ICS example.

1. Is the patient stable for transport?

Airway	Tick
• Airway safe or secured by intubation?	
• Tracheal tube position confirmed on chest x-ray?	
Ventilation	**Tick**
• Adequate spontaneous respiration or ventilation established on transport ventilator?	
• Adequate gas exchange confirmed by arterial blood gas?	
• Sedated and paralysed as appropriate?	
Circulation	**Tick**
• Heart rate, BP optimised?	
• Tissue and organ perfusion adequate?	
• Any obvious blood loss controlled?	
• Circulating blood volume restored?	
• Haemoglobin adequate?	
• Minimum of two routes of venous access?	
• Arterial line and central venous access if appropriate?	
Neurology	**Tick**
• Seizures controlled, metabolic causes excluded?	
• Raised intracranial pressure appropriately managed?	
Trauma	**Tick**
• Cervical spine protected?	
• Pneumothoraces drained?	
• Intra-thoracic and intra-abdominal bleeding controlled?	
• Intra-abdominal injuries adequately investigated and appropriately managed?	
• Long bone/pelvic fractures stabilised?	
Metabolic	**Tick**
• Blood glucose > 4 mmol/L	
• Potassium < 6 mmol/L	
• Ionised calcium > 1 mmol/L	
• Acid-base balance acceptable	
• Temperature maintained	
Monitoring	**Tick**
• ECG	
• Blood pressure	
• Oxygen saturations	
• End-tidal carbon dioxide	
• Temperature	

2. Are you ready for departure?

Patient	Tick
• Stable on transport trolley?	
• Appropriately monitored?	
• All infusions running and lines adequately secured and labelled?	
• Adequately sedated and paralysed?	
• Adequately secured on trolley?	
• Adequately wrapped to prevent heat loss?	

Staff	Tick
• Transfer risk assessment completed?	
• Staff adequately trained and experienced?	
• Received appropriate handover?	
• Adequately clothed and insured?	

Equipment	Tick
• Appropriately equipped ambulance?	
• Appropriate equipment and drugs?	
• Pre-drawn up medication syringes appropriately labelled and capped?	
• Batteries checked (spare batteries available)?	
• Sufficient oxygen supplies for anticipated journey?	
• Portable phone charged and available?	
• Money for emergencies?	

Organisation	Tick
• Case notes, X-rays, results, blood collected?	
• Transfer documentation prepared?	
• Location of bed and receiving doctor known?	
• Receiving unit advised of departure time and estimated time of arrival?	
• Telephone numbers of referring and receiving units available?	
• Relatives informed and information provided?	
• Return travel arrangements in place?	
• Ambulance crew briefed?	

Departure	Tick
• Patient trolley secured?	
• Electrical equipment plugged into ambulance power supply where available?	
• Ventilator transferred to ambulance oxygen supply?	
• All equipment safely mounted and stowed?	
• Staff seated and wearing seatbelts?	

Preparation

A – Patient T has a size 8 tracheostomy in situ. The stoma is 3 days old. Spare tracheostomy tubes the same size and the size below with tracheal dilators should be added to the transfer bag.

B – Patient T should be transferred onto the transfer ventilator at least 30 minutes before the outside transfer and a blood gas taken to confirm adequate ventilation. Monitoring must include $EtCO_2$, saturations, respiratory rate and tidal volumes.

C – Patient T has not required cardiovascular support for 3 days. IV access should be secured and transferring staff aware of where the access is in case of an emergency. Monitoring should include NIBP and continuous ECG.

D – Patient T is recovering from delirium and is calm and co-operative, there is no need to sedate her for this transfer. Her blood glucose should be checked on the blood gas.

E – Patient T's privacy and dignity must be maintained throughout the transfer. Blankets and or sun hats should be considered depending on the weather conditions.

Equipment required

Transfer bag with extra tracheostomy equipment added, transfer monitor, spare tracheostomy tubes, suction.

Staff

A nurse or ODP and a Dr or advanced practitioner who are transfer trained will go on the transfer.

Learning points

- Facilitating critical care patients spending time outside improves their physical and mental health and recovery
- Same principles of patient selection, risk assessment and preparation
- Considerations of transferring a patient with a tracheostomy
- Guidelines on Transfer of Critically Ill Patients to the Outdoors (ICS, 2021)

Snapshot 2

Patient W is a 62-year-old lady who was found collapsed by her neighbor. She was fetched into the Emergency Department by ambulance. Her GCS was 3 and she has been intubated and ventilated. Her CT scan shows a large subarachnoid haemorrhage. She has been accepted by the neurosurgeons at a tertiary centre 45 minutes away.

He past medical history is hypertension and hyperlipidaemia. He takes ramipril 5 mg od and atorvastatin 40 mg on.

Suitability for transfer

Patient W requires life-saving intervention. The transfer is time-critical and needs to happen as soon as possible. A team approach to preparation for transfer is required to achieve this.

Risk assessment

The risks of not doing the transfer immediately outweigh the risks of the transfer. Communication between the two centres and the ambulance service is a key factor of this transfer.

Checklist

Although this transfer is time-critical a checklist should be completed to ensure safety and efficiency.

Preparation

A – Patient W is intubated with a size 7.5 ETT that is 22 cm at the lips. The tube has been taped rather than tied to ensure good venous drainage. A CXR confirming correct position, $EtCO_2$ trace and chest auscultation must be performed prior to transfer.

B – Patient W is on the transfer ventilator. Targets for ventilating a patient with a head injury are a $PaO_2 > 13$ kpa and $PaCO_2$ 4.5–5 kpa. Respiratory rate and tidal volume and FiO_2 should be altered to achieve this.

C – This transfer is time-critical. Insertion of a central line can be time-consuming. A minimum of two large-bore peripheral venous accesses should be secured. Peripheral vasopressors can be bolused as required en route. If central access is obtained it should be femoral rather than internal jugular to ensure good venous drainage. An arterial line should be inserted as NiBP is unreliable in transit, a target MAP of > 80 mmHg should be maintained. Continuous ECG monitoring will be in place.

D – A sedative agent should be infused throughout the transfer. Neuromuscular blockade should be administered prior to transfer and boluses given en route as required. Blood glucose should be checked and be between 6 and 10 mmol/L.

E – Check for signs of other injuries, these should be recorded but not necessarily dealt with if they are not life-threatening. Mrs W should be catheterised for the transfer. The head of the transfer trolley should be raised to > 30 degrees.

Equipment
Transfer trolley, transfer bag, transfer ventilator, infusion of sedation/analgesia, boluses of vasopressors and neuromuscular blockades.

Staff
A nurse or ODP and an advanced practitioner or a Dr with advanced airway skills will transfer the patient.

Learning points
- Time-critical transfers require team working and clear communication.
- Patients with intracranial pathology require tight control of ventilation and blood pressure to prevent secondary brain injury.
- Procedures that are time-consuming should not delay the transfer.
- Ensure scans/X-rays are transferred to the receiving hospital.

Snapshot 3

Patient Z is a 74-year-old man who has been in intensive care for 6 days following an emergency laparotomy for bowel ischaemia with perforation. He has remained on multi-organ support during his ITU stay. Currently he is ventilated, on a noradrenaline infusion and on CVVH due to AKI. His culture results are negative, and a CT scan is required to look for a source of intra-abdominal sepsis. You have received a phone call informing you the scan has been arranged for 20 minutes.

Suitability for transfer
Patient Z is on multi-organ support so the transfer will be complex. However, the transfer can be conducted safely, but the time frame for the CT scan of 20 minutes is unrealistic as Mr Z needs to be disconnected from his CVVH machine. The first consideration is to negotiate a more suitable time slot with the radiology department.

Risk assessment
Discontinuing a patient's renal replacement treatment is not without risk. However, a transfer to CT should be a quick transfer and he can recommence the treatment as soon as he is back on the unit. Communication with the radiology department will also minimise risk and the transfer should be coordinated so he does not have to wait in the radiology department.

Checklist
A transfer checklist should be completed.

Preparation
A – Patient Z is ventilated via an ETT and its correct placement confirmed. The tube should be well secured.

B – Patient Z is ventilated on a volume-controlled mode of ventilation. He should be established on the transfer ventilator on the same settings for 30 minutes before the transfer and an arterial blood as taken to confirm adequate ventilation. ETCO and sats must be continuously monitored.

C – Patient Z is on noradrenaline 4 mg in 50 mL running at 8 mL/hr. There are 35 mL left in the syringe. A piggyback syringe should also be taken on transfer in anticipation of rising noradrenaline requirements. Continuous ECG and invasive blood pressure should be monitored.

D – Sedation and analgesia should continue, taking full syringes of each should be enough for a transfer to CT. A bolus of neuromuscular blockade agent should be administered, and a spare bolus taken on transfer. HIs blood glucose will be checked with the blood gas.

E – Vascath flushed and clearly labelled. Insulin and phosphate infusions discontinued. Patient identification band present. Notes including recent blood results and details of allergies available.

Staff
A nurse or ODP and an advanced practitioner or Doctor with advanced airway skills will go on the transfer.

6Cs: Compassion

Compassion is how care is given through relationships based on empathy, respect and dignity. Compassion can also be described as intelligent kindness and is central to how people perceive their care. All critical care transfers must have compassion at the core of the move. One approach is to ensure patients and their families are kept informed in all stages of the transfer process with appropriate contact numbers and rationale for the transfer.

Conclusion

Intra- and inter-hospital patient transfer is an important aspect of patient care which is often undertaken to improve upon the existing management of the patient and involves multiple professions working in collaboration to achieve a shared goal. That said, transferring critically ill patients is fraught with danger and leaves the patient and the transferring team at their most vulnerable due to limited resources both in terms of manpower, equipment, space and noise. The transferring team should be a team that are well trained in transferring critically ill adults and the patient should continue to receive high-quality care/therapies en route. Preparation is key to a successful transfer, and the use of mnemonics can aid the transferring team in accounting for every aspect of the transfer process. Communication must be of a high quality as failures in communication can hinder ongoing care and can be a detriment to the patient. Structured governance and audit are essential for best practice and to address recurring problems, as is maintaining individual competence through practice and continued professional development.

Take home points

1. Preparation for transfer is one of, if not the most important stage of the patients transfer journey and will determine if the transfer is a safe and successful one.

2. Plan for the unexpected to happen, and discuss contingency plans with the transfer team (including portering staff and or ambulance crew) so that everyone is clear about their roles in the event of them occurring.

3. Always ask yourself, 'Is this transfer needed?' and 'Is the patient safe for transfer in their current state?'

4. If travelling by land ambulance, ensure all equipment is stowed securely, oxygen is attached to the ambulance's oxygen supply, and that all electrical equipment is connected to mains power prior to setting off.

5. As a minimum, the transfer team's equipment should have at least twice the journey time or a minimum of one hour's supply of oxygen/drug infusions.

6. Ensure all patient notes accompany the patient (according to trust policy), including a transfer letter if transferring to a different hospital.

7. Ensure that the receiving unit are aware of your departure and expected time of arrival.

References

Bourn, S., Wijesingha, S., and Nordmann, G. (2018). Transfer of the critically ill adult patient. *British Journal of Anaesthesia Education* 18(3): 63–68.

Critical Care Networks-National Nurse Leads (CC3N) (2015). National Competency Framework for Registered Nurses in Adult Critical Care. Step 2 Competencies. https://www.cc3n.org.uk/uploads/9/8/4/2/98425184/02_new_step_2_final.pdf (accessed 3 August 2021).

Department of Health (UK) (2000). *Comprehensive Critical Care: A Review of Adult Critical Care Services*. London: DH. https://webarchieve.nationalarchives.gov.uk/+http://www.dh.gov.uk/en/PublicationsandStatistics/Publications/PublicationsPolicyAngGuidance/DH_4006585(accessed 31 August 2021).

Droogh, J.M., Smit, M., Hut, J. et al. (2012). Inter-hospital transport of critically ill patients; expect surprises. *Critical Care* 16(1): R26.

Droogh, J.M., Smit, M., Absalom, A.R. et al. (2015). Transferring the critically ill patient: Are we there yet?' *Critical Care* 19(62): 1–7.

Flabouris, A., Runciman, W.B., Levings, B. (2006). Incidents during out-of-hospital patient transportation. *Anaesthesia and Intensive Care* 34(2): 228–236.

Grier, S., Brant, G., and Gould, T.H. (2020). Critical care transfer in an English critical care network: Analysis of 1124 transfers delivered by an ad-hoc system. *Journal of the Intensive Care Society* 21(1): 33–39. doi:10.1177/1751143719832175.

Intensive Care Society (ICS) (2019). *Guidelines for the Transport of the Critically Ill Adult*. London: The Intensive Care Society.

Intensive Care Society (ICS) (2021). *Guidance On: Transfer of Criticaly Ill Patients to the Outdoors*. https://ww.baccn.org/static/uploads/resources/Transfer_outdoors_guidance_final.pdf (accessed 24 August 2021).

Kulshrestha, A. and Singh, J. (2016). Inter-hospital and intra-hospital patient transfer: Recent concepts. *Indian Journal of Anaesthesia* 60(7): 451–457. doi: 10.4103/0019-5049.186012.

Malpass, H.C., Enfield, K.B., and Verghese, G.M. (2012). Interhospital intensive care transfer checklist facilitates early implementation of critical therapies and is associated with improved outcomes. *American Journal of Respiratory and Critical Care Medicine*. 131(23): 1–10.

NICE (2018). *Critical Care Transfers*. https://www.nice.org.uk/guidance/ng94/evidence/34.standardised-systems-of-care-for-intra-and-interhospital-transfers-pdf-172397464673 (accessed 22 May 2021).

Parmentier-Decrucq, E., Poissey, J., Favory, R. et al. (2013). Adverse events during intrahospital transfers of critically ill patients. *Annals of Intensive Care* 3(1): 1–10.

Chapter 31

Rehabilitation after critical illness

Helen Sanger and Clare L. Wade

Aim

This aim of this chapter is to provide the reader with an evidence-based understanding of rehabilitation during and after critical illness.

Learning outcomes

After reading this chapter the reader will be able to:

- Have a basic knowledge of the most common physical, psychological, and cognitive problems that result from critical illness.
- Be able to use a holistic model of functioning, such as the 'International Classification of Functioning, Disability and Health', to describe the complexity of sequelae of critical illness.
- Understand the importance of regular and comprehensive assessment, during and after critical illness.
- Understand the difficulties faced when attempting to treat these sequelae. In particular, the lack of evidence for any specific rehabilitation strategy.
- Have an awareness of the relevant national guidance in the UK, and the key recommendations and standards this contains.

Test your prior knowledge

- Can you describe the most common physical, psychological and cognitive sequelae of critical illness?
- The World Health Organization's International Classification of Functioning, Disability, and Health (ICF) describes a person's functioning in terms of their 'body functions and structures', and which other two domains?
- Why is it important to set rehabilitation goals, and who should set them?
- What are the key timepoints for assessment recommended by National Institute for Health and Care Excellence (NICE)?
- What are the four quality standards set out by the NICE in relation to Rehabilitation after Critical Illness?

Fundamentals of Critical Care: A Textbook for Nursing and Healthcare Students, First Edition. Edited by Ian Peate and Barry Hill.
© 2023 John Wiley & Sons Ltd. Published 2023 by John Wiley & Sons Ltd.
Companion website: www.wiley.com/go/peate/criticalcare

Introduction

This chapter discusses rehabilitation after critical illness (RaCI). That is, the support of physical, psychological, and cognitive problems arising from a period of critical illness.

Critical care mortality has significantly declined over the last decade and is now less than 15% of all admissions (Intensive Care National Audit and Research Centre (ICNARC), 2019). This has resulted in a growing population of individuals who have survived a period of critical illness (Zimmerman et al., 2013). In the United Kingdom (UK) alone, over 140,000 people were discharged alive from critical care in the year to April 2019, in comparison with under 75,000 in the same period to 2009 (ICNARC, 2010, 2019).

This survivorship is frequently characterised by long-term deficits in physical, cognitive and psychological health (Cuthbertson et al., 2010; Herridge et al., 2011; Pandharipande et al., 2013). These can vary from decreased physical function; severe anxiety or post-traumatic stress disorder relating to experiences on critical care; or decreased cognitive capacity, with difficulties concentrating or problem solving. The type and severity of morbidity will depend on various factors, but particularly, how fit and well that person was before their critical illness and the acuity and length of their critical illness (Herridge et al., 2011; Puthucheary et al., 2013).

Step 2 competencies: 2:8.1 contributing factors to rehabilitation needs and patient diaries

You must be able to demonstrate your knowledge using a rationale through discussion, and the application to your practice, the following:

- Reasons why specific health conditions, such as critical illness (of renal, cardiac, respiratory, or other origin), or trauma (including brain and spinal injuries), may cause ongoing rehabilitation needs in the critically ill.
- Demonstrate, understand and complete a short clinical assessment of a critically ill patient with regard to rehabilitation following their illness.
- Make swift referrals to appropriate multidisciplinary team members (on the basis of findings from short or comprehensive clinical assessment).
- Understand diversity issues and how they may impact on the patient's rehabilitation needs.
- Initiate (where used) and understand the benefits of patient diaries following critical illness.
- Be able to signpost to relevant resources available for critical care patients. Such as, rehabilitation teams, step-down follow-up visits, support with ongoing rehabilitation goals, follow-up clinics, local patient and relative information, peer-support groups, such as www.ICUSteps.org.

The impact of critical illness – what do we mean by morbidity?

Physical

The physical sequelae of critical illness are most commonly loss of skeletal muscle strength and endurance, with associated loss of function and independence (Herridge et al., 2011). NICE categorises 'physical morbidity' as: 'problems such as muscle loss, muscle weakness, musculoskeletal problems including contractures, respiratory problems, sensory problems, pain, and swallowing and communication problems' (NICE, 2009). The term 'intensive care unit acquired weakness' (ICU-AW) is used to refer to this presentation of global muscle loss and weakness. ICU-AW is discussed in more detail in Chapter 27. Those with ICU-AW take longer to wean from mechanical ventilation and have poorer long-term functional outcomes than those without (De Jonghe et al., 2002; Dinglas et al., 2017).

Psychological

NICE refers to psychological and cognitive problems together as 'non-physical morbidity', defining this as 'psychological, emotional and psychiatric problems, and cognitive dysfunction' (NICE, 2009). They are considered in turn here.

The psychological diagnoses most commonly reported following critical illness are anxiety, depression and post-traumatic stress disorder (Wade et al., 2012). Their incidence is reported as between 32% and 45% in people who have survived critical illness (Wade et al., 2012; Bein et al., 2019). As with physical health, pre-existing mental health problems are strongly associated with post-critical care psychological morbidity (Hatch et al., 2018; Bein et al., 2019). This psychological morbidity is associated with poorer functional outcomes following critical care, such as rates of returning to work, and even survival (Riddersholm et al., 2018). Individuals with depressive symptoms after critical illness are 47% more likely to die in the 2 years following critical care than those without (Hatch et al., 2018). Unlike ICU-AW, there is no correlation between acuity of illness or ICU length of stay and subsequent incidence of psychological illness.

Cognitive

Cognitive impairment, in the form of compromised global cognition (memory, attention, visuospatial construction and language) or executive functioning (essentially, problem solving), is present in up to 40% of critical care survivors, and can persist for many years (Iwashyna et al., 2010; Pandharipande et al., 2013; Müller et al., 2020). Delirium is associated with more severe cognitive impairment. The longer somebody has been delirious in ICU, the worse their cognition is afterwards (Müller et al., 2020).

Table 31.1   Five conditions that impact on rehabilitation.

5 conditions key to RaCI
Low mood
Dyspnoea
Dysphagia
Dysphonia
Short-term memory problems

In Pandharipande et al.'s seminal study of cognition in 821 patients 1 year after ICU discharge, 40% of them had a cognitive deficit equivalent to a moderate traumatic brain injury (1.5 standard deviations below population average), and 25% equivalent to mild Alzheimer's (2 standard deviations below population average) (Pandharipande et al., 2013).

See Table 31.1 for five conditions that impact on rehabilitation.

Describing physical functioning and morbidity

One of the challenges when considering RaCI, is the need for a holistic rather than individual-systems approach. If rehabilitation is to be person-centred, then it is impracticable to approach it organ system by organ system, as we might other areas of intensive care medicine. Instead, it is useful to consider the sequelae of critical illness in terms of how they impact that person's ability to engage in society, or their family life. There are many different holistic models of physical functioning, we briefly outline two of the most common ones here.

The World Health Organization (WHO) International Classification of Functioning, Disability and Health (ICF)

The ICF is the international standard for describing, recording and measuring functioning and disability created and recommended by the WHO (WHO, 2001). This frames any given health condition in terms of the impact it has on a person's 'body functions and structure' (their impairments), 'activity' (their activity limitations) and 'participation' (their restrictions). It also acknowledges that there will be both environmental and personal factors that influence that person's functioning, in the form of barriers or facilitators to functioning. Each of these factors has the ability to influence the others, and this interplay between environment, person, and disease describe that person's functioning in the context of the health condition considered. This interdependence is illustrated in Figure 31.1.

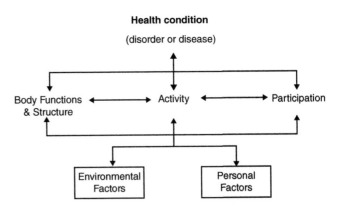

Figure 31.1   The WHO ICF. *Source:* Modified from ICF Education.

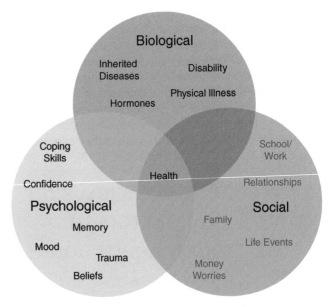

Figure 31.2   The biopsychosocial model. *Source:* Modified from National Health Service.

Biopsychosocial description of functioning

George Engel described an expansion of the traditional 'biomedical' model to include psychological and social factors, making it a 'biopsychosocial' model in the 1970s (Engel, 1977). This formed the basis for more complex models, such as the WHO ICF above, but remains worthy of note in its own right (Wade and Halligan, 2017). It is a simple reminder to all healthcare professionals that a person's functioning, and the impact of disease, must be considered in a holistic way – to include biological, psychological and social factors. It is often depicted visually as in Figure 31.2.

Snapshot

Stephen is a 41-year-old man who is being transferred to a general surgical ward today, following a 154 day stay on critical care.

- Initially admitted with necrotising pancreatitis, requiring necrosectomies.
- Mechanically ventilated for 126 days (initially OETT, then a tracheostomy).

- Weight on admission: 120 kg; weight on critical care discharge: 68 kg.
- Suffered with fluctuant delirium throughout critical care stay
- Has severe ICU-AW.
- Pre-admission Stephen lived with his wife, Tracey (a teacher) and daughter and son (aged 12 and 8), in a two-storey house. Tracey has had to take significant time off work during Stephen's illness.
- Pre-admission worked full-time as an electrician.

Airway: Patent. Tracheostomy stoma still healing;

Breathing: Self-ventilating on 2 L/min O_2 via nasal cannula, SpO2 95%. Weak cough. RR 22.

Circulation: BP 112/73, HR 96, temperature 37.1C, warm peripheries.

Disability: Alert and orientated. Reports distressing and intrusive thoughts on occasion.

Exposure: Sacral pressure sore not fully healed. Pain on sitting 5/10. Catheterised. One abdominal drain in situ. NG tube for ongoing enteral feeding.

Physical function: MRCSS = 50. Bilateral foot-drop with atrophy of tibialis anterior. Requires assistance of one person for bed mobility and standing hoist to stand. Disengaged with rehabilitation over the past week, due to what he perceives as a lack of progress.

- Which symptoms indicate that Stephen has physical and non-physical morbidity?
  - Weakness
  - Limited ability to sit, stand or walk
  - Pain
  - Limited ability to self-care
  - Significant weight loss
  - Intrusive memories/thoughts
  - Disengagement and depressive symptoms
  - Potential complications with tracheostomy wound healing
- Using the WHO ICF as a framework, are you able to consider how Stephen's domains of health are currently impacted by his critical illness?
- What are some of your concerns about his transfer to the ward and how might you deal with them?

Models of post-critical care morbidity

Models such as the ICF, or the biopsychosocial approach, applied to the sequelae of critical illness are commonly used when discussing RaCI (Iwashyna and Netzer, 2012). Hodgson et al.'s study 'The impact of disability in survivors of critical illness' (2017) uses the ICF to describe the many and varied ways in which critical illness affects quality of life. This model can be seen in Figure 31.3.

One well known model for describing the impact of critical illness is that of Needham and colleagues (Needham et al., 2012). They group the physical, psychological (mental health) and cognitive impairments described by NICE together, and describe it as 'Post Intensive Care Syndrome' (PICS). This model does not include the social impact of critical illness specifically, but does incorporate a description of the impact on the mental health of immediate family members and caregivers, PICS-Family. Although it is less comprehensive than the ICF model used by Hodgson et al. (2017), it is more holistic than treating each morbidity in isolation. PICS may be a useful starting point when discussing the complexity of life after critical illness with patients and their loved ones. It is summarised in Figure 31.4.

6Cs: Communication

Although effective communication is essential for all patients, the volume and complexity of information makes it of particular importance to those with a protracted stay.

NICE highlight the importance of communication throughout the RaCI pathway – between professionals in the MDT; between teams at key timepoints, such as transfer from critical care to the ward; through the provision of information and support to each patient and their family (NICE, 2009, 2017).

Assessment

NICE recommends the completion of a 'short clinical assessment as early as clinically possible' following critical care admission. This is defined as 'a brief clinical assessment to identify patients who may be at risk of developing physical and non-physical morbidity' (NICE, 2009). Examples of risk factors are outlined in Box 31.1. If someone is deemed at risk, a comprehensive clinical assessment should be completed. This is 'a more detailed assessment to determine the rehabilitation needs of patients who have been identified as being at risk of developing physical and non-physical morbidity' (NICE, 2009). This should consider both the current status of, and risk factors for future impairments in, all functional domains discussed above. It should include assessments by healthcare professionals experienced in critical care and rehabilitation.

6Cs: Competence

Ensure you have the competence to carry out a comprehensive assessment of your patient's rehabilitation needs, alongside the wider MDT.

A comprehensive clinical assessment can include factors identified in Box 31.2, and may involve the completion of one or more outcome measures, such as the Intensive Care Psychological Assessment Tool (IPAT), Mini Mental State Examination (MMSE) or the Short Physical Performance Battery (SPPB). See Figure 31.5 and Box 31.3.

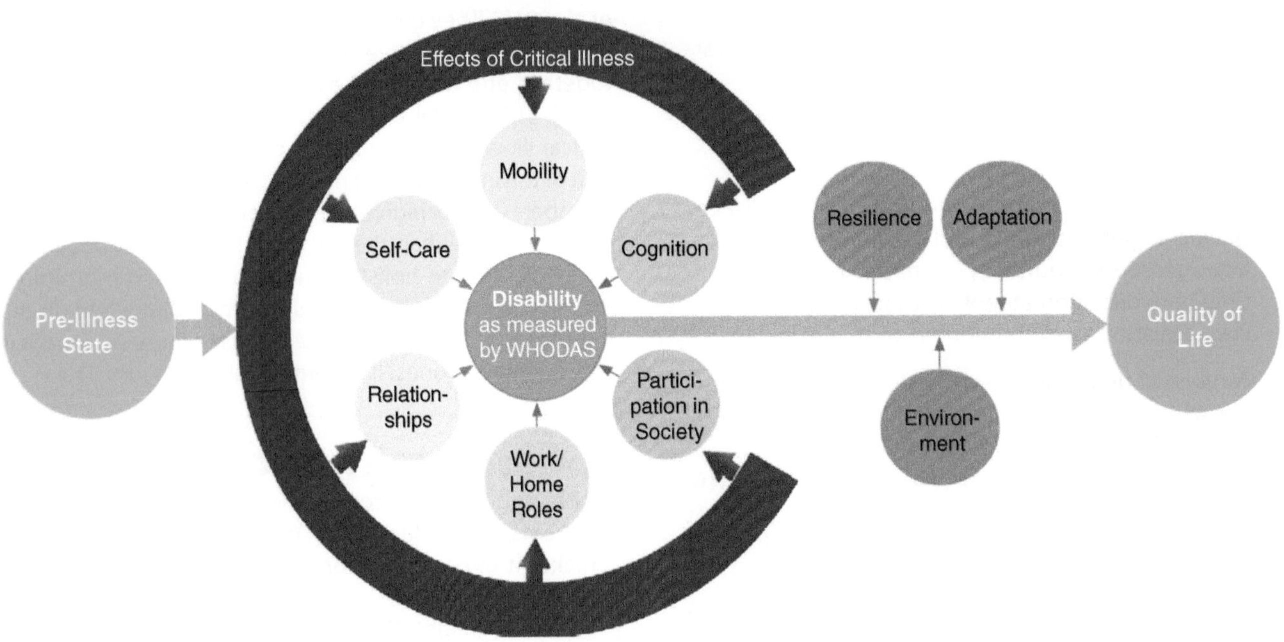

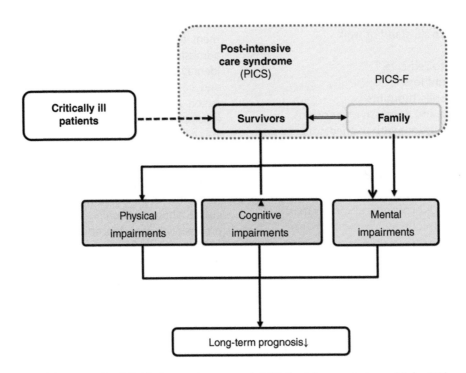

Figure 31.3   Conceptual model of factors that are included in the World Health Organization's Interntational Classification of Functioning after critical illness. Reprinted by permission from Springer Nature: Springer. *Intensive Care Med. The impact of disability in survivors of critical illness*, Hodgson et al., Copyright (2017).

Figure 31.4   Conceptual framework of PICS. *Source:* Inoue et al. (2019) with permission of John Wiley & Sons.

Box 31.1   Examination scenario – Short Clinical Assessment – Examples from short clinical assessment that may indicate a patient at risk of morbidity (NICE, 2009).

Physical dimensions:

- Unable to get out of bed independently
- Anticipated long duration of critical care stay
- Unable to self-ventilate on 35% oxygen or less
- Presence of premorbid respiratory or mobility problems

Non-physical dimensions:

- Insufficient cognitive functioning to exercise independently
- Recurrent nightmares, particularly if these cause a patient to try and stay awake to avoid nightmares
- New and recurrent anxiety or panic attacks
- Expressing their wish not to talk about their illness, or changing the subject quickly off the topic

Box 31.2   Examination Scenario – Comprehensive Clinical Assessment – Symptoms from the functional assessment that may indicate the presence of physical and non-physical morbidity (NICE, 2009).

Physical dimensions:

- Weakness, inability/partial ability to sit, rise to standing, or to walk, fatigue, pain, breathlessness, swallowing difficulties, incontinence, reduce ability to self-care
- Changes in vision, pain, altered sensation
- Difficulties in speaking or using language to communicate, difficulties in writing
- The need for mobility aids, housing benefits, employment and leisure support needs

Non-physical dimensions:

- New or recurrent somatic symptoms, including palpitations, irritability, and sweating; avoidance behaviour; depressive symptoms, including tearfulness and withdrawal; nightmares, delusions, hallucinations, and flashbacks
- Loss of memory, attention deficits, sequencing problems, deficits in organizational skills, confusion, apathy, disinhibition, compromised insight
- Low self-esteem, poor self-image and/or body image issues, relationship difficulties (particularly with family or carers).

475

Medications management: analgesics for neuropathic pain

Patients recovering from ICU-AW may report peripheral neuropathic pain as a result of Critical Illness Polyneuropathy (CIP). Medications such as gabapentin and pregabalin are effective treatments for neuropathic pain. These medications should only be given enterally. Once treatment has commenced, it often takes a few weeks for them to work effectively

Goals

NICE Quality Standard 158, also called RaCI, highlights the importance of setting short- and medium-term rehabilitation goals, based on the comprehensive clinical assessment. This is to ensure the rehabilitation plan is sufficiently structured, individualised, and goal-focused (NICE, 2017). Whenever possible, these should be set by, or at least with, the patient themselves, with the inclusion of their family or carer where appropriate. An ideal might be that a patient provides their functional goal – being able to get dressed independently, say – and the appropriate members of the critical care MDT support them in breaking the goal down into Specific, Measurable, Achievable, Realistic and Timed (SMART) subgoals. In this example, that might be – being able to sit on the edge of the bed unsupported for 3 minutes, lift arms up

Date and time: _____   Patient's hospital number: _____

Patient's name: _____

Intensive Care Psychological Assessment Tool (IPAT)
© University College London Hospitals NHS Foundation Trust

I would like to ask you some questions about your stay in Intensive care, and how you've been feeling in yourself. These feelings can be an important part of your recovery. To answer, please circle the answer that is closest to how you feel, or answer in any way you are able to (e.g. by speaking or pointing.)

	Since you've been in intensive care:	A	B	C
1	Has it been hard to communicate?	No	Yes, a bit	Yes, a lot
2	Has it been difficult to sleep?	No	Yes, a bit	Yes, a lot
3	Have you been feeling tense?	No	Yes, a bit	Yes, a lot
4	Have you been feeling sad?	No	Yes, a bit	Yes, a lot
5	Have you been feeling panicky?	No	Yes, a bit	Yes, a lot
6	Have you been feeling hopeless?	No	Yes, a bit	Yes, a lot
7	Have you felt disorientated (not quite sure where you are)?	No	Yes, a bit	Yes, a lot
8	Have you had hallucinations (seen or heard things you suspect were not really there)?	No	Yes, a bit	Yes, a lot
9	Have you felt that people were *deliberately* trying to harm or hurt you?	No	Yes, a bit	Yes, a lot
10	Do upsetting memories of intensive care keep coming into your mind?	No	Yes, a bit	Yes, a lot

Do you have any comments to add in relation to any of the answers?

_____

SCORING

Any answer in column A = 0 points

Any answer in column B = 1 point

Any answer in column C = 2 points

Sum up the scores of each item for a total I-PAT score out of 20

Cut-off point ≥7 - indicates patient at risk

Figure 31.5   Clinical Investigation – IPAT.

overhead, lift one foot off the floor at a time, sit to stand with supervision – with appropriate timescales.

6Cs: Care
We often associate care with looking after our patients and doing as much for them as we can. Care can also be about empowerment and encouraging independence. Wherever possible, try to empower your patient to be involved in decision making and goal setting. Do what you can to humanise the critical care experience.

Patient-led goal setting can be difficult early in a critical care admission, when many patients are sedated. For this reason, initial goals may need to be set by one or more members of the critical care MDT, with guidance from family/carers, but without input from the patient themselves. Where this is the case, these goals should be discussed and updated as soon as the patient is awake and able to engage.

6Cs: Compassion
Rehabilitation should be compassionate and person-centred, respecting patients' goals and wishes.

Box 31.3 Examination scenario: the SPPB.

The SPPB is a tool to measure physical function after critical illness (Spies et al., 2021). It incorporates three timed tasks:

1. Standing balance tests with progressive reduction in base of support
   a. Feet side-by-side
   b. Semi-tandem
   c. Tandem

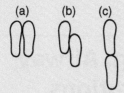

(a)   (b)   (c)

2. Walking speed over a 3-metre or 4-metre course

3. Time to complete five sit-to-stands

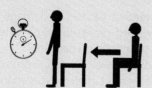

Each task is rated with 0-4, with an aggregate score of between 0 and 12. A lower score indicates greater physical impairment.

Key timepoints in RaCI

The use of a short clinical assessment to triage risk of morbidity following critical illness, followed by a comprehensive assessment and goal setting, should be repeated regularly. Key time points are shown in Figure 31.6. This should be carried out by healthcare professionals with sufficient expertise in critical illness and rehabilitation (NICE, 2009). Therefore, it may be that ongoing support following critical care discharge, both on the ward, and 2–3 months following discharge, is provided by members of the critical care MDT. This would involve reviewing the assessments and goals relating to an individual's critical illness, and be in addition to the care provided by the ward-MDT, and subsequently primary care services. In many hospitals, this takes the form of critical care outreach, then RaCI follow-up clinics, groups, or telephone follow-up, run by one or more members of the critical care MDT (Connolly et al., 2014).

Red Flag: persistent weight loss

Patients with critical illness often lose a significant amount of weight, from both the body's fat and protein stores, and in the form of lost skeletal muscle mass. Failure to gain weight after critical illness is associated with increased morbidity and mortality. Common problems such as loss of appetite, nausea, poor gastric motility, and reduced hand and upper limb function, can all effect calorific intake. Nutritional intake should be closely observed, and proactive referral to the dietetic team should be considered in the case of persistent weight loss or failure to gain weight (van Zanten et al., 2019).

477

During the critical care stay   During ward-based care   2–3 months after discharge from critical care

Before discharge from critical care   Before discharge to home or community care

Information and support

Figure 31.6 NICE CG83 – key principles of care timepoints.

Treatment

Early mobilisation

Early physical rehabilitation has been proposed as a potential treatment, or prophylaxis, for ICU-AW and its associated functional impairments (Morris and Herridge, 2007; Needham, 2008). Confusingly, there are many definitions of 'early mobilisation'. Some specify beginning rehabilitation within a certain number of hours of critical care admission, or commencement of mechanical ventilation; some include passive movements, while other trials of early mobilisation fail to define it at all. A recent systematic review of early mobilisation in mechanically ventilated patients found that only 15 of the 76 included studies defined early mobilisation fully (Clarissa et al., 2019).

'Early mobilisation' is defined here as active exercise of some form, commenced whilst an individual is on critical care. Passive exercises are not included, as there is no evidence for these increasing muscle strength or endurance (Nafziger et al., 1992; Marshall et al., 2011).

It might appear axiomatic that physical rehabilitation should be a treatment option for ICU-AW. Exercise-based interventions have strong evidence for improving strength and function in other clinical populations, such as chronic respiratory disease (McCarthy et al., 2015). However, evidence for early rehabilitation on critical care as a treatment for ICU-AW remains poor. Initial studies demonstrating benefit have been followed by multiple subsequent trials showing no effect of intervention (Castro-Avila et al., 2015; Tipping et al., 2017; Fuke et al., 2018).

One problem with demonstrating effect may be due to a change in usual care on ICU, due to early indications of benefits of rehabilitation. For example, in Schweickert's randomised control trial comparing early physical and occupational therapy on critical care with 'usual care'. The control group was usual care in two North American hospitals at the time. They commented that 'neither site routinely provides physical therapy for patients who are on mechanical ventilation for less than 2 weeks, nor has dedicated physiotherapists for such practice' (Schweickert et al., 2009). Usual care, therefore, was little or no physical rehabilitation on critical care. Subsequent studies, particularly those based in Australia or Europe, have compared 'usual care' – provision of some physical rehabilitation on critical care – with an intervention of either increased dose, earlier commencement, or more prolonged delivery of rehabilitation (Denehy et al., 2013; Walsh et al., 2015). Although these interventions have been shown to be feasible and safe, they have demonstrated little or no improvement in functional outcomes when compared to current usual care (Hodgson and Cuthbertson, 2016; Nydahl et al., 2017).

Another difficulty with the evidence base for rehabilitation is heterogeneity of the patient group, and the interventions themselves. Critical care patients differ both in their individual characteristics, and the way in which they respond to a complex intervention, such as a rehabilitation programme. Unlike trials for drug therapies, rehabilitation interventions are very difficult to 'blind', or to remove con-

founding factors from. Multiple authors have suggested this as a likely confounder when analysing their results (Denehy et al., 2013; Wright et al., 2018).

In summary, the evidence tells us that *some* physical rehabilitation, likely in the form of active mobilisation as early as clinically possible, is better than none. Multiple programmes of physical rehabilitation have been shown to be safe for critical care patients to complete. However, we still do not know which specific interventions, timing, or dose, to use to optimise functional outcomes following critical illness. More evidence is required, although the complex nature of critical illness, and an individual's resulting morbidity, makes generation of this evidence base challenging.

Red Flag: Airway complications

Airway complications, such as laryngeal pathology and tracheal stenosis, can occur after prolonged intubation or tracheostomy.

- The endotracheal tube can cause inflammation and subsequent damage to the vocal cords, leading to reduced cord movement and formation of scar tissue. This may lead to changes to voice, or upper airway obstruction.
- Tracheal stenosis, caused by damage to the tracheal wall, may lead to stridor, persistent cough, or increased dyspnoea on exertion.
- Assessment of airway complications should form part of a comprehensive clinical assessment (NICE, 2009).

Red Flag: pressure damage

Integumentary compromise and pressure damage can occur during prolonged immobility, particularly when accompanied by critical illness. Two of the most common sites for pressure damage are the sacrum and heels. Regular liaison with the tissue viability team is key to a joined-up approach to both rehabilitation and pressure care. The use of specialist seating or ambulatory pressure-relieving footwear may be indicated.

Psychological interventions

The same paucity of evidence for specific interventions, timing, and dose, applies to treatments for psychological morbidity, both during and after critical illness. In one of the largest trials of a psychological intervention delivered on critical care to date, Wade and colleagues assessed a combined intervention of: promotion of a therapeutic environment, three 'stress support sessions', and a relaxation and recovery programme delivered by trained ICU nurses to high-risk (acutely stressed) patients. This randomised trial of almost 1,500 patients found no improvement in PTSD symptoms in the 6 months following discharge (Wade et al., 2019).

Orange Flag: Post-traumatic stress disorder (PTSD)

PTSD screening tools are not always suitable for use in critical care, as many indicators of PTSD in a more general context are confounded by critical illness. For example, 'difficulty concentrating'.

Equally, a PTSD tool may not capture aspects of the critical care experience that commonly trigger distress, such as hallucinations or delusions. A further difficulty is that PTSD measures are often completed with reference to an 'index event'. In critical care it is unclear if this should be the event that resulted in hospitalisation, or the procedures and experiences endured within the hospital itself. It may be more appropriate therefore to use a general measure of critical care distress. (Wade et al., 2014)

Orange Flag: low mood

Critical illness survivors frequently experience low mood and depressive symptoms, both during and following critical illness. Some of the symptoms of depression include a loss of energy, disruptions to sleep patterns, feeling worthless and a loss of interest or pleasure. Patients may feel demotivated or unable to recognise progress. This may have considerable impact on their ongoing rehabilitation and recovery.

Medications management: treating depression

Selective serotonin reuptake inhibitors (SSRIs), such as citalopram and fluoxetine, are commonly used for moderate to severe depression in critical care. Patients on SSRIs should be reviewed regularly to assess for effectiveness and side effects. Appropriate patients should also be offered clinical psychology input.

Snapshot

Micah is a 34-year-old man who has been on critical care for ten days. He was admitted with hypoxic respiratory failure after contracting COVID-19. This was managed with a combination of CPAP and HFO_2, and awake proning. He was not intubated. He has since weaned to nasal cannula oxygen, and is likely to be discharged to the medical ward within the next two days.

Micah's only functional impairment on assessment is reduced exercise tolerance. Whilst on critical care, he has been aware that some of the patients around him have died, and has had recurrent dreams of being suffocated.

- What is Micah at risk of?
- How could you assess Micah?
- What sort of information can you provide to Micah to help him make sense of his critical care stay?

479

One intervention that may help symptoms of anxiety and depression following critical illness is the use of patient diaries. A diary is structured like a personal journal of an individual's stay on critical care – completed by healthcare professionals, family, friends, and the patient themselves when able. These are written with the intention of providing a narrative of the events in critical care to a patient, about themselves. They are written without the use of jargon or medical terminology, and might include photographs, anecdotes, pictures, and so on (Aitken et al., 2013; Ewens et al., 2014). A recent systematic review and meta-analysis by McIlroy and colleagues on the impact of patient diaries on psychological health and quality of life (QoL) following critical illness found that diaries did not improve PTSD symptoms, but did decrease anxiety and depression symptoms, and improve QoL (McIlroy et al., 2019).

Cognitive interventions

As discussed in Chapter 15, delirium is associated with poorer outcomes in all domains – physical, psychological, and cognitive (Pandharipande et al., 2013; Mehta et al., 2015; Salluh et al., 2015). Strategies to reduce rates of delirium in critical care are essential to any rehabilitation pathway.

Bundles of care, such as the 'ABCDEF' discussed in Chapter 15, are an evidence-based approach to reducing incidence and duration of delirium. In particular, early mobility, has been shown to reduce duration of delirium (Schweickert et al., 2009; Devlin et al., 2018). Given the severity of morbidity, and increased mortality, associated with delirium, this makes a strong case for including early mobility in your care of patients on critical care.

Medications management: treating delirium

Many patients in the critical care who experience significant distress due to delirium (delusions, anxiety or agitation) may benefit from short-term use of antipsychotic medications, such as haloperidol or olanzapine. These are not recommended for routine use for patients with delirium, as there is no evidence they reduce its duration.

6Cs: Courage

Providing the recommended individualised information and support during a patient's critical care stay can be challenging. Patients may struggle, or be unable, to communicate their needs and wishes. Have the courage to advocate for your patient and their family.

National guidelines and standards

NICE, FICM and the Intensive Care Society (ICS) all provide guidance relating to rehabilitation during and after critical illness (NICE, 2009, 2017; FICM, 2021; FICM and ICS, 2015, 2019). The NICE Clinical Guideline for RaCI is summarised in Box 31.4. The NICE Quality Standards are shown in Box 31.4. All members of the critical care MDT should contribute to the achievement of these standards (NICE, 2017).

Box 31.4   NICE Quality Standards 158: RaCI (NICE, 2017).

1. Adults in critical care at risk of morbidity have their rehabilitation goals agreed within 4 days of admission to critical care or before discharge from critical care, whichever is sooner.
2. Adults at risk of morbidity have a formal handover of care, including their agreed individualised structured rehabilitation programme, when they transfer from critical care to a general ward.
3. Adults who were in critical care and at risk of morbidity are given information based on their rehabilitation goals before they are discharged from hospital.
4. Adults who stayed in critical care for more than 4 days and were at risk of morbidity have a review 2 to 3 months after discharge from critical care.

The ICS guidance for provision of intensive care services (GPICS) re-iterates the NICE quality standards, and adds standards specifying daily screening for delirium, and assessment of swallow and communication by a speech and language therapist in all patients with a tracheostomy (FICM and ICS, 2019). GPICS also contains eight further recommendations relating to rehabilitation.

Snapshot

Rachael is a 52-year-old woman who was recently discharged from critical care after 42-days, for complications associated with a sub-total oesophagectomy. Despite a prolonged stay, including a period of delirium, she is making good progress with her rehabilitation on the ward. She is able to mobilise short distances with a zimmer frame, and scored 6/12 on the SPPB.

- Balance – 2
- Gait speed – 3
- 5 sit-to stand – 1

She has found her appetite is returning, and has gained 1.5 kg over the past fortnight. She has been keeping a daily activity and recovery diary to chart her progress and keep her family updated. She also finds this useful because recently she has become more forgetful.

Rachael is a full-time secondary school music teacher who enjoys playing the guitar and the piano. She lives with her wife, Karen, a consultant geriatrician, and their two Labradors. Prior to her transfer to the ward, the nurses on the critical care unit were able to arrange to take Rachael outside to meet Karen and the dogs.

- How might you approach goal setting with Rachael?
- Are there any other members of the MDT that you would want to be involved?
- What factors do you consider to have contributed to Rachael's recovery so far?

FICM published guidance on 'life after critical illness' in 2021. They re-iterate the importance of an MDT approach to support both during and after critical illness, and summarise suggested components of a comprehensive assessment, and possible structures for follow-up clinics (FICM, 2021).

Unfortunately, despite this plethora of recommendations and standards relating to RaCI, the limitation on resources in UK critical care units means that achieving these remains aspirational for many (Connolly et al., 2014).

6Cs: Commitment

All those working in critical care should show commitment to improving the survivorship of critical illness survivors.

Learning event

Reflect on your understanding of the lasting impact critical illness and its management can have on a person. Consider in particular the functional impact, and the impact on a survivor's family.

physical, psychological and cognitive functioning. There is currently insufficient evidence to recommend any specific treatment strategies to combat this morbidity. However, this may be due to the challenges of assessing complex rehabilitation strategies using traditional trial design, rather than an absence of efficacy. Early assessment and identification of individuals at risk, goal-focused holistic rehabilitation and information provision and support are clearly essential. These should be undertaken by healthcare professionals with expertise in critical illness and RaCI, and completed throughout both acute illness and the following months.

Conclusion

As the number of people surviving an ICU admission continues to grow, the population of individuals living with the residual effects of critical illness grows also. These span

Take home points

1. There is a need for support of physical, psychological and cognitive problems following critical illness. This will increase as the population of survivors of critical illness grows.
2. As a healthcare professional working in critical care, an understanding of the common sequelae of critical illness is essential. This will allow you to contribute to timely assessment, support patients in goal setting and take part in the creation of structured rehabilitation plans.
3. There is insufficient evidence to support any specific rehabilitation intervention, but many strategies have been shown to be safe.
4. All UK bodies providing guidance and standards for critical care recommend holistic, goal-focused, individualised rehabilitation, provided by the critical care MDT.

Disclaimer

Some of the authors' work in this chapter has previously been published as part of a review in the Journal of the Association of Chartered Physiotherapists in Respiratory Care (Sanger H. (2020). How early is early? When should rehabilitation begin in critical illness? *Journal of ACPRC* 50(1):51–61).

References

Aitken L.M., Rattray, J., Hull, A. et al. (2013). The use of diaries in psychological recovery from intensive care. *Crit Care*, 17:253. doi: 10.1186/cc13164.

Bein, T., Bienvenu, O.J., and Hopkins, R.O. (2019). Focus on long-term cognitive, psychological and physical impairments after critical illness. *Intensive Care Medicine* 45(10): 1466–1468. doi: 10.1007/s00134-019-05718-7.

Castro-Avila, A., Serón, P., Fan, E. et al. (2015). Effect of early rehabilitation during intensive care unit stay on functional status: Systematic review and meta-analysis. doi: 10.1371/journal.pone.0130722.

Clarissa, C., Salisbury, L., Rodgers, S., and Kean, S. (2019). Early mobilisation in mechanically ventilated patients: A systematic integrative review of definitions and activities. *Journal of Intensive Care* 7. doi: 10.1186/ s40560-018-0355-z.

Connolly, B., Douiri, A., Steier, J. et al. (2014). A UK survey of rehabilitation following critical illness: implementation of NICE Clinical Guidance 83 (CG83) following hospital discharge. *BMJ Open* 4(5): e004963. doi: 10.1136/bmjopen-2014-004963.

Cuthbertson, B.H., Rattray, J., Johnston, M. et al. (2007). A pragmatic randomised, controlled trial of intensive care follow up programmes in improving longer-term outcomes from critical illness. The PRACTICAL study. *BMC Health Serv Res* 7: 116. doi: 10.1186/1472-6963-7-116

Cuthbertson, B., Roughton, S., Jenkinson, D. et al. (2010). Quality of life in the five years after intensive care: A cohort study. *Critical Care* 14(1). https://ccforum.biomedcentral.com/articles/10.1186/cc8848 (accessed March 2022).

De Jonghe, B., Sharshar, T.,. Lefaucheur, J.-P. et al. (2002). Paresis acquired in the intensive care unit: A prospective multicenter study. *JAMA* 288(22): 2859–2867. https://jamanetwork.com/journals/jama/fullarticle/195589 (accessed March 2022).

Devlin, J.W., Skrobik, Y., Gélinas, C. et al. (2018). Clinical practice guidelines for the prevention and management of pain, agitation/sedation, delirium, immobility, and sleep disruption in adult patients in the ICU. *Critical Care Medicine* 46(9): e825. doi: 10.1097/CCM.0000000000003299.

Denehy, L., Skinner, E., Edbroooke, L. et al. (2013). Exercise rehabilitation for patients with critical illness: A randomized controlled trial with 12 months of follow-up. *Critical Care* 17(4). https://ccforum.biomedcentral.com/articles/10.1186/cc12835 (accessed March 2022).

Dinglas, V., Friedman, L., Colantuoni, E. et al. (2017). Muscle weakness and 5-year survival in acute respiratory distress syndrome survivors. *Critical Care Medicine* 45(3): 446–453. https://pubmed.ncbi.nlm.nih.gov/28067712/ (accessed March 2022).

Engel, G.L. (1977). The need for a new medical model: a challenge for biomedicine. *Science* 196(4286): 129–136. doi: 10.1126/science.847460.

Ewens B., Chapman, R., Tulloch, A., and Hendricks, J. (2014). ICU survivors' utilisation of diaries post discharge: A qualitative descriptive study. *Aust Crit Care*, 27:28–35. doi: 10.1016/j.aucc.2013.07.001

Faculty of Intensive Care Medicine (FICM) (2021). FICM Position Statement and Provisional Guidance: Recovery and Rehabilitation for Patients Following the Pandemic. https://www.ficm.ac.uk/sites/ficm/files/documents/2021-10/ficm_recovery_and_rehab_provisional_guidance.pdf (accessed March 2022).

Faculty of Intensive Care Medicine (FICM) and Intensive Care Society (ICS) (2015). Guidelines for the Provision of Intensive Care Services, 1e. FICM and ICS.

Faculty of Intensive Care Medicine (FICM) and Intensive Care Society (ICS) (2019). Guidelines for the Provision of Intensive Care Services, 2e. https://www.ficm.ac.uk/sites/default/files/gpics_v2_-_version_for_release_-_final2019.pdf (accessed 20 May 2020).

Fuke, R., Hifumi, T., Kondo, Y. et al. (2018). Early rehabilitation to prevent postintensive care syndrome in patients with critical illness: A systematic review and meta-analysis. *BMJ Open* 8(5). https://bmjopen.bmj.com/content/8/5/e019998 (accessed March 2022).

Hatch, R., Young, D., Barber, V. et al. (2018). Anxiety, depression and post traumatic stress disorder after critical illness: A UK-wide prospective cohort study. *Critical Care (London, England)* 22(1): 310. doi: 10.1186/s13054-018-2223-6.

Herridge, M., Tansey, C., Matté, A. et al. (2011). Functional disability 5 years after acute respiratory distress syndrome. *New England Journal of Medicine* 364(14): 1293–1304. doi: 10.1056/NEJMoa1011802.

Hodgson, C. and Cuthbertson, B. (2016). Improving outcomes after critical illness: Harder than we thought! *Intensive Care Medicine* 42(11): 1772–1774. https://link.springer.com/article/10.1007%2Fs00134-016-4526-x (accessed March 2022).

Hodgson, C.L., Udy, A., Bailey, M. et al. (2017). The impact of disability in survivors of critical illness. *Intensive Care Med* 43: 992–1001. doi: 10.1007/s00134-017-4830-0.

Intensive Care National Audit and Research Centre. (2010). Case mix programme summary statistics 2008–09. https://www.icnarc.org/DataServices/Attachments/Download/9d6ab3e5-86f7-e311-81c1-d48564544b14 (accessed March 2022).

Intensive Care National Audit and Research Centre. (2019). Case mix programme summary statistics 2018–19. https://www.icnarc.org/DataServices/Attachments/Download/fca008ac-9216-ea11-911e-00505601089b (accessed March 2022).

Iwashyna, T., Ely, E., Smith, D. et al. (2010). Long-term cognitive impairment and functional disability among survivors of severe sepsis. *JAMA* 304(16): 1787–1794. https://jamanetwork.com/journals/jama/fullarticle/186769.

Iwashyna, T. and Netzer, G. (2012). The burdens of survivorship: An approach to thinking about long-term outcomes after critical illness. *Seminars in Respiratory and Critical Care Medicine* 33(04): 327–338. doi: 10.1055/s-0032-1321982.

Marshall, P., Cashman, A., and Cheema, B. (2011). A randomized controlled trial for the effect of passive stretching on measures of hamstring extensibility, passive stiffness, strength, and stretch tolerance. *Journal of Science and Medicine in Sport* 14(6): 535–540.

McCarthy, B., Casey, D., Devane, D. et al. (2015). Pulmonary rehabilitation for chronic obstructive pulmonary disease. *Cochrane Database of Systematic Reviews* 2. doi: 10.1002/14651858.CD003793.pub3.

McIlroy, P.A., King, R., Garrouste-Orgeas, M. et al. (2019). The effect of ICU diaries on psychological outcomes and quality of life of survivors of critical illness and their relatives: A systematic review and meta-analysis. *Critical Care Medicine* 47(2): 273–279. doi: 10.1097/CCM.0000000000003547.

Mehta, S., Cook, D., Devlin, J. et al. (2015). Prevalence, risk factors, and outcomes of delirium in mechanically ventilated adults. *Critical Care Medicine* 43(3): 557–566. doi: 10.1097/CCM.0000000000000727.

Morris, P. and Herridge, M. (2007). Early intensive care unit mobility: Future directions. *Critical Care Clinics* 23(1): 97–110. https://www.sciencedirect.com/science/article/abs/pii/S074907040600073X (accessed March 2022).

Müller, A., von Hofen-Hohloch, J., Mende, M. et al. (2020). Long-term cognitive impairment after ICU treatment: a prospective longitudinal cohort study (Cog-I-CU). *Scientific Reports* 10(1): 15518. doi: 10.1038/s41598-020-72109-0.

Nafziger, N., Lee, S., and Huang, S. (1992). Passive exercise system: Effect on muscle activity, strength, and lean body mass. *Archives of Physical Medicine and Rehabilitation* 73(2): 184–189. https://www.archives-pmr.org/article/0003-9993(92)90099-I/pdf (accessed March 2022).

National Institute for Health and Care Excellence. (2009). *Rehabilitation after critical illness in adults (NICE clinical guideline 83)*. https://www.nice.org.uk/guidance/cg83 (accessed March 2022).

National Institute for Health and Care Excellence. (2017). *Rehabilitation after critical illness in adults (NICE Quality Standard 158)*. https://www.nice.org.uk/guidance/qs158 (accessed March 2022).

Needham, D. (2008). Mobilizing patients in the intensive care unit: Improving neuromuscular weakness and physical function. *JAMA* 300(14): 1685–1690. https://jamanetwork.com/journals/jama/article-abstract/182682 (accessed March 2022).

Needham, D.M., Davidson J., Cohen, H. et al. (2012). Improving long-term outcomes after discharge from intensive care unit: Report from a stakeholders' conference. *Critical Care Medicine* 40(2): 502–509. doi: 10.1097/CCM.0b013e318232da75.

Nydahl, P., Sricharoenchai, T., Chandra, S. et al. (2017). Safety of patient mobilization and rehabilitation in the intensive care unit. Systematic review with meta-analysis. *Annals of the American Thoracic Society* 14(5): 766–777. https://www.atsjournals.org/doi/10.1513/AnnalsATS.201611-843SR (accessed March 2022).

Pandharipande, P., Girard, T., Jackson, J. et al. (2013). Long-term cognitive impairment after critical illness. *New England Journal of Medicine* 369(14): 1306–1316. https://www.nejm.org/doi/10.1056/NEJMoa1301372 (accessed March 2022).

Puthucheary, Z., Rawal, J., McPhail, M. et al. (2013). Acute skeletal muscle wasting in critical illness. *JAMA* 310(15): 1591–1600. https://jamanetwork.com/journals/jama/fullarticle/1879857 (accessed March 2022).

Riddersholm, S., Christensen, S., Kragholm, K. et al. (2018). Organ support therapy in the intensive care unit and return to work: a nationwide, register-based cohort study. *Intensive Care Medicine* 44(4): 418–427. doi: 10.1007/s00134-018-5157-1.

Salluh, J.I.F., Wang, H., Schneider, E. et al. (2015). Outcome of delirium in critically ill patients: systematic review and meta-analysis. *BMJ* 350: h2538. doi: 10.1136/bmj.h2538.

Schweickert, W., Phlman, M., Pohlman, A. et al. (2009). Early physical and occupational therapy in mechanically ventilated, critically ill patients: A randomised controlled trial. *Lancet* 373(9678): 1874–1882. https://www.thelancet.com/journals/lancet/article/PIIS0140-6736(09)60658-9/fulltext (accessed March 2022).

Spies, C.D., Krampe, H., Paul, N. et al. (2021). Instruments to measure outcomes of post-intensive care syndrome in outpatient care settings – Results of an expert consensus and feasibility field test. *Journal of the Intensive Care Society* 1751143720923597. doi: 10.1177/1751143720923597.

Tipping, C., Harrold, M., Holland, A. et al. (2017). The effects of active mobilisation and rehabilitation in ICU on mortality and function: A systematic review. *Intensive Care Medicine* 43(2): 171–183. doi: 10.1007/s00134-016-4612-0.

van Zanten, A.R.H., De Waele, E., and Wischmeyer, P.E. (2019). Nutrition therapy and critical illness: practical guidance for the ICU, post-ICU, and long-term convalescence phases. *Critical Care* 23(1): 368. doi: 10.1186/s13054-019-2657-5.

Wade, D.M., Howell, D., Weinman, A. et al. (2012) Investigating risk factors for psychological morbidity three months after intensive care: a prospective cohort study. *Crit Care* 16, R192. doi: 10.1186/cc11677.

Wade, D.M., Hankins, M., Smyth, D. et al. (2014). Detecting acute distress and risk of future psychological morbidity in critically ill patients: validation of the intensive care psychological assessment tool. *Critical Care* 18(5). doi: 10.1186/s13054-014-0519-8.

Wade, D.T. and Halligan, P.W. (2017). The biopsychosocial model of illness: a model whose time has come. *Clinical Rehabilitation* 31(8): 995–1004. doi: 10.1177/0269215517709890.

Wade, D.M., Mouncey, P., Richards-Belle, A. et al. (2019). Effect of a nurse-led preventive psychological intervention on symptoms of posttraumatic stress disorder among critically ill patients: A randomized clinical trial. *JAMA* 321(7): 665–675. doi: 10.1001/jama.2019.0073.

Walsh, T., Salisbury, L., Merriweather, J. et al. (2015). Increased hospital-based physical rehabilitation and information provision after intensive care unit discharge: The RECOVER randomized clinical trial. *JAMA Internal Medicine* 175(6): 901–910. https://jamanetwork.com/journals/jamainternalmedicine/fullarticle/2247164 (accessed March 2022).

World Health Organization. (2001). The International Classification of Functioning, Disability and Health (ICF). Geneva: WHO. http://www.who.int/classifications/icf/en/ (accessed March 2022).

World Health Organisation (2017). WHO Framework on Rehabilitation Services: expert meeting. https://www.who.int/rehabilitation/expert-meeting-june17/en/ (accessed March 2022).

Wright, S., Thomas, K., Watson, G. et al. (2018). Intensive versus standard physical rehabilitation therapy in the critically ill (EPICC): A multicentre, parallel-group, randomised controlled trial. *Thorax* 73(3): 213–221. https://thorax.bmj.com/content/thoraxjnl/early/2017/08/05/thoraxjnl-2016-209858.full.pdf (accessed March 2022).

Zimmerman, J., Kramer, A., and Knaus, W. (2013). Changes in hospital mortality for United States intensive care unit admissions from 1988 to 2012. *Critical Care* 17(2):R81. https://ccforum.biomedcentral.com/articles/10.1186/cc12695 (accessed March 2022).

Chapter 32

Dying and death

Helen Merlane and Leonie Armstrong

Aim

The aim of this chapter is to introduce the reader to the principle of death and dying for people who are critically ill. The 5 Priorities of care will be used as a framework for delivering end-of-life care, and to draw on evidence-based practice to identify the complexities of recognising and caring for a dying patient and their family within the critical care unit and understand the pivotal role of the nurse in facilitating a good death.

Learning outcomes

After reading this chapter the reader will be able to:

1. Understand the difference between Palliative Care, End-of-life care (EoLC) and Dying.
2. Recognise some of the indicators of decline and the difficulty in diagnosing dying within the critical care environment.
3. Recognise the 5 priorities of care and how to incorporate these into patient care.
4. Understand the importance of timely, open and honest communication during death and dying.
5. Discuss the role of the nurse in providing care after death.

Test your prior knowledge

- List some indicators of decline, and discuss why recognising when a patient is dying maybe difficult within critical care.
- What are the benefits of advance care planning?
- What are the five common symptoms at the end of life?
- What are the two ways to diagnose death?
- What are the key issues when planning a discharge for end-of-life care?

Fundamentals of Critical Care: A Textbook for Nursing and Healthcare Students, First Edition. Edited by Ian Peate and Barry Hill.
© 2023 John Wiley & Sons Ltd. Published 2023 by John Wiley & Sons Ltd.
Companion website: www.wiley.com/go/peate/criticalcare

Introduction

The goal of effective critical care is to support and treat reversible causes of critical illness (Pattison, 2011), and patients are admitted to critical care units (usually a combination of high dependency and Intensive care) because the level of care is acute and deteriorating or requires multi-organ support to enable survival (Luckhurst and Clarke, 2017). However, despite advances in medical treatment, over 300,000 people die in hospitals in England, (approximately 60% of all deaths) and whilst some literature suggests that most people would wish to die in familiar surroundings, such as their own home, 22,000 patients die in critical care (Faculty of Intensive Care Medicine (FICM), 2019; Gomes et al., 2012).

With such a high proportion of patients dying within this clinical environment, end-of-life care and caring for dying patients is a core skill required by critical care nurses (Box 32.1). This is so that they can manage the transition of care from acute to end of life, and deliver a high standard of person-centred, holistic care, by acting as the patient's advocate, effectively managing distressing symptoms, educating the family and actively encouraging and supporting their presence in creating positive memories (Arbour & Wiegand, 2014).

6Cs: Competence

Nurses should ensure they are equipped with the knowledge and skills to deliver a high standard of patient-centred end-of-life care, with the support of the multidisciplinary team.

To provide quality care for people dying from a critical illness, it is important to understand the correct usage of dying and death related terminology. Within the literature, and amongst professionals, the terms end of life, palliative care and dying are often used synonymously; however, each term has distinct differences, and prognostic implications (Hui et al., 2014). Therefore, it is essential that nurses and health care professionals understand the distinguishing characteristics of each term, so that they can recognise the phase appropriate for the patient and be able to respond to their care needs in a timely manner.

End-of-life care

The End-of-Life Care Strategy (Department of Health (DH), 2008) suggests that end-of-life care planning should commence for patients who are expected to die within 12 months. However, it goes on to state that identifying the

Box 32.1 End-of-life care (National Competency Framework for Registered Nurses in Critical Care).

2:6.1 Withholding and Withdrawing Treatment
  You must be able to demonstrate your knowledge using a rationale through discussion, and the application to your practice

- Legal constraints, Mental Capacity Act and ethical principles of withdrawal or withholding of treatment
- Procedures for forming and recording agreements on treatment withdrawal
- Best practice procedures for early identification of potential organ/tissue donation according to defined triggers
- How to facilitate access to sources of support within the broader MDT e.g. bereavement support
- Availability of care suitable for patients after withdrawal of treatment e.g. EOL care plan

2:6.2 Assessment, Monitoring and Observation

- You must be able to demonstrate your knowledge using a rationale through discussion, and the application to your practice
- Establish with the MDT that further treatment for the patient is futile and that at some stage, active treatment should be withdrawn in the knowledge that this will result in the patient's death.
- Consider patients and/or family's preference for where care will be delivered after withdrawal of treatment
- Review of end-of-life care options suitable for patients
- Initiate the Specialist Nurse for Organ Donation (SNOD) and participate in the planning and conduct of an MDT approach to families for consent/authorisation for organ and tissue donation according to best practice guidance
- Agree with the patient, where possible and their family and colleagues a plan of care.
- Arrange resources for the delivery of the plan, including liaison with MDT and appropriate support teams
- Evaluate the care plan according to local policy and adapt to patient needs. Initiate individualised treatment plans to ease the effects of illness:
  - Pain
  - Nausea
  - Agitation
  - Dyspnoea
  - Respiratory tract secretions

485

beginning of end-of-life care depends on the person (who may recognise that they are approaching end of life), professional perspective, the disease and the stage that the patient is at within the disease trajectory.

Palliative care

Palliative care is an approach which encompasses comfort-focused, holistic care to patients with a life-limiting illness, including those who are receiving curative treatment. The emphasis is on improving quality of life, by promoting comfort, respect, dignity and supporting the dying person and those important to them and this approach can be used at any point within the patient's disease trajectory. The World Health Organisation (2018) recognises that palliative care is applicable to patients early within their illness, with some people receiving palliative care for years. However, the principles of palliative care are also embedded in end-of-life care, with the focus being on empowering patients with an advanced, progressive, incurable illness to live as well as possible until they die; this includes supporting the needs of the patient and family, and having a management plan to support their holistic needs (Leadership Alliance for the Care of the Dying Person, (LACDP), 2014).

Dying

The term 'dying' is sometimes used in the same context as end-of-life and palliative care. However, where end-of-life care is a phase within a patient's illness trajectory, and palliative care is an approach, Hui et al. (2014) define dying as the hours or days preceding imminent death.

The LACDP (2014) published the One Chance to Get it Right document, highlighting five 'Priorities of Care' (Table 32.1) which are based on the wishes of the patient.

A key consideration is that these priorities can be applied in any environment, with the focus being on the provision of a high standard of end-of-life care. This framework will be explored throughout this chapter in identifying the role of the nurse in meeting the needs of the dying patient and family within the critical care unit.

Recognising Dying

Coombs et al. (2012) refer to three phases of care within the critical care unit; Admission with Hope of Recovery, Transition from Intervention to End-of-life care and Controlled Death.

Defining the point at which a patient may be nearing the end of their lives or dying is dependent on several factors (Box 32.2) such as the illness itself, the stage the patient is at in the disease trajectory and there should be a continuum of care including an ongoing assessment of the patient and family needs and responding in an appropriate and timely manner (LACDP, 2014). However, identifying when someone may be transitioning from intervention to end-of-life care can be more complex in the critical care setting as technological and medical advances such as invasive ventilation and complex drug regimens can sustain life when vital organs are failing, and death may also be unexpected during the period of care. In addition, there may also be a conflict of opinion amongst health care professionals regarding the goals of

Box 32.2   General indicators of decline and increasing needs (Gold Standards Framework, 2016).

- General physical decline, increasing dependence and need for support
- Repeated unplanned hospital admissions
- Advanced disease – unstable, deteriorating, complex symptom burden
- Presence of significant multi-morbidities
- Decreasing activity – functional performance status declining (e.g. Barthel score) limited selfcare, in bed or chair 50% of day and increasing dependence in most activities of daily living
- Decreasing response to treatments, decreasing reversibility
- Patient choice for no further active treatment and focus on quality of life
- Progressive weight loss (>10%) in past 6 months
- Sentinel event e.g. serious fall, bereavement, transfer to nursing home
- Serum albumin <25g/litre
- Considered eligible for DS1500 payment

Table 32.1   Priorities of care. *Source:* LACDP, 2014.

Priority 1: Recognise	This possibility is recognised and communicated clearly, decisions made, and actions taken in accordance with the person's needs and wishes, and these are regularly reviewed, and decisions revised accordingly.
Priority 2: Communicate	Sensitive communication takes place between staff and the dying person, and those identified as important to them.
Priority 3: Involve	The dying person, and those identified as important to them, are involved in decisions about treatment and care to the extent that the dying person wants.
Priority 4: Support	The needs of families and others identified as important to the dying person are actively explored, respected and met as far as possible.
Priority 5: Plan and Do	An individual plan of care, which includes food and drink, symptom control and psychological, social, and spiritual support, is agreed, co-ordinated and delivered with compassion.

end-of-life care and patients may not be involved in any decision making or be able to communicate their wishes regarding their care and ongoing treatment (Festic et al., 2011).

The LACDP (2014) suggests that the point at which treatment ends, and care becomes palliative should be a continuum, where the patients' needs are constantly assessed by a senior clinician and responded to in a timely and sensitive manner. This is in line with the General Medical Council (GMC) (2018), who state that clinicians must recognise when a patient is dying, and this may be in response to a patient's condition continuing to deteriorate despite optimising interventions.

6Cs: Courage

To express your view that a patient may be transitioning to end-of-life care and advocate for the patient and family requires and exhibits courage.

Snapshot

Jane is a 37-year-old lady who was admitted to critical care direct from the Accident & Emergency department 5 days ago. She was found at home unconscious by her husband. There was evidence of a suicide attempt, as a note, a packet of tablets, and used insulin needles were found next to her.

She is currently intubated and ventilated, and recent investigations have detected evidence of worsening sepsis, and a recent EEG has identified poor neurological outcome.

Jane is unconscious.

Airway: Intubated.
Breathing: RR 20, (NEWS2 = 2); Oxygen Saturations 94% (NEWS2 = 1).
Circulation: BP 100/60 (NEWS2 = 2); Pulse 110bpm (NEWS2 = 2) Capillary refill 4 seconds (She is cool to touch).
Disability: T 38.9c (NEWS2 = 1), CVPU (NEWS2 =3).
Exposure: Tattoos, dry lips. No abnormalities seen.
Total NEW2 Score: 11.

Diagnosis

Despite being in the unit for 5 days and attempts at optimising her treatment which included intubation, ventilation and dialysis, Jane did not respond well to ventilation weaning attempts. An electroencephalogram (EEG) was arranged, and this showed minimal continuous, irregular and low-amplitude slow activity. It was evaluated that there was no chance of neurological recovery.

Nursing actions:
- Ensure that husband is aware of Jane's deterioration and allow him the opportunity to ask questions.
- Ensure that plan of care is communicated clearly to the husband, and reassurance given that the focus of care to promote comfort.
- Check if any Advance Care Plan in place.
- Ascertain preferred place of care/death.
- Carry out a holistic assessment.

Clinical investigation

It is essential to assess the patient recognised to be dying for any indwelling devices. Review medical notes, past medical history, and correspondence from other healthcare facilities regarding indwelling devices. Observe the patient's upper chest both left and right for evidence of an implantable cardiac defibrillator (ICD)

The ICD should be deactivated if the patient is diagnosed as dying, to prevent any distressing firing episodes that could occur as the patient dies. It is imperative that mortuary and funeral staff are aware of any devices left in situ. Refer to local policies regarding deactivation process and documentation of decision.

(FICM, 2019; Resuscitation Council, British Cardiovascular Society, National Council Palliative Care, 2015)

6Cs: Communication

Effective communication is a key requisite in end-of-life care because open and transparent communication with patients and their families is vital in enabling and supporting patients to consider what is important to them.

Pattison et al. (2013) suggest that initiating end-of-life care in the critical care unit can be challenging and any delays may affect the dying experience. Therefore, once a decision has been made that the focus of care has changed from hope of recovery to end-of-life care, this needs to be clearly communicated to the patient and those important to them. In some cases, critical care settings can allow time to adjust, particularly time for a family to make sense of a situation. Being open and transparent with patients and their families is vital in enabling and supporting patients to consider what is important to them, therefore, is imperative that during these discussions, that the uncertainty of prognosis is also acknowledged and communicated to the patient and family (Walter et al., 2016). If we do not tell someone that they are near the end of their life or dying, we can prevent someone who has openly talked about their end-of-life care wishes from being able to express their preferences, as well as making provisions for their loved ones.

Shared decision making involving patients and those close to them in the decision processes can reduce confusion and conflict. It can support complex decisions not to escalate interventions, not to resuscitate, to withdraw life-sustaining treatment and support patients' end-of-life care preferences. This should lead to improved individualised care, patient, and staff experiences, aid the allocation of scarce resources and reduce complicated grief of relatives and loved ones (FICM, 2019).

Discussing the preferred place of care is important particularly at the point of withdrawal of Level 3 and Level 2 interventions, as the patient may no longer require the support of the critical care unit. Ethical issues such as resource allocation are prominent in critical care, and decisions to move a patient away from the high-level care environment at the end of life requires a personalised approach. Issues to be considered may include the cause of dying, how long the dying process is anticipated, organ donation and previously expressed wishes of the patient, as this may provide an understanding of the impact of the patient's situation on choice of preferred place of care. The way that this is communicated to the patient and their family should be sensitive, whilst being honest about what support needs the patient has, and where that care can be provided without the patient and their family feeling abandoned or that the professionals are giving up. Whilst it is acknowledged that the patient should be at the centre of all communication, this can be difficult within critical care as often the patients are unconscious or sedated. It is also important to consider whether the patient has capacity as set out in the Mental Capacity Act (MCA) (2005). More than 80% of critical care patients lack capacity to make important decisions about their care and management at a time when consideration is being given to withholding or withdrawing life-sustaining treatments, and only 13% of patients dying in critical care have made any pre-emptive statement (Sprung et al., 2018.)

In this instance, the MCA and best interest processes support patients/individuals who lack capacity whether that is temporary or permanent. This can result in decisions regarding futility and withdrawal of treatment being made through a best interest process which would involve key members of the multidisciplinary team (MDT). The nurse is in a pivotal position as having developed a therapeutic relationship with the patient and family, this allows the nurse to act as an advocate and convey the wishes or concerns to the medical staff and members of the MDT on their behalf.

Advance care planning

One way to ensure that a patient's wishes and preferences are known is to have an Advance Care Plan (ACP). An ACP is a continuous process, involving many conversations with the patient and the people important to them, and is a means of extending a patient's autonomy by planning their

Box 32.3   Definition of advance care planning (NHS Improving Quality, 2014).

Advance care planning is a voluntary process of discussion and review to help an individual who has capacity to anticipate how their condition may affect them in the future and, if they wish, set on record: choices about their care and treatment and/or an advance decision to refuse a treatment in specific circumstances, so that these can be referred to by those responsible for their care or treatment (whether professional staff or family carers) in the event that they lose capacity to decide once their illness progresses.

future care should they become unable to do so in the future (Brinkman-Stoppelenburg et al., 2014; Izumi, 2017) (Box 32.3). Nurses should have the necessary skills and qualities to engage and facilitate these conversations, and it is a requirement stipulated in the Nursing and Midwifery Code (2018).

The key components that are required by nurses to be able to effectively facilitate ACP conversations focus around effective communication, instilling hope, being approachable, ensuring 'timeliness' (not leaving it too late) and being equipped with the right skills.

At the end of a futility conversation with a patient or patients' family, there will be a decision and an individualised plan established to support the patients end-of-life care. That could result in an organ donation situation, withdrawal of life-sustaining treatment on the critical care unit and end-of-life care or discharge to another environment including the patient's home for end-of-life care (Merlane and Armstrong, 2020).

Table 32.2 Documentation to support advance care planning. *Source:* FICM, 2019; MCA, 2005; Merlane & Armstrong, 2020; Paes, 2019.

Do Not Attempt Cardiopulmonary Resuscitation (DNACPR)	Legally binding document.
Emergency health care plan (EHCP)	Information-sharing document – how to respond in specific situations relating to an individual patient, for example a catastrophic bleed for a patient with a head and neck cancer.
Advance Decision to Refuse Treatment (ADRT)	Legally binding document. Setting out an individual's requests to refuse specific treatments in specific situations, for example a patient with MND refusing to have non-invasive ventilation with respiratory failure.

(Continued)

Table 32.2 (Continued)

Lasting power of attorney LPA (health and welfare or finance)	Legally binding documents. An individual appoints persons to act on their behalf some specific areas (health and welfare or finance). There is an application and registering process.
Advance statement	Not legally binding. A document that provides information about a patient's preferences and wishes, usually including end-of-life preferences.

Involve and support

It is important to ascertain the extent to which the patient and those important to the patient want to be involved in any decisions about their ongoing care, and then regularly check this as the level of involvement will vary from person to person. Once this has been established the dying patient and their family, must be given the names of the senior doctor and nurse responsible for leading their care (LACDP, 2014). Families and those important to the dying person have their own needs, which can be overlooked by themselves and others during this difficult period (Broom and Kirby, 2013). Nurses and other health care professionals must regularly assess and meet the needs of families and those important to the dying person, as the family's experience of a loved one's final illness and death impacts on their own responses to future health care (Sykes, 2015). Some ways in which the nurse can do this include ensuring that hospital car parking fees are waived or reduced, comfort packs are provided – this will vary from trust to trust but some include meal tokens, refreshments and toiletries. Referral to the hospital chaplain or faith leader may also be done at this stage to offer spiritual and pastoral support. From a staff perspective, McAree and Doherty (2010) suggest that the most challenging phase is when it is recognised that treatment is not effective and acknowledgement that the patient may be dying. Caring for dying patients can evoke strong emotions, therefore it is important to consider what your own needs are and identify where to seek appropriate support from. This support may be through formal and informal debriefing sessions, clinical supervision or through a period of self-reflection.

6Cs: Commitment

Being committed to providing high-quality and safe patient care demonstrates that you are aware of the professional values that underpin practice.

Orange Flag

Caring for patients who are end of life or dying, although a rewarding experience can also be stressful and anxiety provoking. It is important that you identify key services and professionals who can seek support. This may include your academic assessor or supervisor, Specialist Palliative Care Team, Hospital Chaplaincy team, personal tutor or the university support and wellbeing services.

Nursing the dying patient

6Cs: Compassion

Compassion concerns how care is given through relationships that are founded on empathy, respect and dignity.

Once the decision has been made that the delivery of care has changed from aiming for a cure to promoting a comfortable death within the critical care unit, which Coombs et al. (2012) refer to as Phase 3: Controlled Death, in line with the fifth priority of care, 'Plan and Do' the role of the nurse is to ensure that the death takes place in a dignified way through ensuring that there is an individualised plan of care, which includes food and drink, symptom control and psychological, social, and spiritual support, should be agreed, co-ordinated and delivered with compassion (LACDP, 2014).

The critical care environment

It is important to think about where the patient is positioned within the critical care unit, as if in an open plan layout, then following a conversation with the patient (if able to) and the family, one consideration would be to move the patient into a single room. When this is not possible, the curtains need to be drawn around the bed space to ensure privacy and dignity, but also to create a space for the family to grieve and pay their last respects. Attention should also be given to any monitoring equipment. Where possible, these may be removed, or the alarms silenced. Coombs et al. (2012) suggest that removing equipment and machinery returns the person to the family and allows the family to be closer to the patient without the monitors acting as a barrier.

Snapshot

On assessment, Jane appears agitated and uncomfortable. She has a syringe driver with morphine sulphate 50 mg and cyclizine 150 mg continuously over 24 hours subcutaneously, and this is infusing as prescribed. On reviewing the care plan, you notice that she has not been agitated before. She is nursed in a side room, with the lights on and door open. She has a urinary catheter in situ, and there is no urine in the bag. It was last emptied 4 hours ago.

What factors may be causing her to be agitated?

Medicine management: distress, agitation, and delirium

At end of life, midazolam is used to treat distress and agitation with haloperidol used to treat delirium. Alternatively, levomepromazine can be used to treat delirium, however, is more sedating. Terminal agitation and restlessness can be very distressing for the patient, family and carers, therefore it is important that the patient is regularly assessed, and if symptoms persist, specialist advice is sought.

Orange Flag: memory making

It is important to take the opportunity when it is recognised that the patient is dying, to offer family members time and resources to make memory mementos, such as handprints, locks of hair, memory boxes and provide knitted hearts. These activities can support discussions about the individual and initiate appropriate grief reactions in a supportive environment (FICM, 2019).

Symptom management

The dying patient is at a very unstable point in their life trajectory; therefore, it is important that their condition and symptoms are monitored and assessed frequently, and any changes are made as required (see Table 32.3). The principles of symptom management at the end of life remain the same irrespective of the environment, and include a thorough assessment of the patients' physical, emotional, psychological, social, spiritual, cultural and religious needs. Nurses should utilise a range of skills and tools to support the assessment, particularly when the patient is not able to engage or offer feedback themselves.

All necessary medications should be prescribed and available in a form or route that is appropriate for the patient. Palliative care would usually advocate the least invasive but the most effective route possible and often discourages the intravenous route. However, if a patient has intravenous or central access then this may be an appropriate and effective route for that patient. What is important is that each individual patient has a medication regime that is specific to their individual needs and symptoms and should also include anticipatory prescribing. This is the process of prescribing potential needed medications to be available 'if' and 'when' a patient should develop symptoms.

Key symptoms to consider and assess at end of life are:

- Pain
- Breathlessness
- Upper respiratory tract secretions
- Nausea
- Agitation, delirium and or distress

Assessment of such symptoms in a critical care setting may differ slightly to a ward or patients' home environment, as it is likely that the patient in critical care is sedated or having level 3 support to help with their breathing. It is therefore vital to incorporate critical care assessments such as the Respiratory Distress Scale (RDOS) Critical Care Pain Observation Tool (CPOT), Richmond Agitation-Sedation Scale (RASS) in the holistic assessment of end-of-life care.

Table 32.3   Symptom management overview (FICM, 2019; Frew and Snell, 2019; Paes, 2019).

Symptoms	Observation	Management/medication
Breathing: Breathlessness	Oxygen saturation Respiratory rate RDOS scales – respiratory distress scale	Opioids: morphine, oxycodone, alfentanil to reduce the sensation perception of breathlessness. Benzodiazepine: midazolam to reduce associated distress associated with breathlessness
Breathing: Secretions	Listening (for audible secretions)	Anticholinergic drugs: hyoscine hydrobromide/hyoscine butylbromide to reduce amount of secretions The position of the patient: consider nursing on their side to allow postural drainage. Suction of secretions: if appropriate and not going to increase patient distress
Pain	Critical Care Pain Observation Tools (CPOT) for sedated patients	Opioids: morphine, oxycodone, alfentanil should be prescribed and available if required.

(Continued)

Table 32.2 (Continued)

Symptoms	Observation	Management/medication
	Visual Analogue Pain scale for conscious/awake patients	Consider any underlying conditions and long-term analgesic requirements.
	Observe for verbal and non-verbal signs of pain/distress in the non-sedated patients	Paracetamol and non-steroidal anti-inflammatory drugs can also be considered in rectal or injectable forms.
Agitation/distress/delirium	Richmond agitation-sedation scale (RASS) Confusion Assessment Method for the Intensive Care unit (CAM-ICU) Observe for verbal and non-verbal signs of agitation/distress in the non-sedated patients	Benzodiazepine: midazolam Antipsychotic: haloperidol, levomepromazine. Consider the environment, make changes to promote calm, lighting, noise, comfort items and family attendance.
Nausea	Observation of non-verbal signs of nausea Retching Triggers to nausea: often chemical, medication driven or biochemical	Anti-emetics: cyclizine, haloperidol NB: not all patients experience nausea, therefore may only require medication to be prescribed and available. Anticipatory prescribing.

Medicine Management

Unless contraindicated, Morphine is the injectable first-line choice of opiate prescribed to help control pain. Morphine can also be prescribed to manage breathlessness. Morphine is excreted renally, therefore caution should be taken when prescribing morphine if a patient has impaired or no renal function.

End-of-life care discharges from a critical care setting

Transferring critically ill patients to their home for end-of-life care is a complex, multi-professional process that requires knowledge of care and resources available in both primary and secondary care (Coombs et al., 2015). Discharge home should only be explored if achievable and safe. Discharge home directly from a critical care

Clinical Examination: mouth care

Where there is high flow oxygen or CPAP, patients can experience dryness or oxygen 'burning' of the tongue causing pain. In intubated patients, it is important to observe for signs of pressure damage of the tube and securing device on skin.

To promote comfort, the oral mucosa, tongue, and lips should be clean, moist, soft, and intact.

To check a patients' mouth you will need a

- Tongue depressor
- Tissues
- A pen torch
- Personal Protective Equipment (PPE).

Correct PPE should be worn, and local infection control policies adhered to. Figure 32.1 shows the structures to examine.

You will need to seek consent from the patient. If this is not possible, explain to the patient what you are going to do to minimise any distress.

Any dentures or palates should be removed.

Using a gloved finger or tongue depressor, the lips including the upper and lower labial sulci should be inspected

The left and right buccal mucosa should be clean, moist, and soft.

The dorsal surface of the tongue should be free from debris, and not dry or coated.

The floor of the mouth should be clean, moist, and pink with saliva present

The patient's own teeth should be clean and debris free, and dentures should be well fitting.

Observe the patient's mouth regularly, paying attention to the lips and mucous membranes.

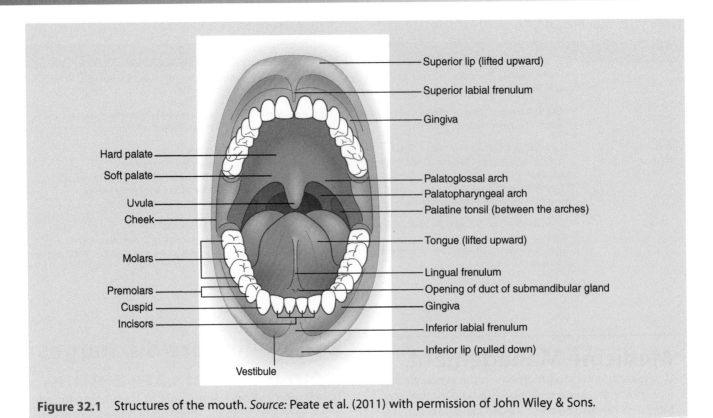

Figure 32.1   Structures of the mouth. *Source:* Peate et al. (2011) with permission of John Wiley & Sons.

setting is low at 6% (Intensive Care National Audit, 2018) with only a small proportion of which are for end-of-life care. In the case when a patient is dying and time is measured in days rather than hours, discharge from critical care could include settings such as general wards, hospices, palliative care units or even the patient's own home. Nurses must support the family by preparing them for the likelihood that the patient will die at home, and in the case of a quickly deteriorating patient, the possibility that the patient may die in transit. The fears and concerns of the family must also be explored and listened to, as the incidence of a patient dying at home is reduced by two thirds if carers are reluctant to support on discharge (Alonso-Babarro et al., 2011).

Some of the key considerations to ensure a safe discharge home are highlighted in Box 32.4.

Box 32.4   Key considerations for discharge home (Merlane and Booth, 2020).

- An urgent referral should be made to the hospital specialist palliative care team and occupational therapy
- Completion of continuing healthcare fast-track funding application
- Inform District nurses (DNs) of pending discharge
- Ensure that discharge medications are ordered by doctors, including end-of-life anticipatory medications.
- Liaise with pharmacy to prioritise prescription
- Home oxygen ordered and delivery time arranged with family
- Ensure that a Case manager is identified, and care package arranged to meet the identified needs of the patient and family
- Equipment is ordered and delivered – this includes hospital bed, commode, pressure-relieving mattress

On day of discharge:

- Reassessment and exploration of any concerns with the patient and family regarding preferred place of death
- Ensure that there is effective communication with key professionals to confirm equipment and services are ready to receive patient in place
- Transport arranged – ambulance service contacted and informed of discharge for end of-life care

- GP contacted by ward doctors and pending discharge discussed
- Medication checked and discussed with patient and family
- Relevant documents including do-not-attempt cardiopulmonary resuscitation, emergency healthcare plan, discharge letter, discharge medication list, relevant trust documentation to support caring for the dying patient and DN letter given to family
- Contact details for DN and care providers including out-of-hours support given to patient and family DN, care providers and family contacted when patient has left the unit

Medications management

Anticipatory prescribing at the end of life should include anti-emetics. Not all patients dying will experience nausea or vomiting, but biochemical changes that occur because of organ failure, and pharmacological side effects of increased opiates and antimuscarinic drugs, can lead to chemically driven nausea. Therefore, ensuring that either cyclizine or haloperidol are prescribed is important. Cyclizine requires water for injections to be used as a diluent for syringe driver use, as sodium chloride can cause precipitation. Cyclizine should not be mixed with more than one other medication in a syringe driver without seeking advice from pharmacy or specialist palliative care teams.

Red Flag

Caution is required when extubating a patient at end of life. Observe for signs of obstructive breathing, this could be perceived to be distressing to the patient and the family could be left with memories of distress or uncontrolled symptoms at the end of life. If obstructive breathing is noticed then positioning the patient in the lateral position may improve airway patency, drainage of excess secretions and reduce audible stridor (Frew and Snell 2019).

Snapshot

Jane has been diagnosed by the MDT as dying within days. She has an individualised end-of-life care plan and the family have requested that she dies in the critical care unit. Her condition is assessed regularly by the bedside nurse. As she is dying, no observations are monitored. The nurse uses her observation skills and knowledge to assess, diagnose and manage Jane's end-of-life symptoms.

Airway: No tubes. Secretions can be heard in back of throat and upper airway. Often known as the 'death rattle'.

Breathing: shallow and laboured. Some apnoea episodes.

Circulation: Jane is pale and cool to the touch, she has signs of cyanosis – lips and fingertips are blue in colour.

Conscious level: Jane is not responsive to voice or touch.

Hydration: Subcutaneous fluids are prescribed and running. The fluids are pooling in subcutaneous tissues, and not effectively being absorbed. If the fluids are not discontinued, pain could develop at the site of infusion.

Pain: No nonverbal signs of pain.

Nursing actions:
- Place Jane on her on side, to allow natural drainage of secretions.
- Suction secretions if position change is not enough to ease the impact of secretions.
- Consider reducing or stopping SC fluids. SC fluids could be driving or contributing to excess secretions. Patients who are near to death will not require the same amount of hydration or nutrition.
- Reassure her husband, that Jane is unlikely to be aware of the secretions as she is unconscious

Medication management

Secretions are common in the very latter stages of dying. If the non-pharmacological methods are not sufficient in reducing or managing the secretions, give as required antimuscarinic drugs – such as hyoscine hydrobromide. If two or three as required doses have been administered, then good practice would be to start a continuous subcutaneous infusion including the antimuscarinic.

Death: clinical investigations

Circulatory death – after the heart has stopped. The most common method to pronounce death. The NMC Registered Nurse should observe the patient for 5 minutes to establish death has occurred and documented on the verification of death form. Before undertaking

493

verification, ensure equipment available including a stethoscope, torch, clean gauze or tissue and a watch with second's hand.

- Absence of carotid pulse after palpation for 1 minute
- Absence of heart sounds using a stethoscope for 1 minute
- Absence of respiratory movements and breath sounds for 1 minute
- Both pupils fixed and dilated not reacting to light using a torch
- No corneal reflex in both eyes, using a piece of gauze or tissue gently touch the iris of the eye to ensure no blink response
- No response to painful stimuli, using a finger and thumb, performs a trapezius squeeze

These checks need to be repeated and documented again after 5 minutes.

Neurological death – after the brain has died but when the other organs of the body remain functioning.

- Evidence of irreversible brain damage of known aetiology
- Exclusion of reversible causes of coma and apnoea
- Tests for absence of brain-stem reflexes
- Apnoea test
- Document completion of diagnosis
- Two doctors perform two sets of tests at least five minutes apart.
- One of the doctors should have been registered more than five years.
- Legal time of death documented at first confirmed tests
- Death is confirmed at the second set of tests.

(Academy of Medical Royal Colleges (AOMRC), 2008)

Red Flag: neurological death test

The first set of tests should not be performed with family members present. There is a chance of a Lazarus reflex even in the event of neurological death. There is potential for the neurologically dead patient to move their arms above their head and drop them, goosebumps and shivers can also occur following the arm movements. The reflex is a neural pathway response through the spinal column not the brain. It can be exceedingly difficult for a family member who witnesses this response to accept that their loved one is dead. Therefore, the first neurological death tests should be performed without family present to establish if the reflex will occur, so that it can then be fully explained to the family.

(AOMRC, 2008; FICM, 2019; Moon and Dong, 2017)

Care after death

6Cs: Care

The care that dying and deceased patients receive should be individualised and person-centred. For example, whilst carrying out personal care on a deceased patient, the patient's own nightwear is worn, hair washed or brushed as they would like it to be.

Care after death involves meeting the holistic care needs of not just the deceased patient, but also their family, significant others and health professionals (Wilson, 2015). The Nursing and Midwifery Council (2018) supports the holistic approach to caring for deceased patients, stipulating that duty of care should include the care of the deceased and bereaved while respecting cultural requirements and protocols. It is important that the family and carers of the person who has died feel that the body has been cared for in a dignified and culturally sensitive manner (National Institute for Health and Care Excellence (NICE), 2011). Nurses need to be aware of any cultural or religious considerations when carrying out the procedure and where possible, religious, spiritual, and cultural should have been discussed with the patient and family prior to death or be aware of any advance statements where the patient may have made their wishes and preferences clear (Wilson, 2015; Gold Standards Framework, 2018).

Ensuring that the family and significant others have time to be with the patient is a crucial step in facilitating the grieving process, and where possible they should be allowed to assist in performing the personal care and can carry out any cultural, religious or spiritual rituals. Health and safety guidelines are adhered to, to prevent any risk to the staff, family, mortuary staff or funeral directors (Health & Safety Executive (HSE), 2018) and Personal Protective Equipment should be worn and local infection control and moving and handling guidelines adhered to (Merlane and Armstrong, 2019).

Reflection

Do you understand the cultural and religious sensitivities and processes for people of different faiths? How would you care for a person who is Jewish or Muslim when they die in the critical care unit?

It is important to be aware of legal consideration. For example, determining whether the deceased patient requires a coroner's referral (see Box 32.5), to comply with the correct personal care, and allow the family time to prepare for the possibility of a post-mortem examination (Gov.uk, 2019). Personal care cannot commence until death has been verified. If the death is unexpected, a doctor will

Box 32.5 Circumstances requiring a referral to the Coroner (Gov.UK, 2019)

- Cause of death is unknown
- Death was violent or unnatural
- Death was sudden or unexplained
- Person who died was not visited by a medical practitioner during their final illness
- Person who died was not seen by the medical practitioner who signed the medical certificate within 14 days before death or after they died
- Death occurred during surgery or before the person came round from anaesthetic
- Medical certificate suggests the death may have been caused by an industrial disease or industrial poisoning

usually conduct the verification of death. If the death is expected, then depending on local trust policy, a registered nurse who has received additional training may be able to verify the death (Royal College of Nursing (RCN), 2018; Wilson et al., 2019).

The patient's preferences in relation to organ and tissue donation should be recorded, ideally before death has occurred. Further advice and information regarding consent should be sought from NHS Blood & Transplant (NHSBT) Specialist Nurses in Organ Donation (SNOD).

Conclusion

End-of-life care is an integral part of the nurse's role. Within the critical care unit, knowing when a patient may be dying is complex, and involves a multidisciplinary decision. It is imperative that when patients are thought to be dying, this is recognised and communicated in a sensitive and timely manner, involving the patient, family and key members of the multidisciplinary team. An appropriate plan of care and support should be implemented and regularly reviewed, which also includes care after death. National and local guidelines should be adhered to when planning care, and nurses should act with compassion and empathy in providing this care.

Take home points

1. You only get one chance to get dying right.
2. Care for a dying patient as you would want your loved one to be cared for.
3. Encourage open and honest conversations about uncertainty and potential of dying.
4. Support patients and their families to explore end-of-life care preferences and wishes.
5. Care for a dying patient requires a senior medical review and individualised care plan.
6. Consider preferred place of care for all dying patients but only offer realistic options for highly dependent patients.
7. Remember all potential end-of-life care symptoms that patients can experience, even for ventilated and sedated patients.
8. Ensure that all dying patients and their families have access to appropriate spiritual and religious support.
9. Care for the dying patient always includes care after death and memory making for loved ones.
10. Think about your own needs, and look after yourself, as caring for dying patients is emotional for us all.

References

Academy of Medical Royal Colleges (2008). *A Code of Practice for the Diagnosis and Confirmation of Death*. http://aomrc.org.uk/wp-content/uploads/2016/04/Code_Practice_Confirmation_Diagnosis_Death_1008-4.pdf (accessed November 2020).

Alonso-Babarro, A., Bruera, E., Varela-Cerdeira, M. et al. (2011). Can this patient be discharged home? Factors associated with at home death among patients with cancer. *Journal of Clinical Oncology* 29(9): 1159–1167.

Arbour, R. and Wiegand, D. (2014). Self-described nursing roles experienced during care of dying patients and their families: a phenomenological study. *Intensive & Critical Care Nursing*, 30: 211–218.

Brinkman-Stoppelenburg, A., Rietjens, J., and van der Heide, A. (2014). The effects of advance care planning on end of life care: A systematic review. *Palliative Medicine* 28(8) 1000–1025.

Broom, A. and Kirby, E. (2013). The end of life and the family: hospice patients' views on dying as relational. *Social Health Illness*. 35(4): 499–513.

Coombs, M., Darlington, A., Long-Sutehall, T., and Richardson, A. (2012). Transferring Critically ill patients home to die: developing a clinical guidance document. *Nursing in Critical Care*, 20(5):p264–270.

Department of Health. (2008). *End of Life Care Strategy: Promoting High Quality Care for All Adults at the End of Life*. https://assets.publishing.service.gov.uk/government/uploads/system/uploads/attachment_data/file/136431/End_of_life_strategy.pdf (accessed November 2020).

Dougherty, L and Lister, S. (2015). *The Royal Marsden Manual of Clinical Nursing Procedures*, 9e. Oxford: Wiley-Blackwell.

Faculty of Intensive Care Medicine (2013). *Core Standards for Intensive Care Units*. https://ukclinicalpharmacy.org/wp-content/uploads/2017/07/Core-Standards-for-ICUs.pdf (accessed 1 March 2022).

Faculty of Intensive Care Medicine (2019). *Care at the End of Life: A guide to best practice, discussion and decision making in and around critical care*. https://www.ficm.ac.uk/sites/default/files/ficm_care_end_of_life.pdf (accessed October 2020).

Festic, E., Wilson, M.E., Gajic, O., Divertie, G.D., and Rabatin, J.T., (2011). Perspectives of physicians and nurses regarding end-of-life care in the intensive care unit. *Journal of Intensive Care Medicine*. doi:10.1177/0885066610393465.

Frew, K.E. and Snell, D. (2019). Palliative care in the critical care unit. In: *Integrated Palliative Care of Respiratory Disease*, 2e (ed. S.J. Bourke and T. Peel), 199–209. Springer.

Gold Standards Framework (2016). *The Gold Standards Framework Proactive Identification Guidance*. https://www.goldstandardsframework.org.uk/cdcontent/uploads/files/PIG/NEW%20PIG%20-%20%20%202020.1.17%20KT%20vs17.pdf (accessed November 2020).

Gomes, B., Calanzani, N., and Higginson, I (2012). Reversal of the British trends in place of death: Time series analysis 2004–2010. *Palliative Medicine*. 23(2): 102–107.

Gov.uk. (2019). *When a death is reported to a coroner*. https://www.gov.uk/after-a-death/when-a-death-is-reported-to-a-coroner (accessed December 2020).

Health and Safety Executive (2018). Managing infection risks when handling the deceased. https://www.hse.gov.uk/pubns/priced/hsg283.pdf (accessed November 2020).

Hui D., Nooruddin, M., Didwaniya, Z. et al. (2014). Concepts and definitions for 'actively dying', 'end of life care', 'terminally ill', 'terminal care' and 'transition care': A systematic review. *Journal of Pain & Symptom Management*. 47(1): 77–89.

Izumi, S. (2017). Advance care planning: The nurses role. *AJN* 117(6): 56–61.

Leadership Alliance for the Care of Dying People (2014). *One Chance to Get it Right*. https://assets.publishing.service.gov.uk//government/uploads/system/uploads/attachment_data/file/323188/One_chance_to_get_it_right.pdf (accessed 1 November 2020).

Luckhurst, H. and Clarke, C. (2017). Palliative & end of life care in a critical care setting. In: *Palliative and End of Life Nursing*, 2e (ed. B. Nyatanga and J. Nicol), 120–136. London: Sage.

McCree, S.J. and Doherty, P.A. (2010). A survey regarding physician preferences in end of life practices in intensive care across Scotland. *Journal of the Intensive Care Society*. 11(3): 182–185.

Mental Capacity Act (MCA) (2005) *Code of Practice*. https://assets.publishing.service.gov.uk/government/uploads/system/uploads/attachment_data/file/921428/Mental-capacity-act-code-of-practice.pdf (accessed October 2020).

Merlane, H. and Armstrong, L. (2019). Care after death. *British Journal of Nursing* 28(6): 342–343.

Merlane, H. and Armstrong, L. (2020). Advance care planning. *British Journal of Nursing* 20(2): 2–3.

Merlane, H. and Booth, Z. (2020). Discharge Planning in End of Life Care. *British Journal of Nursing* 29(4): 202–203.

Moon, J.W. and Dong, K.H. (2017). Chronic brain-dead patients who exhibit Lazarus sign. *Korean Journal of Neurotrauma* 13(2): 153–157.

National Competency Framework for Registered Nurses in Adult Critical Care (2015). https://www.cc3n.org.uk/uploads/9/8/4/2/98425184/02_new_step_2_final.pdf (accessed November 2020).

National Competency Framework for Registered Nurses in Adult Critical Care (2015). https://www.cc3n.org.uk/uploads/9/8/4/2/98425184/03_new_step_3_final.pdf (accessed November 2020).

National Institute for Health & Clinical Excellence (NICE) (2007). *Acutely ill patients in hospital. Recognition of and response to acute illness in adults in hospital*. https://www.nice.org.uk/guidance/cg50/evidence/full-guideline-pdf-195219037 (accessed October 2020).

National Institute for Clinical Excellence (NICE) (2011) *Quality Statement 12: Care afer death – Care of the Body*. https://www.nice.org.uk/guidance/qs13/chapter/Quality-statement-12-Care-after-death-care-of-the-body (accessed October 2020).

National Institute for Clinical Excellence (NICE) (2017). *Quality Statement 12: Care after death – Care of the Body*. https://www.nice.org.uk/guidance/qs13/chapter/Quality-statement-12-Care-after-death-care-of-the-body (accessed October 2020).

NHS Improving Quality (2014). Capacity, care planning and advance care planning in life limiting illness. https://www.england.nhs.uk/improvement-hub/wp-content/uploads/sites/44/2017/11/ACP_Booklet_2014.pdf (accessed October 2020).

Nursing & Midwifery Council (NMC) (2018). *Standards of Proficiency for registered Nurses*. https://www.nmc.org.uk (accessed September, 2020).

Paes, P. (2019). End-of-life care. In: Bourke, S. J and Peel, T. (eds) *Integrated Palliative Care of Respiratory Disease*, 2e (ed. S.J. Bourke and T. Peel), 225–251. Springer.

Pattison, N. (2011). End of life in critical care: an emphasis on care. *Nursing in Critical Care* 16(3): 113–115.

Pattison, N., Carr, S.M., Turnock.C., and Dolan, S. (2013). 'Viewing in slow motion': patients' families', nurses and doctors perspectives of end of life care in critical care. *Journal of Clinical Nursing*, 22: 1442–1454.

Resuscitation Council, British Cardiovascular Cociety, National Council Palliative Care (2015), *Deactivation of implantable cardioverter-defibrillators towards end of life*. https://www.resus.org.uk/library/publications/publication-cardiovascular-implanted-electronic-devices (accessed November 2020).

Royal College of Nursing (2018) *Confirmation or Verification of Death by Registered Nurses*. https://www.rcn.org.uk/get-help/rcn-advice/confirmation-of-death (accessed November 2020).

Sprung, C.L., Somerville, M.A., Radbruch, L. et al. (2018). Physician-Assisted Suicide and Euthanasia: Emerging Issues from a Global Perspective. *Journal of Palliative Care*, 33(4): 197–203.

Sykes, N. (2015). *One Chance to get it Right*: understanding the new guidance for care of the dying person. *British Medical Bulletin* 115(1): 143–150.

Wilson, J. (2015). *Hospice UK and National Nurse Consultant Group (Palliative Care). Guidance for Staff Responsible for Care After Death*, 2e. Hospice UK.

World Health Organisation (WHO) (2018). *Definition of Palliative Care*. http://www.who.int/cancer/palliative/definition/en (accessed November 2020).

Index

Abandonment, 28–29
Abbreviated Injury Scale (AIS), 412
ABCDE approach, 60–62, 94, 95, 160, 281, 282
  airway
    burn injury, 432
    during critical care transfer, 458, 462
    emergencies, 282, 286–290
    musculoskeletal impairment/injury, 420
  breathing
    burn injury, 433
    during critical care transfer, 459–460, 462
    emergencies, 290–292
    musculoskeletal impairment/injury, 420
  circulation/ cardiovascular
    burn injury, 433
    during critical care transfer, 460–462
    emergencies, 291, 293–297
    musculoskeletal impairment/injury, 420–421
  disability
    burn injury, 434
    during critical care transfer, 461, 462
    emergencies, 298–300
    musculoskeletal impairment/injury, 421, 422
  exposure/environment
    burn injury, 434
    during critical care transfer, 461–462
    emergencies, 301–307
    musculoskeletal impairment/injury, 421
Abdominal examination, 321–322
Abdominal surgical drains, 326
Absent breath sounds, 221
Acetylcholine (ACh), 143
Acetylcholinesterase (AChE) inhibitors, 117
Acid-base balance, 352

ACS. See Acute coronary syndrome (ACS)
Action potential, 168
Acute abdomen, in critical care, 322
Acute brain injuries (ABI), 168, 182, 183
Acute coronary syndrome (ACS), 91, 92, 236
Acute glomerulonephritis, 357
Acute kidney injury (AKI), 93, 352
  acute glomerulonephritis, 357
  classification of, 353, 355
  clinical features and examination, 355, 359, 361
  definition of, 353
  glomerular disease, 357
  hepatorenal syndrome, 357
  life-threatening emergencies, 359–361
  management, 361–362
  organ cross-talk, 354–355
  pathophysiology of, 353–354
  rhabdomyolysis, 357
  risk factors for, 355
Acute liver failure, 324–325
Acute pancreatitis, 323–324
Acute respiratory distress syndrome (ARDS), 209
Acute severe pancreatitis, 376
Acute tubular necrosis (ATN), 353–354
Addison's disease, 348
Adenosine, 249
Adenosine triphosphate (ATP), 173, 218
Admission process, standards of care for, 59–60
Adrenal cortex, 380, 382–383
Adrenal glands, 382
  adrenal cortex, 380, 382–383
  adrenal crisis, 383
  adrenaline, 382–383
  adrenal medulla, 382
  aldosterone, 381, 382
  glucocorticoids, 381–382
  gonadocorticoids, 382
  mineralocorticoids, 380
  noradrenaline, 382–383

Adrenaline, 92, 96, 382–383, 460
Adrenal medulla, 382
Adrenocorticotrophic hormone (ACTH), 381
Adrenoreceptors, 238, 239
Adult in-hospital resuscitation algorithm, 281, 283–285
Advance care planning (ACP), 488–489
Advance Decision to Refuse Treatment (ADRT), 27
Advanced haemodynamic monitoring, 260–262
Advanced life support (ALS) algorithms, 281, 284, 285
Aerosolisation medication administration, 155
Agency for Healthcare Research and Quality (AHRQ), 309
Agitation, 490
Airway obstruction, 286
AKI. See Acute kidney injury (AKI)
Alanine aminotransferase (ALT), 317
Alarm settings, 62–63
Albumin, 268
Aldosterone, 381, 382
Alkaline phosphatase (ALP), 317
Altered mental status (AMS), 190
Alveolar-capillary membrane, 217
Alveolar dead space, 199
Alveolar gas, 215
American Society for Parenteral and Enteral Nutrition (ASPEN) guidelines, 334, 335, 339
Aminoglycosides, 358
Aminophylline, 224
Amiodarone, 254
Anaesthesia
  defined, 139
  indications for, 139–141
  medications, 142
Anaesthetics, 139, 326
Analgesia, 419
Analgesia first, 147
Analgesics, 130
Anaphylactic shock, 95–96
Anaphylaxis, 160, 286

Fundamentals of Critical Care: A Textbook for Nursing and Healthcare Students, First Edition. Edited by Ian Peate and Barry Hill.
© 2023 John Wiley & Sons Ltd. Published 2023 by John Wiley & Sons Ltd.
Companion website: www.wiley.com/go/peate/criticalcare

Anatomical dead space, 199
Anatomical shunt, 199
Angina pectoris, 234
Angiotensin-converting enzyme (ACE), 380
Antenatal corticosteroid, 442
Antenatal pneumonia, 443
Antepartum haemorrhage, 444
Anti-arrhythmics and anti-anginal drugs, 124
Anticoagulant drugs, 126, 420
Anticonvulsants, 132
Antideliriogenics, 132
Anti-diarrhoeal drugs, 130
Antidiuretic hormone (ADH), 277
Antiemetics, 129, 327
Antifungals, 133–134
Antihistamine chlorphenamine, 117
Antihypertensive drugs, 125
Antimicrobial resistance, 132–133
Antipsychotic drugs, 193
Antiviral drugs, 134
Anxiolytics, 131
Aortic dissection, 242
Aortic stenosis, 232
Apneustic area, 218
ARDS. See Acute respiratory distress syndrome (ARDS)
Arterial blood gas (ABG) analysis, 90, 200–201
Arterial blood pressure monitoring, 124
Arterial waveform, 255
Artificial ventilation, 198, 207
Aseptic non-touch technique (ANTT), 151, 255
Asthma, 223–224
Asystole, 251, 253
ATN. See Acute tubular necrosis (ATN)
Atracurium, 144, 168
Atrial fibrillation, 250, 252
Atrial flutter, 250, 252
Atrioventricular heart valves, 230, 232
Auscultation, 221
    of heart sounds, 232
Autonomic nervous system (ANS), 122, 123, 169, 170
Axonal degeneration, 417

Bacterial translocation, 324
Baroreceptors, 241
Basal metabolic rate (BMR), 173
Basophils, 387
BDNF. See Brain-derived neurotrophic factor (BDNF)
Benzodiazepines, 142
Betamethasone, 442
Biliary sepsis, 324
Bilirubin, 317
Biochemistry monitoring, 338–339
Biopsychosocial model, 472–473
BIPAP, mask options for, 202

Bisacodyl, 66
blood cancer, types of, 390
Blood coagulation pathways, 390, 391
Blood components, 388
    plasma, 386
    platelets, 387
    red blood cells, 386
    white blood cells, 386–387
Blood glucose monitoring, 301–303, 375
Blood groups, 398–399
Blood pressure (BP), 238, 254
    monitoring of, 254–255
    regulation of, 241–242
Blood Safety and Quality Regulations (BSQR), 399
Blood sample collections, 398
Blood transfusion
    in adults, 397–398
    indications for, 399
Boolean operators, 48, 49
Bowel care, 65–66, 182, 320
    constipation, 320
    diarrhoea, 320
    faecal management systems, 320–321
Bowel obstruction, 324
Bowel sounds, 335
Bradycardia
    algorithm, 291, 295
    with haemodynamic instability, 294, 305
Brain
    cerebral blood flow, 173
    cerebrospinal fluid, 171
    CPP, regulation of, 173
    herniation of, 173, 174
    ICP, regulation of, 173
    meninges, 170–171
    Monro-Kellie hypothesis, 173
    primary brain injury, 180
    secondary brain injury, 180
    structure and function of, 169–172
Brain-derived neurotrophic factor (BDNF), 193–194
Breastfeeding, 447
Breath dysynchrony stacking (BDS), 208
Breathing, voluntary control of, 218
British Society for Haematology (BSH), 397–398
British Thoracic Society, 120
Bronchial sounds, 221
Bronchodilators, 121–122
Bronchospasm, 292
B-type natriuretic peptide (NT-pro BNP), 240
Buffer system, 200–201
Burn injury
    burn size estimation, 430–432
    classification of, 427, 428

deep dermal, 428–429
erythema, 427, 428
first aid considerations, 427
full thickness, 429
normothermia, 427
pathological considerations, 429–430
psychological support, 434–436
SKIN, 427
superficial dermal, 428
Burns response, 429, 430
Burn wound progression, 429
B12 vitamin deficiency, 387–389

Cadaveric organ donation, 33
Calcitonin, 371
Calcium, 349
Can't Intubate, Can't Oxygenate (CICO), 205, 211, 287
Capillaries, 215, 243
    exchange, 244–245
    shunt, 199
Capillary refill time (CRT), 258
Carbon dioxide, 217–218
Carboxyhaemoglobin (COHb), 433
Cardiac arrest (CA), 293, 304
Cardiac arrhythmias, 248–253
Cardiac conduction system, 234–237
Cardiac contractility, 239
Cardiac cycle, 236–238
Cardiac output (CO), 87–88, 238
Cardiac tamponade, 94
Cardiogenic shock (CS), 293, 305
    causes of, 91, 92
    defined, 91
    management, 93, 94
    pathophysiology, 92
    pulmonary embolism, 94
    symptoms, 92–93
Cardiomyopathies, 242–243
Cardiopulmonary resuscitation (CPR), 440
Cardiotocograph (CTG), 442
Cardiovascular assessment, 248
    advanced haemodynamic monitoring, 260–262
    atrial ectopic beats, 249, 252–254
    blood pressure, 254–255
    blood tests, 258–260
    cardiac pacing, 260, 262–263
    CVC and CVP, 256–257
    heart rate and rhythm, 248–253
    neurological status, 258
    nursing considerations and recommendations, 263
    organ and tissue perfusion, 258
    urine output, 258
Cardiovascular drugs
    anti-arrhythmics and anti-anginal, 124
    antihypertensive drugs, 125

autonomic nervous system, receptors of, 122, 123
 inodilators, 123
 inotropic drugs, 123
Cardiovascular dysfunction, 248
Cardiovascular instability, 421
Cardiovascular system (CVS), 122, 228
 capillary exchange, 244–245
 functions of, 228
 heart (See Heart)
 maternal critical care, 439–440, 444
 microcirculation, 243–244
 ventilation effects on, 245
Care after death, 494–495
Care Quality Commission (CQC), 15, 20
Catecholamines, 461
Catheter-associated urinary tract infection (CAUTI), 65
Catheter-related blood stream infections (CRBSIs), 256
CCUs. See Critical care units (CCUs)
Cellular respiration, 218
Central chemoreceptors, 220
Central line-associated blood stream infection (CLABSI), 106
Central nervous system (CNS), 168–170
 brain
  cerebral blood flow, 173
  cerebrospinal fluid, 171
  CPP, regulation of, 173
  herniation of, 173, 174
  ICP, regulation of, 173
  meninges, 170–171
  Monro-Kellie hypothesis, 173
  primary and secondary injury, 180
  structure and function of, 169–172
 drugs, 130, 131
Central venous catheters (CVCs), 256–257
Central venous oxygen saturation (ScVO$_2$), 258
Central venous pressure (CVP), 256–257
Centre for Evidence-Based Medicine (CEBM), 51
Centre for Reviews and Dissemination (CRD), 51
Cerebral blood flow, 173
Cerebral perfusion pressure (CPP), 173, 181
Cerebrospinal fluid (CSF), 171, 173
Chemoreceptors, 218, 220, 241
Chest trauma, 413
Chlorhexidine gluconate mouthwash, 65
Cholecystokinin (CCK), 314
Chromaffin cells, 382
Chronic kidney disease (CKD), 352
 classification of, 363
 clinical manifestations of, 364

complications of, 362
 definition of, 362
 management of, 362
Chronic obstructive pulmonary disease (COPD), 4, 220
Chronic respiratory disease, 222
CIS. See Clinical Information Systems (CIS)
Clinical audit, 53–55
 electronic health records, 110–111
Clinical dexterity, 151
Clinical Information Systems (CIS), 106, 107, 109, 112
Clinical Practice Guidelines, 359
Clinical Research Network (CRN), 55
Clustering care, 182
CNS. See Central nervous system (CNS)
Cognition, 151
Cognitive impairment (CI)
 causes of, 187
 defined, 187
 delirium, 188–190
  diagnosis of, 192
  management of, 191–193
  risk factors, 190–191
 morbidity, 471–472
 signs of, 188
 sleep, 193–195
Colectomy, 325
Colonoscopy, 319
Communication
 during COVID-19 pandemic, 100–101
 description of, 99–100
 with families, 102–103
 with patients, 100
 during resuscitation, 307
 through EHRs, 112
Competency frameworks, 41–42
Complete heart block, 250, 252
Compliance, 222
Comprehensive assessment, 60–61
Confidentiality, 17
Confusion Assessment Method for the ICU (CAM-ICU), 61, 146, 190, 191
Consensus-based algorithm, 298
Consent, SaBTO recommendations on, 403–408
Consent, for organ donation, 30–31
 deemed, 31–32
 first person consent, 30, 31
 hierarchy of relationships, 32–33
 nominated/appointed representative, 31
Consolidated framework for implementation research (CFIR), 52
Constipation, 130, 320
Continuous positive airway pressure (CPAP), 202, 204, 210, 224

Continuous renal replacement therapy (CRRT), 364
 anticoagulation, 364, 366
 dosing of, 364, 367
 indications of, 365
 principles of, 364, 366
COPD. See Chronic obstructive pulmonary disease (COPD)
Corticosteroids, 134
Corticotropin releasing hormone (CRH), 381
COVID-19 pandemic, 8
 communication during, 100–101
 EHRs, 111
 NICE guidelines, 20
 prone positioning in, 209–210
CPAP. See Continuous positive airway pressure (CPAP)
Cricoid pressure (CP), 205
Critical Appraisal Skills Programme (CASP), 51
Critical care emergencies (CCE), 307, 309
Critical Care National Network of Nurses (CC3N) competencies, 19, 47, 71
Critical Care Network (2016), 41, 44
Critical Care Outreach Team (CCOT), 4, 5, 7
Critical Care Pain Observation Tool (CPOT), 418
Critical Care Registered Nurses (CCRNs), 59, 60, 62. See also Nursing care
Critical Care Service Specification, 19
Critical care units (CCUs)
 adult, 2
 challenges, 11
 communication, 7
 competence, 5–6
 death in, 9
 defined, 2
 environment, 2–3
 healthcare professions, 6–7
 humanisation, 8
 levels of care, 2, 4–5
 nursing considerations and recommendations, 11
 patients, 3–4
 philosophy of care, 8
 professional issues in (See Professional issues, in CCU)
 regional anaesthesia, 140
 resilience, 9–11
 sedative medications in, 141
 survival, 9
 working ways, 7
Critical illness neuromyopathy (CINM), 416
Critical illness polyneuropathy (CIP), 416
Critical thinking, in healthcare, 42, 43

CRRT. *See* Continuous renal replacement therapy (CRRT)
Cryoprecipitate, 400
Crystalloids and colloids, 267–268
CS. *See* Cardiogenic shock (CS)
Cushing's triad, 459
Cyanosis, 221

Data extraction tool, 52
Data protection, 107
Data Protection Act (DPA) (2018), 17
Data security, 106, 107–108
Dead space, 199
Deemed consent, for organ donation, 31–32
Deep dermal burn injury, 428–429
Delirium, 132, 188–190, 471, 480, 490
    diagnosis of, 192
    management of, 191–193
    risk factors, 190–191
Delirium Detection Score (DDS), 190
Department of Defense (DoD), 309
Department of Health (DH), 2, 15, 18
Department of Health and Social Care (DHSC), 2, 15, 19
Dermis skin layer, 71
Desensitisation, 119
Device for indirect non-invasive automatic mean arterial pressure (DINAMAP), 254
Device-related pressure ulcers, 75
Dexamethasone, 442
Dexmedetomidine, 143, 193
Dextran, 276
Diabetes insipidus (DI), 374
Diabetes mellitus (DM), 129, 375
Diabetic ketoacidosis (DKA), 129, 376–378
Diabetic nephropathy, 362–363
Diagnostic imaging, in pregnancy, 443–444
Dialysis, drugs and, 120
Diarrhoea, 320
DIC. *See* Disseminated intravascular coagulation (DIC)
Difficult Airway Society (DAS), 205, 282
Digitisation, within healthcare, 106
Disseminated intravascular coagulation (DIC), 89, 407
    care and treatment of, 394
    defined, 393
    diagnosis of, 394
    pathophysiology of, 393
    process of, 393
    signs and symptoms of, 393–394
Distress, 490
Distributive shock
    anaphylactic shock, 95–96
    defined, 95
    neurogenic shock, 96
    septic shock, 95
Disuse atrophy, 417

Diuretics, 126, 127
DKA. *See* Diabetic ketoacidosis (DKA)
Dobutamine, 240
Do not attempt cardiopulmonary resuscitation (DNACPR), 17, 309
Drug-induced anaphylaxis (DIA), 160
Drug therapy, 116–119
    analgesics, 130
    anticonvulsants, 132
    anti-diarrhoeal drugs, 130
    anti-emetics, 129
    cardiovascular drugs, 122–125
    core drugs, with critical care, 120
    and dialysis, 120
    electrolyte disorder, 128
    epidural and regional anaesthesia, 130–131
    fluids, 127–128
    gastrointestinal drugs, 128
    haematological drugs, 126
    H_2-histamine antagonists, 129
    immunomodulatory drugs, 132–134
    insulin, 129
    laxatives, 130
    medication safety, in critical care, 119–120
    muscle relaxants, 131
    neurological drugs, 130
    opioids, 130
    PPIs, 129
    renal drugs, 126–127
    respiratory drugs, 120–122
    sedatives and anxiolytics, 131
    toxicology, 134
Dying and death. *See* End-of-life care
Dynamic measurements, 260
Dysphagia, 339

Early enteral nutrition (EEN), 334
Early mobilisation, 420, 478
EBP. *See* Evidence-based practice (EBP)
EHRs. *See* Electronic health records (EHRs)
e-learning modules (e-ICM), 281
Electrocardiogram (ECG)
    demonstrating atrial fibrillation, 254
    peaked T waves on, 253
    3-5 leads, 248
    12-lead, 297
Electrolyte balance, 346, 348, 349, 351
Electrolyte disorders, 127, 128
Electrolytes, fluids and. *See* Fluids and electrolytes
Electronic clinical documentation systems, 109
Electronic health records (EHRs)
    barriers, 106
    barriers to implementation, 112–113
    benefits, 112
    buy-in from clinicians, 113
    clinical audit and research, 110–111

clinical documentation, 109
critical care bed space, 109–110
data security, 106
defined, 106
errors and personal responsibility, 106
imaging systems, 108
Intensive Care Society guidelines, 107–108
in monitoring performance, 111
NHS Long Term Plan and technology, 106
responsibility, for record keeping, 107
test and result systems, 108–109
Emergencies, within critical care environment
    ABCDE approach, 281, 282
        airway emergencies, 282, 286–290
        breathing emergencies, 290–292
        circulation/cardiovascular emergencies, 291, 293–297
        disability emergencies, 298–300
        everything else emergencies, 301–307
    adult in-hospital resuscitation algorithm, 281, 283–285
    CCE and human factors, 307, 309
    debriefing, 309
    DNACPR, 309
    life-threatening, 281
    ReSPECT, 309
    return of spontaneous circulation, 307, 308
Emphysema, 222–223
End-diastolic volume (EDV), 239
Endocrine system, 371
    adrenals (*See* Adrenal glands)
    diabetes insipidus, 374
    diabetic ketoacidosis, 376–378
    hyperglycaemia, 376
    hyperosmolar, hyperglycaemic states, 379–380
    pancreas, 375–376
    parathyroid glands, 372–373
    pituitary gland, 373–374
    thyroid gland, 371–372
End-of-life care, 17–18, 485
    advance care planning, 488–489
    care after death, 494–495
    critical care environment, 489–490
    discharges, from critical care setting, 491–493
    ethics
        abandonment, 28–29
        confidentiality, 25–26
        decisions, 26–27
        ethical themes, 27
        euthanasia, 28
        organ donation (*See* Organ donation)
        principles of, 25

involve and support, 489
nursing dying patient, 489
priorities of care, 486
recognition, 486–488
symptom management, 490–491
Endoscopy, 319
Endotracheal complications, 287
Endotracheal tube (ETT), 4, 182,
204, 205
England
Care Quality Commission, 20
health and social care, 15
NICE guidelines, 20
Enteral medication administration,
155–156
Enteral nutrition (EN), 334–335
Environmental emergencies, 301–307
Enzyme inhibitors, 117
Eosinophils, 387
Epicardial cardiac pacing, 262
Epic3 guidelines, 20
Epidermis skin layer, 71
Epidural anaesthesia, 130–131
Epinephrine. See Adrenaline
Epstein-Barr virus, 391
Ergometrine maleate, 447
Erythema burn injury, 427, 428
Erythrocytes. See Red blood cells
(RBCs)
Erythrocytes, disorders of, 387
Essence of Care benchmarking, 20
Etomidate, 143
European Society of Intensive Care
Medicine, 260
Euthanasia, 28
Evidence-based guidelines, 20
Evidence-based practice (EBP)
clinical audit, 53–55
critical appraisal, 49, 51
description of, 47–48
formulating clinical question, 48
hierarchy of evidence, 49, 51, 52
implementation, 52–54
inclusion/exclusion criteria, 49, 50
locate research/evidence, 48–50
outcomes, 51–52
quality assurance and clinical
governance, 53
quality improvement, 53–55
research and development, 55
translational research, 52
Expiratory reserve volume (ERV), 216
External respiration, 217
Extracellular fluid (ECF), 277
Extracorporeal membrane
oxygenation (ECMO), 111
Eye care, 64

Faculty of Intensive Care Medicine
(FICM), 2, 28, 209, 331, 480
Faecal incontinence-associated
dermatitis, 66

Family-centred care, 8
Feeding tubes, 336–337
Fentanyl, 143
Fetal wellbeing, assessment of,
441–442
Fick's Law, 217
FICM. See Faculty of Intensive Care
Medicine (FICM)
First person consent, for organ
donation, 30, 31
Fluid balance, 180–181, 348
Fluid resuscitation, 91, 93, 269, 270
Fluids and electrolytes, 127–128, 266
critical care nurses role in, 266
de-escalation, 277
dosing, 276
drugs, 276
duration, 276
fluid overload, 276
imbalance, parenteral preparations
for, 273–275
intravenous (See Intravenous (IV)
fluids)
plasma and plasma substitutes, 276
replacement therapy, 271
hyperkalaemia, 272
oral preparations, 271
oral rehydration therapy, 272
potassium loss, 271–272
sodium bicarbonate, 273
sodium chloride, 272
Focused assessment, 62
Focused Assessment with Sonography
for Trauma (FAST) scan,
318–319
Fraction of inspired oxygen (FiO$_2$), 207
Frank-Starling relationship, 240
Freedom of Information Act (FOIA)
(2000), 17
Free nerve endings, 72
Fresh frozen plasma (FFP), 268, 400
Full thickness burn injury, 429
Functional residual capacity (FRC), 440
Fundus post-birth assessment, 446

Gastric Residual Volume (GRV),
334, 335
Gastrointestinal (GI) system
abdominal surgical drains, 326
acute abdomen, 322
acute liver failure, 324–325
acute pancreatitis, 323–324
anaesthetics, 326
anatomy and physiology of,
314–316
bacterial translocation, 324
biliary sepsis, 324
bowel care, 320–322
bowel obstruction, 324
in critically ill
blood tests, 316–317
computer tomography (CT), 319

endoscopy, 319
ultrasound (USS), 318–319
X-ray, 317, 318
description of, 314
drugs, 128
gastrointestinal tract lining, 314, 316
haemorrhage, 322–323
ischaemic colitis, 323
maternal critical care, 440
perforation, 322
peritonitis, 324
pharmacology, 327–328
post-operative complications,
326–327
post-operative monitoring, 325
surgical procedures, 325
wound dehiscence, 327
GCS. See Glasgow Coma Scale (GCS)
Gelatin, 276
General Data Protection Regulation
(GDPR), 17, 107
General Medical Council (GMC), 6,
16, 487
Genetic haemochromatosis, 389–390
Gentamicin, 358
Gestation, 441
GI system. See Gastrointestinal (GI)
system
Glasgow Coma Scale (GCS), 60,
174, 177
Glomerular disease, 357
Glomerular filtration rate (GFR), 353
Glucagon, 375
Glucocorticoids, 381–382
Glucose solutions, 275
Glycaemic control, 337–338
Glyceryl trinitrate (GTN), 119,
234–235, 239
Goal-directed therapy, 180
Gonadocorticoids, 382
Good Clinical Practice (GCP), 55
Granulocytes, 400
Graves' disease, 372
Great Britain (GB), health and social
care provision, 15
GTN. See Glyceryl trinitrate (GTN)
Guidance for provision of intensive
care services (GPICS), 20, 53,
143, 480

Haematemesis, 322
Haematological disorders, 386, 391
administration, of blood product,
400–401
blood groups, 398–399
blood sample collections, 398
blood transfusion
in adults, 397–398
alternatives to, 403
indications for, 399
B12 vitamin deficiency, 387–389
compatibility, 399

Haematological disorders (cont'd)
  disseminated intravascular
    coagulation, 393–394
  erythrocytes, disorders of, 387
  fresh frozen plasma, 400
  genetic haemochromatosis,
    389–390
  haematopoiesis, 387
  haemostasis, 390, 391
  lymphoma, 390–391
    Hodgkin lymphoma, 391–392
    non-Hodgkin lymphoma,
      392–393
  neutropenia, 394–395
  patient information, 402–403
  physiology, 386
  platelets, 400
  post-procedural care, 401
  procedural safety, 400
  SaBTO recommendations, on
    consent, 403–408
  sepsis, 395
  sickle cell anaemia, 388–389
  thrombocytopenia, 394
  traceability, 401–402
  transfusion reactions, 401, 402
  vasculitis, 396, 397
Haematological drugs, 126
Haematopoiesis, 387
Haemodynamic therapy, 181
Haemoglobin, 387
Haemolysis, Elevated Liver enzymes
    and Low Platelets (HELLP)
    syndrome, 445
Haemostasis, 390, 391
Hair follicle and muscle, 72
Haloperidol, 193
Handover, of patient care
    information, 62
Hartmann's procedure, 325
HCW. See Healthcare worker (HCW)
Health and Care Professions Council
    (HCPC), 6, 16
Health and Safety Executive (HSE), 18
Healthcare Improvement Scotland
    (HIS), 20
Healthcare Inspectorate Wales, 20
Healthcare worker (HCW), 154,
    157, 159
Health Education England, 15
Heart
  anatomy of, 228–229
  blood pressure, 238, 241–242
  cardiac conduction system,
    234–237
  cardiac cycle, 236–238
  cardiac output, 238
  chambers of, 230
  coronary circulation, 232–234
  heart rate, regulation of, 238
  internal structures of, 231–232
  layers of, 229

  pericardium, 229, 230
  stroke volume, 238–241
  valves, 230, 232–234
Heart failure, 241
Heart rate and rhythm, 248–251
Heart rate, regulation of, 238
Heart sounds, 232
Heel offloading device, 78
Helicobacter pylori, 392
Hemicolectomy, 325
Hepatic encephalopathy, 324–325
Hepatic system, anatomy and
    physiology of, 316, 317
Hepatorenal syndrome (HRS), 357, 361
H₂-histamine antagonists, 129
HHS. See Hyperosmolar,
    hyperglycaemic states (HHS)
High flow nasal cannula (HFNC), 204
Hodgkin lymphoma (HL), 391–392
Homoeostasis, 266
Hormone inhibitors, 117
HRS. See Hepatorenal syndrome
    (HRS)
Human Rights Act (1998), 18, 33
Human Tissue Act (2004), 30, 32
Human Tissue Authority (HTA), 30
Humidification, 208
Hydroxyethyl starch, 276
Hyperactive form, delirium, 188–189
Hypercalcaemia, 372–373
Hyperchloraemic acidosis, 273
Hyperglycaemia, 129, 337, 376
Hyperkalaemia, 275, 349
  management of, 272
  treatment algorithm for, 359–361
Hypernatraemia, 277
Hyperosmolar, hyperglycaemic states
    (HHS), 129, 379–380
Hyperoxaemia, 120–122
Hypertensive crisis, 294, 305
Hyperthyroidism, 372
Hypertonic saline (HS), 275
Hypoactive form, delirium, 189
Hypocalcaemia, 278, 373
Hypoglycaemia, 129, 307, 380
Hypokalaemia, 277, 349
Hypomagnesaemia, 278
Hyponatraemia, 277
Hypophosphataemia, 278
Hypotension, 421
Hypothyroidism, 371–372
Hypoventilation, 198–199
Hypovolaemia, 181, 266
Hypovolaemic shock, 294, 305
  aetiology, 88
  blood analysis, 88–89
  clinical features of, 88
  complications of, 90
  description of, 87
  fluid resuscitation, 91
  gastrointestinal (GI) losses, 88
  investigations table, 89

  management of, 90
  multiple organ dysfunction
    syndrome, 89
  pathophysiology and symptoms, 87
  renal losses, 88
  risk factors, 88
  skin losses, 88
  stages of, 90
  third-space sequestration, 88
  training and education, 91
Hypoxaemia, 459

ICO statutory Data Sharing Code of
    Practice, 17
ICP. See Intracranial pressure (ICP)
ICS. See Intensive Care Society (ICS)
ICUAW. See Intensive care unit-
    acquired weakness (ICUAW)
Ileus, 327
Immune system, maternal critical
    care, 440
Immunoglobulins, 134, 386
Immunological problems, burn
    injury, 429
Immunomodulatory drugs, 132, 133
  antibacterial agents, 132–133
  antifungals, 133–134
  antiviral drugs, 134
  corticosteroids, 134
  immunoglobulins, 134
Independent mental capacity
    advocate (IMCA), 27
Indirect calorimetry (IC), 333
Infection in Critical Care Quality
    Improvement Programme
    (ICCQIP), 111
Inflammation phase, wound
    healing, 79
Inhalation injury, 433
Inoconstrictors, 122
Inodilators, 123
Inotropic drugs, 4, 123
Inspiratory:expiratory (I:E) ratio, 208
Inspiratory reserve volume (IRV), 216
Insulin, 129, 328, 375
Insulin dextrose, 259
Insulin infusion, 338
Integrated Care Systems (ICS), 19
Intensive Care Delirium Screening
    Checklist (ICDSC), 61, 190
Intensive Care National Audit and
    Research Centre (ICNARC), 228
Intensive Care Psychological
    Assessment Tool (IPAT), 475
Intensive Care Society (ICS), 2,
    107–108, 339, 480
Intensive care unit (ICU)
  delirium management in, 191
  maternal critical care, 439
  Mobility Scale, 421, 423
  psychosis, 188
  sleep assessment in, 193–195

Intensive care unit-acquired weakness (ICUAW), 419, 423, 471, 478
  axonal degeneration, 417
  bioenergetic disturbance, 417
  clinical presentation, 417
  diagnosis and assessment of, 417
  disuse atrophy, 417
  muscle protein homeostasis, 416
  muscle weakness, 415
  pathophysiological processes and risk factors in, 415
Internal respiration, 218–220
International Classification of Functioning, Disability and Health (ICF), 472, 474
International critical care organisations, 18
InterTASC Information Specialists' Sub-Group Search Filter Resource database, 48–49
Intestinal anastomosis, 327
Intestinal motility disorders, 335
Intra-abdominal pressure (IAP), 326
Intra-and inter-hospital transfer, 452–454
  ABCDE process, 458–462
  bed and repatriation, 456
  checklist handover, 464–468
  of critically ill adult, 452, 454–455
  flow chart, 463
  preparation for, 458
  risks of, 457
  roles and responsibilities, 457–458
  transfer process, 457
  transfer terms, 456
Intracranial pressure (ICP), 173, 298–299
  fluid balance, 180–181
  goal-directed therapy, 180
  haemodynamic therapy, 181
  oncotic therapy, 181
  signs and symptoms of increasing, 179
Intramuscular medication administration, 155
Intravenous (IV) fluids, 266–267
  assessment and monitoring, 269–270
  crystalloids and colloids, 267–268
  electrolyte concentrations in, 278
  5 Rs of, 270
  management strategies, 268–269
  overload, 276
  third spacing, 269
  training and education, 271
Intravenous (IV) medication administration, 156–157
Intubation, 204–206
  complications, 287
Invasive mechanical ventilation, 198
Inverse ratio, 208
Involuntary pathway, 218

Ion-exchange resins, 272
Ischaemic colitis, 323
Isoprenaline, 460–461

Joint British Diabetes Societies Inpatient Care Group (2013), 377, 379
Joint range of motion (ROM), 417–418

Ketamine, 143
Kidney
  drugs, adverse effects of, 358
  functions of, 344
  internal structure of, 349
  transplantation, 367
Kleihauer test, 444–445

LACDP. See Leadership Alliance for the Care of the Dying Person, (LACDP)
Lactate, 95, 258
Langerhans cells, 72
Lasting power of attorney (LPA), 26, 31
Laxatives, 130, 328
Leadership Alliance for the Care of the Dying Person, (LACDP), 486, 487
Left ventricular failure, 240
Legal and ethical issues. See End-of-life care ethics
Leukaemia, 390
Leukocytes. See White blood cells
Levine technique, 81, 83
Levothyroxine, 373
Life-sustaining treatments, 27, 28
Life-threatening emergencies, 281, 359–361
Liver, maternal critical care, 440
Liver function test (LFT), 317
Local anaesthetic drugs, 131
Local Clinical Research Networks (LCRNs), 55
Local policies, in critical care, 21
Long-term cognitive impairment (LTCI), 187
Look-listen-feel assessment, lungs, 220
Loss phase, third spacing, 269
Low molecular weight heparins (LMWH), 126
LPA. See Lasting power of attorney (LPA)
Lund and Browder chart, 430, 431
Lung function, 214
Lungs
  absent breath sounds, 221
  air composition, 215, 216
  anatomy and physiology of, 214–215
  assessment of, 220–221
  asthma, 223–224
  breathing, 222
  bronchial sounds, 221

  compliance, 222
  crackles, 222
  emphysema, 222–223
  expired air, 216
  external respiration, 217
  gas exchange, 215
  internal respiration, 218–220
  obstructive sleep apnoea, 224
  prone positioning, 225
  psychological implications of, 225
  pulmonary ventilation, 216–217
  resistance, 222
  transport of gases, 217–218
  ventilation/perfusion, 217
  volumes, 216
  wheeze, 222
Lymphocytes, 387
Lymphoma, 390–391
  Hodgkin lymphoma, 391–392
  non-Hodgkin lymphoma, 392–393

Magnesium sulphate, 445
Mannitol, 275
Manual muscle testing algorithm, 418
Manual pulse, 253
Maternal critical care, 439
  adapted physiology, 439
    cardiovascular system, 439–440
    immune system, 440
    liver and gastro-intestinal system, 440
    placenta, 441
    renal system, 440
    respiratory system, 440
  breastfeeding, 447
  epidemiology, 439
  maternal-infant bond, 448
  physiological changes, of pregnancy, 441
  recognising clinical deterioration, 441–442
  specialist knowledge and skills, 442–443
  vital signs, in pregnancy, 441
Maternal Early Warning Score (MEWS), 441
Maternal sepsis, 443
Mathematical drug calculations, in adult CCU, 160–161
  converting from one unit to another, 161, 162
  decimals and rounding, 161, 162
  drip rate, 163–164
  expressed in percentage, 164
  expressed in ratio, 164
  flow rate, 164–165
  rate, time and volume, 162–163
  stated rate, 163
  volume and dose, 162
Mean arterial pressure (MAP), 173, 254, 396
Mechanical bowel obstruction, 324

Mechanical circulatory support (MCS), 92
Mechanical ventilation, 206–207
  artificial ventilation, 207
  benefits of, 208
  fraction of inspired oxygen, 207
  humidification, 208
  inspiratory:expiratory ratio, 208
  inverse ratio, 208
  minute ventilation, 207
  positive end-expiratory pressure, 207
  pressure control, 207
  prone position, 209
  risks of, 208–209
  synchronisation, 208
  ventilator-associated pneumonia, 209
  volume control, 207
  weaning from, 210
Medical Research Council (MRC) system, 418
Medication administration
  anaphylaxis, 160
  collaborative multidisciplinary team working, 154
  displacement, 165
  drug-induced anaphylaxis, 160
  legal and professional issues, 152–153
  mathematical drug calculations, 160–165
  medication errors, 154, 159–160
  pharmacological interventions, for adult, 152
  rights of, 158–159
  routes and methods for, 155–157
  skills, 151
Medicines management, defined, 151
Medullary rhythmicity area, 218
Melanocytes, 72
Melatonin, 194
Meninges, 170–171
Mental Capacity Act (MCA) (2005), 16, 26–28, 488
Merkel cells, 72
Metabolic acidosis, 91, 352
Metabolic problems, burn injury, 429
Microcirculation, 243–244
Midazolam, 142
Mineralocorticoids, 380
Minute ventilation, 207
Minute volume (MV), 216
Mitochondrial dysfunction, in skeletal muscle, 417
Mixed delirium, 189
Mixed venous oxygen saturation (SvO$_2$), 258
Mobilisation, in critical care, 66–67
Modified Early Obstetric Warning Score (MEOWS), 441

Monocytes, 387
Monro-Kellie hypothesis, 173
Moral balance, 28
Morphine, 143, 491
  for acute pain, 80
Motor Activity Assessment Scale (MAAS), 190
Mouth care, 491–492
MRC sum score (MRC-SS), 417
Mucolytics, 122
Multidisciplinary team (MDT), 339, 488
Multiple myeloma, 390
Multiple organ dysfunction syndrome (MODS), 89
Muscle protein homeostasis, 416
Muscle relaxants, 131
Musculoskeletal impairment/injury
  airway, 420
  assessment of, 417–419
  breathing, 420
  circulation, 420–421
  disability, 421, 422
  early mobilisation, 420
  exposure/environment, 421
  ICUAW, 415–417
  joint positioning and passive movements, 419
  measuring mobility and function, 421–423
  trauma (See Traumatic injury)
Myxoedema coma. See Hypothyroidism

Naloxone, 122
Nasogastric tube (NG), 337
National Competency Framework, 25
  for registered nurses (RNs), 151, 152
National Confidential Enquiry into Patient Outcome and Death (NCEPOD), 55
National critical care organisations, 18
National early warning scores (NEWS), 55, 110, 394
National Health Service (NHS), 99
  critical care units in, 19
  England, 15, 19
  Long Term Plan, 106
  Scotland, 15
  Wales, 15
National Institute for Health and Care Excellence (NICE), 3, 30, 55, 91, 119, 333, 338, 339
  guidelines, 20, 127, 398
  Quality Standards, 480
National Institute for Health Research (NIHR), 55
National Tracheostomy Project, 290
Neostigmine, 144
Nephrons, 345, 348, 349
Nervous system

CNS (See Central nervous system (CNS))
  functions of, 168, 169
  peripheral nervous system, 168–170
Network for Investigation of Delirium: Unifying Scientists (NIDUS), 187
Neurogenic shock, 96
Neurological death
  organ donation, 33
  test, 494
Neurological drugs, 130
Neurological emergencies. See Disability emergencies
Neurological system, 168
  Glasgow Coma Scale, 174, 177
  limb movement, 176, 177
  nervous system (See Nervous system)
  nursing care, 181–183
  observation chart, 174–176
  pupillary assessment, 178
  transfer and interventions, 183
Neuromuscular blocking agents (NMBAs), 143–145, 210, 416
Neurone, 168, 169
Neuropathic pain, 475
Neurovascular assessment, 419
Neutropenia, 394–395
Neutrophils, 387
NHS Blood and Transplant (NHSBT), 30, 34
NHS Commissioning Board (NHS CB), 456
NHS Organ Donor Register (NHS ODR), 31, 32
Nimodipine, 183
NIV. See Non-invasive ventilation (NIV)
NMBAs. See Neuromuscular blocking agents (NMBAs)
Nominated/appointed representative consent, for organ donation, 31
Non-healing wounds, management of, 83, 84
Non-Hodgkin lymphoma (NHL), 392–393
Non-invasive ventilation (NIV), 201–203
Non-opioid analgesics, 130
Non-steroidal anti-inflammatory drugs (NSAIDs), 130, 357–358
Noradrenaline, 382–383, 460
Norepinephrine, 93, 244
Northern Ireland (NI)
  health and social care in, 15
  NICE guidelines, 20
  Regulation and Quality Improvement Authority, 20
Numerical rating scale (NRS), 418
Nurse-patient relationship, 102
Nursing and Midwifery Council (NMC), 16, 18, 107, 151, 336, 494

Code, 59, 100
code of conduct, 25, 38–41
standards, 71
Nursing care
critical care bundles, 67
mobility, 66–67
physical care, 63
bowel care, 65–66
eye care, 64
oral care, 64–65
patient hygiene, 63
perineum and elimination care, 65
skin care, 63–64
urinary incontinence, 65
standards of care, 59
admission process, 59–60
alarm settings, 62–63
comprehensive assessment, 60–61
focused assessment, 62
handover, 62
preadmission phase, 59
safety assessment, 62
Nutrition
discontinuing feed, 339
enteral nutrition, 334–335
exhaustion phase, 332
feeding tubes, 336–337
fight/flight phase, 332
glycaemic control, 337–338
indirect calorimetry, 333
nursing considerations and recommendations, 336
nutritional guidance, 339–340
nutritional support, 331
parenteral nutrition, 335–336
pathophysiology, 331–332
refeeding syndrome, 338–339
resistance phase, 332
screening and assessment, 333

Obstructive shock, 93–94
Obstructive sleep apnoea, 224
Oedema, 245
Oesophagectomy, 325
Oesophago-Gastro-Duodenoscopy (OGD), 319
Omeprazole, 334
Oncotic therapy, 181
Ondansetron, 327
Open reduction and internal fixation (ORIF), 413
Operational Delivery Networks (ODNs), 456
Opioids, 130, 143
Optimal osmolality, 346
Oral care, 64–65
Oral medication administration, 155
Oral rehydration therapy (ORT), 272
Organ and tissue perfusion, 258

Organ cross-talk, 354–355
Organ donation, 29–30
cadaveric, 33
consent for, 30–33
guiding principle of, 33–34
organ allocation, 34–35
post organ retrieval, 34
Organisational influences, 15
confidentiality, 17
end-of-life care, 17–18
England, 15
international influences, 18
legislation, 15
local policies, 21
national guidelines, 20
national influences, 18
networks, 19
Northern Ireland, 15
nursing considerations and recommendations, 21
Professional Statutory Regulatory Bodies, 15–16
quality assurance, 20
risk management, 18
Scotland, 15
shared decision making, 16–17
UK government, 18–19
Wales, 15
Organisational resilience, 10–11
Overdrive pacing, 260
Oxygen, 198, 217
calculations
for spontaneously breathing patient, 459
for ventilated patient, 459–460
respiratory drugs, 120–122
Oxygen saturation (SaO$_2$), 217
Oxytocin, 446–447

Pabrinex. See Thiamine
Pain, Agitation, Delirium, Immobility, and Sleep Disruption (PADIS) Guidelines, 191
Palliative care, 486
Pancreas, 375–376
Paradoxical breathing, 218
Paralytic ileus, 324
Parasympathetic neurones, 238
Parathyroid gland, 372
hypercalcaemia, 372–373
hypocalcaemia, 373
Parathyroid hormone (PTH), 351, 372
Parenteral nutrition (PN), 335–336
Partial colectomy, 325
Partial thromboplastin time (PTT), 394
Passive range of motion (PROM), 66
Pathogenesis, 394
Patient-centred care, 8
Patient hygiene, 63
Patient positioning, 182

Pelvic trauma, 412–413
Perineum and elimination care, 65
Peripheral chemoreceptors, 219, 220
Peripheral nervous system (PNS), 168–170
Peristalsis, 314
Peritonitis, 324
Pernicious anaemia, 387
PERSONAL mnemonic, 461, 462
Personal protective equipment (PPE), 100, 253
Personal resilience, 9
Phaeochromocytoma, 382
Pharmaceutical process, 117
Pharmacodynamic process, 117
Pharmacokinetic process, 117
Pharmacology, principles of, 116
Pharmacotherapy
description of, 116
drug therapy (See Drug therapy)
principles of, 116
processes of, 117
Phenothiazines, 327
Phenytoin, 183
Philosophy of care, 8
Phosphate, 349
Physical care, 63
bowel care, 65–66
eye care, 64
oral care, 64–65
patient hygiene, 63
perineum and elimination care, 65
skin care, 63–64
urinary incontinence, 65
Physical morbidity, 471
PICO model, 48, 49
PICS. See Post-intensive care syndrome (PICS)
Pitting oedema, 268
Pituitary gland, 373–374
Placenta, maternal critical care, 441
Plan Do Study Act (PDSA) cycle, 54
Plasma, 386
osmolality, 346, 350
and plasma substitutes, 276
Platelets, 387, 400
Pneumothorax, 214–215
PNS. See Peripheral nervous system (PNS)
Pnuemotaxic area, 218
Point-of-Care (PoC) testing, 378
Positive end-expiratory pressure (PEEP), 206, 207
Post-intensive care syndrome (PICS), 59, 67, 188, 473, 474
Post organ retrieval, 34
Postpartum haemorrhage, 446
Post-resuscitation care algorithm, 308
Post-traumatic stress disorder (PTSD), 3, 448, 479
Potassium, 259, 349

PPE. *See* Personal protective equipment (PPE)
Preadmission phase, 59
Prednisolone, 223
Preeclampsia, 445
Pressure control, 207
Pressure damage, 478
Pressure support ventilation (PSV), 210
Pressure ulcers, 71–75
  management of, 79
  people with darker skin tones, 76
  prevention of, 76–78
  redistribution, 77
  risk assessments, 75
Primary brain injury, 180
Prioritising process, 42–43
  multidisciplinary interaction, 43–44
  resource constraints, 43
  time, 43
Proctocolectomy, 325
Professional issues, in CCU, 38
  competency frameworks, 41–42
  core principles
    practise effectively, 40
    preserve safety, 40
    prioritise people, 39
    promote professionalism and trust, 40–41
  critical thinking, 42, 43
  learning opportunities, 38
  NMC Code, 38–39
  prioritisation, 42–44
  support systems, 44
Professional Statutory Regulatory Bodies (PSRBs), 15–16
Proliferation phase, wound healing, 79
Propofol, 142, 183
Protocolised sedation, 147
Proton pump inhibitors (PPIs), 129, 327
Pseudo-obstruction, 324
PSRBs. *See* Professional Statutory Regulatory Bodies (PSRBs)
Psychological distress, 419
Psychological morbidity, 471
Psychological safety, 7
Psychomotor skills, 151
PTSD. *See* Post-traumatic stress disorder (PTSD)
Pulmonary embolism (PE), 94, 292
Pulmonary shunt, 199
Pulmonary ventilation, 216–217
Pulse oximetry, 220
Pulsus paradoxus, 241
Pupillary assessment, 178

Quality assurance, 20
Quality improvement (QI), 53–55
Quick Sequential (Sepsis-related) Organ Failure Assessment (qSOFA), 396

RaCl. *See* Rehabilitation after critical illness (RaCl)
Radial pulse, 253
Radiocontrast-induced nephropathy, 358
Radiology information systems (RISs), 108
Randomised control trial (RCT), 111
Ranitidine, 198
Rapid Sequence Induction (RSI), 204, 205
  of anaesthesia, 140
  drug administration in, 140
RASS. *See* Richmond Agitation-Sedation Score (RASS)
Reabsorption phase, third spacing, 269
Recommended Summary Plan for Emergency Care and Treatment (ReSPECT), 309
Rectal medication administration, 155
Red blood cells (RBCs), 386–389, 398, 399
Reed-Sternberg cells, 391
Refeeding syndrome, 338–339
Regional anaesthesia (RA), 130–131, 140
Registered nurse (RN), 157
  medication error, 159, 160
  with NMC, 152
Regulation and Quality Improvement Authority (RQIA), 20
Rehabilitation after critical illness (RaCl), 471
  conditions impact on, 472
  goals, 475–477
  key timepoints in, 477
  morbidity
    biopsychosocial model, 472–473
    clinical assessment, 473, 475, 476
    cognitive impairment, 471–472
    physical, 471, 472
    post intensive care syndrome, 473, 474
    psychological, 471
  national guidelines and standards, 480
  treatment
    cognitive interventions, 479–480
    early mobilisation, 478
    psychological interventions, 478–479
Remifentanil, 143
Renal drugs, 126–127
Renal replacement therapy (RRT), 120
Renal system
  acid-base balance, 352
  AKI (*See* Acute kidney injury (AKI))
  anatomy and physiology of, 344, 345
  biochemical investigations, 355–356
  chronic kidney disease, 352, 362–364

continuous renal replacement therapy, 364–367
  diabetic nephropathy, 362–363
  drug-induced renal damage, 357–358
  electrolyte balance, 346, 348, 349, 351
  kidney transplantation, 367
  maternal critical care, 440
  nephrons, 345, 348, 349
  plasma osmolality, 346, 350
  RAAS, 344, 347
  vascular supply, 344
Renal tubulointerstitial disease, 348
Renin-angiotensin-aldosterone system (RASS), 344, 347
Renin-angiotensin pathway, 380
Renin-producing granular cells (RPGC), 344
Residual volume (RV), 216
Resilience
  description of, 9
  in nurses, 10
  organisational, 10–11
  personal, 9
  team, 9–10
  workplace stressors, 10, 11
Resistance, 222
Respiratory centre, 219
Respiratory drugs
  bronchodilators, 121–122
  classes of, 120, 121
  mucolytics, 122
  oxygen, 120–122
  stimulants, 122
Respiratory failure, 198, 292
  arterial blood gas analysis, 200–201
  continuous positive airway pressure, 204
  and gas exchange, 198, 199
  high flow nasal cannula, 204
  hypoventilation, 198–199
  intubation, 204–206
  mechanical ventilation, 206–210
  non-invasive ventilation, 201–203
  V/Q mismatch, 199
  work of breathing, 199–200
Respiratory problems, burn injury, 429
Respiratory system, maternal critical care, 440
Respiratory zone, 215
Resuscitation Council (UK), 95, 96, 291, 307
Return of spontaneous circulation (ROSC), 307, 308
Rhabdomyolysis, 357
Richmond Agitation-Sedation Score (RASS), 60–61, 182, 190, 191, 146, 147
Riker Sedation-Agitation Scale (SAS), 60–61

Risk management, in critical care, 18
Rocuronium, 144
Royal College of Nursing (RCN), 151, 152
Royal Pharmaceutical Society (RPS), 116, 151, 152
    guidelines, in CCU clinical practice, 152, 153

SaBTO. *See* Safety of Blood, Tissues and Organs (SaBTO)
Safety assessment, 62
Safety of Blood, Tissues and Organs (SaBTO), 403–408
Salbutamol, 208, 222
SBAR tool, 309
Scotland
    health and social care in, 15
    Healthcare Improvement Scotland, 20
    SIGN guidelines, 20
Scotland Act (1998), 15
Scottish Intensive Care Society (SICS), 339
Scottish Intercollegiate Guidelines Network (SIGN), 20
Sebaceous glands, 72
Secondary brain injury, 180
Secondary diabetes, 375–376
Sedation, 131, 182
    analgesia first, 147
    defined, 139
    drugs, 142–143
    indications for, 139–142
    interruption, 147
    medications, 142
    protocolised, 147
    targeted, 145–147
Sedation-Agitation Scale (SAS), 190
Selective serotonin reuptake inhibitors (SSRIs), 479
Semilunar heart valves, 230, 232
Sensitisation, 399
Sepsis, 81, 395
    campaign guidelines 2021, 396
    management of, 396
    pathophysiology of, 395
    risk factors of, 395
    signs and symptoms of, 395–396
Septic shock, 95, 395, 396
Serious Hazards of Transfusion (SHOT), 398
Service Specification for Adult Critical Care, 19
Shared decision making, 16–17
Shock
    cardiogenic shock, 91–93
    defined, 87
    distributive, 95–96
    hypovolaemic, 87–91
    obstructive, 93–94

septic, 95, 395, 396
    types of, 396
Short-acting insulin, 375
Short Physical Performance Battery (SPPB) tool, 475, 477
Shunt, 199
Sickle cell anaemia, 388–389
Silver trauma, 412, 415
Sinus bradycardia, 250, 252
Sinus tachycardia, 250, 252
Skills for Care & Skills for Health (2013), 6
Skin care, 63–64
Skin integrity, 71
    age-related changes in, 71, 73
    anatomy and physiology of, 71, 72
    nursing assessment, 75
    pressure ulcers (*See* Pressure ulcers)
    specialised cells and appendages, 71, 72
    wound healing (*See* Wound healing)
Skin turgor, 272
Sleep assessment, in ICU, 193–195
Sleep/wake cycle, 194
SMART goals, 41
Socialisation, in healthcare, 7
Sodium bicarbonate, 273
Sodium chloride, 274
Sodium-glucose co-transporter 2 (SGLT2) inhibitors, 129
Somatic nervous system (SNS), 169
Specific, Measurable, Achievable, Realistic and Timed (SMART) subgoals, 475
Spinal injury, 413
Spontaneous breathing trial (SBT), 210
Standards of care, 59
    admission process, 59–60
    alarm settings, 62–63
    comprehensive assessment, 60–61
    focused assessment, 62
    handover, 62
    preadmission phase, 59
    safety assessment, 62
Status epilepticus (SE), 132
Steroids, 373, 383
Stroke volume, 238
    afterload, 239–240
    contractility, 239
    preload, 239
Subcutaneous fat layer, 71
Subcutaneous medication administration, 155
Sublingual medication administration, 155
Sub-optimal sedation, 145, 146
Sugammadex, 144
Superficial dermal burn injury, 428
Supernumerary status, 44
Supraventricular tachycardia (SVT), 250, 252

Surgical intensive care unit (SICU), 106
Suxamethonium, 143–144
Sweat glands, 72
Sympathetic neurones, 238
Sympathomimetic drugs, 124, 125
Synchronisation, 208
Syndrome of Inappropriate Antidiuretic Hormone Secretion (SIADH), 373–374
Systemic inflammatory response syndrome (SIRS), 95
Systolic blood pressure (SBP), 181

Tachycardia
    algorithm, 291, 296
    with haemodynamic instability, 294, 305
Tachyphylaxis, 118
Targeted sedation, 145–147
Team resilience, 9–10
TeamSTEPPS® 2.0, 309
Tension pneumothorax, 94, 290, 292
Test and result systems, 108–109
Thalassaemia, 389
Therapeutic drug monitoring (TDM), 119
Therapeutic process, 117
Thiamine, 339
Thiopentone (thiopental sodium), 142
Thrombocytes, 387
Thrombocytopenia, 394
Thyroid gland, 371
    crisis, 372
    hyperthyroidism, 372
    hypothyroidism, 371–372
Thyroid-stimulating hormone (TSH), 371
Thyrotoxicosis. *See* Hyperthyroidism
Thyroxine, 373
Ticagrelor, 237
Tidal volume (TV), 216
TIMERS framework, 83, 84
Tolerance, drug therapy, 117, 119
Tonic influences, 218
Topical medication administration, 155
`Top-to-toe' approach, 301
Total Body Surface Area (TBSA) burned, 430
Total colectomy, 325
Total lung capacity (TLC), 216
Toxicology, 134
Toxidromes, 192
Tracheostomy, 205
    complications, 288
    tube, 4
Transcutaneous cardiac pacing, 262
Transducer system, 255
Transthoracic echocardiography, 260
Transvenous cardiac pacing, 262
Traumatic brain injury (TBI), 459

Traumatic injury, 412
   chest, 413
   conservative management, 413–415
   external fixation, 413
   management of, 413
   mechanism of, 412
   musculoskeletal injuries, 412
   pelvic injury, 412–413
   surgical fixation, 413, 414
Treitz, ligament of, 322, 323
Tripartite model, 42
12-lead electrocardiogram (ECG), 236, 297

UK
   government organisations, 18–19
   organ donation in, 29–30
UK Blood Services, 403
UK National Competency Framework. *See* Competency frameworks
UK Organ Donor Register, 30
Unfractionated heparin (UFH), 126
United Kingdom General Data Protection Regulation (UK GDPR), 17
United Kingdom Resuscitation Council (UKRC), 249, 253

Universal Declaration of Human Rights, 99
Uptake blockers, 116
Urinalysis, 356, 377
Urinary incontinence, 65

Vasculitis, 396, 397
Vasoconstrictors, 122
Vasopressin, 374
Vasopressors, 4
Venous thromboembolism (VTE), 238
Ventilation, defined, 198
Ventilation/perfusion (V/Q) mismatch, 199
Ventilator-associated pneumonia (VAP), 208, 209
Ventilator-induced lung injury (VILI), 209
Ventricular fibrillation (VF), 250, 252
Ventricular tachycardia (VT), 250, 252
Vital capacity (VC), 216
Volume control, 207
Voluntary pathway, 218

Wales health system, 15
   Healthcare Inspectorate Wales, 20
   NICE guidelines, 20

Waveform capnography, 205
Welsh healthcare, 15
White blood cells (WBCs), 386–387
Work of breathing (WOB), 199–200
World Health Organization (WHO), 18, 472, 474
Worldwide healthcare, 52
Wound dehiscence, 327
Wound healing, 79
   inflammation and proliferation phase, 79
   non-healing wounds management, 83, 84
   nursing assessment, 79–80
   patient factors, 79, 80
   recognising infection, 81–83
   wound bed, 81
Wound photography, 80
Wrong blood in tube (WBIT) errors, 398

Zone of coagulation, 429
Zone of hypernatraemia, 429
Zone of stasis, 429
Zopiclone, 194